Calculate with Confidence

DEBORAH C. GRAY, RN, BSN, MA
Associate Professor of Nursing
Bronx Community College
Bronx, New York

Second Edition

With 680 illustrations

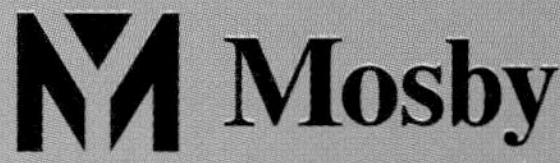

A Harcourt Health Sciences Company
St. Louis London Philadelphia Sydney Toronto

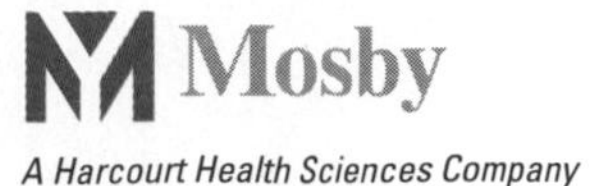

A Harcourt Health Sciences Company

A NOTE TO THE READER

The author and publisher have made every attempt to check dosages and nursing content for accuracy. Because the science of pharmacology is continually advancing, our knowledge base continues to expand. Therefore we recommend that the reader always check product information for changes in dosage or administration before administering any medication. This is particularly important with new or rarely used drugs.

Second Edition
Copyright © 1998 by Mosby, Inc.

Previous edition copyrighted 1994.

All rights reserved. No part of this publication may be reproduced, stored in a retrieval system, or transmitted, in any form or by any means, electronic, mechanical, photocopying, recording, or otherwise, without prior written permission from the publisher.

Permission to photocopy or reproduce solely for internal or personal use is permitted for libraries or other users registered with the Copyright Clearance Center, provided that the base fee of $4.00 per chapter plus $.10 per page is paid directly to the Copyright Clearance Center, 222 Rosewood Drive, Danvers, MA 01923. This consent does not extend to other kinds of copying, such as copying for general distribution, for advertising or promotional purposes, for creating new collected works, or for resale.

Printed in the United States of America

Mosby, Inc.
11830 Westline Industrial Drive
St. Louis, Missouri 63146

Library of Congress Cataloging-in-Publication Data

Gray, Deborah, RN.
Calculate with confidence / Deborah C. Gray. —2nd ed.
p. cm.
Includes bibliographical references and index.
ISBN 0-8151-2607-7
1. Nursing—Mathematics. 2. Pharmaceutical arithmetic.
I. Title.
[DNLM: 1. Drugs—administration & dosage—problems. 2. Drugs—administration & dosage—nurses' instruction. 3. Mathematics—nurses' instruction. 4. Mathematics—problems. QV 18.2 G778c 1997]
RT68.G43 1997
615'.4 dc21
DNLM/DLC

97-21619

01 02 / 9 8 7 6 5 4

Calculate with Confidence

Preface

Calculate with Confidence is written to meet the needs of current and potential practitioners of nursing at any level. This book can be used for inservice education programs and as a reference for the inactive nurse returning to the work world. It is also suitable for courses of instruction whose content reflects the calculation of dosage and solutions for any health care professional whose responsibilities include safe administration of medications and solutions to clients in diverse clinical settings.

Despite the advent of what is called a *unit dose* in some institutions, this procedure does not completely absolve health care professionals from the responsibility of calculation. With the increasing focus on providing health care outside the hospital, it becomes even more imperative that calculations be precise, done with thought, and correct to ensure the safe administration of medications to clients. A working knowledge in the area of dosage calculation is necessary, regardless of the medication system used in an institution or in settings outside the institution.

Calculate with Confidence offers a simplified approach to the calculation and administration of drug dosages. The book includes theoretical and mathematical concepts related to the administration of medications. An increased need for competency in basic math continues to be an essential prerequisite for dosage calculation and demands a review of basic math skills. A step-by-step approach to dosage calculation by the various rates of administration is also included.

Information related to systems of measurement and conversion is discussed in detail. Numerous illustrations, including full-color drug labels, syringes, and equipment used in medication administration, have been included to enhance learning and application to the clinical setting. Practice problems have been offered in each section to test the mastery of the content presented. In the area of basic math, a pretest and posttest have been included. The pretest will allow students to identify areas that need or do not need review. "Objectives" and "Points to Remember" are listed to guide students in learning the material in each chapter. Shading of syringes has been used to allow for visualization of dosages. Rationale for answers to dosage calculation problems has been included to enhance understanding of principles and answers related to dosages. Formulas that are simplified and encourage understanding of the dynamics in calculation are also presented. Alternative vocabulary has been used in certain areas to enhance the learning of some material presented.

Calculate with Confidence is acknowledged for its simplicity in presenting material relevant to dosage calculation and for enhancing the needs of the learner at different curricular levels. The book is also known for making content relevant to the needs of the student and for its use of realistic problems to enhance learning and to make material clinically applicable.

The second edition of *Calculate with Confidence* has maintained a style similar to the first. Revision of this edition is based on feedback from reviewers and on instructors' suggestions. It has been made more current to reflect the increasing responsibility of the nurse in medication administration and presents material necessary to reflect the current scope of practice. In addition to the revisions mentioned, the second edition, like the first, is organized in a progression of basic to more complex information.

New features in the second edition include:

- Addition of new drug labels and discussion of equipment used in medication administration.
- Content about issues related to medication administration in home care settings.
- Color throughout the book to highlight and visually enhance material presented.
- Many new practice problems to help students apply and evaluate learning in different types of calculations.
- An explanation of SI units and their use consistently throughout the book.
- Expanded content in the areas of I.V. calculation and pediatric dosages, using the body-surface area (BSA) method and formula method; I.V. calculation chapter expanded to include methods of administering I.V. medications specific to the child.
- A comprehensive posttest at the end of the book, giving additional practice and serving as an overall evaluation of learning.
- Perforated and three-hole punched pages for a more user-friendly book.

It is my hope that use of this book will help nurses and potential nurses calculate dosages accurately and with confidence, ensuring administration of medications safely to all clients in all settings, which is the primary responsibility of the nurse.

Deborah C. Gray

To my family, friends, colleagues, and students past and present, but especially with love to my children, Cameron, Kimberly, Kanin, and Cory, who had to be patient and understanding while I worked on this text. You light up my life and have supported me in whatever I had to do.

To current practitioners of nursing and future nurses, I hope this book will be valuable in teaching the basic principles of medication administration and will ensure safe administration of medication to all clients regardless of the setting.

Acknowledgments

I wish to extend sincere gratitude and appreciation to my family, friends, and colleagues for their support and encouragement during the writing of this second edition. I am indebted to the Nursing Department at Bronx Community College, who listened to me, made pertinent suggestions, helped with validation of content used in the text, and brought me problems from the clinical situation. Special thanks to the reviewers of this text; their comments and suggestions were invaluable. Particular thanks to the math reviewer, Donna S. Thomas, R.N., M.S.N, Nursing Instructor, Lutheran Medical Center, School of Nursing, St. Louis, Missouri. Thanks to students past and present at Bronx Community College who brought practice problems and gave valuable feedback for revisions.

I am sincerely grateful to the following people: Arlene Levey, a former and late colleague, who told me "I could fly" and whose encouragement helped me to "soar like an eagle"; Professor Marie-Louise Nickerson of the English Department at Bronx Community College who nurtured and encouraged me to first consider publication and worked closely with me on a project that resulted in the development of the text for publication; and the late Dr. Gerald S. Lieblich, former Chairperson of the Department of Mathematics at Bronx Community College, who took the time to review and validate content, as well as to make pertinent suggestions for the unit on Basic Math.

Thanks to the following companies and hospitals for permission to reproduce records used in this text: TDS Health Care Systems Corporation, St. Barnabas Hospital (Bronx, New York), and Jack D. Weiler Hospital of the Albert Einstein College of Medicine, a division of Montefiore Medical Center.

Thanks to the Research Foundation of New York for giving permission to use the I.V. formulas and formula for dosage calculations from the computer-assisted programs in pharmacology, which are copyrighted by the foundation.

I am especially grateful to the staff at Mosby, Beverly Copland, Susan Epstein, and Shannon Canty, for their support and help in planning, writing, and producing the first edition of this text. Thanks for all of your encouragement, nurturing, and support at times when I felt I wasn't going to complete the project. Your support helped me tremendously. A special thanks to Jeff Burnham and especially Lisa P. Newton for her time, support, patience, and understanding with the revisions of the second edition. Thanks for your encouragement and sincere concerns at times when I needed it most. I would also like to thank Helen Hudlin, who worked closely with me making corrections and pertinent suggestions, for her patience.

To Reginald B. Morris, my husband, thanks for your help, encouragement, support, and understanding while I revised this text. Thanks for the long hours you spent at the computer inputting the revisions and doing whatever to help complete the manuscript.

Finally I wish to thank all of the pharmaceutical companies that allowed me to reproduce their medication labels in the book to provide a more realistic picture for the student.

Rhone-Poulenc Rorer Pharmacueticals, Inc.
Hoechst Marion Roussel
Burroughs Wellcome Co.
GlaxoWellcome, Inc.
Merck & Co., Inc.
Bayer Corporation
SmithKline Beecham
Bristol Meyers Squibb
Apothecon—a Bristol Meyers Squibb Company
The Upjohn Company
Dista—a division of Eli Lilly Corporation
Squibb
Astra USA, Inc.
Parke-Davis Division of Warner Lambert
Eli Lilly and Company

Introduction to the Student

The nursing profession is undergoing profound changes. Today's nurses face many technological advances not only in the hospital setting, but in settings outside of the hospital in the community and home. The nurse has to be competent and able to use critical thinking skills because application of dosage calculations appears in a variety of settings. The accurate calculation of drug dosages is a critical and necessary skill in health care. Serious harm can come to clients from mathematical errors in calculating a drug dosage. Therefore it is a major responsibility of those administering drugs to ensure safe administration of medications by having the ability to accurately calculate a dosage. This text is intended to provide you with the skills to calculate a dosage with accuracy. Errors can be avoided if dosage calculation is approached in a logical fashion, and consideration is given to the reasonableness of the answer based on the principles presented. It is hoped that this text will help to emphasize the importance of accurate medication administration to clients and will assist nurses to feel more confident in mastering the skill of dosage calculation.

Deborah C. Gray

Contents

UNIT ONE
Math Review

This unit contains a review of basic math skills that are essential for the calculation of dosage and solutions, regardless of the problem-solving method used in calculation. Knowledge of basic math is a necessary component of dosage calculation that nurses need to know to prevent medication errors and to ensure the safe administration of medications. Although calculators are accessible for basic math operations, the nurse needs to be able to perform the processes involved in basic math. Performing basic math operations enables the nurse to think logically and critically about the dose that is ordered and the dosage calculated.

A pretest and a posttest have been included in this unit, offering an opportunity for students to assess their skills.

Pretest

This test is designed to test your ability in the basic math areas reviewed in Unit One. The test consists of 50 questions that are worth 2 points each. The passing score is 70 or better. If you miss three or more questions in any section, review the chapter relating to the content. (See pp. 325-326 for answers.)

Express the following in Roman numerals.

1. 9 __________
2. 16 __________
3. 23 __________
4. $10\frac{1}{2}$ __________
5. 22 __________

Express the following in Arabic numbers.

6. $\overline{\text{xiss}}$ __________
7. $\overline{\text{xii}}$ __________
8. $\overline{\text{xviii}}$ __________
9. $\overline{\text{xxiv}}$ __________
10. $\overline{\text{vi}}$ __________

Reduce the following fractions to lowest terms.

11. $\frac{14}{21}$ __________
12. $\frac{25}{100}$ __________
13. $\frac{2}{150}$ __________
14. $\frac{24}{30}$ __________
15. $\frac{24}{36}$ __________

Perform the indicated operations; reduce to lowest terms where necessary.

16. $\frac{2}{3} \div \frac{3}{9} =$ ____________

17. $4 \div \frac{3}{4} =$ ____________

18. $\frac{2}{5} + \frac{1}{9} =$ ____________

19. $7\frac{1}{7} - 2\frac{5}{6} =$ ____________

20. $4\frac{2}{3} \times 4 =$ ____________

Change the following fractions to decimals; express your answer to the nearest tenth.

21. $\frac{6}{7}$ ____________

22. $\frac{6}{20}$ ____________

23. $\frac{2}{3}$ ____________

24. $\frac{7}{8}$ ____________

Indicate the largest fraction in each group.

25. $\frac{3}{4}, \frac{4}{5}, \frac{7}{8}$ ____________

26. $\frac{7}{12}, \frac{11}{12}, \frac{4}{12}$ ____________

Perform the indicated operations with decimals.

27. $20.1 + 67.35 =$ ____________

28. $0.008 + 5.0 =$ ____________

29. $4.6 \times 8.72 =$ ____________

30. $56.47 - 8.7 =$ ____________

Divide the following decimals; express your answer to the nearest tenth.

31. $7.5 \div 0.004 =$ ____________

32. $45 \div 1.9 =$ ____________

33. $84.7 \div 2.3 =$ ____________

Indicate the larger decimal in each group.

34. 0.674, 0.659 ____________

35. 0.375, 0.37, 0.038 ____________

36. 0.25, 0.6, 0.175 ____________

Solve for x, the unknown value.

37. $8 : 2 = 48 : x,\ x =$ ____________

38. $x : 300 = 1 : 150,\ x =$ ____________

39. $\frac{1}{10} : x = \frac{1}{2} : 15,\ x =$ ____________

40. $0.4 : 1 = 0.2 : x,\ x =$ ____________

Round off to the nearest tenth.

41. $0.43 =$ ____________

42. $0.66 =$ ____________

43. $1.47 =$ ____________

Round off to the nearest hundredth.

44. 0.735 = ____________ 46. 1.227 = ____________

45. 0.834 = ____________

Complete the table below, expressing the measures in their equivalents where indicated. Reduce to lowest terms where necessary.

	Percent	Decimal	Ratio	Fraction
47.	6%	________	________	________
48.	35%	________	________	________
49.	________	________	________	$5\frac{1}{4}$
50.	________	0.015	________	________

Chapter 1

Roman Numerals

Objectives

After reviewing this chapter the student will be able to do the following:

1. **Change Roman numerals to Arabic numbers**
2. **Change Arabic numbers to Roman numerals**

The Roman numeral system dates back to ancient Roman times and uses letters to designate amounts. Roman numerals are used a great deal, especially in the **apothecaries' system** of measurement. Roman numerals may sometimes be used with apothecary weights and measure.

Example: **grx**

Apothecary measure unit of weight (gr) — Roman numeral (Arabic equivalent 10) (x)

Roman numerals are also still used on objects that indicate time (i.e., watches, clocks).

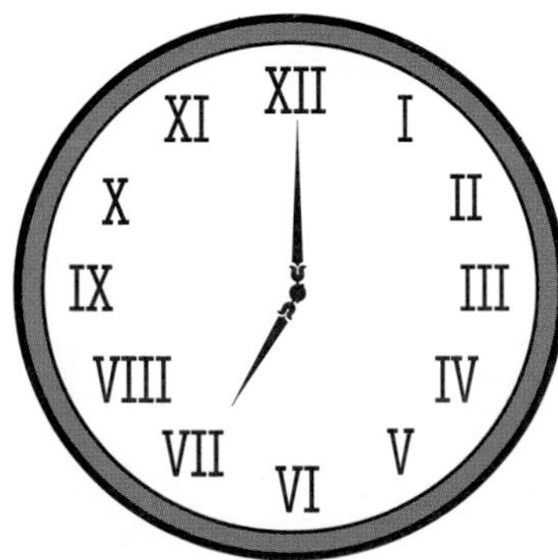

In the Arabic system, numbers, not letters, are used to express amounts. The Arabic system also uses fractions (1/2) and decimals (0.5).

To calculate drug dosages the nurse needs to know both Roman numerals and Arabic numbers. Lower case letters are usually used to express Roman numerals. The Roman numerals that you will see most often in the calculation of dosages are built on the basic symbols *i*, *v*, and *x*. To prevent errors in interpretation a line is sometimes drawn over the symbol. If this line is used, the lower case "i" is dotted above the line, not below.

Example 1: Aspirin gr$\overline{\text{x}}$

Example 2: two = $\dot{\overline{\text{ii}}}$

When the symbol for 1/2 is used in conjunction with Roman numerals, the symbol (ss) is placed at the end.

Example 1: $3\frac{1}{2} = \overline{\text{iiiss}}$

Example 2: $1\frac{1}{2}$ grains = gr$\overline{\text{iss}}$

The following box shows the common Arabic equivalents for Roman numerals. Review this list before proceeding to the rules pertaining to Roman numerals.

Arabic number	Roman numeral
1/2	ss or $\overline{\text{ss}}$
1	i or $\overline{\dot{\text{i}}}$, I
2	ii or $\overline{\dot{\text{i}}\dot{\text{i}}}$, II
3	iii or $\overline{\dot{\text{i}}\dot{\text{i}}\dot{\text{i}}}$, III
4	iv or $\overline{\dot{\text{i}}\text{v}}$, IV
5	v or $\overline{\text{v}}$, V
6	vi or $\overline{\text{v}\dot{\text{i}}}$, VI
7	vii or $\overline{\text{v}\dot{\text{i}}\dot{\text{i}}}$, VII
8	viii or $\overline{\text{v}\dot{\text{i}}\dot{\text{i}}\dot{\text{i}}}$, VIII
9	ix or $\overline{\dot{\text{i}}\text{x}}$, IX
10	x or $\overline{\text{x}}$, X
15	xv or $\overline{\text{xv}}$, XV
20	xx or $\overline{\text{xx}}$, XX
30	xxx or $\overline{\text{xxx}}$, XXX

To add, place a Roman numeral that is of lesser value after one of greater value. The numeral of lesser value is then added to the one of greater value. The same numeral is never repeated more than three times.

Example: 25 = $\overline{\text{xxv}}$

16 = $\overline{\text{xv}\dot{\text{i}}}$

To subtract, place a Roman numeral of lesser value before a numeral of greater value. The numeral of lesser value is then subtracted from the one of greater value.

Example: $\overline{\dot{\text{i}}\text{x}}$ = 9

Example: $\overline{\text{xx}\dot{\text{i}}\text{v}}$ = 24

$\overline{\text{xx}}$ = 20, $\overline{\dot{\text{i}}\text{v}}$ = 4

$\overline{\text{v}}$ being placed after $\overline{\dot{\text{i}}}$ is 5 − 1 or 4

10 + 10 and 5 − 1 = 20 + 4 = 24

Practice Problems (p. 326)

Practice addition and write the following in Roman numerals.

1. 15 ____________
2. 13 ____________
3. 30 ____________
4. 11 ____________
5. 17 ____________

Practice subtraction and write the following in Roman numerals.

6. 14 ____________
7. 29 ____________
8. 4 ____________
9. 19 ____________
10. 34 ____________

Chapter Review (p. 326)

Write the following Arabic numbers as Roman numerals.

1. 6 ____________
2. 30 ____________
3. $1\frac{1}{2}$ ____________
4. 27 ____________
5. 12 ____________
6. 18 ____________

7. 20 ____________

8. 3 ____________

9. 21 ____________

10. 26 ____________

Write the following Roman numerals as Arabic numbers.

11. v$\overline{\text{ii}}$ss ____________

12. $\overline{\text{xix}}$ ____________

13. $\overline{\text{xv}}$ ____________

14. $\overline{\text{xxx}}$ ____________

15. $\overline{\text{ss}}$ ____________

16. $\overline{\text{iii}}$ ____________

17. $\overline{\text{xxii}}$ ____________

18. $\overline{\text{xvi}}$ ____________

19. $\overline{\text{v}}$ ____________

20. $\overline{\text{xxvii}}$ ____________

Chapter 2

Fractions

Objectives

After reviewing this chapter the student will be able to do the following:

1. Compare the size of fractions
2. Add and subtract fractions
3. Divide and multiply fractions
4. Reduce fractions to lowest terms

> Understanding fractions is necessary because the nurse often encounters fractions when dealing with apothecaries' measures in dosage calculation.

A fraction is a part of a whole number (Figure 2-1). It is a division of a whole into units or parts (Figure 2-2).

Example: $\frac{1}{2}$ is a whole divided into two parts.

Fractions are composed of two parts: a **numerator,** which is the top number, and a **denominator,** which is the bottom number.

$$\frac{\text{Numerator}}{\text{Denominator}} : \frac{\text{how many parts of the whole you are taking}}{\text{how many equal parts the whole is divided into}}$$

Example: In the fraction $\frac{5}{6}$, 5 is the numerator, and 6 is the denominator.

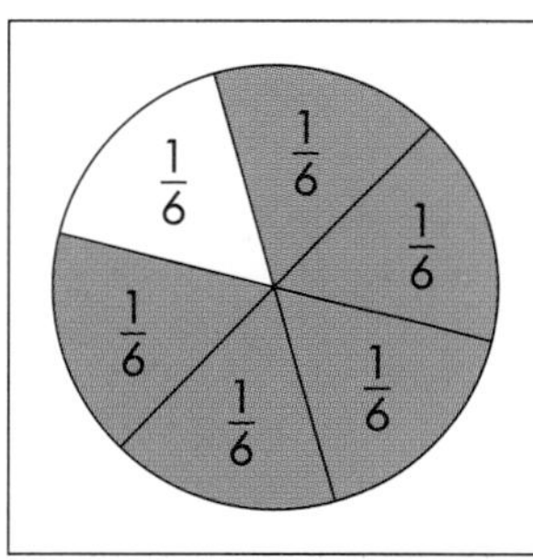

Figure 2-1 Diagram representing fractions of a whole. Five parts shaded out of six parts represents:

$$\frac{5 \quad \text{Numerator}}{6 \quad \text{Denominator}}$$

Types of Fractions

Proper Fraction: Numerator is less than the denominator.

Examples: $\frac{1}{8}, \frac{5}{6}, \frac{7}{8}, \frac{1}{150}$

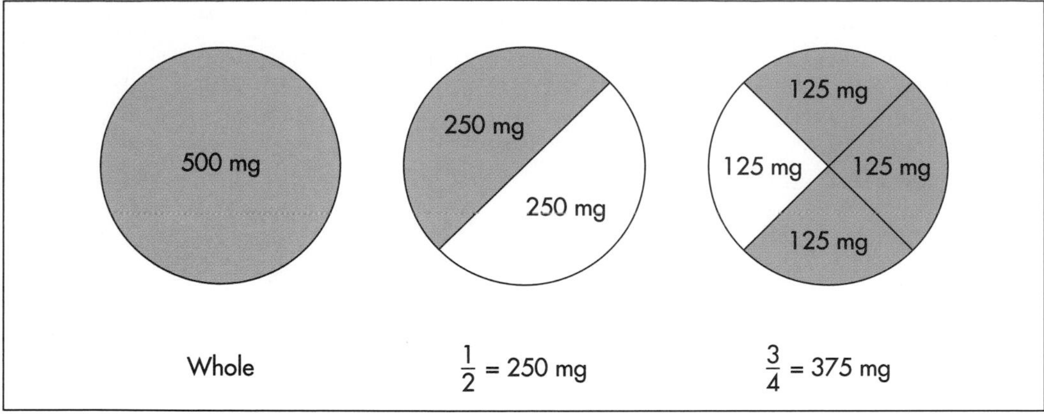

Figure 2-2. Fraction pie charts.

Improper Fraction: Numerator is larger than, or equal to, the denominator.

Examples: $\frac{3}{2}, \frac{7}{5}, \frac{300}{150}, \frac{4}{4}$

Mixed Number: Whole number and a fraction.

Examples: $3\frac{1}{3}, 5\frac{1}{8}, 9\frac{1}{6}, 25\frac{7}{8}$

Complex Fraction: Numerator, denominator, or both, are fractions.

Examples: $\frac{3\frac{1}{2}}{2}, \frac{\frac{1}{3}}{\frac{1}{2}}, \frac{2}{1\frac{1}{4}}, \frac{2}{\frac{1}{150}}$

Whole Numbers: Have an unexpressed denominator of one (1).

Examples: $1 = \frac{1}{1}, 3 = \frac{3}{1}, 6 = \frac{6}{1}, 100 = \frac{100}{1}$

An improper fraction can be changed to a mixed number or whole number by dividing the numerator by the denominator.

Examples:

$$\frac{6}{5} = 6 \div 5 = 1\frac{1}{5}, \frac{100}{25} = 100 \div 25 = 4$$

A mixed number can be changed to an improper fraction by multiplying the whole number by the denominator, adding it to the numerator, and placing the sum over the denominator.

Example: $5\frac{1}{8} = (5 \times 8) + \frac{1}{8} = \frac{41}{8}$

Fractions with different denominators can be compared by changing both fractions to fractions with the same denominator. This is done by finding the lowest common denominator (LCD) or the lowest number evenly divisible by the denominators of the fractions being compared.

Example: Which is larger, $\frac{3}{4}$ or $\frac{4}{5}$?

Solution: The lowest common denominator is 20, because it is the smallest number that can be divided by both denominators evenly. Change

Comparing the size of fractions is important in the administration of medications. Here are some basic rules to keep in mind when comparing fractions.

1. If the numerators are the same, the fraction with the smaller denominator has the larger value.

   Example 1: $\frac{1}{2}$ is larger than $\frac{1}{3}$

   Example 2: $\frac{1}{150}$ is larger than $\frac{1}{300}$

2. If the denominators are the same, the fraction with the larger numerator has the larger value.

   Example 1: $\frac{3}{4}$ is larger than $\frac{1}{4}$

   Example 2: $\frac{3}{100}$ is larger than $\frac{1}{100}$

each fraction to the same terms by dividing the lowest common denominator by the denominator and multiplying that answer by the numerator. The answer obtained from this is the new numerator. The numerators are then placed over the lowest common denominator.

For the fraction $\frac{3}{4}$: $20 \div 4 = 5; 5 \times 3 = 15;$

therefore $\frac{3}{4}$ becomes $\frac{15}{20}$.

For the fraction $\frac{4}{5}$: $20 \div 5 = 4; 4 \times 4 = 16;$

therefore $\frac{4}{5}$ becomes $\frac{16}{20}$.

Practice Problems (pp. 326-327)

Circle the fraction with the lesser value in each of the following sets.

1. $\frac{6}{30}, \frac{4}{5}$ ____________
2. $\frac{5}{4}, \frac{6}{8}$ ____________
3. $\frac{1}{75}, \frac{1}{100}, \frac{1}{150}$ ____________
4. $\frac{6}{18}, \frac{7}{18}, \frac{8}{18}$ ____________
5. $\frac{4}{5}, \frac{7}{5}, \frac{3}{5}$ ____________
6. $\frac{4}{8}, \frac{1}{8}, \frac{3}{8}$ ____________
7. $\frac{1}{40}, \frac{1}{10}, \frac{1}{5}$ ____________
8. $\frac{1}{300}, \frac{1}{200}, \frac{1}{175}$ ____________
9. $\frac{4}{24}, \frac{5}{24}, \frac{10}{24}$ ____________
10. $\frac{4}{3}, \frac{1}{2}, \frac{1}{6}$ ____________

Circle the fraction with the higher value in each of the following sets.

11. $\frac{6}{8}, \frac{5}{9}$ ____________
12. $\frac{7}{6}, \frac{2}{3}$ ____________
13. $\frac{1}{72}, \frac{6}{12}, \frac{1}{24}$ ____________
14. $\frac{1}{10}, \frac{1}{6}, \frac{1}{8}$ ____________
15. $\frac{1}{75}, \frac{1}{125}, \frac{1}{225}$ ____________
16. $\frac{2}{5}, \frac{6}{5}, \frac{3}{5}$ ____________
17. $\frac{1}{8}, \frac{4}{6}, \frac{1}{4}$ ____________
18. $\frac{7}{9}, \frac{5}{9}, \frac{8}{9}$ ____________
19. $\frac{1}{10}, \frac{1}{50}, \frac{1}{150}$ ____________
20. $\frac{2}{15}, \frac{1}{15}, \frac{6}{15}$ ____________

Reducing Fractions

Fractions should always be reduced to their lowest terms.

> To reduce a fraction to its lowest terms, the numerator and denominator are each divided by the largest number by which they are both evenly divisible.

Example 1: Reduce the fraction $\frac{6}{20}$

Solution: Both numerator and denominator are evenly divisible by 2.

$6 \div 2 = 3; 20 \div 2 = 10$

$$\frac{6}{20} = \frac{3}{10}$$

Example 2: Reduce the fraction $\frac{75}{100}$

Solution: Both numerator and denominator are evenly divisible by 25.

$75 \div 25 = 3; 100 \div 25 = 4$

$$\frac{75}{100} = \frac{3}{4}$$

Practice Problems (p. 327)

Reduce the following fractions to their lowest terms.

21. $\frac{10}{15} =$ __________

22. $\frac{7}{49} =$ __________

23. $\frac{64}{128} =$ __________

24. $\frac{100}{150} =$ __________

25. $\frac{20}{28} =$ __________

26. $\frac{14}{98} =$ __________

27. $\frac{10}{18} =$ __________

28. $\frac{24}{36} =$ __________

29. $\frac{10}{50} =$ __________

30. $\frac{9}{27} =$ __________

31. $\frac{9}{9} =$ __________

32. $\frac{15}{45} =$ __________

33. $\frac{124}{155} =$ __________

34. $\frac{12}{18} =$ __________

35. $\frac{36}{64} =$ __________

Adding Fractions

> To add fractions with the same denominator, add the numerators, place the sum over the denominator, and reduce to lowest terms.

Example 1: $\frac{1}{6} + \frac{4}{6} = \frac{5}{6}$

Example 2: $\frac{1}{6} + \frac{3}{6} + \frac{4}{6} = \frac{8}{6}$

$$\frac{8}{6} = \frac{4}{3} = 1\frac{1}{3}$$

(*Note:* In addition to reducing to lowest terms in example 2, the improper fraction was changed to a mixed number.)

> To add fractions with different denominators, change fractions to their equivalent fraction with the least common denominator, add the numerators, write the sum over the common denominator, and reduce if necessary.

Example 1: $\frac{1}{4} + \frac{1}{3}$

Solution: The least common denominator is 12. Change to equivalent fractions.

$$\frac{1}{4} = \frac{3}{12}$$
$$+\frac{1}{3} = \frac{4}{12}$$
$$\frac{7}{12}$$

Example 2: $\frac{1}{2} + 1\frac{1}{3} + \frac{2}{4}$

Solution: Change the mixed number 1 1/3 to 4/3. Find the lowest common denominator, change fractions to equivalent fractions, add, and reduce if necessary. The lowest common denominator is 12.

$$\frac{1}{2} = \frac{6}{12}$$
$$\frac{4}{3} = \frac{16}{12}$$
$$+\frac{2}{4} = \frac{6}{12}$$

$$\frac{28}{12} = 2\frac{4}{12} = 2\frac{1}{3}$$

Subtracting Fractions

> To subtract fractions with the same denominator, subtract the numerators, and place this amount over the denominator. Reduce to lowest terms, if necessary.

Example 1: $\frac{5}{4} - \frac{3}{4} = \frac{2}{4} = \frac{1}{2}$

Example 2: $2\frac{1}{6} - \frac{5}{6}$

Solution: Change the mixed number 2 1/6 to 13/6

$$\frac{13}{6} - \frac{5}{6} = \frac{8}{6} = \frac{4}{3} = 1\frac{1}{3}$$

> To subtract fractions with different denominators, find the lowest common denominator, change to equivalent fractions, subtract the numerators, and place the sum over the common denominator. Reduce to lowest terms, if necessary.

Example 1: $\frac{15}{6} - \frac{3}{5}$

Solution: The lowest common denominator is 30. Change to equivalent fractions and subtract.

$$\frac{15}{6} = \frac{75}{30}$$
$$-\frac{3}{5} = \frac{18}{30}$$
$$\frac{57}{30} = 1\frac{27}{30} = 1\frac{9}{10}$$

Example 2: $2\frac{1}{5} - \frac{4}{3}$

Solution: Change the mixed number 2 1/5 to 11/5. Find the lowest common denominator, change to equivalent fractions, subtract, and reduce if necessary. The lowest common denominator is 15.

$$\frac{11}{5} = \frac{33}{15}$$
$$-\frac{4}{3} = \frac{20}{15}$$
$$\frac{13}{15}$$

Multiplying Fractions

> To multiply fractions, multiply the numerators, multiply the denominators, and reduce, if necessary.

Example 1: $\frac{3}{4} \times \frac{2}{5} = \frac{6}{20} = \frac{3}{10}$

(*Note:* If fractions are not in lowest terms, reduction can be done before multiplication.)

Example 2: $6 \times \frac{5}{6}$

$$\frac{6 \times 5}{6} = \frac{30}{6} = 5$$

or

$$\frac{6}{1} \times \frac{5}{6} = \frac{30}{6} = 5$$

(*Note:* The whole number 6 is expressed as a fraction here, by placing one (1) as the denominator.)

Example 3: $3\frac{1}{3} \times 2\frac{1}{2}$

Solution: Change the mixed numbers to improper fractions. Proceed with multiplication.

$$3\frac{1}{3} = \frac{10}{3}; 2\frac{1}{2} = \frac{5}{2}$$

$$\frac{10}{3} \times \frac{5}{2} = \frac{50}{6} = 8\frac{2}{6} = 8\frac{1}{3}$$

Dividing Fractions

> To divide fractions, invert (turn upside down) the second fraction (divisor), and multiply. Reduce where necessary.

Example 1: $\frac{3}{4} \div \frac{2}{3}$

Solution: $\frac{3}{4} \times \frac{3}{2} = \frac{9}{8} = 1\frac{1}{8}$

Example 2: $1\frac{3}{5} \div 2\frac{1}{10}$

Solution: Change mixed numbers to improper fractions. Proceed with steps of division.

$$1\frac{3}{5} = \frac{8}{5}; 2\frac{1}{10} = \frac{21}{10}$$

$$\frac{8}{5} \times \frac{10}{21} = \frac{80}{105} = \frac{16}{21}$$

Example 3: $5 \div \frac{1}{2}$

Solution: $5 \times \frac{2}{1} = \frac{10}{1}$

or

$$\frac{5}{1} \times \frac{2}{1} = \frac{10}{1} = 10$$

(*Note:* When doing dosage calculations that involve division, the fractions may be written as follows: $\frac{\frac{1}{4}}{\frac{1}{2}}$. In this case $\frac{1}{4}$ is the numerator, and $\frac{1}{2}$ is the denominator. Therefore the problem is set up as: $\frac{1}{4} \div \frac{1}{2}$, which becomes $\frac{1}{4} \times \frac{2}{1} = \frac{2}{4} = \frac{1}{2}$.)

Chapter Review (pp. 327-328)

Change the following improper fractions to mixed numbers and reduce to lowest terms.

1. $\frac{10}{8} =$ ____________
2. $\frac{30}{4} =$ ____________
3. $\frac{22}{6} =$ ____________
4. $\frac{11}{4} =$ ____________
5. $\frac{59}{14} =$ ____________
6. $\frac{67}{10} =$ ____________
7. $\frac{9}{2} =$ ____________
8. $\frac{11}{5} =$ ____________
9. $\frac{64}{15} =$ ____________
10. $\frac{100}{13} =$ ____________

Change the following mixed numbers to improper fractions.

11. $2\frac{1}{2} =$ ____________
12. $7\frac{3}{8} =$ ____________
13. $8\frac{3}{5} =$ ____________
14. $16\frac{1}{4} =$ ____________

15. $3\frac{1}{5} =$ __________

16. $2\frac{3}{5} =$ __________

17. $8\frac{4}{10} =$ __________

18. $9\frac{1}{4} =$ __________

19. $12\frac{3}{4} =$ __________

20. $6\frac{5}{7} =$ __________

Add the following fractions and mixed numbers. Reduce to lowest terms.

21. $\frac{2}{5} + \frac{1}{3} + \frac{7}{10} =$ __________

22. $\frac{1}{4} + \frac{1}{6} + \frac{1}{8} =$ __________

23. $20\frac{1}{2} + \frac{1}{4} + \frac{5}{4} =$ __________

24. $\frac{1}{2} + \frac{1}{5} =$ __________

25. $6\frac{1}{4} + \frac{2}{9} + \frac{1}{36} =$ __________

Subtract the following fractions and mixed numbers. Reduce to lowest terms.

26. $\frac{6}{4} - \frac{1}{2} =$ __________

27. $2\frac{1}{4} - 1\frac{1}{2} =$ __________

28. $2\frac{3}{4} - \frac{1}{4} =$ __________

29. $\frac{4}{5} - \frac{1}{6} =$ __________

30. $\frac{4}{9} - \frac{3}{9} =$ __________

31. $\frac{4}{5} - \frac{1}{4} =$ __________

32. $\frac{4}{6} - \frac{3}{8} =$ __________

33. $4\frac{1}{6} - 1\frac{1}{3} =$ __________

34. $\frac{8}{5} - \frac{1}{3} =$ __________

35. $\frac{4}{7} - \frac{1}{3} =$ __________

Multiply the following fractions and mixed numbers. Reduce to lowest terms.

36. $\frac{1}{3} \times \frac{4}{12} =$ __________

37. $2\frac{7}{8} \times 3\frac{1}{4} =$ __________

38. $8 \times 1\frac{3}{4} =$ __________

39. $15 \times \frac{2}{3} =$ __________

40. $36 \times \frac{3}{4} =$ __________

41. $\frac{5}{4} \times \frac{2}{4} =$ __________

42. $\frac{2}{5} \times \frac{1}{6} =$ __________

43. $\frac{3}{10} \times \frac{4}{12} =$ __________

44. $\frac{1}{9} \times \frac{7}{3} =$ __________

45. $\frac{10}{25} \times \frac{5}{3} =$ __________

Divide the following fractions and mixed numbers. Reduce to lowest terms.

46. $2\frac{1}{3} \div 4\frac{1}{6} =$ ____________

47. $\frac{1}{3} \div \frac{1}{2} =$ ____________

48. $25 \div 12\frac{1}{2} =$ ____________

49. $\frac{7}{8} \div 2\frac{1}{4} =$ ____________

50. $\frac{6}{2} \div \frac{3}{4} =$ ____________

51. $\frac{4}{6} \div \frac{1}{2} =$ ____________

52. $\frac{3}{10} \div \frac{5}{25} =$ ____________

53. $3 \div \frac{2}{5} =$ ____________

54. $\frac{15}{30} \div 10 =$ ____________

55. $\frac{8}{3} \div \frac{8}{3} =$ ____________

Chapter 3

Decimals

Objectives

After reviewing this chapter the student will be able to do the following:

1. Read and write decimals
2. Compare the size of decimals
3. Change fractions to decimals and decimals to fractions
4. Add, subtract, multiply, and divide decimals
5. Round off decimals to the nearest tenth or hundredth

An understanding of decimals is crucial to the calculation of dosages. Most medications are ordered in metric measures that use decimals.

Example 1: Digoxin 0.125 mg

Example 2: Capoten 6.25 mg

A decimal is a fraction that has a denominator that is a multiple of 10. A decimal fraction is written as a decimal by the use of a decimal point (.). The decimal point is used to indicate place value. Some examples are as follows:

Fraction	Decimal number
$\frac{3}{10}$	0.3
$\frac{18}{100}$	0.18
$\frac{175}{1000}$	0.175

The decimal point represents the center. Notice that the numbers written to the right of the decimal point are decimal fractions with a denominator of 10, or a multiple of 10, and represent a value that is less than one (1) or part of one (1). Numbers written to the left of the decimal point are whole numbers, or have a value of one (1) or greater.

The easiest way to understand decimals is to memorize the place values (see box on p. 20).

The **first** place to the right of the decimal is tenths.

The **second** place to the right of the decimal is hundredths.

The **third** place to the right of the decimal is thousandths.

The **fourth** place to the right of the decimal is ten-thousandths.

In the calculation of medication dosages it is only necessary to **consider three figures after the decimal point (thousandths) (e.g., 0.375 mg). It is important to place a zero (0)**

The decimal value is determined by its position to the right of the decimal point.

Hundred-thousands (100,000)	Ten-thousands (10,000)	Thousands (1000)	Hundreds (100)	Tens (10)	Ones (Units) (1)		Tenths (.1)	Hundredths (.01)	Thousandths (.001)	Ten-thousandths (.0001)	Hundred-thousandths (.00001)
6	5	4	3	2	1	.	1	2	3	4	5
			Whole numbers to left			Decimal point	Decimal numbers to right				

in front of the decimal point to indicate that it is a fraction, when there is no whole number before it. This will emphasize its value and prevent errors in interpretation. *The source for many medication errors is misplacement of a decimal point or incorrect interpretation of a decimal value.*

Reading and Writing Decimals

Once you have an understanding of the place value of decimals, reading and writing them is simple.

To read the decimal numbers read:

1. The whole number,
2. the decimal point as "and", and
3. the decimal fraction.

Example 1: The number 8.3 is read as "eight and three tenths."
Example 2: The number 0.4 is read as "four tenths."
Example 3: The decimal 4.06 is read as "four and six hundredths."

Decimals can be read as "point" instead of "and" to indicate a decimal point. When there is only a zero (0) to the left of the decimal, as in example 2, the zero is not read aloud.

An exception to this is in an emergency situation where a nurse has to take a verbal order over the phone from a doctor. When repeating back an order for a medication involving a decimal, the zero should be read aloud to prevent a medication error.

To write a decimal number write the following:

1. The whole number. (If there is no whole number, write zero [0].)
2. The decimal point to indicate the place value of the rightmost number.
3. The decimal portion of the number.

Example 1: Written, seven and five tenths = 7.5
Example 2: Written, one-hundred and twenty-five thousandths = 0.125
Example 3: Written, five tenths = 0.5

Practice Problems (p. 328)

Write each of the following numbers in word form.

1. 8.35 ____________________
2. 11.001 ____________________
3. 4.57 ____________________
4. 5.0007 ____________________
5. 10.5 ____________________
6. 0.163 ____________________

Write each of the following in decimal form.

7. four tenths ____________

8. eighty-four and seven hundredths ____________

9. seven hundredths ____________

10. two and twenty-three hundredths ____________

11. five hundredths ____________

12. nine thousandths ____________

Comparing the Value of Decimals

Understanding which decimal is larger or smaller is important in the calculation of dosage problems.

When decimal numbers contain whole numbers, the whole numbers are compared to determine which is greater.

Example 1: 4.8 is larger than 2.9
Example 2: 11.5 is larger than 7.5
Example 3: 7.37 is larger than 6.94

If the whole numbers being compared are the **same** (e.g., 5.6 and 5.2) or if there is **no whole number** (e.g., 0.45 and 0.37), then the number in the **tenths** place determines which decimal is larger.

Example 1: 0.45 is larger than 0.37
Example 2: 1.75 is larger than 1.25

If the whole numbers are the same or zero and the numbers in the **tenths place** are the **same,** then the decimal with the higher number in the **hundredths place** has the larger value, and so forth.

Example 1: 0.67 is larger than 0.66
Example 2: 0.17 is larger than 0.14

Note: The addition of zeros at the end of a decimal does not alter its value; they are therefore unnecessary and could result in a calculation error.

Example 1: 0.2 is the same as 0.2000, 0.20
Example 2: 4.4 is the same as 4.40, 4.400

Practice Problems (p. 328)

Circle the decimal with the largest value in the following:

13. 0.5, 0.15, 0.05 ____________

14. 2.66, 2.36, 2.87 ____________

15. 0.125, 0.375, 0.25 ____________

16. 0.175, 0.1, 0.05 ____________

17. 7.02, 7.15, 7.35 ____________

18. 0.067, 0.087, 0.077 ____________

Addition and Subtraction of Decimals

To add or subtract decimals, place the numbers in columns so that the decimal points are lined up directly under one another and add or subtract from right to left.

Example 1: Add 16.4 + 21.8 + 13.2

$$\begin{array}{r} 16.4 \\ 21.8 \\ +13.2 \\ \hline 51.4 \end{array}$$

Example 2: Add 11.2 + 16

```
 11.2
+16.0
 27.2
```

Note the addition of a zero to make the columns the same length.

Example 3: Subtract 3.78 from 12.84

```
 12.84
 -3.78
  9.06
```

Example 4: Subtract 0.007 from 0.05

```
 0.050
-0.007
 0.043
```

Note the addition of a zero to make the columns the same length.

Practice Problems (p. 328)

Add the following decimals.

19. 4.7 + 5.3 + 8.4 = ____________

20. 38.52 + 0.029 + 1.90 = ____________

21. 0.7 + 3.25 = ____________

22. 2.2 + 1.67 = ____________

Subtract the following decimals.

23. 3.67 − 0.75 = ____________

24. 64.3 − 21.2 = ____________

25. 0.08 − 0.045 = ____________

26. 6.75 − 0.87 = ____________

Multiplying Decimals

When multiplying decimals, be sure the decimal is placed in the correct position in the answer (product).

> To multiply decimals, multiply as with whole numbers. In the answer (product), count off from right to left as many decimal places as there are in the numbers being multiplied.

Example 1: 1.2 × 3.2

```
  1.2
 ×3.2
   24
  36
  384
```

Answer: 384 = 3.84

In example 1, 1.2 has one number after the decimal, and 3.2 also has one. Therefore you will need to place the decimal point 2 places to the left in the answer (product). Addition of a zero is not necessary (3 is a whole number).

> When there is insufficient numbers in the answer for correct placement of the decimal point, add as many zeros as needed to the left of the answer.

Example 2: 1.35 × 0.65

```
  1.35
 ×0.65
   675
  810
  8775
```

Answer: 8775 = 0.8775

In example 2, 1.35 has two numbers after the decimal, and 0.65 also has two. Therefore you will need to place the decimal point 4 places to the left in the answer (product), and add a zero in front.

Example 3: 0.11×0.33

$$\begin{array}{r} 0.11 \\ \underline{\times 0.33} \\ 33 \\ \underline{33} \\ 363 \end{array}$$

Answer: 363 = 0.0363

In example 3, there are four decimal places needed (two numbers after each decimal in 0.11 and 0.33), but there are only three numbers in the product. A zero must be placed to the left of these numbers for correct placement of the decimal point.

Multiplication by Decimal Movement

> This method may be preferred when doing metric conversions because it is based on the decimal system.

> Multiplying by 10, 100, 1000, and so forth can be done by moving the decimal point to the right the same number of places as there are zeros in the number by which you are multiplying.

Example: When multiplying by 10, move the decimal one place to the right; by 100, two places to the right; by 1000, three places to the right, and so forth.

Example 1: $1.6 \times 10 = 16$ (decimal moved two places to the right)

Example 2: $5.2 \times 100 = 520$ (decimal moved two places to the right)

Example 3: $0.463 \times 1000 = 463$ (decimal moved three places to the right)

Example 4: $6.64 \times 10 = 66.4$ (decimal moved one place to right and remains in the answer)

Practice Problems (p. 328)

Multiply the following decimals.

27. $3.15 \times 0.015 =$ __________

28. $3.65 \times 0.25 =$ __________

29. $9.65 \times 1000 =$ __________

30. $8.9 \times 0.2 =$ __________

31. $14.001 \times 7.2 =$ __________

Division of Decimals

> The division of decimals is done in the same manner as dividing whole numbers except for placement of the decimal point. Incorrect placement of the decimal point changes the numerical value and can cause error in calculation. Errors made in the division of decimals are commonly due to improper placement of the decimal point, incorrect placement of numbers in the quotient, and omission of necessary zeros in the quotient.

The parts of a division problem are as follows:

$$\text{Divisor}\overline{)\text{Dividend}}^{\text{Quotient}}$$

The number being divided is called the **dividend,** the number used for the division is the **divisor,** and the answer is the **quotient.**

Symbols used to indicate division are as follows:

1. $\overline{)}$

   Example: $9\overline{)27}$

2. ÷

   Example: 27 ÷ 9

3. The horizontal bar with the dividend on the top and the divisor on the bottom.

   Example: $\frac{27}{9}$

4. The slanted bar with the dividend to the left and the divisor to the right.

   Example: 27/9

Dividing a Decimal by a Whole Number

> To divide a decimal by a whole number, place the decimal point in the quotient directly above the decimal point in the dividend. Proceed to divide as with whole numbers.

Example:

$$\begin{array}{r} 3.5 \\ 5\overline{)17.5} \\ \underline{-15} \\ 25 \\ \underline{-25} \\ 0 \end{array}$$

Dividing a Decimal or a Whole Number by a Decimal

> To divide by a decimal, the decimal point in the divisor is moved to the right until the number is a whole number. The decimal point in the dividend is moved the same number of places to the right, and zeros are added as necessary. Proceed to divide as with whole numbers.

Example: Divide 6.96 by 0.3

$6.96 \div 0.3 = 0.3\overline{)6.96}$

Step 1: $3\overline{)69.6}$ (After moving decimals in the divisor the same number of places as the dividend.)

Step 2:

$$\begin{array}{r} 23.2 \\ 3\overline{)69.6} \\ \underline{-6} \\ 9 \\ \underline{-9} \\ 6 \\ \underline{-6} \\ 0 \end{array}$$

Division by Decimal Movement

> To divide a decimal by 10, 100, or 1000, move the decimal point to the **left** the same number of places as there are zeros in the divisor.

Example 1: $0.46 \div 10 = 0.046$ (The decimal is moved one place to the left.)

Example 2: $0.07 \div 100 = 0.0007$ (The decimal is moved two places to the left.)

Example 3: $0.75 \div 1000 = 0.00075$ (The decimal is moved three places to the left.)

Rounding Off Decimals

The determination of how many places to carry your division in calculation of dosages is based on the materials being used. Some syringes are marked in **tenths,** some in **hundredths.** As you become familiar with the materials used in dosage calculation, you will learn how far to carry your division and when to round off. To ensure accuracy, most calculation problems require that you carry your division at least **two decimal places (hundredths place)** and **round off to the nearest tenth.**

> To express an answer to the nearest tenth, carry the division to the hundredths place (two places after the decimal). If the number in the hundredths place **is 5 or greater, add** one to the tenths place. If the number **is less than 5, drop** the number to the right of the desired decimal place.

Example 1: Express 4.15 to the nearest tenth.
Answer: 4.2 (The number in the hundredths place is 5, so the number in the tenths place is **increased by one.** 4.1 becomes 4.2.)

Example 2: Express 1.24 to the nearest tenth.
Answer: 1.2 (The number in the hundredths place is less than 5, so the number in the **tenths place does not change.**)

> To express an answer to the nearest hundredth, carry the division to the thousandths place (three places after the decimal). If the number in the thousandths place is 5 or greater, add one to the hundredths place. If the number is less than 5, drop the number to the right of the desired decimal place.

Example 1: Express 0.176 to the nearest hundredth.

Answer: 0.18 (The number in the thousandths place is 6, so the number in the hundredths place is increased by one. 0.17 becomes 0.18.)

Example 2: Express 0.554 to the nearest hundredth.

Answer: 0.55 (The number in the thousandths place is less than 5, so the number in the hundredths place does not change.)

Practice Problems (p. 328)

Divide the following decimals. Carry division to the hundredths place where necessary.

32. $2 \div 0.5 =$ ____________

33. $1.4 \div 1.2 =$ ____________

34. $63.8 \div 0.9 =$ ____________

35. $39.6 \div 1.3 =$ ____________

36. $1.9 \div 3.2 =$ ____________

Express the following decimals to the nearest tenth.

37. 3.57 ____________

38. 0.95 ____________

39. 1.98 ____________

Express the following decimals to the nearest hundredth.

40. 3.550 ____________

41. 0.607 ____________

42. 0.738 ____________

Divide the following decimals.

43. $0.005 \div 10 =$ ____________

44. $0.004 \div 100 =$ ____________

Multiply the following decimals.

45. $58.4 \times 10 =$ ____________

46. $0.5 \times 1000 =$ ____________

Changing Fractions to Decimals

> To change a fraction to a decimal, divide the numerator by the denominator and add zeros as needed. If the numerator doesn't divide evenly into the denominator, carry division three places.

Example 1: $\frac{2}{5} = 5\overline{)2} = 5\overline{)2.0}$ (quotient 0.4)

Example 2: $\frac{3}{8} = 8\overline{)3} = 8\overline{)3.000}$ (quotient 0.375)

Changing fractions to decimals can also be a method of comparing fraction size. The fractions being compared are changed to decimals, and the rules relating to comparing decimals are then applied. (See Comparing the Value of Decimals, p. 21.)

Example: Which fraction is larger, $\frac{1}{3}$ or $\frac{1}{6}$?

Solution: $\frac{1}{3} = 0.333$ as a decimal

$\frac{1}{6} = 0.166$

$\frac{1}{3}$ would therefore be the larger fraction.

Changing Decimals to Fractions

> To change a decimal to a fraction, simply read the decimal as a fraction and write it as it is read. Reduce if necessary. (*Note:* See Reading and Writing Decimals, p. 20.)

Example 1: 0.4 is read "four tenths" and written $\frac{4}{10}$, which $= \frac{2}{5}$ when reduced.

Example 2: 0.65 is read "sixty-five hundredths" and written $\frac{65}{100}$, which $= \frac{13}{20}$ when reduced.

Practice Problems (p. 328)

Change the following fractions to decimals and carry the division three places as indicated.

47. $\frac{3}{4}$ __________

48. $\frac{5}{9}$ __________

49. $\frac{1}{2}$ __________

Change the following decimals to fractions and reduce to lowest terms.

50. 0.75 __________

51. 0.0005 __________

52. 0.04 __________

Points to Remember

- Read decimals carefully.
- When the decimal fraction is **not** preceded by a whole number (e.g., 12), **always place a "0"** to the left of the decimal (0.12) to avoid interpretation errors.
- Add zeros to the right as needed for making decimals of equal spacing for addition and subtraction. These zeros do not change the value.
- Double-check work to avoid errors.

Chapter Review (pp. 328-329)

Identify the decimal with the largest value in the following sets.

1. 0.4, 0.44, 0.444 __________

2. 0.8, 0.7, 0.12 __________

3. 1.32, 1.12, 1.5 __________

4. 0.1, 0.05, 0.2 __________

5. 0.725, 0.357, 0.125 __________

Perform the indicated operations.

6. 3.005 + 4.308 + 2.47 = __________

7. 20.3 + 8.57 + 0.03 = __________

8. $5.886 - 3.143 =$ ______________

10. $3.8 - 1.3 =$ ______________

9. $8.17 - 3.05 =$ ______________

Solve the following. Carry division to the hundredths place where necessary.

11. $5.7 \div 0.9 =$ ______________

12. $3.75 \div 2.5 =$ ______________

13. $1.125 \div 0.75 =$ ______________

14. $0.15 \times 100 =$ ______________

15. $15 \times 2.08 =$ ______________

16. $472.4 \times 0.002 =$ ______________

Express the following decimals to the nearest tenth.

17. 1.75 ______________

18. 0.13 ______________

Express the following decimals to the nearest hundredth.

19. 1.427 ______________

20. 0.147 ______________

Change the following fractions to decimals. Carry division three decimal places as necessary.

21. $\frac{8}{64}$ ______________

22. $\frac{3}{50}$ ______________

23. $6\frac{1}{2}$ ______________

Change the following decimals to fractions and reduce to lowest terms.

24. 1.01 ______________

25. 0.065 ______________

Chapter 4

Ratio and Proportion

Objectives

After reviewing this chapter the student will be able to do the following:

1. Define ratio and proportion
2. Define means and extremes
3. Use ratio and proportion to calculate problems for a missing term (x)

Ratio and proportion is one logical method for calculating medication dosages. It can be used to calculate all types of calculation problems. To use this method it is necessary to have an understanding of the concept of ratio and proportion.

Ratios

A ratio is used to indicate a relationship between two numbers. These numbers are separated by a colon (:).

Example: 3 : 4

The colon indicates division; therefore a ratio is a fraction and the numbers or terms of the ratio are the numerator and denominator. The numerator is always to the left of the colon, and the denominator is always to the right of the colon.

Example: 3 : 4 (3 is the numerator, 4 is the denominator, and the expression can be written as $\frac{3}{4}$.)

Proportions

A proportion is an equation of two ratios of equal value. The terms of the first ratio have a relationship to the terms of the second ratio. A proportion can be written in any of the following formats:

Example 1: 3 : 4 = 6 : 8 (separated with an equal sign)

Example 2: 3 : 4 :: 6 : 8 (separated with a double colon)

Example 3: $\frac{3}{4} = \frac{6}{8}$ (written as a fraction)

Read as follows: 3 is to 4 equals 6 is to 8; 3 is to 4 as 6 is to 8; or, as a fraction, three fourths equals six eighths.

Proving that ratios are equal and that the proportion is true can be done mathematically.

Example: 5 : 25 = 10 : 50

or

5 : 25 :: 10 : 50

The terms in a proportion are called the means and extremes. Confusion of these terms can result in an incorrect answer. To avoid confusion of terms in proportions remember **m** for middle terms **(means)** and **e** for the end terms **(extremes)** of the proportion. Let's refer to our example to identify these terms.

The extremes are the outer or end numbers (previous example 5, 50), and the means are the inner or middle numbers (previous example 25, 10).

Example:

means

$$5 : 25 = 10 : 50$$

extremes

> In a proportion the product of the means equals the product of the extremes.

In other words, the answers obtained when you multiply the means and extremes are equal.

Example: $5 : 25 = 10 : 50$

$$25 \times 10 = 50 \times 5$$

means extremes

$$250 = 250$$

Note: The product of the means, 250, equals the product of the extremes, 250, proving the ratios are equal and the proportion is true.

To verify that the two ratios in a proportion expressed as a fraction are equal and that it is a true proportion, multiply the numerator of each ratio by its opposite denominator. The sum of the products are equal. The numerator of the first fraction and the denominator of the second fraction are the extremes. The numerator of the second fraction and denominator of the first fraction are the means.

Example: $5 : 25 = 10 : 50$

$$\frac{5}{25} = \frac{10}{50}$$ (proportion written as a fraction)

$$\frac{\textbf{5 (extreme)}}{\textbf{25 (mean)}} = \frac{\textbf{10 (mean)}}{\textbf{50 (extreme)}}$$

Note: When stated as a fraction, the proportion is solved by cross multiplication.

$$5 \times 50 = 25 \times 10$$

$$250 = 250$$

Solving for *x* in Ratio-Proportion

Because the product of the means is always equal to the product of the extremes, if three numbers of the two ratios are known the fourth number can be found. In a proportion problem, the unknown quantity is represented by x.

Example: $12 : 9 = 8 : x$

Steps: $72 = 12x$ 1. Multiply the means and extremes.

$\frac{72}{12} = \frac{12x}{12}$ 2. Divide both sides of the equation by the number in front of x to obtain the value for x.

$$x = 6$$

Proof: Place the answer obtained for x in the equation and multiply to be certain that the product of the means equals the product of the extremes.

$$12 : 9 = 8 : 6$$

$$9 \times 8 = 12 \times 6$$

$$72 = 72$$

Solving for x with a proportion in a fraction format can be done by cross multiplication to determine the value of x.

Example: $\frac{4}{3} = \frac{12}{x}$

Steps: $4x = 36$ 1. Cross multiply to obtain the product of the means and extremes.

$\frac{4x}{4} = \frac{36}{4}$ 2. Divide by the number in front of x to obtain the value for x.

$$x = 9$$

Proof: Place the value obtained for x in the equation; the cross products should be equal.

$$\frac{4}{3} = \frac{12}{9}$$

$$4 \times 9 = 12 \times 3$$

$$36 = 36$$

Solving for x in proportions that involve decimals in the equation can be done by the same process.

Example: $25 : 5 = 1.5 : x$

Steps: $5 \times 1.5 = 25x$ 1. Multiply the means and extremes.

$$\frac{7.5}{25} = \frac{25x}{25}$$ 2. Divide by the number in front of x to solve for x.

$$x = 0.3$$

Proof:

$$25 : 5 = 1.5 : 0.3$$
$$5 \times 1.5 = 25 \times 0.3$$
$$7.5 = 7.5$$

Proportions with unknowns that also involve fractions may be solved by the same method.

Example: $\frac{1}{5} : 1 = \frac{1}{2} : x$

Steps:

$$\frac{1}{2} = \frac{1}{5} \times x$$ 1. Multiply the means and extremes.

$$\frac{1}{2} = \frac{1}{5x}$$

$$x = \frac{1}{2} \div \frac{1}{5}$$ 2. Divide both sides by the number in front of x. Division of two fractions becomes multiplication, and the second fraction is inverted. Multiply numerators and denominators.

$$x = \frac{1}{2} \times \frac{5}{1}$$

$$x = \frac{5}{2} = 2.5 \text{ or } 2\frac{1}{2}$$

3. Divide the final fraction to solve for x.

Proof:

$$\frac{1}{5} : 1 = \frac{1}{2} : 2\frac{1}{2}$$
$$1 \times \frac{1}{2} = \frac{1}{5} \times 2\frac{1}{2} = \frac{1}{5} \times \frac{5}{2}$$
$$\frac{1}{2} = \frac{5}{10} = \frac{1}{2}$$
$$\frac{1}{2} = \frac{1}{2}$$

Note: If the answer is expressed in fraction format for x, it must be reduced to **lowest terms.** Division should be carried **two decimal places** when an answer does not work out evenly and may have to be **rounded to the nearest tenth** to prove the answer correct.

Applying Ratio-Proportion to Dosage Calculation

Now that we have reviewed the basic definitions and concepts relating to ratio and proportion, let's look at how this might be applied in dosage calculation.

In dosage calculation, ratio proportion may be used to represent **the weight of a drug that is in tablet or capsule form.**

Example 1: 1 tab : 0.125 mg or $\frac{\text{1 tab}}{\text{0.125 mg}}$

This may also be expressed stating the weight of the drug first:

0.125 mg : 1 tab or $\frac{\text{0.125 mg}}{\text{1 tab}}$

This means that 1 tablet contains 0.125 mg or is equal to 0.125 mg of drug.

Example 2: If a capsule contains a dosage of 500 mg, this could be represented by a ratio as follows:

1 cap : 500 mg or $\frac{\text{1 cap}}{\text{500 mg}}$

This may also be expressed stating the weight of the drug first:

500 mg : 1 cap or $\frac{\text{500 mg}}{\text{1 cap}}$

Another use of ratio and proportion in dosage calculation is to express dosages of liquid medications used for oral administration and for injection. When stating a dosage of a liquid medication, a ratio expresses the **weight (strength) of a drug in a certain volume of solution.**

Example 3: A solution that contains 250 mg of drug in each **1 mL** would be written as:

1 mL : 250 mg or $\frac{\textbf{1 mL}}{\text{250 mg}}$

1 mL contains 250 mg of drug

This may also be written as:

250 mg : **1 mL** or $\frac{\text{250 mg}}{\textbf{1 mL}}$

Example 4: A solution that contains 80 mg of drug in each **2 mL** would be written as:

$$\mathbf{2\ mL} : 80\text{ mg or } \frac{\mathbf{2\ mL}}{80\text{ mg}}$$

2 mL contains 80 mg of drug

This may also be written as:

$$80\text{ mg} : \mathbf{2\ mL} \text{ or } \frac{80\text{ mg}}{\mathbf{2\ mL}}$$

Proving mathematically that ratios are equal and the proportion is true is important with medications. This can be illustrated by using our previous drug strength examples.

Example 1: 1 cap : 500 mg = 2 cap : 1000 mg

If 1 cap contains 500 mg, 2 cap will contain 1000 mg

extremes

1 cap : 500 mg = 2 cap : 1000 mg

means

$$500 \times 2 = 1000 \times 1$$

$$1000 = 1000$$

(In true proportion, the product of means equals product of extremes.)

Example 2: 2 mL : 80 mg = 1 mL : 40 mg

$$80 \times 1 = 2 \times 40$$

$$80 = 80$$

(In true proportion, the product of means equals product of extremes.)

Points to Remember

- Proportions represent two ratios that are equal and have a relationship to each other.
- When 3 values are known, the fourth can be easily calculated with this method.
- Proportions can be stated using an (=) sign, a double colon (::), or in a fraction format.
- Ratio can be used to state the amount of drug contained in a volume of solution, tablet, or capsule.
- Proportions are solved by multiplying the means and extremes.
- Ratios are always stated in their lowest terms.
- Double-check work.

Chapter Review (p. 329)

Express the following fractions as ratios. Reduce to lowest terms.

1. $\frac{2}{3}$ 2:3
2. $\frac{1}{9}$ 1:9
3. $\frac{6}{8}$ 6:8; 3:4
4. $\frac{1}{5}$ 1:5
5. $\frac{5}{10}$ 5:10; 1:5
6. $\frac{2}{10}$ 2:10

Express the following ratios as fractions. Reduce to lowest terms.

7. 3 : 7 3/7
8. 4 : 6 4/6
9. 1 : 7 1/7
10. 8 : 6 8/6
11. 3 : 4 3/4

Solve for x in the following proportions. Carry division two decimal places as necessary.

12. $20 : 40 = x : 10$ __________

13. $\frac{1}{4} : \frac{1}{2} = 1 : x$ __________

14. $0.12 : 0.8 = 0.6 : x$ __________

15. $\frac{1}{250} : 2 = \frac{1}{150} : x$ __________

16. $x : 9 = 5 : 10$ __________

17. $\frac{1}{4} : 1.6 = \frac{1}{8} : x$ __________

18. $\frac{1}{2} : 2 = \frac{1}{3} : x$ __________

19. $125 : 0.4 = 50 : x$ __________

20. $x : 1 = 0.5 : 5$ __________

Express the following dosages as ratios. Be sure to include the units of measure and numerical value.

21. An injectable solution that contains 1000 units (U) in each mL. __________

22. A tablet that contains 0.2 mg of drug. __________

23. A capsule that contains 250 mg of drug. __________

24. An oral solution that contains 125 mg in each 5 mL. __________

25. An injectable solution that contains 40 mg in each mL. __________

Chapter 5

Percentages

Objectives

After reviewing this chapter the student will be able to do the following:

1. Define percent
2. Convert percents to fractions, decimals, and ratios
3. Convert decimals to percents
4. Convert fractions to percents and ratios

Percentage is a commonly used word. Common things such as sale taxes are a *percentage* of the sale price; a final examination is a certain *percentage* of the final grade; interest on a home mortgage represents the balance owed; interest on a savings account is expressed as a *percentage*. **Health care professionals see percentages written with medications** (e.g., magnesium sulfate 50%).

Doctors prescribe solutions that are expressed in percentages for external as well as internal use.

Example: Hydrocortisone cream, Burrow's solution, and intravenous solutions

In current practice most percentage solutions are prepared by the pharmacy; however, there are still some institutions that require nurses to prepare these solutions. Understanding percentages provides the foundation for preparation and calculation of dosages for medications that are ordered in percentages.

The term *percent (%)* means hundredths. A percentage is the same as a fraction in which the denominator is 100, and the numerator indicates the part of 100 that is being considered.

Example: $4\% = \dfrac{4}{100}$

Intravenous solutions are ordered in percentage strengths, and nurses need to be familiar with their meaning (e.g., 1000 mL/cc 5% dextrose and water). **Percentage solution means the number of grams of solute per 100 mL/cc of diluent.**

Example 1: 1000 mL IV of 5% dextrose and water contains 50 g (grams) of dextrose

Example 2: 250 mL IV of 10% dextrose contains 25 g (grams) of dextrose

A point to remember with percentage solutions such as intravenous fluids is the higher the percentage strength the more drug/solute it contains, and the more potent the solution will be.

Example: 10% I.V. solution is more potent than 5%. **Always check the percentage of I.V. solution ordered by the doctor.**

Practice Problems (p. 329)

1. How many grams of drug will 500 mL of a 10% solution contain? ____________
2. How many grams of dextrose will 1000 mL of a 10% solution contain? ____________
3. How many grams of dextrose will 250 mL of a 5% solution contain? ____________
4. How many grams of drug will 100 mL of a 50% solution contain? ____________
5. How many grams of dextrose will 150 mL of 5% solution contain? ____________

Changing Percentages to Fractions, Decimals, and Ratios

The percent symbol may be used with a whole number (15%), a fraction (1/2%), a mixed number (14 1/2%), or a decimal (0.6%). Percentages therefore can be expressed in different forms without changing the value.

> To change a percent to a fraction, drop the % sign, place the number over 100, and reduce to lowest terms.

Example 1: $8\% = \frac{8}{100}$, reduced is $\frac{2}{25}$

Example 2: $\frac{1}{4}\% = \frac{1}{4} \div 100 = \frac{1}{4} \times \frac{1}{100} = \frac{1}{400}$

Practice Problems (p. 329)

Change the following percents to fractions and reduce to lowest terms.

6. 1% ____________
7. 2% ____________
8. 50% ____________
9. 80% ____________
10. 3% ____________

> To change a percent to a decimal, drop the % sign, and move the decimal point two places to the left (add zeros as needed).

Example 1: 25% = 0.25

Example 2: 1.4% = 0.014

Note: An alternate method is to drop the % sign, express the percent as a fraction in its lowest terms, and divide the numerator by the denominator to obtain a decimal.

Example: $75\% = \frac{3}{4}$ (lowest terms). Divide the numerator of the fraction (3) by the denominator (4).

$$4\overline{)3.00} = 0.75$$

Practice Problems (pp. 329-330)

Change the following percents to decimals.

11. 10% ____________
12. 35% ____________
13. 50% ____________
14. 14.2% ____________
15. $\frac{1}{4}\%$ ____________

> To change a percent to a ratio, change it to a fraction and reduce to lowest terms, then place the numerator as the first term of the ratio and the denominator as the second term. Separate the two terms with a colon (:).

Example: $10\% = \frac{10}{100} = \frac{1}{10} = 1:10$

Practice Problems (p. 330)

Change the following percents to a ratio. Express in lowest terms:

16. 25% ____________
17. 11% ____________
18. 75% ____________
19. 4.5% ____________
20. $\frac{2}{5}\%$ ____________

Changing Fractions, Decimals, and Ratios to Percentages

> To change a fraction to a percent, multiply the fraction by 100, reduce if necessary, and add the percent sign.

Example 1: $\frac{3}{4}$ changed to a percent is

$$\frac{3}{4} \times \frac{100}{1} = \frac{300}{4} = \frac{75}{1} = 75$$

Add symbol for percent: 75%

Example 2: $5\frac{1}{2}$ changed to a percent is

$5\frac{1}{2}$: change to an improper fraction $\frac{11}{2}$

$$\frac{11}{2} \times \frac{100}{1} = \frac{1{,}100}{2} = \frac{550}{1} = 550$$

Add symbol for percent: 550%

Practice Problems (p. 330)

Change the following fractions to percents.

21. $\frac{2}{5}$ ____________
22. $\frac{11}{4}$ ____________
23. $\frac{1}{2}$ ____________
24. $\frac{1}{4}$ ____________
25. $\frac{7}{10}$ ____________

> To change a decimal to a percent, move the decimal point two places to the right (multiply), add zeros if necessary, and add the percent symbol.

Example 1: Change 0.45 to %

Move the decimal point two places to the right.

Add the symbol for percent: 45%

Example 2: Change 2.35 to %

Move the decimal point two places to the right.

Add the symbol for percent: 235%

Note: A decimal may also be changed to a percent by changing the decimal to a fraction and following the steps to change a fraction to a percent. If the percentage does not end in a whole number, express the percentage with the remainder as a fraction, to the nearest whole percent, or to the nearest tenth of a percent.

Example: $0.625 = \frac{5}{8} = 62\frac{1}{2}\%$, 63%, or 62.5%.

$$\frac{625}{1000} = \frac{5}{8}; \frac{5}{8} \times \frac{100}{1} = \frac{500}{8} = 62.5\%$$

> To change a ratio to percent, change the ratio to a fraction, and proceed with steps for changing a fraction to percent.

Example: $1:4 = \frac{1}{4}, \frac{1}{4} \times \frac{100}{1} = 25$

Add the symbol for percent: 25%

Practice Problems (p. 330)

Change the following ratios to percent.

26. 1 : 25 ____________
27. 3 : 4 ____________
28. 1 : 10 ____________
29. 1 : 100 ____________
30. 1 : 2 ____________

Chapter Review (p. 330)

Complete the table below. Express each of the following measures in their equivalents where indicated. Reduce to lowest terms where necessary.

	Percent	Ratio	Fraction	Decimal
1.	0.25%	________	________	________
2.	71%	________	________	________
3.	________	________	$\frac{7}{100}$	________
4.	________	1 : 50	________	________
5.	________	________	________	0.06
6.	________	________	$\frac{1}{30}$	________
7.	________	________	$\frac{61}{100}$	________
8.	________	7 : 1000	________	________
9.	5%	________	________	________
10.	2.5%	________	________	________

Posttest

After completing Unit One of this text, you should be able to complete this test. The test consists of a total of 50 questions that are worth 2 points each. The passing score is 70 or better. If you miss three or more questions in any section, review the chapter relating to that content. (See pp. 330-331 for answers).

Express the following in Roman numerals.

1. 5 ______________
2. 17 ______________
3. 27 ______________
4. 29 ______________
5. 30 ______________

Express the following in Arabic numbers.

6. $\overline{\text{viss}}$ ______________
7. $\overline{\text{xxiv}}$ ______________
8. $\overline{\text{xix}}$ ______________
9. $\overline{\text{xxv}}$ ______________
10. $\overline{\text{xv}}$ ______________

Reduce the following fractions to lowest terms.

11. $\frac{8}{6}$ ______________
12. $\frac{22}{33}$ ______________
13. $\frac{27}{63}$ ______________
14. $\frac{10}{15}$ ______________
15. $\frac{16}{10}$ ______________

Perform the indicated operations with fractions; reduce to lowest terms where needed.

16. $\frac{5}{6} \div \frac{7}{10} =$ ______________

17. $5\frac{1}{2} \div 4\frac{1}{2} =$ ______________

18. $6\frac{1}{3} \times 4 =$ ______________

19. $5\frac{1}{5} - 3\frac{4}{7} =$ ______________

20. $\frac{5}{4} + \frac{2}{9} =$ ______________

Change the following fractions to decimals; express your answer to the nearest tenth.

21. $\frac{8}{7}$ ______________

22. $\frac{1}{8}$ ______________

23. $\frac{1}{15}$ ______________

24. $\frac{12}{13}$ ______________

Indicate the largest fraction in each group.

25. $\frac{1}{2}, \frac{2}{3}, \frac{5}{9}$ ______________

26. $\frac{3}{4}, \frac{7}{10}, \frac{5}{8}$ ______________

Perform the indicated operations with decimals.

27. $16.7 + 21.0 =$ ______________

28. $0.007 + 17.4 =$ ______________

29. $10.57 \times 10 =$ ______________

30. $36.8 - 3.86 =$ ______________

Divide the following decimals; express your answer to the nearest tenth.

31. $67.8 \div 0.8 =$ ______________

32. $9 \div 0.4 =$ ______________

33. $5.01 \div 10 =$ ______________

Indicate the largest decimal in each group.

34. 0.850, 0.085 ______________

35. 3.002, 0.390, 0.399 ______________

36. 0.478, 0.445, 0.493 ______________

Solve for x, the unknown value.

37. $10 : 20 = x : 8, x =$ ______________

38. $500 : x = 200 : 1, x =$ ______________

39. $0.3 : x = 1.8 : 0.6, x =$ ______________

40. $\frac{1}{4} : x = \frac{1}{8} : 2, x =$ ______________

Round off to the nearest tenth.

41. $0.57 =$ ______________

42. $0.99 =$ ______________

43. $1.42 =$ ______________

Round off to the nearest hundredth.

44. 0.677 = ____________

45. 0.832 = ____________

46. 1.222 = ____________

Complete the table below. Express each of the measures in their equivalents where indicated. Reduce to lowest terms where necessary or round off to nearest hundredth.

	Percent	Decimal	Ratio	Fraction
47.	________	________	1 : 10	________
48.	60%	________	________	________
49.	$66\frac{2}{3}\%$	________	________	________
50.	25%	________	________	________

UNIT TWO

Systems of Measurement

Three systems of measurement are used in the computation of medication doses: metric, apothecaries', and household. To be competent in the administration of medications, it is essential that the nurse be familiar with all three systems and the measures used in the computation of doses.

Chapter 6

Metric System

Objectives

After reviewing this chapter the student will be able to do the following:

1. Express metric measures correctly using rules of the metric system.
2. State from memory common equivalents in the metric system that are used for medication administration.
3. Convert metric measures to their equivalents in metric.

The metric system is an international decimal system of weights and measures that was introduced in France in the late 17th and 18th centuries. The system is also referred to as the International System of Units (SI). SI is the abbreviation for the French *Système International d'Unités.* Although the system was rooted in the late 17th and 18th centuries, the standard system of abbreviations was not adopted until 1960. The metric system is more precise than the apothecaries' and household systems. Apothecaries' and household measures are gradually being replaced with the metric system. More and more in everyday situations we are encountering the use of metric measures. For example, soft drinks come in bottles labeled in liters; engine sizes are also expressed in liters.

Most medications and measurements used in the health care field are calibrated and calculated using the metric system. For example, newborn weights are recorded in grams and kilograms, and adult weights are expressed in kilograms, as opposed to pounds and ounces. In obstetrics we express fundal height (upper portion of the uterus) in centimeters. While some medications are still prescribed in apothecaries' and household terms, the nurse will find the majority of medication calculation and administration skills involve **accurate** use of the metric system.

Particulars of the Metric System

1. The metric system is based on the decimal system, in which divisions and multiples of ten are used. Therefore a lot of math can be done by decimal point movement. (Refer to pp. 47-48.)
2. Three basic units of measure are used:
   a) **Gram**—the basic unit for weight
   b) **Liter**—the basic unit for volume
   c) **Meter**—the basic unit for length

   Doses are calculated using measurements from the metric system that relate to weight and volume. Meter, which is used for linear (length) measurement, is not used in the calculation of doses. Linear measurements (meter, centimeter) are commonly used to measure the height of an individual and to determine growth patterns.

3. Common prefixes in this system denote the numerical value of the unit being discussed. Memorization of these prefixes is necessary for quick and accurate calculations.

Prefix	Numerical value	Meaning
Kilo	1000	One thousand times
Centi	0.01	One hundredth part of
Milli	0.001	One thousandth part of
Micro	0.000001	One millionth part of

Let's look at the following example to see how the prefix can tell us something about a measure.

Example: 67 milligrams

Prefix—*milli*—means measure in thousandths of a unit.

Gram is a unit of weight.

Therefore 67 milligrams = 67 thousandths of a gram.

4. Regardless of the size of the unit, the name of the **basic unit** is incorporated into the measure. This allows easy recognition of the unit of measure.

Example 1: Milli**liter**—The word **liter** indicates that you are measuring **volume.** (*Milli* indicates 1/1000 of that volume.)

Example 2: Kilo**gram**—The word **gram** indicates that you are measuring **weight.** (*Kilo* indicates 1000 of that weight.)

5. The abbreviation for a unit of measure in the metric system is often the first letter of the word. Lower case letters are used more often than capital letters.

Example: Liter = **L** (This is the one abbreviation that still uses a capital letter.)

6. When prefixes are used in combination with the basic unit, the first letter of the prefix and the first letter of the unit of measure are written together in lower case letters.

Example 1: Milligram—Abbreviated as **mg.** The *m* is taken from the prefix *milli* and the *g* from *gram,* the unit of weight.

Example 2: Microgram—Abbreviated as **mcg.** Microgram is also written using the symbol (μ) in combination with the letter *g* from the basic unit *gram.* **However, using the symbol μg should be avoided when transcribing orders, because it might be interpreted as mg.**

Example 3: Milliliter—Abbreviated as **mL.** Note that when *L (liter)* is used in combination with a prefix, it **remains capitalized.**

Common Metric Abbreviations

gram = g
milligram = mg
kilogram = kg
liter = L
milliliter = mL
microgram = mcg

Rules of Metric System

There are rules that are specific to the metric system and important to remember.

Metric System Rules

1. Arabic numbers are used to express quantities in this system.

   Example: 1; 1000; 0.5

2. Parts of a unit or fractions of a unit are expressed as decimals.

   Example: 0.4 g, 0.5 L $\left(\text{not } \frac{2}{5}\text{ g, } \frac{1}{2}\text{ L}\right)$

3. The quantity, whether in whole numbers or in decimals, is always written before the abbreviation or symbol for a unit of measure.

   Example: 1000 mg, 0.75 mL (not mg 1000, mL 0.75)

Note: **A zero should always be placed in front of the decimal when the quantity is not a whole number. When the quantity expressed is preceded by a whole number, a zero is not necessary.**

Example 1: .52 mL is written as 0.52 mL to **reinforce the decimal** and avoid being misread as 52 mL.

Example 2: 2.5 mL is written as 2.5 mL, not 2.50 mL. **Addition of unnecessary zeros can lead to errors in reading;** 2.50 mL may be misread as 250 mL instead of 2.5 mL.

Units of Measure

Weight

The gram is the basic unit of weight. Some medications are ordered as fractions of grams.

1. The milligram is 1000 times smaller than a gram; medications may be ordered in milligrams.

   1000 mg = 1 g

2. The microgram is 1000 times smaller than a milligram and 1 million times smaller than a gram. The word *micro* also means tiny or small. Micrograms are tiny parts of a gram: 1000 mcg = 1 mg. A milligram is 1000 times larger than a microgram. It takes 1 million mcg to make 1 g.
3. The kilogram is very large and is not used for measuring medications. A kilogram is 1000 times larger than a gram: 1 kg = 1000 g. This measure is frequently used to denote weights of clients, upon which medication doses are based.

Units of Weight to Memorize

1 kilogram (kg) = 1000 grams (g)
1 gram (g) = 1000 milligrams (mg)
1 milligram (mg) = 1000 micrograms (mcg)

Volume

1. The **liter** is the basic unit.

   1000 mL (cc) = 1 L

2. The **milliliter** is 1000 times smaller than a liter. It is abbreviated as mL.

   1 mL = 0.001 L

3. The **cubic centimeter** is the amount of space that 1 mL of liquid occupies. It is abbreviated as cc.

   1 cc = 0.001 L = 1 mL or
   1 L = 1000 cc = 1000 mL

Cubic centimeter (cc) and milliliter (mL) are considered to be the **same** and are used **interchangeably** (Figure 6-1 illustrates metric measures).

Units of Volume to Memorize

1 liter = 1000 milliliters (mL) or
1000 cubic centimeters (cc)
1 milliliter (mL) = 1 cubic centimeter (cc)

Although pint and quart are not metric measures, they have metric equivalents. For example, a quart is approximately the size of a liter: 1 quart = 1000 mL or cc, and 1 pint = 500 mL or cc. Pint and quart are not measures used in medication administration.

Conversions between Metric Units

Since the metric system is based on the decimal, system conversions between one metric system unit and another can be done by moving the decimal point. To **convert** or make a **conversion** means to change from one form to another. This converting can be simply changing a measure to its equivalent in the same system. Changing from grams to milligrams illustrates a metric measure changed to another metric measure. Each unit in the metric system differs from the next by a factor of 1000. Metric conversions can therefore be made by dividing or multiplying by **1000.** Knowledge concerning the size of a unit is important when converting by moving the decimal since this determines whether division or multiplication is necessary to make the conversion.

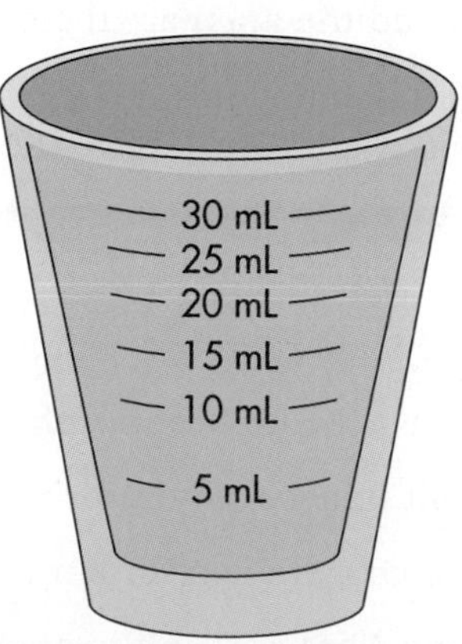

Figure 6-1. Medicine cup showing volume measures in milliliters.

> Nurses frequently make conversions within the metric system when administering medications; for example, g to mg.

To make conversions within the metric system remember the common conversion factors (1 kg = 1000 g, 1 g = 1000 mg, 1 mg = 1000 mcg, and 1 L = 1000 mL (1000 cc) and the following rules:

1. To convert a **smaller** unit to a **larger** one, **divide** by moving the decimal point **three places to the left.**

Example 1:

100 mL = _____ L (smaller) (larger) (conversion factor 1000 mL = 1 L)

100 mL = .100 = 0.1 L (Placing zero in front of the decimal is important.)

Example 2:

50 mg = _____ g (smaller) (larger) (conversion factor 1000 mg = 1 g)

50 mg = .050 = 0.05 g (Placing zero in front of the decimal is important.)

2. To convert a **larger** unit to a **smaller** one, **multiply** by moving the decimal **three places to the right.**

Example 1:

0.75 g = _____ mg (larger) (smaller) (conversion factor 1 g = 1000 mg)

0.75 g = 0.750 = 750 mg

Example 2:

0.04 kg = _____ g (larger) (smaller) (conversion factor 1 kg = 1000 g)

0.04 kg = 0.040 = 40 g

Practice Problems (p. 331)

Convert the following metric measures

1. 300 mg = _____ g
2. 6 mg = _____ mcg
3. 0.7 L = _____ mL
4. 180 mcg = _____ mg
5. 0.02 mg = _____ mcg
6. 4.5 L = _____ mL
7. 4.2 g = _____ mg
8. 0.9 g = _____ mg
9. 3,250 mL = _____ L
10. 42 g = _____ kg

Points to Remember

- The liter and the gram are the basic units used for medication administration.
- Conversion factors must be memorized to do conversions. The common conversion factors in the metric system are 1 kg = 1000 g, 1 g = 1000 mg, 1 mg = 1000 mcg, and 1 L = 1000 mL (1000 cc).
- Express answers using rules of the metric system.
  1. Fractional parts are expressed as a decimal.
  2. Place a zero in front of the decimal point when it is not preceded by a whole number.
  3. Omit unnecessary zeros to avoid misreading of a value.
  4. The abbreviation for a measure is placed after the quantity.
- Converting from one unit to another within the metric system is done by moving the decimal point three places.

Chapter Review (p. 331)

1. List the three units of measurement used in the metric system.

   a) ____________

   b) ____________

   c) ____________

2. Which is larger, kilogram or milligram? ____________

3. 1 mL = ____________ L

4. What units of measure are used in the metric system for:

   a. liquid capacity? ____________

   b. weight? ____________

5. 1000 mg = ____________ g

6. 1 mL = ____________ cc

7. 1000 mcg = ____________ mg

8. 1000 mL = ____________ L

9. 10 cc = ____________ mL

10. The abbreviation for microgram is ____________

11. The abbreviation for milliliter is ____________

12. The abbreviation for gram is ____________

13. mL is the same as ____________

14. The prefix *kilo* means ____________

15. The prefix *milli* means ____________

Using abbreviations and the rules of the metric system, express the following quantities correctly:

16. Six tenths of a gram ____________

17. Fifty kilograms ____________

18. Four tenths of a milligram ____________

19. Four hundredths of a liter ____________

20. Four and two tenths micrograms ____________

21. Five thousandths of a gram ____________

22. Six hundredths of a gram ____________

23. Two and six tenths milliliters ____________

24. One hundred milliliters ____________

25. Three hundredths of a milliliter ____________

Convert the following metric measures:

26. 950 mcg = ____________ mg

27. 58.5 L = ____________ mL

28. 130 mL = ____________ cc

29. 276 g = ____________ mg

30. 550 mL = ____________ L

31. 56.5 L = ____________ mL

32. 205 g = ____________ kg

33. 0.025 kg = ____________ g

34. 1 L = ____________ mL

35. 0.015 g = ____________ mg

Chapter 7

Apothecaries' and Household Systems

Objectives

After reviewing this chapter the student will be able to do the following:

1. **State the common apothecaries' and household equivalents**
2. **State specific rules that relate to the apothecaries' and household systems**
3. **Identify symbols and interpret measures in the apothecaries' and household systems**

Apothecaries' System

The apothecaries' system is one of the oldest systems of measurement. It was brought to this country from England during the colonial period. In the European countries, the apothecaries' system has been totally replaced by the metric system. This transition in the United States has been a gradual and slow process, with the apothecaries' system still used in dose calculation.

Doctors employ this system to order medications that have been in use for many years (morphine, codeine, atropine, aspirin). An example of this would be an order such as "aspirin grains ten." Pharmaceutical companies often label drugs using the apothecaries' system as well as the metric. For example, if we look at a bottle of nitroglycerin tablets we see that while the tablets may be labeled grains 1/150, which is an apothecaries' measure, the label may have 0.4 mg in parentheses, which is a metric measure.

Other medications that illustrate the use of both apothecaries' and metric measures include atropine sulfate, morphine sulfate, and phenobarbital sodium. (Figure 7-1 illustrates the use of metric and apothecaries' measures on drug labels.) Since the apothecaries' system is still in use, it is necessary for those involved in the administration of medications to be familiar with the basics relating to it.

Particulars of the Apothecaries' System

1. The measures used in this system are **approximations;** however, they have become acceptable in the preparation and administration of medications.
2. Roman numerals, as well as Arabic numbers, are often used in this system.
3. Fractions are used to express quantities that are less than one, as opposed to the use of decimals in the metric system.

A

NDC 0002-0313-02
100 TABLETS No. 1571
Lilly
FERROUS SULFATE TABLETS USP
5 grs (324 mg)
For Iron Deficiency in Hypochromic Anemias.

B

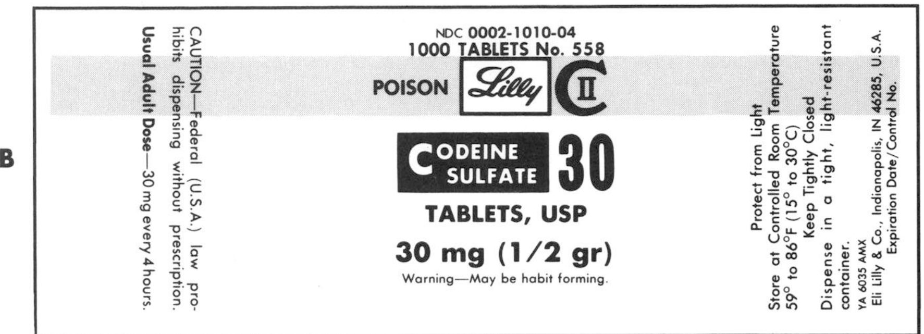

Figure 7-1. **A,** Drug label showing apothecaries' and metric measures (*gr,* apothecaries'; *mg,* metric). **B,** Drug label showing metric and apothecaries' measures (*mg,* metric; *gr,* apothecaries). (From Radcliff R, Ogden S: *Calculation of drug dosages,* ed 5, St Louis, 1995, Mosby.)

4. The symbol *ss* is used for the fraction 1/2. When used it can be written ss or $\overline{\text{ss}}$.

   Example: half of a grain in abbreviated form would be gr ss or gr $\overline{\text{ss}}$.

   The symbol *ss* can also be used with Roman numerals. When used with Roman numerals, it is placed at the end.

   Example: seven and a half grains = gr $\overline{\text{viiss}}$.

5. Unlike the metric system, in the apothecaries' system the abbreviation or symbol for a unit of measure is written **before** the amount or quantity.

   Example: twelve drams. The symbol for dram is ʒ, or it is abbreviated dr. Therefore twelve drams would be written as ʒ xii, ʒ 12, dr xii, or dr 12.

6. A combination of Arabic numerals and fractions can also be used in this system to express units of measure.

   Example: gr $7\frac{1}{2}$

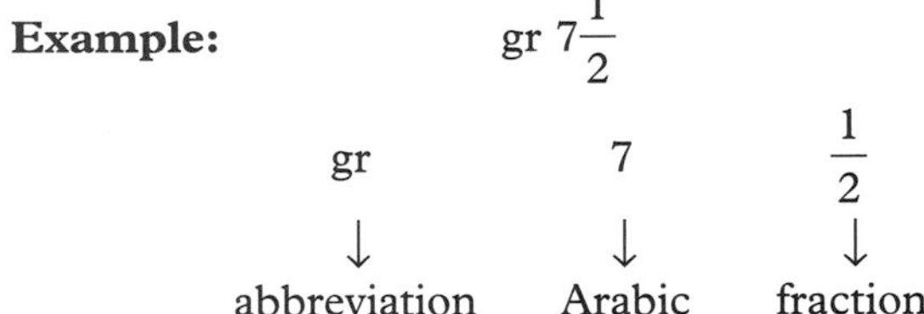

Apothecaries' Units of Measure

The units of measure used for medication administration are few.

Weight

The basic unit for weight is the **grain.**

1. Grain is abbreviated in lower case letters as gr. The abbreviations for grain and gram are often confused. Remember **grain** is abbreviated as **gr,** and **gram** is abbreviated as **g.** Grain, which is an apothecaries' measure for weight, has some metric equivalents. Two important conversions to remember are **gr 15 = 1 g** and **60 mg = gr 1.** Another way to remember common apothecaries' and metric conversions is to remember the **conversion clock.**

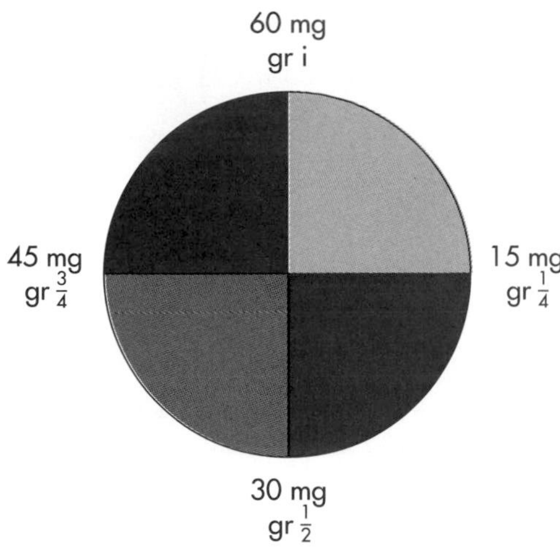

2. Dram is also a unit of weight; 1 dram is equal to 60 grains. The symbol for dram is a single-headed z with a tail (ʒ). Dram is also abbreviated as dr.
3. Ounce—the symbol for ounce is a **double-headed** z with a tail (℥). Note: The extra loop on the z differentiates it from the symbol for dram. It is important not to confuse the symbols for dram and ounce because of the large difference in measures. A way to avoid confusion is to remember that an ounce is larger than a dram, thus the symbol is bigger. Another cue to remember to differentiate an ounce from a dram is to remember that the **"ounce (symbol) has the extra bounce."** Ounce is also abbreviated as oz.

Volume

The basic unit for volume is the **minim.**

1. The most current abbreviation for minim is a lower case m. A minim is extremely small (the size of one drop), and minims are therefore always expressed as whole numbers. A way to remember the size of a minim is to think about the beginning three letters of the word (min) and think of words such as minute and minimal.
2. Volume can also be measured by dram and ounce. To differentiate liquid measures from solid measures, an f may be seen before the measure. F = fluid; it is abbreviated with a lower case f. When it is obvious that the measure is a liquid, f is omitted.

Example: fʒ = fluid dram; f℥ = fluid ounce

1 fluid dram = 60 minims
(fʒ i = m 60), or fʒ i = m lx

1 fluid ounce = 8 fluid drams
(f℥ i = fʒ viii)

3. The pint and quart are also apothecaries' measures.

Pint is abbreviated as pt*

1 pint = 16 fluid ounces

Quart is abbreviated as qt*

1 quart = 32 fluid ounces or 2 pints

4. Some apothecaries' measures have equivalents in the metric system that must be memorized:

1 dram = 4 mL or 5 mL

1 ounce = 30 mL

1 pint = 500 mL

1 quart = 1000 mL

Discrepancies in Apothecaries' Equivalents

Discrepancies in the apothecaries' system exist because of the inaccuracy and approximation within this system. A table of equivalents may state that **gr 1 equals 60 mg** and **also 64 mg**; both are correct. The equivalent used for most medications is gr 1 = 60 mg (for example, aspirin 300 mg = gr 5). In some instances labels may indicate gr 5 is equivalent to 325 mg or 324 mg. It is important for the nurse to realize discrepancies do exist. An example of a discrepancy is Figure 7-1, *A,* a ferrous sulfate label that shows 5 grains equaling 324 mg, and Figure 7-2, an aspirin label that shows 5 grains equaling 325 mg.

For medication administration it is necessary to be familiar with the following units from the apothecaries' system.

Units of the Apothecaries' System

Weight: grain (gr)
Volume: minim (m)
dram (dr) (ʒ)
ounce (oz) (℥)

*Abbreviation used most often.

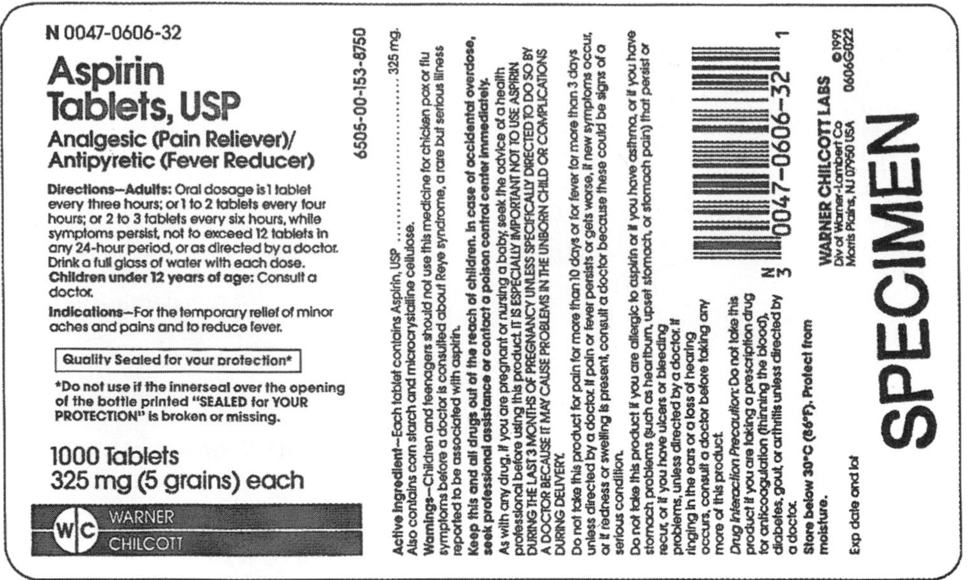

Figure 7-2. Label from aspirin. (From Radcliff R, Ogden S: *Calculation of drug dosages,* ed 5, St Louis, 1995, Mosby.)

Household System

The household system is still in use for doses given primarily at home, as indicated by the name. The nurse needs to be familiar with household measures since clients frequently use utensils in the home to take prescribed medications. The household system is the **least accurate** of the three systems of measure. Capacities of utensils such as teaspoon, tablespoon, and cup vary from one house to another; therefore liquid measures are approximate. With the increase in nursing being provided at home (home care, visiting nurse) it is imperative that nurses become adept in converting from one system to another. When calculating doses or interpreting physicians' instructions for the client at home, the nurse must remember that household measures are used at home. Consequently the nurse must be able to change equivalents for adaptation in the home, even though medication administration spoons, droppers, and medication measuring cups are available.

Common household measures to memorize are the following:

1 teaspoon (tsp) = 5 mL (cc)

1 tablespoon (tbs) = 15 mL (cc)

1 teaspoon = 60 drops (gtt)

1 measuring cup = 8 oz

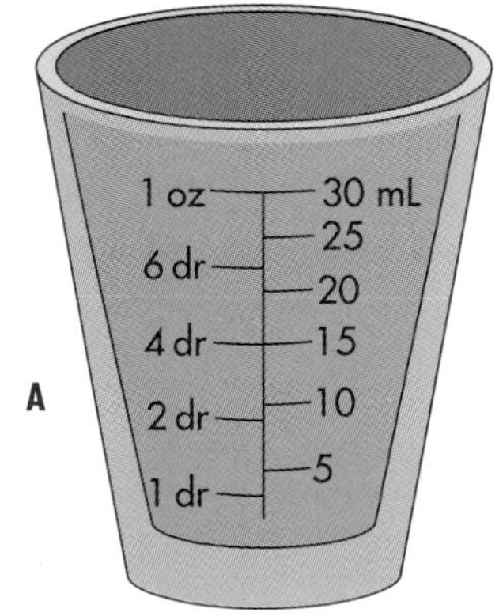

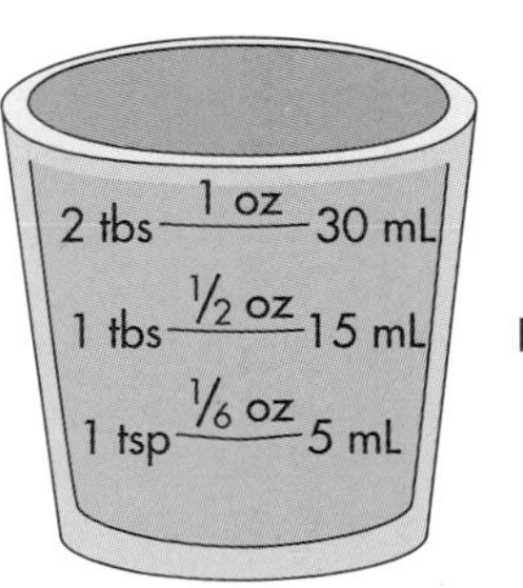

Figure 7-3. Apothecaries' fluid measures. **A,** drams. **B,** ounces.

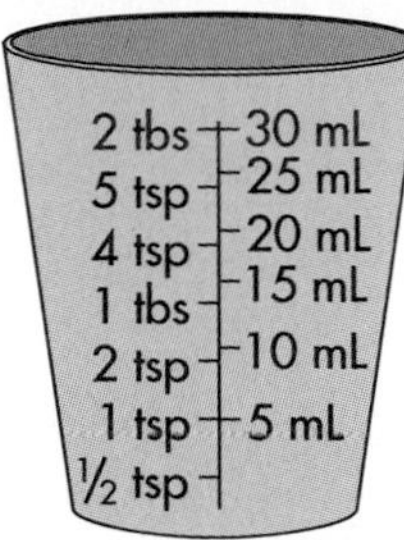

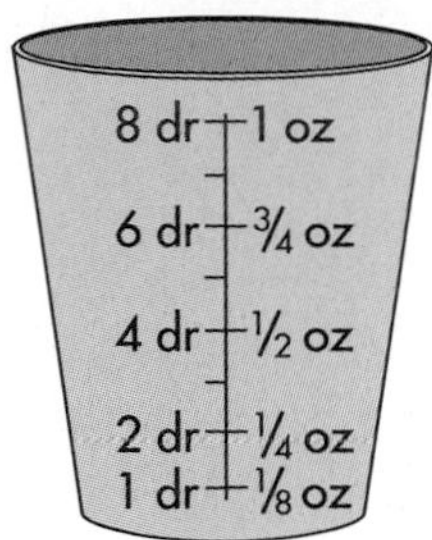

One Ounce Medicine Cups (30 mL)

Figure 7-4. Medicine cups showing household/metric and apothecaries'/household measurements.

Particulars of the Household System

1. Some of the units for liquid measures are the same as those in the apothecaries' system, for example, pint and quart.
2. There are no standard rules for expressing household measures, which accounts for variety in their use.
3. Standard cookbook abbreviations are used in this system.
4. Arabic numerals and fractions are used to express quantities.
5. The basic unit in the household system is the **drop (gtt).**
   Note: Drops should never be used as a measure for medications since the size of drops varies and therefore can be inaccurate. When drops are used as a measure for medications, they should be calibrated or used only when associated with a dropper size, as in intravenous (I.V.) flow rates.
6. Common household measures and conversions within this system are as follows. See also Table 7-1.

   Drop (gtt)

   Teaspoon (t, tsp) (60 gtt = 1 tsp)

   Tablespoon (T, tbs) (3 tsp = 1 tbs)

   Cup (C) (16 tbs = 1 C)

   Pint (pt) (2 C = 1 pt)

   Quart (qt) (2 pt = 1 qt)

Table 7-1 Approximate Equivalents of Metric, Apothecaries', and Household Measures

Household	Apothecaries'	Metric
60 drops (gtt)	1 teaspoon (tsp)	5 mL (or cc)*
1 teaspoon (tsp)	1 fluidram (f℥)	5 mL
1 tablespoon (tbs)	4 fluidrams	15 mL
2 tablespoons (tbs)	8 fluidrams = 1 ounce (℥)	30 mL
1 measuring cup	8 ounces	240 mL
1 pint	16 ounces	500 mL
1 quart	32 ounces	1000 mL

*The abbreviations *mL* and *cc* are used interchangeably; however, *mL* is generally used for liquids, *cc* for solids and gases, and *g* for solids.

Brown M, Mulholland J: *Drug calculations: process and problems for clinical practice,* ed 5, St Louis, 1995, Mosby.

Points to Remember

- In the apothecaries' system, the abbreviation or symbol is placed before the quantity.
- Apothecaries' measures are approximate.
- The apothecaries' system uses fractions, Roman numerals, and Arabic numerals.
- Teaspoon, tablespoon, and drop are common measures used in the household system.
- There are no rules for stating household measures.
- The household system uses fractions and Arabic numerals.
- Conversions between metric, apothecaries', and household are not equal measures.

Chapter Review (pp. 331-332)

Using the rules of the apothecaries' system, write the following using the correct abbreviations or symbols.

1. Eight and one-half grains __________
2. Three minims __________
3. Five drams __________
4. Eight ounces __________
5. Quart __________
6. Pint __________
7. One hundred twenty-fifth of a grain __________
8. Six and a half fluid drams __________
9. Two fluid ounces __________
10. Five ounces __________

Complete the following.

11. The volume of one drop equals __________
12. ʒ i = m __________
13. f℥ i = fʒ __________
14. 1 pt = f℥ __________
15. 1 qt = f℥ __________
16. 1 tbs = f℥ __________
17. The abbreviation for drop is __________ .
18. T is the abbreviation for __________ .
19. The abbreviation t is used for __________ .
20. 1 t = __________ mL
21. 1 tsp = __________ gtt
22. 1 cup = __________ ounces
23. 1 tbs = __________ mL
24. 1 pt = __________ ounces
25. 1 qt = __________ ounces

Chapter 8

Converting Within and Between Systems

Objectives

After reviewing this chapter the student will be able to do the following:

1. Recall equivalents/conversions from metric, apothecaries', and household systems to convert a given measure
2. Convert a unit of measure to its equivalent within the same system
3. Convert a unit of measure to its equivalent in another system of measure (for example, metric to apothecaries')

Equivalents among Metric, Apothecaries', and Household Systems

As already discussed in the previous chapters dealing with the systems of measure, some equivalents in one system have equivalents in another system; however, equivalents are not exact measures, and there are discrepancies. Several tables have been developed illustrating conversions/equivalents. Sometimes drug companies use different equivalents for a measure. As mentioned previously, a common discrepancy is with grains, which is an apothecaries' measure. In some tables 65 mg = gr 1, and in others 60 mg = gr 1. Both of these equivalents are correct. However, remember that **60 mg = gr 1** is most often used in medication administration.

In the health care system it is imperative that nurses be proficient in converting between all three systems of measure (metric, apothecaries', and household). Nurses are becoming increasingly responsible for administration of medications to clients outside of the conventional hospital setting (for example, home care). Nurses have become more involved in discharge planning and are responsible for ensuring that the client can safely self-administer medications in the correct dosage. Table 8-1 lists some of the equivalents that exist between systems. Memorize these common equivalents!

Converting

The term *convert* means to change from one form to another. Converting can mean changing a measure to its equivalent in the same system or changing a measurement from one system to another system, which is called converting between sys-

Table 8-1 Approximate Equivalents of Metric, Apothecaries', and Household Measures

Household	Apothecaries'	Metric
	m 15 or m 16*	1 mL (cc)†
1 t, 1 tsp	ʒ i	4 or 5* mL (cc)
1 T, 1 tbs	ʒ iv	15* or 16 mL (cc)
	gr 15	1 g (1000 mg)
	gr 1	60 mg
	1 oz (℥ i)	30 mL
	1 pt (16 oz)	500 mL (cc)
	1 qt (32 oz)	1000 mL (cc), 1 L
	2.2 lb	1 kg (1000 g)

*Equivalent used most often.
†mL and cc are used interchangeably; mL is preferred when used for liquids.

tems. The measurement obtained when converting between systems is approximate, not exact. Thus certain equivalents have been established to ensure continuity.

It is important for nurses to be able to make conversions, since they are often called upon to convert medication doses between metric, apothecaries', and household systems. The nurse therefore must understand the systems of measurement and be able to convert within the same system, as well as from one to another, with accuracy.

Before beginning the actual process of converting, the nurse should remember the following important points that can make converting simple.

Points for Converting

1. Memorization of the equivalents/conversions is essential.
2. Think of memorized equivalents/conversions as essential conversion factors.

   Example: 1000 mg = 1 g is called a conversion factor.

3. Follow basic math principles regardless of the conversion method used.
4. Answers should be expressed applying specific rules that relate to the system to which you are converting.

   Example: The metric system uses decimals; the apothecaries' system uses fractions.

5. Ratio-proportion is the easiest method to use, and this method can also be used for the calculation of doses.

Methods of Converting

Moving the Decimal Point

This method was discussed in Chapter 6. Because the metric system is based on the decimal system, conversions within the metric system can be done easily by movement of the decimal point. Conversely, this method cannot be applied in the apothecaries' or household system since decimal points are not used in either system. **Remember the two rules in moving decimal points:**

1. To convert a smaller unit to a larger one, divide or move the decimal point to the left.

   Example: 350 mg = _____ g
   (smaller) (larger)

   Solution: After determining that mg is the smaller unit and you are converting to a larger unit (g), recall the conversion factor that allows you to change milligrams to grams: 1 g = 1000 mg. Therefore 350 is divided by 1000 by moving the decimal point three places to the left, indicating 350 mg = 0.35 g.

   350. = 0.35 g

   Note: The final answer is expressed in decimal format. Remember to always place a (0) in front of the decimal point to indicate a value that is less than one.

2. To convert a larger unit to a smaller one, multiply or move the decimal point to the right.

   Example: 0.85 L = _____ mL
   (larger) (smaller)

   Solution: After determining that L is the larger unit and you are converting to a smaller unit (mL), recall the conversion factor that allows you to change liters to milliliters: 1 L = 1000 mL. Therefore 0.85 is multiplied by 1000 by moving the decimal point three places to the right, indicating 0.85 L = 850 mL.

   0.850 = 850 mL

   Note the addition of a zero here to allow movement of the decimal point the correct number of places.

Practice Problems (p. 332)

Convert the following metric measures to the equivalent units indicated for additional practice in converting by decimal movement.

1. 600 cc = ______________ L
2. 0.016 g = ______________ mg
3. 4 kg = ______________ g
4. 3 mcg = ______________ mg
5. 0.3 mg = ______________ g
6. 0.01 kg = ______________ g
7. 1.9 L = ______________ mL
8. 0.5 g = ______________ kg
9. 0.07 mg = ______________ mcg
10. 650 cc = ______________ L
11. 0.04 g = ______________ mg
12. 0.12 g = ______________ kg
13. 180 mg = ______________ g
14. 1,700 mL = ______________ L
15. 15 kg = ______________ g

Using Ratio-Proportion

This is one of the easiest ways to make conversions, whether they are within the same system or between systems. The basics on how to state ratio-proportions and how to solve them when looking for one unknown are presented in Chapter 4. To make conversions using ratio-proportion, a proportion must be set up that expresses a numerical relationship between the two systems. A proportion may be written in a colon format or as a fraction when making conversions. Regardless of the format used, there are some basic rules to follow when using this method.

Rules for Ratio-Proportion

1. State the known equivalent first (memorized equivalent).
2. Add the incomplete ratio on the other side of the equal sign, making sure the units of measurement are written in the same sequence.

   Example: mg : g = mg : g

3. Label all terms in the proportion including x (These labels are ignored when multiplying or dividing.)
4. Solve the problem by using the principles for solving ratio-proportions. (The product of the means equals the product of the extremes.)
5. The final answer for x should be labeled with the appropriate unit of measure or desired unit.

When using the method of ratio-proportion to make conversions, as with any method used, the known equivalents must be memorized. Stating the proportion in the fraction format may be a way of avoiding confusion with the terms (means and extremes). However, regardless of the format used, the terms must correspond to each other in value and have a relationship. Division should always be carried at least two decimal places to ensure accuracy.

Example: 8 mg = ______ g

Solution: State the known equivalent first; add the incomplete ratio, making sure the units are in the same sequence. Label all the terms in the proportion including x.

1000 mg : 1 g	=	8 mg : x g
(known equivalent)		(unknown)

Read as "1000 mg is to 1 g as 8 mg is to x g."

Note: The terms of the proportion are in the same sequence, (mg : g = mg : g), and there is a correspondence in the ratio: small : large = small : large.

Once the proportion is stated, solve it by multiplying the means (inner terms) and the extremes (outer terms).

Result:

means (1 g and 8 mg); extremes (1000 mg and x g)

1000 mg : 1 g = 8 mg : x g

$$1 \times 8 = 1000 \times (x)$$

$$\frac{8}{1000} = \frac{1000\,x}{1000}$$

$$x = \frac{8}{1000}$$

Since the measure you are converting to is metric, the fraction is changed to a decimal by dividing 8 by 1000 to obtain an answer of 0.008 g.

However, because the measures are metric in this example, perhaps moving the decimal point would be the preferred method as opposed to actual division.

Example: 8 mg = _____ g

1. Note that conversion is going from smaller to larger, thus division or moving the decimal point to the left is indicated.
2. Note that the unit is going from mg to g thus changing by a factor of 1000.
3. The decimal point will be moved three places to the left to complete this conversion: 8 mg = 0.008.

An alternate way of stating the problem illustrated in the previous example would be stating it as a fraction and cross multiplying to solve for *x*.

$$\frac{1000 \text{ mg}}{1 \text{ g}} = \frac{8 \text{ mg}}{x \text{ g}}$$

$$\frac{1000\,x}{1000} = \frac{8}{1000}$$

$$x = 0.008 \text{ g}$$

The remainder of this chapter will show examples of the methods used in converting within the same system and between systems.

Converting Within the Same System

Converting within the same system is frequently seen with metric measures; however it can be done using the other systems of measurement, such as one apothecaries' measure being converted to an equivalent within the apothecaries' system. Any one of the methods discussed can be used, but movement of decimal points is limited to the metric system. Ratio-proportion can be used for all systems.

Example 1: (metric) (metric)

0.6 mg = _____ mcg

Solution: Equivalent: 1000 mcg = 1 mg

A milligram is larger than a microgram; the answer is obtained by moving the decimal point three places to the right (multiply).

Answer: 600 mcg

Alternate: Set up as a proportion following the rules presented, as a fraction or using the colon.

Example 2: (apothecaries') (apothecaries')

fʒ iv = m _____

Solution: m 60 = fʒ i

A dram is larger than a minim; the answer is obtained by multiplying 4 by 60.

Answer: m 240

Alternate: Set up as a proportion using the colon format or as a fraction.

Note: Since it may be confusing to write using apothecaries' symbols when stating the proportion, it can be written as follows:

1 fluid dram : 60 minims = 4 fluid dram : *x* minims

OR

$$\frac{1 \text{ fluid dram}}{60 \text{ minims}} = \frac{4 \text{ fluid dram}}{x \text{ minims}}$$

The principles presented for solving ratio-proportion problems are used to solve for *x*, when presented in colon format or fraction.

Practice Problems (p. 332)

Convert the following to the equivalent measures indicated.

16. 500 cc = _____________ L
17. 4 kg = _____________ g
18. 1.4 L = _____________ cc
19. ʒ vi = ℥ _____________
20. m 120 = ʒ _____________
21. ℥ ss = ʒ _____________
22. 10 gtt = _____________ tsp
23. 60 g = _____________ kg

24. 600 mg = ____________ g

25. 0.736 mg = ____________ mcg

26. 1,600 mL = ____________ L

27. 15 cc = ____________ mL

28. 0.18 g = ____________ mg

29. 25 mcg = ____________ mg

30. 5.2 g = ____________ kg

Converting Between Systems

The methods presented previously can be used to change a measure in one system to its equivalent in another.

Example 1: (apothecaries') (metric)

$$\text{gr } \frac{1}{100} = \_\_\_\_ \text{ mg}$$

Solution: Equivalent: gr 1 = 60 mg

A grain is larger than a milligram.

Multiply 1/100 by 60 to obtain 60/100.

Since the final answer is a metric measure, 60/100 is changed to a decimal by dividing 100 into 60. The fraction could also be reduced first to lowest terms 3/5 then changed to a decimal by dividing 5 into 3.

Answer: 0.6 mg

Alternate: Express the conversion in proportion format and solve for x.

$$\text{gr } 1 : 60 \text{ mg} = \text{gr } \frac{1}{100} : x \text{ mg}$$

$$60 \times \frac{1}{100} = x$$

$$\frac{60}{100} = x$$

$$x = 0.6 \text{ mg}$$

OR

$$\frac{\text{gr } 1}{60 \text{ mg}} = \frac{\text{gr } 1/100}{x \text{ mg}}$$

$$x = \frac{1}{100} \times 60$$

$$x = \frac{60}{100}$$

$$x = 0.6 \text{ mg}$$

Example 2: (apothecaries') (metric)

110 lb = ____ kg

Solution: Equivalent: 1 kg = 2.2 lbs

A pound is smaller than a kilogram; 110 is divided by 2.2.

Answer: 50 kg

Calculating Intake and Output

The nurse frequently converts between systems to calculate a client's **intake and output.** Intake and output is abbreviated **I & O.** Intake refers to the monitoring of fluid that a client takes orally (p.o.), by feeding tube, or parenterally. Oral intake includes fluids and solids that become liquid at body and room temperature, such as jello and popsicles. Intake also includes water, broth, and juice. Intake does not include solids such as bread, cereal, or meats. Liquid output refers to fluids that exit the body, such as diarrhea, vomitus, gastric suction, and urine. A client's intake and output are usually recorded on a special form called an intake and output sheet, which varies from institution to institution. A variety of clients require I & O monitoring, such as clients whose fluids are restricted, clients receiving diuretic therapy, and clients receiving I.V. therapy.

Intake and output are recorded using cubic centimeters or milliliters. When measuring output, the nurse uses a graduated receptacle that is calibrated in metric measures (mL and cc), and conversions are not necessary. Oral intake usually must be converted from household measures to metric measures before it can be recorded. Some agencies have cups that are calibrated to facilitate easy measuring and accurate recording of intake and output. Each time a client takes oral liquids, even those administered with medications, the amount is recorded on the appropriate form along with the time. The total intake and output are recorded at the end of each shift and also for a 24-hr period.

Conversion of a client's intake is usually required when recording measurements such as a bowl or coffee cup. Each agency usually has an

Juice Glass	– 180 cc	Jello Cup	– 150 cc		Addressograph with Client Information
Water Glass	– 190 cc	Ice Cream	– 120 cc		
Coffee Cup	– 240 cc	Creamer	– 30 cc		
Soup Bowl	– 180 cc				
Small Water Cup	– 120 cc				

Date July 16, 1996

INTAKE						OUTPUT				
ORAL			IV						OTHER	
TIME	TYPE	AMT	TIME	TYPE	AMOUNT ABSORBED	TIME	URINE	STOOL		
8A	Juice	60cc								
	Coffee	120cc								
	Milk	250cc								

Figure 8-1. Sample I & O sheet.

I & O sheet with a ledger that indicates the standard measurement for the utensils used in its facility. For example, it may indicate a standard cup is 6 oz or a coffee cup is 180 cc. A client's oral intake is calculated in the same manner as other conversion problems. After each item is converted, the items are added together for the total intake.

Sample Problem: Calculate the client's intake for breakfast in cubic centimeters. Assume the glass holds 6 oz and the cup 8 oz. The client had the following for breakfast at 8 AM:

Items	**Conversion factors**
1/3 glass of apple juice	1 oz = 30 cc (mL)
2 sausages	1 pint = 500 cc (mL)
1 boiled egg	1 cup = 8 oz
1/2 cup of coffee	1 glass = 6 oz
1/2 pint of milk	

Note: 2 sausages and 1 boiled egg are not part of fluid intake.

Solution:

1. 1/3 glass of apple juice

   1 glass = 6 oz; 1/3 of 6 oz = 2 oz

   Therefore 1 oz = 30 cc, 2 oz × 30 cc = 60 cc
   OR 1 oz : 30 cc = 2 oz : x cc, 60 cc = x

2. 1/2 cup of coffee

   1 cup = 8 oz; 1/2 of 8 oz = 4 oz

   Therefore 4 oz × 30 = 120 cc
   OR 1 oz : 30 cc = 4 oz : x cc, 120 cc = x

3. 1 pint of milk

   1 pint = 500 cc; 1/2 of 500 cc = 250 cc

   Total cc = 60 cc + 120 cc + 250 cc = 430 cc

Another solution could have been to total the number of ounces, which in this example is 6 ounces, convert that amount to cubic centimeters, and add the half pint of milk (expressed in cubic centimeters).

1 oz : 30 cc = 6 oz : x cc

180 cc = x

180 cc + 250 cc (1/2 pint) = 430 cc

The conversions are recorded on an I & O sheet next to time ingested. The I & O sheet in Figure 8-1 is filled out with the data for this sample problem.

8:00 AM	juice, 60 cc
	coffee, 120 cc
	milk, 250 cc

I & O sheets usually have a place on them for recording p.o. intake, I.V. intake, and a column or columns for output. Figure 8-2 shows a sample 24-hr I & O sheet illustrating the charting of the intake.

ST. BARNABAS HOSPITAL
BRONX, NEW YORK

DEPARTMENT OF NURSING

8 HR INTAKE AND OUTPUT RECORD

Addressograph with Client Identification

DATE: July 16, 1996.

INTAKE					OUTPUT				
TIME					TIME				
6A-2P	ORAL/TUBE FEEDING TYPE	AMOUNT	I.V. / BLOOD TYPE	AMOUNT	6A-2P	URINE (**CBI)	LIQUID STOOLS	EMESIS	DRAINAGE
8A	juice	240cc	LIB* D5W 1000cc	850cc	8A	300cc			
	milk	120cc			10A	200cc			
	coffee	200cc			1³⁰P	425cc			
9³⁰A	water	60cc							
12p	broth	180cc							
	juice	120cc							
1p	water	120cc							
TOTAL		1,040cc		850cc	**TOTAL**	925cc			
2P-10P			LIB* D5W 150cc	150cc	2P-10P				
5p	tea	100cc	1000cc D5W	750cc	4p	425cc			
	broth	360cc			7p	350cc			
	ice-cream	120cc			9³⁰P	200cc			
9p	water	240cc							
TOTAL		820cc		900cc	**TOTAL**	975cc			
10P-6A			LIB* D5W 250cc	250cc	10P-6A				
1A	water	120cc	1000cc D5W	600cc	2A	350cc			
5A	tea	200cc			5A	150cc			
TOTAL		320cc		850cc	**TOTAL**	500cc			

24 HR TOTAL SHIFT	INTAKE	OUTPUT	RN / LPN SIGNATURES
DAY	1,890cc	925cc	Deborah C. Gray, RN
EVE.	1,720cc	975cc	Mary Jones, RN
NIGHT	1,170cc	500cc	Sandra Jenkins, LPN
TOTALS	4,780cc	2,400cc	

*LIB - LEFT IN BOTTLE
**CBI - CONTINUOUS BLADDER IRRIGATION

MEASUREMENT GUIDE

MILK CARTON = 240cc
PLASTIC DRINK CUPS = 210cc
SOUP BOWL = 180cc
CEREAL BOWL = 180cc
ICES / ICE CREAM = 120cc
STYROFOAM CUP = 240cc
TEA / COFFEE CUP = 200cc
JUICE GLASS = 120cc
MEDICINE CUP = 30cc

Figure 8-2. I & O sheet (completed 24 hours). (Used with permission from St. Barnabas Hospital, Bronx, New York.)

Practice Problems (p. 332)

Convert the following to the equivalent measures indicated.

31. 60 lb = ____________ kg
32. 15 mg = gr ____________
33. ʒ v = ____________ cc
34. gr v = ____________ mg
35. ℥ vii = ____________ cc
36. 250 cc = ____________ qt
37. 45 mL = ____________ tbs
38. gr 45 = ____________ g
39. gr iss = ____________ mg
40. m 45 = ____________ mL
41. gr 15 = ____________ mg
42. 4 qt = ____________ mL
43. 72 kg = ____________ lb
44. gr $\frac{1}{125}$ = ____________ mg
45. 2.4 L = ____________ cc

Points to Remember

- Regardless of the method used for converting, **memorizing equivalents** is a necessity.
- Answers stated in fraction format should be **reduced** as necessary.
- When more than one equivalent is learned for a unit, use the **most common equivalent** for the measure or use the number that divides equally without a remainder.
- The apothecaries' system does not convert exactly to metric.
- Division should be carried out **two decimal** places to ensure accuracy.
- Decimal point movement as a method for converting is limited to the metric system; ratio-proportion can be used for all systems of measure.
- Conversion of oral intake is done before placing on an I & O sheet.

Chapter Review (pp. 332-333)

Convert the following to the equivalent measures indicated.

1. 0.007 g = ____________ mg
2. 1 mg = ____________ g
3. 6,000 g = ____________ kg
4. 5 mL = ____________ L
5. 0.45 L = ____________ cc
6. 60 mL = ℥ ____________
7. gr $\frac{1}{300}$ = ____________ mg
8. 1 mg = gr ____________
9. 12 mL = ʒ ____________
10. gr ii = ____________ mg
11. $1\frac{1}{2}$ qt = ____________ mL
12. 30 mg = gr ____________
13. 1.6 L = ____________ mL
14. 47 kg = ____________ lb

15. 1 mL = m ______________

16. 75 lb = ______________ kg

17. 0.008 g = ______________ mg

18. 3 mL = m ______________

19. gr $\frac{1}{2}$ = ______________ mg

20. gr $\frac{1}{150}$ = ______________ mg

21. 6,172 g = ______________ kg

22. 200 mL = ______________ tsp

23. 102 lb = ______________ kg

24. 204 g = ______________ kg

25. 1.5 L = ______________ cc

26. 200 mcg = ______________ mg

27. 48.6 L = ______________ cc

28. 0.7 L = ______________ cc

29. ℥ vss = ______________ mL

30. 4 tsp = ______________ cc

31. gr iv = ______________ mg

32. 2 tbs = ______________ mL

33. ʒ ii = ______________ mL

34. 45 mg = gr ______________

35. gr 45 = ______________ g

36. ℥ xx = ______________ mL

37. gr iiss = ______________ mg

38. gr $\frac{3}{8}$ = ______________ mg

39. gr x = ______________ mg

40. 4 kg = ______________ lb

41. 3.25 mg = ______________ mcg

42. 75 mL = ℥ ______________

43. gr $\frac{1}{120}$ = ______________ mg

44. 6.653 g = ______________ mg

45. 4 g = ______________ mg

46. 36 mg = ______________ g

47. 0.8 g = ______________ mg

48. 9 g = gr ______________

49. 0.5 mg = gr ______________

50. 2 qt = ______________ L

Calculate the fluid intake.

(Assume that a cup holds 8 oz and a glass holds 4 oz for the following problems. Calculate the number of cubic centimeters.)

51. Ms. Jones had the following at lunch:

    4 oz fruit cocktail, 1 tunafish sandwich,

    1/2 cup of tea, 1/4 pt of milk.

    Total cc = ______

52. Calculate the following individual items and give the total number of cubic centimeters:

    3 popsicles (3 oz each), 1/2 qt iced tea,

    1 1/2 glasses water, 12 oz soft drink

    Total cc = _____

UNIT THREE

Methods of Administration and Calculation

The safe and accurate administration of medications to a client is an important and primary responsibility of a nurse. Being able to read and calculate medication orders is necessary for accurate administration.

Chapter 9

Medication Administration

Objectives

After reviewing this chapter the student will be able to do the following:

1. State the six "rights" of safe medication administration
2. Identify factors that influence medication doses
3. Identify the common routes for medication administration
4. Define *critical thinking*
5. Explain the importance of critical thinking in medication administration
6. Identify important critical thinking skills necessary in medication administration
7. Discuss the importance of client teaching
8. Identify special considerations relating to the elderly and medication administration
9. Identify home care considerations in relation to medication administration

Medications are therapeutic measures for a client; however, when administered haphazardly they can cause harmful effects. When a medication error is made, it is often caused by multiple factors. Some causes of medication errors are as follows:

1. **The way in which a drug is ordered**
2. **Errors in the mathematical calculation of doses**
3. **Incorrect reading of labels on medications**
4. **Poor labeling and/or packaging of drugs by the pharmaceutical companies**
5. **Lack of knowledge concerning the medication to be administered**
6. **Use of improper abbreviations, incorrect expression of drug dosages, or illegible and incorrect preparation of medication records**
7. **Failure to properly identify a client before administering medications or failure to listen to a client and to double-check when a client raises questions regarding a medication**
8. **Failure to educate clients properly about medications they are taking**

9. **Administration of medications without any thought**

The reasons for medication errors are not limited to those listed and are not limited to nursing errors alone. The best solution for medication errors is prevention. One way to prevent medication errors is for personnel involved in the administration of medications to perform the task properly.

The administration of medications is more than just giving the medication ordered or giving it merely because it is what the doctor ordered. The doctor orders the medication, but the nurse should know the action, uses, side effects, expected response, and the range of dosage for the medication being administered. Nurses must be accountable when administering medications. This includes preparation and administration.

Medication administration is a process that includes assessment, nursing diagnosis, planning, intervention, evaluation, and teaching clients about safe administration. Failure to think about what you are doing and why you are doing it and failure to assess a client can result in errors.

Critical Thinking and Medication Administration

There are numerous definitions for *critical thinking*. The best way to define critical thinking is to identify it as a process of thinking that includes being reasonable and rational. Thinking is based on reason. Critical thinking involves all phases of nursing but is particularly relevant in the discussion of medication administration.

Critical thinking encompasses several skills. Skills in critical thinking that are relevant to medication administration include identification of an organized approach. An example of this in medication administration involves the calculation of doses in an organized systematic manner (formula, ratio-proportion) to decrease the likelihood of errors in determining a client's dose.

A second skill characteristic of critical thinking is the ability to be an autonomous thinker, which includes thinking independently—for example, challenging a medication order that is written incorrectly and not just passively accepting the order. Critical thinking also involves the ability to distinguish irrelevant data from that which is relevant. For example, when reading a medication label, the nurse is able to decipher the information from the label that is necessary for calculating the correct dose to administer. Critical thinking involves using reasoning and application of concepts—for example, choosing the correct type of syringe to administer a dose, and using concepts learned to decide the appropriateness of a dose. Asking for clarification of what you don't understand and not making assumptions also involves critical thinking. Clarification of a medication order and dosage indicates critical thinking. Checking the accuracy and reliability of information decreases the chance of medication errors. The ability to validate information requires a high level of thinking and decreases the chance of medication errors that could be harmful to the client.

Critical thinking is essential to the safe administration of medications. This process fosters a nurse who thinks before doing, translates knowledge into practice, and makes appropriate judgments. To be safe in medication administration the nurse must be able to base decisions on knowledge regarding medication administration and rational thinking. A nurse who administers medications in a routine manner rather than with thought and reasoning is not using critical thinking skills.

Factors that Influence Drug Doses and Action

Several factors influence drug doses and the way they act, including the following:

1. Route of administration
2. Time of administration
3. Age of the client
4. Nutritional status of the client
5. Absorption and excretion of the drug
6. Health status of the client
7. Sex of the client

All of the above factors affect how clients react to a medication and the dose they receive. All of these factors must be considered when medications are prescribed and administered. Due to differences in the actions and the types of drugs, clients also respond in various ways, and therefore dosages must be individualized. No two clients will respond to a medication in the same manner. Nurses must bear these factors in mind when administering medications.

Special Considerations for the Elderly

Elderly individuals can be considered high-risk drug consumers. As a person grows older there is a tendency to consume more medications. According to an article entitled "The Effect of Medication on Older Adults" by Cervantes et al in *Caring Magazine,* March 1996, "People over 65 consume four times more health care products than those under 65, and take 25% of the medications." The article also indicated that older people account for taking 30% of prescribed and 40% to 50% of over-the-counter (OTC) medications.

People are now living longer; therefore the elderly person is a constant user of the health care system. As with children (see Chapter 19), special consideration should be given to the client who is over 65 years of age. With the aging process come physiological changes that have a direct effect on medications and their action in the elderly individual. Aging causes the slowing down of the body's functions. Other physiological changes include a decrease in circulation, slower absorption, slower metabolism, a decrease in excretory functions, and a decrease in the ability to respond to stress such as the stress of drugs on the system. Other changes with aging include a decrease in body weight, which can affect the dose of medications, and changes in mental status that may be due to the effects of physical illness or physiological changes in the neurological system that can occur with aging. These physiological changes can cause unexpected drug reactions and cause the elderly person to be more sensitive to the effects of many drugs. Oftentimes the elderly client is taking more than one medication at a time (the average is four or more), which causes problems such as drug interactions, severe adverse reactions, drug and food interactions, and an increase in medication errors. Many elderly persons are hospitalized each year for problems caused by medications.

As a rule the elderly client will require smaller doses of medications (as dose size increases, the number of side effects and their severity increase), and the doses should be given farther apart to prevent accumulation of drugs and toxicity. With aging, visual and hearing problems may develop. Special attention must be given when teaching clients about their medications to avoid medication errors. Develop a relationship with the client; building rapport and trust is important for the elderly. Take time and talk to the elderly, listen to what they say, and never assume they don't know how much or what medications they are taking. Ascertain that all instructions are written as clearly as possible. Make sure the client has appropriate measuring devices (for example, calibrated dropper or measuring cup). Try to establish specific times for taking medications that are compatible with the client's routine to lessen the chance of taking too much medication or forgetting a dose. Help the client to recognize pills by the name on the bottle, not by color. If the print on medications is too small for the client to read, encourage the use of a magnifying glass. Other measures might include a simple chart that outlines the medications to be taken, time they are to be taken, and special instructions if needed. These charts should be geared to the client's visual ability and comprehension level. Encourage the elderly client to request that childproof containers not be used; some will have difficulty opening child-resistant containers. Recommend medication aids for the client such as special medication containers that are divided into separate compartments for storing daily or weekly drug doses. (See Figure 9-1 below showing examples of medication containers.)

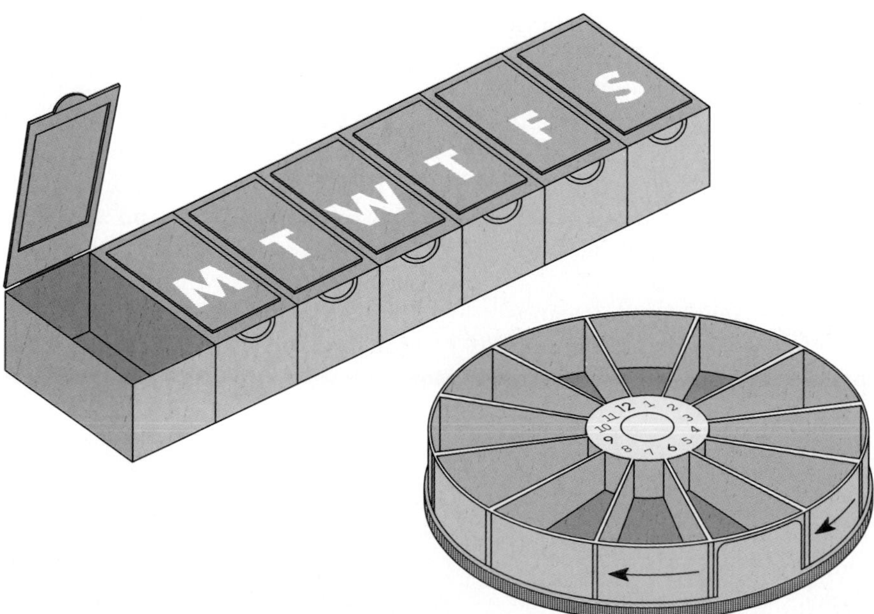

Figure 9-1. Medication containers. (From Radcliff R, Ogden S: *Calculation of drug dosages,* ed 5, St Louis, 1995, Mosby.)

In teaching elderly clients it is important to remember that the elderly are mature adults who are capable of learning and deserve time for learning to take place. Be patient, use simple language, and maintain the independence of the elderly as much as possible.

The Six Rights of Medication Administration

When the nurse is administering medications to a client, the six rights of medication administration should serve as guidelines. Failure to achieve any of these "rights" constitutes a medication error. The six rights should be checked before administering any medication to avoid errors and to ensure client safety.

The Six Rights

1. The right drug
2. The right dose
3. The right client
4. The right route
5. The right time
6. The right documentation

1. **The right drug**—When medications are ordered, the nurse should compare them with the written order. When administering medications, the nurse should check the label on the medication container against the Medication Administration Record (MAR) or medication ticket. Medications should be checked three times: before pouring, after pouring, and before replacing the container. With unit dose (each drug dose is prepared in the prescribed dose, packaged, labeled, and ready to use), the label should still be checked three times.
2. **The right dose**—Always perform and check calculations carefully, without ignoring decimal points. Have someone else double-check a dose that causes concern. In some agencies certain medication doses are always checked by another nurse (for example, insulin and heparin). After doses are calculated, they should be given using standard measurement devices such as calibrated medicine droppers and cups.
3. **The right client**—Always make sure you are administering medications to the right client. Ask for the client's name, and check the client's identification bracelet against the MAR. If a client does not have an identification bracelet, obtain one; secure the help of a staff member in establishing proper identification. Never go by room number or last name only.
4. **The right route**—Medications should be given by the correct route (for example, orally or by injection). The route of the medication should be stated on the order. Do not assume which route is appropriate.
5. **The right time**—Drugs should be given at the correct time of day and interval (for example, three times a day [t.i.d.] or every 6 hr [q6h]). Judgment should be used as to when medications should be given or not given. If several medications are ordered, set priorities and administer medications that must act at a certain time. For example, insulin should be given at an exact time before meals.
6. **The right documentation**—Medications should be charted accurately as soon as they are given—on the right client's medication record, under the right date, and next to the right time. If a medication is refused, it should be documented as such with a notation on the medication record or in the nurse's notes. Never chart a medication as given before administering it or without documentation as to why it was not given. Follow the policy of the institution when documenting. All documentation should be legible. Correct documentation has also been included in the rights of medication administration and is referred to as the sixth right.

In addition to the six rights of medications, **a client has the right to refuse medications**. When this occurs the nurse needs to document the refusal correctly and make appropriate persons aware of the refusal. Another important right has to do with educating the client. **All clients have a right to be educated regarding the medication they are taking**.

Teaching the Client

One of the most important nursing functions is teaching the client. Teaching clients about their medications is imperative in preventing errors and improving the quality of health care. Educating clients regarding medications plays a role in preventing adverse reactions and achieving adherence to prescribed therapy; taking the correct dose of the right medication at the right time helps to prevent problems with medication administration. Remember, clients cannot be expected to follow a medication regimen—taking the correct dose of the right medication at the right time—if they haven't been taught. Not knowing what to do results in noncompliance, inaccurate dosages, and other problems. Nurses are in a unique position to teach the client, and this has been a traditional activity of nursing practice. Teaching should begin in the hospital and be a major part of discharge planning because, once discharged, clients need to have been educated about their medications to continue taking them safely and correctly at home. With today's emphasis on outpatient treatment and early discharge, a thorough client education regarding medications is necessary.

When the nurse is teaching clients, it is important to thoroughly assess the client's needs. Determine what the client knows about the medication prescribed, how to take the medication, and the frequency, time, and dose. Identify the client's learning needs, which should include literacy level and language most easily and clearly understood. Identify relevant ethnic, cultural, and socioeconomic factors that may influence medication use; consider factors such as age and physical capabilities. A variety of teaching techniques may have to be used to facilitate and enhance learning. Return demonstrations on proper use of medication equipment and reading dosages, in addition to repeated instructions and directions, may be necessary, especially regarding management at home.

What a client needs to know about a medication varies with the drug. There may be numerous pieces of information that clients should learn regarding their medications. The items discussed here relate particularly to dosage administration. To ensure that the client takes the right medication in the right dose, by the right route at the right time, the teaching of the client should include the following:

- Both the brand and generic names of the drug.
- Clear explanation of the amount of the drug to be taken (for example, one tablet or 1/2 tablet).
- Clear explanation of when to take the drug. (Prepare a chart created with the client's lifestyle in mind. For example, if the medication is to be taken with meals, perhaps the chart can indicate the client's mealtime and the medication scheduled accordingly.)
- Clear demonstration of measuring oral doses such as liquids. (Encourage the use of measuring devices.)
- Clear explanation of the route of administration (for example, place under tongue).

Although nurses cannot ensure clients will act on or retain everything they are taught, we are responsible for providing information to the client that will prevent error-prone situations and will enable safe drug administration.

Home Care Considerations

Home health nursing has become a large part of the health care delivery system because of the emphasis on early discharge. Home health nursing provides nursing care to clients in their homes. Home care nursing may involve many activities, such as providing treatments, dressing changes, hospice care, client/family teaching, and medication administration. Medication administration involves administration of medications in various ways (for example, I.V., p.o., and injection). With the increased movement of nursing into the home of the client, which is not a controlled setting, this has some important nursing implications. The nurse has to be able to do a thorough assessment, communicate effectively, problem solve, and use expert critical thinking skills. Thinking must be rational, reasonable, and based on knowledge.

The principles regarding medication administration are the same as in a structured setting (for example, hospital, acute care facility, or nursing home). It is imperative that the client be well educated about safe administration. Depending on the client's condition, home nursing services can be scheduled visits or intermittent visits to monitor the status of a client. Not all clients have a health aide, family member, or continuous nursing services in the home (around the clock). It is essential that the nurse perform calculations of medication administration in a systematic, organized manner and adhere to the six rights of medication administration. Correct interpretation of medication orders and validation are imperative. Proper education of the client concerning the medication, dose, and route of administration is crucial in order for the client to manage in the home environment. Some may look at it as "the client being totally at your mercy." Clients depend on the nurse to provide direction for them to ensure safe home administration. The nurse has to be able to teach the client to use home utensils for measuring doses and determining the accuracy of the dose. (As discussed in the chapters on systems of measure, the nurse has to be able to convert doses between the various systems.) The nurse providing services to the client in the home has to be innovative and knowledgeable and demonstrate excellent critical thinking skills.

Routes of Medication Administration

Route refers to how a drug is administered. Medications come in a number of forms for administration.

Oral (p.o.). Oral medication is administered by mouth (for example, tablets, capsules, and liquid solutions). Some medications are sublingual (placed under the tongue) or buccal (placed against the cheek).

Parenteral. This is medication administered by a route other than by mouth or gastrointestinal tract. Parenteral routes include intravenous (I.V.), intramuscular (I.M.), subcutaneous (s.c.), and intradermal.

Insertion. Medication is placed into a body cavity, where the medication dissolves at body temperature (for example, suppositories).

Instillation. Medication is introduced in liquid form into a body cavity. It can also include placing an ointment into a body cavity, such as erythromycin eye ointment, which is placed in the conjunctiva of the eye. Instillation medications also include nose drops and ear drops.

Inhalation. Medication is administered into the respiratory tract, via for example, nebulizers used by clients for asthma. In some institutions these medications are administered to the client by special equipment, such as positive pressure breathing equipment or the aerosol mask. Other drugs in inhalation form include pentamidine, which is used to treat *Pneumocystis carinii,* a type of pneumonia found in acquired immunodeficiency syndrome (AIDS) clients.

Topical. The medication is applied to the external surface of the skin. It may include aerosol powders, liquids, ointments, or pastes that have a local effect and transdermal medications. Transdermal medication is contained in a patch applied to skin and is slowly released and absorbed through the skin and enters the systemic circulation. The patch may be effective for hours or days at a time. Examples include nitroglycerine for chest pain and nicotine for the purpose of stopping smoking.

Forms of oral medications (tablets, capsules), oral solutions, and routes for parenteral medications will be discussed in more detail in later chapters.

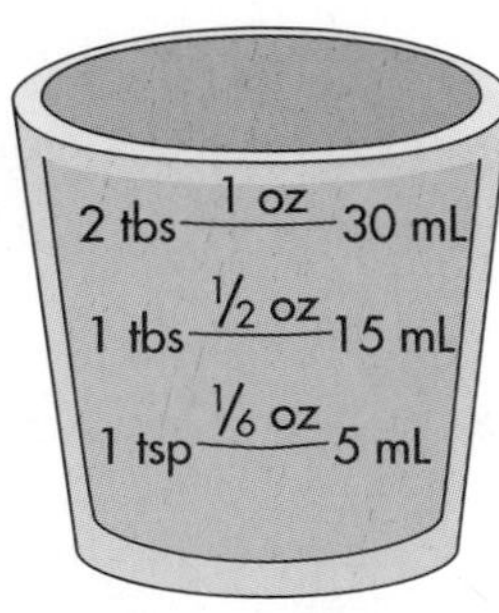

Figure 9-2. Medicine cup.

Equipment Used in Dose Calculation

Medicine cup. Equipment used for oral administration includes a 30-mL or 1-oz medication cup made of plastic that is used to measure most liquid medications. The cup has measurements in all three systems of measure (Figure 9-2).

Souffle cup. This is a small paper or plastic cup used for solid forms of medication such as tablets and capsules (Figure 9-3).

Calibrated dropper. This may be used to administer small amounts of medication to an adult or child (Figure 9-4). It is usually marked in milliliters or cubic centimeters. The size of the drops varies and depends on the dropper. Since the size of drops varies it is important to remember that drops should not be used as a medication

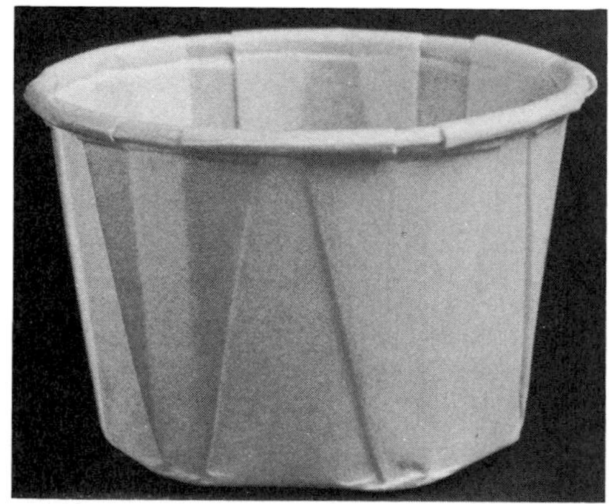

Figure 9-3. Souffle cup. (From Clayton B, Stock Y: *Basic pharmacology for nurses,* ed 10, St Louis, 1993, Mosby.)

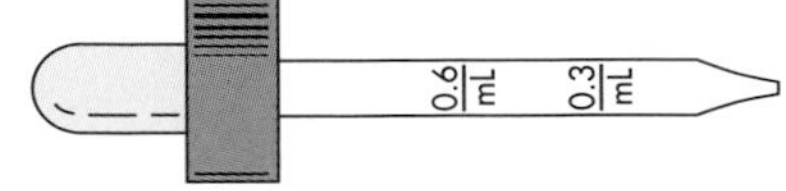

Figure 9-4. Medicine dropper. (From Brown M, Mulholland JL: *Drug calculations: process and problems for clinical practice,* ed 5, St Louis, 1996, Mosby.)

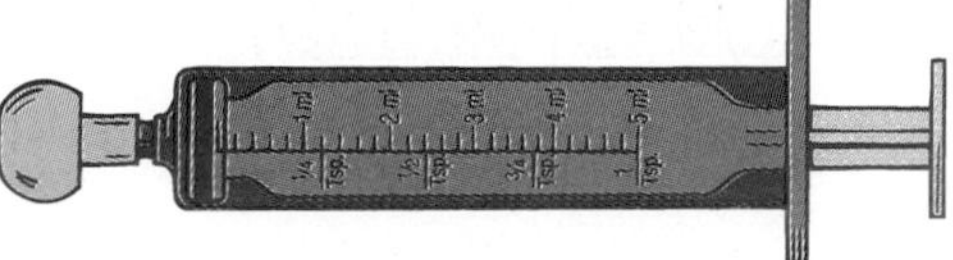

Figure 9-5. Plastic oral syringe. (From Brown M, Mulholland JL: *Drug calculations process and problems for clinical practice,* ed 5, St Louis, 1996, Mosby.)

measure unless the dropper is calibrated. Droppers used for the administration of eye, nose, and ear medications are designed for that purpose. Certain medications come with a dropper that is calibrated according to the medication. Examples include children's vitamins and nystatin oral solutions.

Oral syringe. This may be used for the administration of liquid medications to adults and children. This type of syringe is designed for the purpose of administering medications orally. No needle is attached (Figure 9-5).

Parenteral syringe. This type of syringe is used for I.M., s.c., intradermal, and I.V. drugs. These syringes come in various sizes and are marked in minims and cubic centimeters. Some are marked in units. The specific types of syringes are discussed in more detail in the chapter on parenteral medications. The barrel of the syringe holds the medication and has calibrations on it. The needle is attached to the tip. The plunger pushes the medication out (Figure 9-6). The size of the needle depends on how the medication is given (for example, s.c. or I.M.), the viscosity of the drug, and the size of the client.

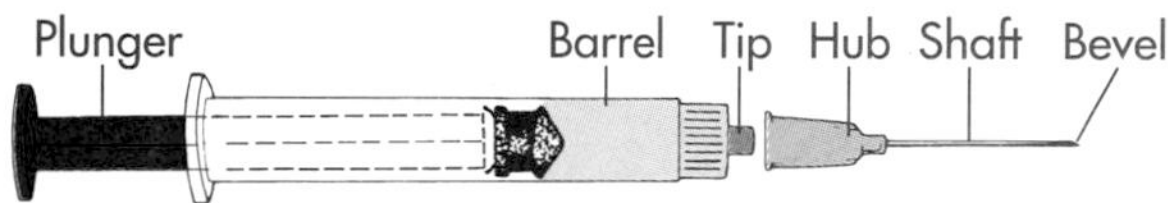

Figure 9-6. Parts of a syringe. (From Lilley LL, Audler RS, Albanese JA: *Pharmacology and the nursing process,* St Louis, 1996, Mosby.)

Chapter Review (p. 333)

1. Name the six rights of medication administration

   Right ______________

   Right ______________

   Right ______________

   Right ______________

   Right ______________

   Right ______________

2. Two ways of administering medications to the right client are the following:

   a) ______________

   b) ______________

3. A medication label should be read ______________ times.

4. Medications should be charted ______________ you have given them.

5. The administration of medications outside the gastrointestinal tract is termed ______________.

Chapter 10

Understanding Medication Orders

Objectives

After reviewing this chapter the student will be able to do the following:

1. Identify the components of a medication order
2. Identify the meanings of standard abbreviations used in medication administration
3. Interpret a given medication order

Physicians communicate to the nurse or designated health care worker which medication or medications to administer to a client by giving a medication order. The terms medication orders and doctor's orders are used interchangeably. Medication orders can be verbal or written. Verbal orders should be taken only in an emergency situation; however, the verbal order should then be written and signed by the doctor as soon as possible. Doctors are usually the only persons allowed to prescribe medications, although in some institutions individuals such as nurse practitioners, midwives, and physician's assistants may have this privilege as well. Some institutions may require that medication orders written by persons other than a doctor be countersigned by designated personnel. It is important to be familiar with the specific policies regarding doctor's orders since they vary according to the institution or health care facility.

The doctor's order indicates the drug plan or medication a doctor has ordered for a client. After a medication order has been written, the nurse has the responsibility of transcribing the order. This means the order is written on the MAR (Medication Administration Record) or entered into a computer system and communicated to the hospital pharmacy. Once the medication is received on the unit, the medication order is implemented and the client receives the drug. Before transcribing an order or preparing a dose, the nurse must be familiar with reading and interpreting an order. To interpret a medication order the nurse must be knowledgeable in the components of a medication order and the standard abbreviations and symbols used in writing a medication order. The nurse therefore must memorize the abbreviations and symbols frequently used in medication orders. The abbreviations include units of measure, route, and frequency for the medication ordered. The common abbreviations and symbols used in medication administration are listed on the inside of the back cover.

In writing medication orders, some doctors may use capital letters, others may use lower case letters; some may place a period after an abbreviation or symbol, others do not. These variations often reflect writing styles. It is important for you to concentrate on understanding what the abbreviation or symbol means in the context of the order.

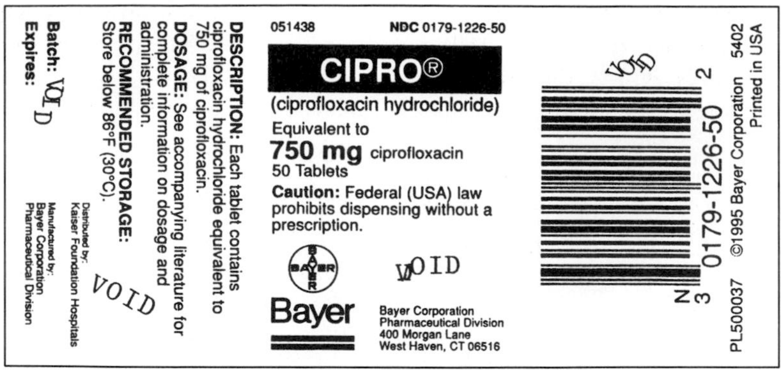

Figure 10-1. Cipro label. Notice the two names. The first, *Cipro,* is the trade name, identified by the registration symbol, ®. The name in smaller and different print is *ciprofloxacin hydrochloride,* the generic or official name.

Some abbreviations may be capitalized to indicate different meanings. For example: o.d. lower case letters means once a day, every day; OD in capital letters indicates right eye.

Writing a Medication Order

A doctor writes a medication order in a special book for doctor's orders or on a form called the *doctor's order sheet* in the client's chart or hospital record. Doctor's order sheets vary from institution to institution. The order sheet should have the client's name on it. A prescription blank is used to write medication orders for clients who are being discharged from the hospital or are seeing the doctor in an outpatient facility. Nurses frequently have to explain these orders to clients so they understand the dosages they will be taking.

Components of a Medication Order

When a medication order is written, it must contain the following seven important parts or it is considered invalid or incomplete.

Client's full name. This avoids confusion of the client with another, thereby preventing error in administering the wrong medication to the wrong client. Many institutions use a nameplate to imprint the client's name and record number on the order sheet. In institutions that use computers, the computer screen will show identifying information for the client, such as age and known drug allergies.

Date and time the order was written. This includes the month, day, year, and the time the order was written. This will help in determining the start and stop of the medication order. In many institutions the doctor is required to include the length of time the medication is to be given (for example, 7 days) or he may use the abbreviation LOS (length of stay), which means the client is to receive the medication during the entire stay in the hospital. Even when not written as part of the order, LOS is implied unless stated otherwise. In some institutions there are automatic cutoff times for certain medications even if not specified (for example, 5 to 7 days for a specific antibiotic.)

Note: A record of the time the order was written is preferred in many institutions, but omission does not invalidate the order.

Name of the medication. The medication may be ordered by the generic or brand name (Figures 10-1 and 10-2). To avoid confusion with another medication, the medication should be written clearly and spelled correctly.

generic name—the proper name, or chemical compound. It is usually designated in lower case letters or a different typeface. Occasionally only the generic name will appear on the label. Each medication has only one generic name.

trade name—the brand name, or the name under which a manufacturer markets the drug. This is usually designated by capital letters and indicated first on a drug label. The trade name is followed by the registration symbol, ®. A drug may have several trade names, based on the manufacturer.

Note: Nurses must be familiar with both the generic name and the trade name for a drug. To ensure correct drug identification nurses should cross-check trade and generic names as needed.

Dose of the medication. The amount of the medication as well as the strength should be written clearly to avoid confusion.

Example: In some institutions when the medication ordered is expressed in units, which is abbreviated U, the order is written without abbreviating units to avoid confusion with the U being read as a zero (0). When abbreviations for measure are used, only standard abbreviations should be used.

Route of administration. This is a very important part of a medication order since medications can be administered by several routes. Never assume that you know which route is appropriate. Standard abbreviations should be used to indicate the route.

Example: p.o. (oral, by mouth)

Time and/or frequency of administration. This uses standard abbreviations to indicate the times a medication is to be given.

Example: q.i.d. (four times a day), stat (immediately)

The time intervals at which a medication is administered are determined by the institution, and most health care facilities have routine times for administering medications.

Example: t.i.d. (three times a day) may be 9 AM, 1 PM, and 5 PM or 10 AM, 2 PM, and 6 PM

Factors such as the purpose of the drug, drug interactions, absorption of the drug, and side effects should be considered when scheduling medication times.

Signature of the person writing the order. For a medication order to be legal it must be signed by the doctor. The doctor writing the order must include his or her signature on the order, and it should be legible. In some institutions, depending on the rank of the doctor, an order may have to be cosigned by a senior doctor.

Example: Residents' or interns' orders may require the signature of an attending doctor.

In addition to the seven items listed, any special instructions for certain medications need to be clearly written.

Example: Hold if blood pressure is below 100 systolic; administer a half hour before meals.

Medications ordered as needed or whenever necessary (p.r.n.) should indicate the purpose of administration as well.

Example: For chest pain, temperature above 101° F, or blood pressure greater than 140 systolic and 90 diastolic.

In instances where specific instructions are not stated, nursing judgment must be used to determine whether it is appropriate or not to administer a medication.

For dosage calculations the nurse is usually concerned with the drug name, dose of the drug, route, and time or frequency of administration. This information is necessary in determining a safe and reasonable dosage for a client.

Interpreting a Medication Order

Medication orders are written in the following order:

1. The name of the drug
2. The dose expressed in standard abbreviations or symbols
3. The route
4. The frequency

Figure 10-2. Carafate label. Notice the two names. The first, *Carafate,* is the trade name, identified by the registration symbol, ®. The name in smaller and different print is *sucralfate,* the generic or official name.

Example: Colace 100 mg p.o. t.i.d.

Colace	100 mg	p.o.	t.i.d.
↓	↓	↓	↓
name	dose	route	frequency

This order means the doctor wants the client to receive 100 milligrams of a stool softener named Colace by mouth three times a day. The use of abbreviations in a medication order is like a form of shorthand; it shortens the amount of writing to give a specific order.

Depending on the policy of the institution, the nurse or trained personnel such as the unit secretary (ward clerk) transcribes the medication order to the appropriate MAR or ticket. In facilities where personnel other than the nurse transcribe orders, the nurse still has the responsibility for double-checking and cosigning the order, indicating it has been correctly transcribed.

Transcribing of orders has decreased in institutions where the unit dose is used, resulting in fewer errors. In some institutions that use unit dose, however, more transcribing may be necessary because the MAR may have the capacity to be used for only a 5-day period. Therefore it is necessary to transcribe orders again at the end of the designated time period.

In facilities that use computers, the medication order is placed into the computer, and a printout is generated that lists the currently ordered medications. The use of the computer therefore eliminates the need for transcribing orders. The charting of the medications administered is also done directly into the computer. Computerized charting does not eliminate the responsibility of the nurse to double-check medication orders.

Points to Remember

- A primary responsibility of the nurse is the safe administration of medications to a client.
- The seven components of a medication order are as follows:
  1. The full name of the client
  2. Date and time the order was written
  3. Name of the medication to be administered
  4. Dose of the medication
  5. Route of administration
  6. Time or frequency of administration
  7. Signature of the person writing the order.
- All medication orders must be legible and use standard abbreviations and/or symbols.
- If any of the seven components of a medication order is missing or seems incorrect, don't assume—clarify the order!

Chapter Review (pp. 333-334)

List the seven components of a medication order.

1. ______________________________
2. ______________________________
3. ______________________________
4. ______________________________
5. ______________________________
6. ______________________________
7. ______________________________

Write the meaning of the following abbreviations.

8. b.i.d. ____________
9. OU ____________
10. ad.lib. ____________
11. s.c. ____________
12. c̄ ____________
13. a.c. ____________
14. q.i.d. ____________
15. b.i.w. ____________
16. h.s. ____________
17. o.d. ____________
18. elix. ____________
19. OS ____________
20. syr ____________
21. n.p.o. ____________
22. sl ____________

Give the abbreviations for the following.

23. after meals ____________
24. three times a day ____________
25. intramuscular ____________
26. every eight hours ____________
27. suppository ____________
28. intravenous ____________
29. once if necessary ____________
30. without ____________
31. immediately ____________
32. right eye ____________
33. ointment ____________
34. one half ____________
35. milliequivalents ____________
36. every night at bedtime ____________
37. by rectum ____________

Interpret the following orders.

38. Methergine 0.2 mg p.o. q4h × 6 doses. ____________________________________

____

39. Digoxin 0.125 mg p.o. o.d. ____________________________________

____

40. Regular Humulin Insulin 14 U. s.c. q.d. 7:30 A.M. ____________________________________

____

41. Demerol 50 mg I.M. and atropine gr 1/150 I.M. on call to the operating room. ____________

____

42. Ampicillin 500 mg p.o. stat, and then 250 mg p.o. q.i.d. thereafter. ______

43. Lasix 40 mg I.M. stat. ______

44. Librium 50 mg p.o. q4h p.r.n. for agitation. ______

45. Potassium chloride 20 mEq I.V. × 2 L. ______

46. Tylenol gr × p.o. q4h p.r.n. for pain. ______

47. Mylicon 80 mg p.o. pc and hs. ______

48. Folic acid 1 mg p.o. o.d. ______

49. Nembutal 100 mg p.o. h.s. p.r.n. ______

50. Aspirin gr × p.o. q4h p.r.n. for temperature >101° F. ______

51. Dilantin 100 mg p.o. t.i.d. ______

52. Minipress 2 mg p.o. b.i.d.; hold for systolic b/p (blood pressure) <120. ______

53. Compazine 10 mg I.M. q4h p.r.n. for nausea and vomiting. ______

54. Ampicillin 1 g I.V.P.B. q6h × 4 doses. ______

55. Heparin 5,000 U. s.c. q12h. ______

56. Dilantin susp 200 mg per NGT q a.m. and 300 mg per NGT h.s. ______________________

____

57. Benadryl 50 mg p.o. stat. ____

____

58. Vitamin B_{12} 1000 mcg IM t.i.w. ____

____

59. Milk of magnesia 1 oz p.o. h.s. prn. ____

____

60. Septra DS tab 1 p.o. qd. ____

____

61. Neomycin ophthalmic ointment 1% OD tid. ______________________________________

____

62. Carafate 1 g via NGT qid. ____

____

63. Morphine sulfate 15 mg s.c. stat and 10 mg s.c. q4h prn. ___________________________

____

64. Ampicillin 120 mg ivss q6h × 7 days. ____

____

65. Prednisone 10 mg po qod. ____

____

Identify the missing part from the following medication orders. Assume the date, time, and signature are included on the orders.

66. Dicloxacillin 250 mg q.i.d. ____________

67. Synthroid 0.05 mg p.o. ____________

68. Nitrofurantoin p.o. q6h × 10 days. ____________

69. 25 mg p.o. q12h, hold if B/P <100 systolic. ____________

70. Solu-Cortef 100 q6h. ____________

Chapter 11

Medication Administration Records

Objectives

After reviewing this chapter the student will be able to do the following:

1. Identify the necessary information that must be transcribed to an MAR
2. Read an MAR and identify medications that are given on a routine basis, including the name of the medication, the dose, the route of administration, and the time of administration
3. Transcribe medication orders to a MAR (Medication Administration Record)

The medication record system is the most widely used system for drug administration. The medication record is a way of keeping track of medications that a client has received and is currently receiving. The name of each medication, as well as the dose, route, and frequency, is written on the client's medication record. A complete schedule is written out of all the administration times for medications that are given on a continuous or routine basis. Each time a dose is given the nurse initials it next to the time. In some institutions separate records are maintained for routine, I.V., and p.r.n. medications, and medications administered on a one-time basis, while in others these are kept on the same record in a designated area. The medication record system is the same as the Medication Administration Record (MAR).

For medication records and charting, some institutions use a Kardex, a MAR, or a combination of both. Other institutions use a computerized system in which medication-charting information is entered into the computer, which automatically generates a list of all the medications to be given and the times.

After a doctor's order has been verified, the order is transcribed to the official record used at the institution. As we examine the various medication records presented in this chapter, you will notice that despite the difference in forms, there is essential information that is common to all.

Essential Information on a Medication Record

All of the information that appears on the medication record must be legible and transcribed carefully to avoid a medication error. In addition to client information, the following information is necessary on all medication forms:

1. **Dates.** This information usually includes the date the order was written and the date the medication is to be started (if different from the order date).
2. **Medication Information.** This includes the drug's full name, the dose, the route, and the frequency. Abbreviations used on the medication record should be standard abbreviations.
3. **Time of Administration.** This will be based on the desired administration schedule stated on the order, such as "t.i.d." The desired administration time is placed on the medication record and converted to time periods based on the institution's time intervals for scheduled or routine medications. (Thus t.i.d. may mean 9 AM, 1 PM, and 5 PM at one institution and 10 AM, 2 PM and 6 PM at another.) Medication times for p.r.n. and one-time doses are recorded at the time they are administered.
4. **Initials.** Most medication records have a place for the initials of the person transcribing the medication to the MAR and the person administering the medication (see Figure 11-6).
5. **Special Instructions.** Any special instructions relating to a medication should be indicated on the medication record. For example, "Hold if blood pressure <100 systolic" or "p.r.n. for pain."

In addition to the above information, some medication records may include space for charting information such as injection site, pulse, and blood pressure if this information is relevant to the medication.

Documentation of Medications Administered

Medication records include an area for documenting medications administered. After administering the medication, the nurse or other qualified personnel must sign his or her initials next to the time the drug was given. For scheduled medications, a complete schedule is written out, and the initials are recorded next to each given time. With one-time doses and p.r.n. medication, *the time of administration* is written and again initialed by the person administering it. The medication form has a place for the full name of each person administering medications, along with the identifying initials. This allows for immediate identification of the person's initials if necessary. When medications are not administered, some records have notations, such as an asterisk (*), that indicate this or there is an area on the back or at the bottom of the MAR for charting medications not given (see Figure 11-6). The type of notations used will depend on the institution. In addition to the notations made on the medication record, most institutions require documentation in the nurse's notes.

Explanation of Medication Administration Records

There are a variety of medication records in existence and they vary from institution to institution. However, despite the variety, there is essential information contained on them that is common to all and to their purpose. The MAR is used to determine what medications are ordered, the dose, route, and when each is to be given. The MAR is also verified with the doctor's orders. Any MAR requiring transcription of orders should always be checked against the doctor's orders. In institutions where personnel other than the nurse transcribe orders, the nurse should double-check the transcription to make sure there are no discrepancies. Regardless of the variation in format for MARs, the information common to all is:

a) The name of the client
b) Medication (the dose, route)

```
MEDICATIONS:
INDERAL, PROPRANOLOL TAB 40MG,
 09/12 09:00AM #1, PO,GIV          MCKINNEY,PATRICIA
 09/12 05:00PM #1, PO,GIV          MCKINNEY,PATRICIA
DIGOXIN TAB 0.25MG,
 09/12 09:00AM #1, PO,GIV          MCKINNEY,PATRICIA
LASIX, FUROSEMIDE TAB 20MG,
 09/12 09:00AM #1, PO,GIV          MCKINNEY,PATRICIA
 09/12 09:00PM #1, PO,GIV          MCKINNEY,PATRICIA
```

Figure 11-1. Sample computer printout relating to medication administration. (Used with permission from TDS-Hospital Information Systems, Atlanta, Georgia.)

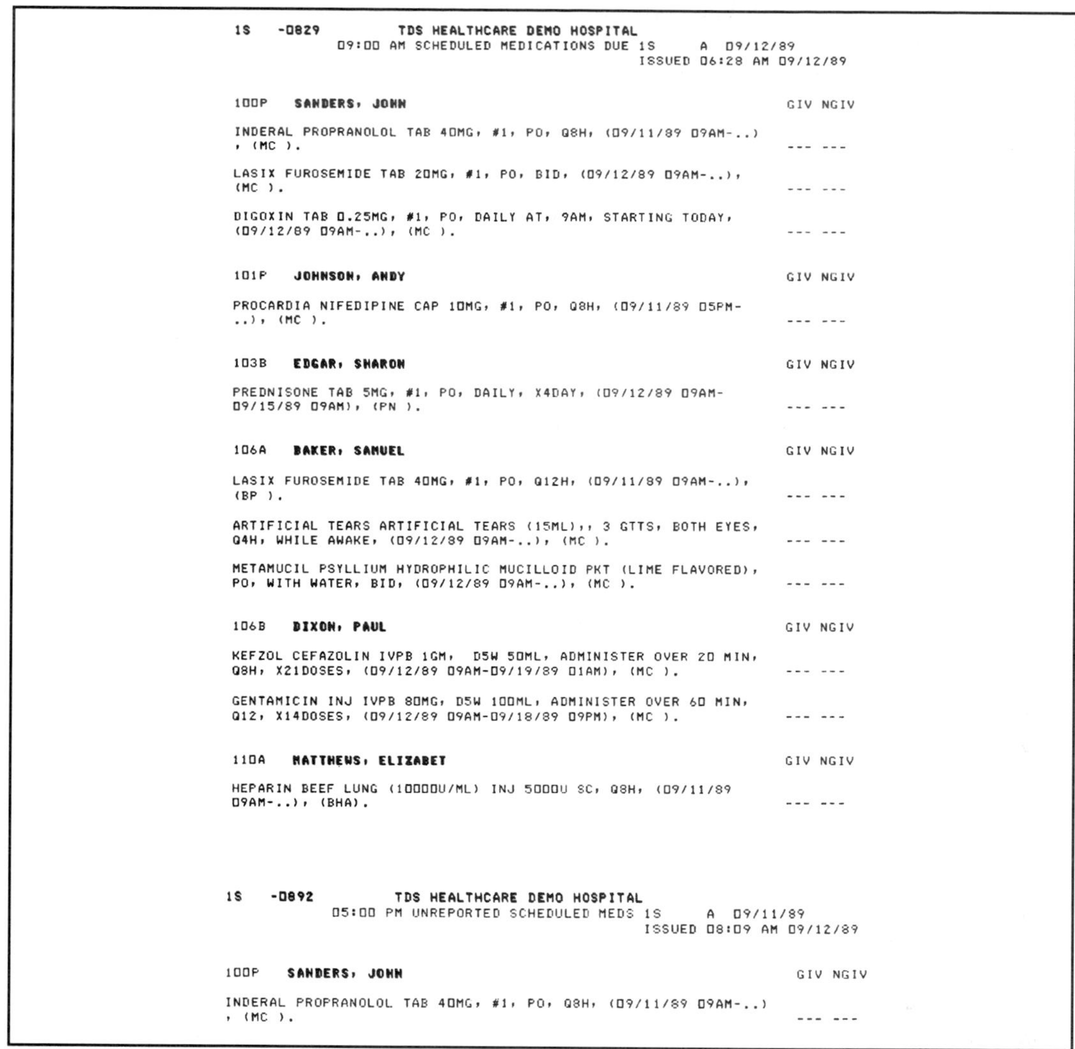

```
1S    -0829           TDS HEALTHCARE DEMO HOSPITAL
         09:00 AM SCHEDULED MEDICATIONS DUE 1S      A  09/12/89
                                          ISSUED 06:28 AM 09/12/89

100P    SANDERS, JOHN                                          GIV NGIV

INDERAL PROPRANOLOL TAB 40MG, #1, PO, Q8H, (09/11/89 09AM-..)
, (MC ).                                                       --- ---

LASIX FUROSEMIDE TAB 20MG, #1, PO, BID, (09/12/89 09AM-..),
(MC ).                                                         --- ---

DIGOXIN TAB 0.25MG, #1, PO, DAILY AT, 9AM, STARTING TODAY,
(09/12/89 09AM-..), (MC ).                                     --- ---

101P    JOHNSON, ANDY                                          GIV NGIV

PROCARDIA NIFEDIPINE CAP 10MG, #1, PO, Q8H, (09/11/89 05PM-
..), (MC ).                                                    --- ---

103B    EDGAR, SHARON                                          GIV NGIV

PREDNISONE TAB 5MG, #1, PO, DAILY, X4DAY, (09/12/89 09AM-
09/15/89 09AM), (PN ).                                         --- ---

106A    BAKER, SAMUEL                                          GIV NGIV

LASIX FUROSEMIDE TAB 40MG, #1, PO, Q12H, (09/11/89 09AM-..),
(BP ).                                                         --- ---

ARTIFICIAL TEARS ARTIFICIAL TEARS (15ML),, 3 GTTS, BOTH EYES,
Q4H, WHILE AWAKE, (09/12/89 09AM-..), (MC ).                   --- ---

METAMUCIL PSYLLIUM HYDROPHILIC MUCILLOID PKT (LIME FLAVORED),
PO, WITH WATER, BID, (09/12/89 09AM-..), (MC ).                --- ---

106B    DIXON, PAUL                                            GIV NGIV

KEFZOL CEFAZOLIN IVPB 1GM,  D5W 50ML, ADMINISTER OVER 20 MIN,
Q8H, X21DOSES, (09/12/89 09AM-09/19/89 01AM), (MC ).           --- ---

GENTAMICIN INJ IVPB 80MG, D5W 100ML, ADMINISTER OVER 60 MIN,
Q12, X14DOSES, (09/12/89 09AM-09/18/89 09PM), (MC ).           --- ---

110A    MATTHEWS, ELIZABET                                     GIV NGIV

HEPARIN BEEF LUNG (10000U/ML) INJ 5000U SC, Q8H, (09/11/89
09AM-..), (BHA).                                               --- ---


1S    -0892           TDS HEALTHCARE DEMO HOSPITAL
         05:00 PM UNREPORTED SCHEDULED MEDS 1S      A  09/11/89
                                          ISSUED 08:09 AM 09/12/89

100P    SANDERS, JOHN                                          GIV NGIV

INDERAL PROPRANOLOL TAB 40MG, #1, PO, Q8H, (09/11/89 09AM-..)
, (MC ).                                                       --- ---
```

Figure 11-2. Printout of medications for unit. (Used with permission from TDS-Hospital Information Systems, Atlanta, Georgia.)

c) Time/frequency desired for administration
d) A place to indicate allergies
e) A place for date, the initials of the person who administers the medication, and a section to identify the initials of the person administering the medication

Samples of the various MARs are included in this chapter. As you look at the sample records, it is important to locate and identify the information common to all with focus on medications that are given on a continuous basis.

Computerized Medication Records

In institutions that use a computerized system, orders are entered directly into the computer by the doctor along with all other essential information relating to the client. The institution generates its own medication record, following a specific format. Figure 11-1 shows the charting of the medications, which is done directly into the computer. The abbreviation GIV next to the medications means that the medications were given. The full name of the nurse administering the medications is listed on the right of the printout. In addition to the printout for an individual, a printout is generated that shows the scheduled medications that are due on the various units (Figure 11-2). Each client's name and room number are also included on the printout.

Unit Dose System

Many institutions have adopted a system of medication administration referred to as *unit dose.* This system has decreased medication preparation

ST. BARNABAS HOSPITAL
BRONX, NY• DEPARTMENT OF NURSING
MEDICATION ADMINISTRATION RECORD

DIAGNOSES: Bipolar Disorder

ALLERGIC TO: Aspirin | DATE 5/7/96

Legend — Omitted doses (use red pen): 1. NPO 2. Off-Unit 3. I.V. Out 4. Pt. Refused 5. Other
Document in Medication Omission Record

PAGE 1 **OF** 1

R.N. INIT.	ORDER DATE / EXP. DATE	STANDING MEDICATIONS (MED-DOSE-FREQ-ROUTE)	DATE / HOUR	5/7 INIT.	5/8 INIT.	5/9 INIT.	5/10 INIT.	5/11 INIT.	5/12 INIT.	5/13 INIT.	5/14 INIT.	5/15 INIT.
Dg	5/7/96 / 6/7/96	Thorazine 200mg p o tid	9a 1p 5p	Dg								
Dg	5/7/96 / 6/7/96	Multi-vitamin 1 tab p.o. od	9a	Dg								
Dg	5/7/96 / 6/7/96	Ensure 1 can po tid	9a 1p 5p	Dg								
Dg	5/7/96 / 5/14/96	Clonazepam 0.25 mg p.o. tid	9a 1p 5p	Dg								
Dg	5/7/96 / 5/9/96	Benadryl 25mg p.o. H.S. x 3 nights	9p	ms ①	②	③						

PHR-002

INJECTION CODES: RT = RIGHT THIGH; LT = LEFT THIGH; RA = RIGHT ARM; LA = LEFT ARM; LU = LEFT UPPER GLUTEAL; RU = RIGHT UPPER GLUTEAL; RAB = UPPER RIGHT ABDOMEN; RAB = LOWER RIGHT ABDOMEN; LAB = UPPER LEFT ABDOMEN; LAB = LOWER LEFT ABDOMEN

Figure 11-3. MAR showing transcription of medication orders to medication administration record. (Used with permission from St Barnabas Hospital, Bronx, New York.)

time since the medications are prepared in the pharmacy on a daily basis and sent to the unit. The type of medication forms used for this system varies from one institution to another. In some instances this system has decreased the amount of transcription of orders. In other institutions using unit dose, however, transcription of medication orders to the MAR is required. The doctor's orders are therefore written on a separate order sheet. Figure 11-3 illustrates the transcription of orders to the MAR.

At some institutions the original doctor's order is attached to the left side of the medication record, eliminating the need for transcription of the order. Copies of the order remain in the client's chart, and one is sent to the pharmacy (Figure 11-4).

THE JACK D. WEILER HOSPITAL
OF THE
ALBERT EINSTEIN COLLEGE OF MEDICINE

A DIVISION OF
MONTEFIORE MEDICAL CENTER
BRONX, NEW YORK, 10461

NR7976E (REV. 7/92) DOCTOR'S ORDER SHEET NURSING COPY

DRUG SENSITIVITY: ☒NONE

Addressograph with Client Identification	MEDICATION: Colace DOSE / ROUTE: 100 mg p.o FREQUENCY / DURATION: tid SPECIAL INSTRUCTIONS: PRACTITIONER'S SIGNATURE: M Smith MD DATE/TIME: 5/8/96 8[10] A.M. M.D. COUNTER SIGNATURE DATE/TIME A.M. P.M. ① NOTED BY: Deborah C Morris DATE/TIME: 5/8/96 9[20] A.M.	Admit to Postpartum Dx - Intrauterine Pregnancy - Delivered - NSD Vital Signs - as per policy Diet - Regular Activity OOB ad lib PRACTITIONER'S SIGNATURE: M Smith MD DATE/TIME: 5/8/96 8[10] A.M. R.N. SIGNATURE: Deborah C Morris RN DATE/TIME: 5/8/96 9[20] A.M. M.D. COUNTER SIGNATURE DATE/TIME A.M. P.M. U.S./LPN SIGNATURE DATE/TIME A.M. P.M.
Addressograph with Client Identification	MEDICATION: Ferrous Sulfate DOSE / ROUTE: 325 mg p.o. FREQUENCY / DURATION: tid SPECIAL INSTRUCTIONS: PRACTITIONER'S SIGNATURE: M Smith MD DATE/TIME: 5/8/96 8[10] A.M. M.D. COUNTER SIGNATURE DATE/TIME A.M. P.M. ② NOTED BY: Deborah C Morris DATE/TIME: 5/8/96 9[20] A.M.	Ice packs to perineum 1st 24 hours p.r.n Sitz bath to perineum TID after 1st 24 hours prn Witch Hazel Pads to perineum prn CBC in AM of Postpartum day # 1 PRACTITIONER'S SIGNATURE: M. Smith MD DATE/TIME: 5/8/96 8[10] A.M. R.N. SIGNATURE: Deborah C Morris RN DATE/TIME: 5/8/96 9[20] A.M. M.D. COUNTER SIGNATURE DATE/TIME A.M. P.M. U.S./LPN SIGNATURE DATE/TIME A.M. P.M.

A

WEILER HOSPITAL
BRONX, NEW YORK 10461

MEDICATION ADMINISTRATION RECORD

ALLERGY: ☒NONE

		TIME	DATE 5/8/96 INIT.	DATE 5/9/96 INIT.
Addressograph with Client Identification	MEDICATION: Colace DOSE / ROUTE: 100mg p.o FREQUENCY / DURATION: tid SPECIAL INSTRUCTIONS: PRACTITIONER'S SIGNATURE: M. Smith MD DATE/TIME: 5/8/96 8[10] A.M. M.D. COUNTER SIGNATURE DATE/TIME A.M. P.M. ③ NOTED BY: Deborah C Morris RN DATE/TIME: 5/8/96 9[20] A.M.	10A	DM	
		2P		
		6P		
Addressograph with Client Identification	MEDICATION: Ferrous Sulfate DOSE / ROUTE: 325mg p.o. FREQUENCY / DURATION: tid SPECIAL INSTRUCTIONS: PRACTITIONER'S SIGNATURE: M Smith MD DATE/TIME: 5/8/96 8[10] A.M. M.D. COUNTER SIGNATURE DATE/TIME A.M. P.M. ④ NOTED BY: Deborah C. Morris RN DATE/TIME: 5/8/96 9[20] A.M.	10A	DM	
		2P		
		6P		

B

Figure 11-4. Doctor's order sheet **(A)** and placement of med orders on MAR **(B)**. (Used with permission from Montefiore Medical Center, Jack D. Weiler Hospital of the Albert Einstein College of Medicine Division, Bronx, New York.)

WEILER HOSPITAL BRONX, NEW YORK 10461		**PRN MEDICATION ADMINISTRATION RECORD**		
		DATE 5/11/96	DATE 5/12/96	DATE
ALLERGY:	☒ NONE	TIME/INIT.	TIME/INIT.	TIME/INIT.
Addressograph with Client Identification	MEDICATION: Demerol	9:30 P DJ	2:30 A BS	
	DOSE / ROUTE: 75mg IM			
	FREQUENCY / DURATION: Q4h prn x 72 hrs			
	SPECIAL INSTRUCTIONS: for moderate pain			
	PRACTITIONER'S SIGNATURE: M. Johnson MD — DATE/TIME 5/11/96 5:40 A.M. (P.M.)			
	M.D. COUNTER SIGNATURE — DATE/TIME A.M. P.M.			
③	NOTED BY: Dolores Jenkins RN — DATE/TIME 5/11/96 6:00 A.M. (P.M.)			
Addressograph with Client Identification.	MEDICATION: Phenergan	9:30 P DJ	2:30 A BS.	
	DOSE / ROUTE: 25mg IM			
	FREQUENCY / DURATION: Q4h prn x 72hrs.			
	SPECIAL INSTRUCTIONS			
	PRACTITIONER'S SIGNATURE: M. Johnson MD — DATE/TIME 5/11/96 5:40 A.M. (P.M.)			
	M.D. COUNTER SIGNATURE — DATE/TIME A.M. P.M.			
④	NOTED BY: Dolores Jenkins RN — DATE/TIME 5/11/96 6:00 A.M. (P.M.)			

Figure 11-5. MAR showing p.r.n. medications. (Used with permission from Montefiore Medical Center, Jack D. Weiler Hospital of the Albert Einstein College of Medicine Division, Bronx, New York.)

Military Time

In some institutions military time may be used on MARs. Military time is a 24-hr clock. The main advantage of using military time is it helps to prevent errors in time since numbers are not repeated. In military time the colon and AM and PM are omitted. It starts at 1 AM, or 0100 in the morning, and ends at 12 midnight, or 2400. Remember the following rules for conversion.

Rules for Conversion

To convert AM time: omit the colon and AM.

Example: 8:45 AM = 0845

To convert PM time: omit the colon and PM; add 1200 to time.

Example: 7:50 PM = 1950

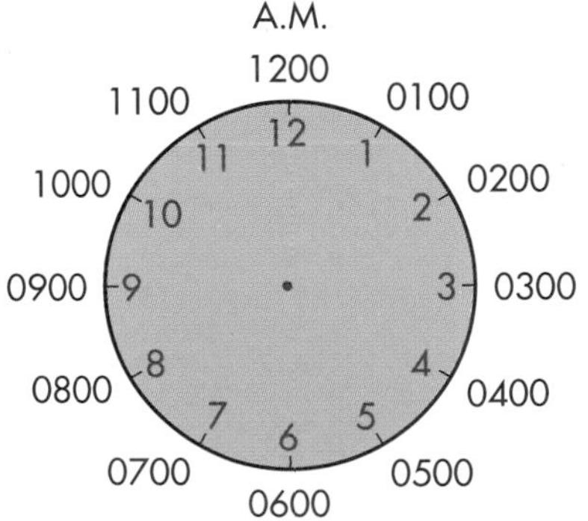

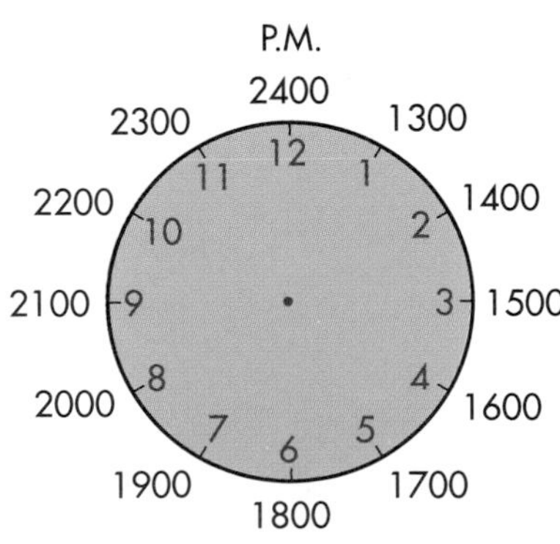

Points to Remember

- The system used for medication administration plays a role in determining the type of medication record used and whether transcription of orders is necessary.
- Regardless of the type of medication record used at an institution, the nurse should know the data that is essential for the medication record and understand the importance of determining accuracy and clarity of medication orders.
- Persons transcribing orders should transcribe them in ink and write legibly to avoid medication errors. All essential notations or instructions should be clearly written on the medication record.
- Documentation of medications administered should be done accurately and only by the person administering them.
- To avoid errors in administration, always check transcribed orders against the doctor's orders.

Practice Problems (p. 334)

Convert the following to military time.

1. 7:30 AM ______________
2. 10:30 AM ______________
3. 8:10 PM ______________
4. 5:45 PM ______________
5. 12:16 AM ______________

Convert the following military times to ordinary time.

6. 0207 ______________
7. 1743 ______________
8. 0004 ______________

Practice Exercise 1 (p. 335)

Using the MAR in Figure 11-6, list the medication, dosage, route, and time for the medications given by DG (Deborah C. Gray) on 4/6/92 and 4/8/92.

Date 4/6/92	Medication	Dosage	Route	Time
1.	______	______	______	______

Date 4/8/92	Medication	Dosage	Route	Time
1.	______	______	______	______
2.	______	______	______	______
3.	______	______	______	______
4.	______	______	______	______
5.	______	______	______	______

Date 4/8/92	Medication	Dosage	Route	Time
6.				
7.				
8.				
9.				

MONTEFIORE MEDICAL CENTER
JACK D. WEILER HOSPITAL OF THE ALBERT EINSTEIN COLLEGE OF MEDICINE DIVISION

STANDING ORDERS MEDICATION RECORD

INIT.	SIGNATURE	INIT.	SIGNATURE	INIT.	SIGNATURE
Dg	Deborah C. Gray				
MB.	Mary Brown				
AS.	ann smith				

Addressograph with Client Identification

ADDRESSOGRAPH

DRUG SENSITIVITIES ☐ NONE KNOWN
PCN, Sulfa

	MEDICATIONS	DATE 4/6/92 TIME AND INITIALS	DATE 4/7/92 TIME AND INITIALS	DATE 4/8/92 TIME AND INITIALS	DATE 4/9/92 TIME AND INITIALS	DATE 4/10/92 TIME AND INITIALS	DATE 4/11/92 TIME AND INITIALS	DATE 4/12/92 TIME AND INITIALS
1	DRUG Digoxin; DOSE 0.25 mg; FREQUENCY o.d.; ADMINISTRATION TIMES 9A; ROUTE PO; DATE ORDERED 4/6/92	9A MB ap 76	9A AS. ap 72	9a Dg ap 88				
2	DRUG Lasix; DOSE 20 mg; FREQUENCY bid; ADMINISTRATION TIMES 9A - 5P; ROUTE PO; DATE ORDERED 4/6/92	9A MB 5p MB	9A AS. 5p AS	9A Dg 5p Dg				
3	DRUG Procardia; DOSE 10 mg; FREQUENCY tid; ADMINISTRATION TIMES 9A - 1P - 5P; ROUTE PO; DATE ORDERED 4/6/92	9A MB 1p MB 5p Dg	9A AS 1p AS 5p. MB	9A Dg 1p Dg 5p Dg				
	DRUG Colace; DOSE 100 mg; FREQUENCY bid; ADMINISTRATION TIMES 9A - 5P; ROUTE PO; DATE ORDERED 4/6/92	9A MB 5p MB	9A AS 5p AS	9A Dg 5p Dg				
5	DRUG Heparin; DOSE 5,000 U; FREQUENCY od; ADMINISTRATION TIMES 9A; ROUTE S.C.; DATE ORDERED 4/6/92	9A MB	9A AS	9A Dg				
	DRUG; DOSE; FREQUENCY; ADMINISTRATION TIMES; ROUTE; DATE ORDERED							
7	DRUG; DOSE; FREQUENCY; ADMINISTRATION TIMES; ROUTE; DATE ORDERED							

☐ PATIENT DISCHARGED

STANDING ORDERS

DATE	TIME	DRUG	REASON NOT GIVEN	DATE	TIME	DRUG	REASON NOT GIVEN

NR 1586E 1/89

CHART COPY

Figure 11-6. MAR for practice exercise 1. (Used with permission from Montefiore Medical Center, Jack D. Weiler Hospital of the Albert Einstein College of Medicine Division, Bronx, New York.)

Practice Exercise 2 (pp. 335-336)

Transcribe the following orders to the practice medication sheet (Figure 11-7). When you have completed this, place your initials and signature in the appropriate space on the medication form. Use the times indicated and the date 4/9/92. Indicate client has no known allergies.

1. Potassium chloride 20 mEq p.o. o.d. (10A)
2. Digoxin 0.125 mg p.o. o.d. (10A)
3. Lasix 30 mg p.o. b.i.d. (10A and 6P)
4. Aldomet 500 mg p.o. b.i.d. (10A and 6P)
5. Restoril 30 mg p.o. HS (10P)

Continued.

MONTEFIORE MEDICAL CENTER
JACK D. WEILER HOSPITAL OF THE ALBERT EINSTEIN COLLEGE OF MEDICINE DIVISION

STANDING ORDERS MEDICATION RECORD

INIT.	SIGNATURE	INIT.	SIGNATURE	INIT.	SIGNATURE

	DRUG SENSITIVITIES ☐ NONE KNOWN	DATE	DATE	DATE	DATE	DATE	DATE	DATE	☐ PATIENT DISCHARGED
	MEDICATIONS	TIME AND INITIALS	TIME AND INITIALS	TIME AND INITIALS	TIME AND INITIALS	TIME AND INITIALS	TIME AND INITIALS	TIME AND INITIALS	
1	DRUG / DOSE / FREQUENCY / ADMINISTRATION TIMES / ROUTE / DATE ORDERED								
2	DRUG / DOSE / FREQUENCY / ADMINISTRATION TIMES / ROUTE / DATE ORDERED								
3	DRUG / DOSE / FREQUENCY / ADMINISTRATION TIMES / ROUTE / DATE ORDERED								STANDING
4	DRUG / DOSE / FREQUENCY / ADMINISTRATION TIMES / ROUTE / DATE ORDERED								
5	DRUG / DOSE / FREQUENCY / ADMINISTRATION TIMES / ROUTE / DATE ORDERED								ORDERS
6	DRUG / DOSE / FREQUENCY / ADMINISTRATION TIMES / ROUTE / DATE ORDERED								
7	DRUG / DOSE / FREQUENCY / ADMINISTRATION TIMES / ROUTE / DATE ORDERED								

DATE	TIME	DRUG	REASON NOT GIVEN	DATE	TIME	DRUG	REASON NOT GIVEN

Figure 11-7. MAR for practice exercise 2. (Used with permission from Montefiore Medical Center, Jack D. Weiler Hospital of the Albert Einstein College of Medicine Division, Bronx, New York.)

Use Figure 11-8 Stat and PRN Medication Record for orders 6 and 7.

6. Percocet 2 tabs p.o. q3-4h p.r.n. for pain × 2 days. Chart that you administered it on 4/9/92 at 2 PM.
7. Tylenol 650 mg p.o. q4h p.r.n. temp > 38.2° C.

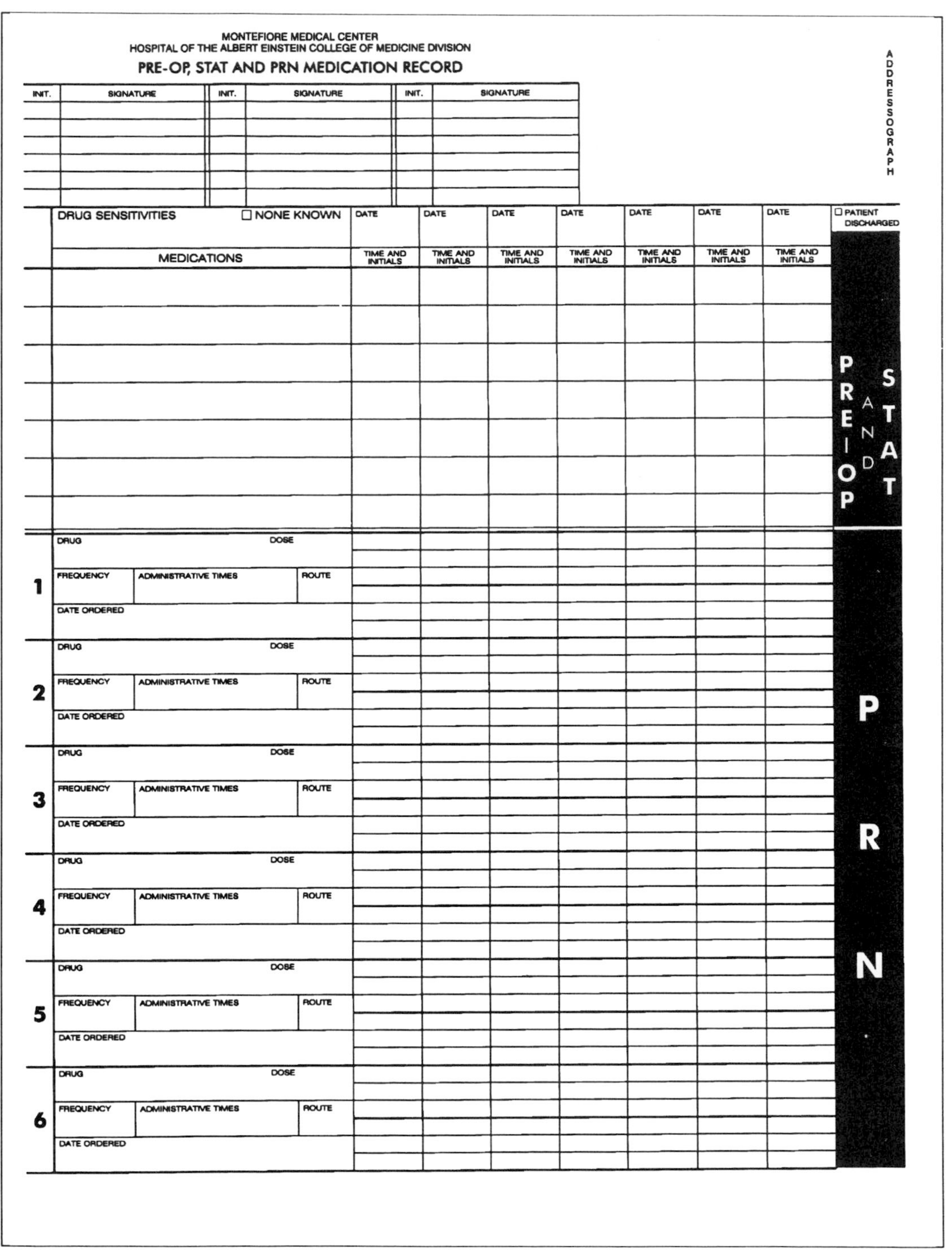

MONTEFIORE MEDICAL CENTER
HOSPITAL OF THE ALBERT EINSTEIN COLLEGE OF MEDICINE DIVISION

PRE-OP, STAT AND PRN MEDICATION RECORD

ADDRESSOGRAPH

INIT.	SIGNATURE	INIT.	SIGNATURE	INIT.	SIGNATURE

DRUG SENSITIVITIES ☐ NONE KNOWN	DATE	DATE	DATE	DATE	DATE	DATE	DATE	☐ PATIENT DISCHARGED
MEDICATIONS	TIME AND INITIALS	TIME AND INITIALS	TIME AND INITIALS	TIME AND INITIALS	TIME AND INITIALS	TIME AND INITIALS	TIME AND INITIALS	PRE-OP AND STAT
1 DRUG / DOSE / FREQUENCY / ADMINISTRATIVE TIMES / ROUTE / DATE ORDERED								PRN.
2 DRUG / DOSE / FREQUENCY / ADMINISTRATIVE TIMES / ROUTE / DATE ORDERED								
3 DRUG / DOSE / FREQUENCY / ADMINISTRATIVE TIMES / ROUTE / DATE ORDERED								
4 DRUG / DOSE / FREQUENCY / ADMINISTRATIVE TIMES / ROUTE / DATE ORDERED								
5 DRUG / DOSE / FREQUENCY / ADMINISTRATIVE TIMES / ROUTE / DATE ORDERED								
6 DRUG / DOSE / FREQUENCY / ADMINISTRATIVE TIMES / ROUTE / DATE ORDERED								

Figure 11-8. MAR for practice exercise 2. (Used with permission from Montefiore Medical Center, Jack D. Weiler Hospital of the Albert Einstein College of Medicine Division, Bronx, New York.)

Chapter 12

Reading Medication Labels

Objectives

After reviewing this chapter the student will be able to do the following:

1. Identify the trade and generic names of medications
2. Identify the dosage strength of medications
3. Identify the form in which a medication is supplied
4. Identify the total volume of a medication container where indicated
5. Identify directions for mixing or preparing a drug where necessary

To administer medications safely to a client, nurses must be able to read and interpret the information on a medication label. Medication labels indicate the dose contained in the package. It is important to read the label carefully and recognize essential information.

Reading Medication Labels

The nurse should be able to recognize the following information on a medication label.

Generic Name

This is a name given by the manufacturer that first develops the medication. Medications have only one generic name. Doctors are ordering medications more often by the generic name, so nurses need to know the generic name, as well as the trade name. Pharmacists in many institutions are dispensing medications by generic name to decrease costs. Sometimes only the generic name may appear on a medication label or package. This is common for drugs that have been used for many years and are well known and do not require marketing under a different trade name. See sample labels illustrating this.

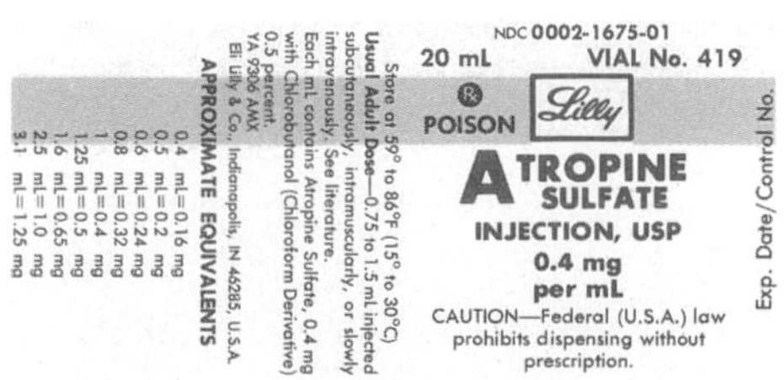

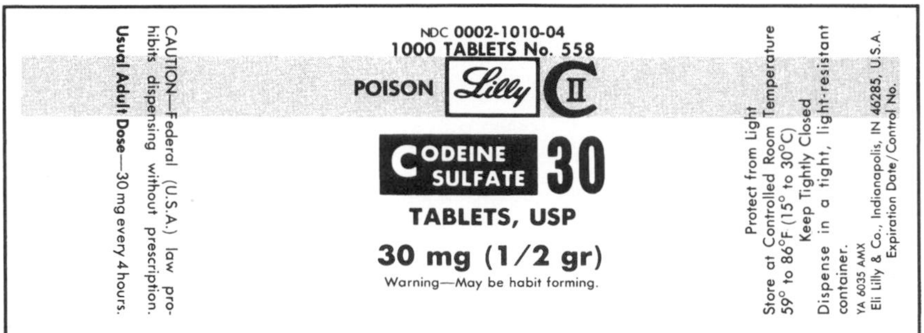

Notice on both labels the abbreviation USP appears after the name of the drug. USP is the abbreviation for United States Pharmacopeia, which is an official national listing for drugs.

Trade Name

This is also referred to as the brand name. It is important to remember that a drug may be marketed under different trade names by different manufacturers. The trade name is followed by an ®, which is the registration symbol. Some medications may have the abbreviation ™ after the trade name, which stands for trademark. See the illustrations of the labels for Epivir oral solution, manufactured by GlaxoWellcome Inc. and Corvert, manufactured by The Upjohn Company.

NDC 0173-0471-00

GlaxoWellcome

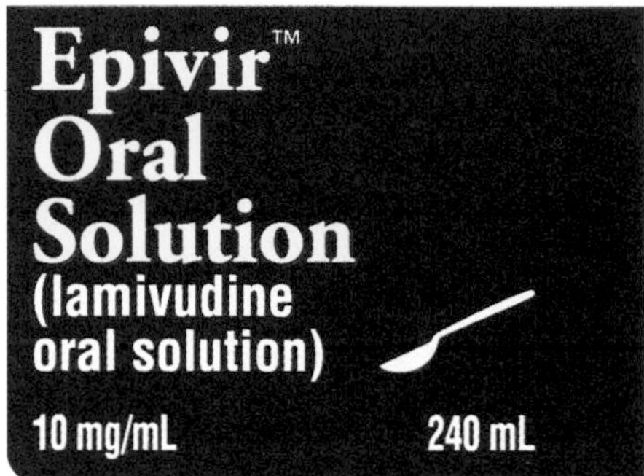

Caution: Federal law prohibits dispensing without prescription.

See package insert for Dosage and Administration.

Store between 2° and 25°C (36° and 77°F) in tightly closed bottles. Contains 6% alcohol.

4 058895

Glaxo Wellcome Inc.
Research Triangle Park,
NC 27709
Manufactured in England under agreement from BioChem Pharma Inc.
Laval, Quebec, Canada
Rev. 10/95

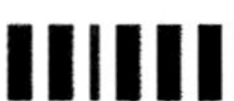

Caution: Federal law prohibits dispensing without prescription. See package insert for complete product information. Store at controlled room temperature (20° to 25° C or 68° to 77° F) [see USP]. Each mL contains: Ibutilide fumarate, 0.1 mg; sodium chloride, 8.90 mg; sodium acetate trihydrate, 0.189 mg; water for injection. When necessary, pH was adjusted with sodium hydroxide and/or hydrochloric acid.
816 416 000
The Upjohn Company
Kalamazoo, MI 49001, USA

NDC 0009-3794-01 10 mL
Corvert™
Injection
ibutilide fumarate injection
0.1 mg per mL
For IV use only

Notice ™ appears after the names *Epivir* and *Corvert.* The trade name is the name given to the drug by the manufacturer and therefore cannot be used by any other company. The drug name is a trademark for that company. Once the trademark is formally registered by the Patent and Trademark Office, the symbol ® then appears on the medication label.

Think Critically to Avoid Errors in Administration

Always read a drug label carefully to avoid errors. Drug names can be deceptively similar. Similarity in name doesn't mean the same action. For example, *Inderal* and *Inderide* are similar names, but the action and the contents of the medication are different. Inderal delivers a certain dose of propranolol hydrochloride; Inderide combines two antihypertensive agents (propranolol hydrochloride and hydrochlorothiazide, a diuretic-antihypertensive).

Dose Strength

This refers to the weight of the medication per unit of measure (the weight per tablet, capsule, milliliter, etc.). In solutions, the medication may be stated as 80 mg/2 mL or in solid forms, such as tablets, the strength per tablet may be indicated.

Example: 50 mg per tablet

Form

This specifies the type of preparation available.

Example: Tablets, capsules. For solutions it may indicate milliliters (mL) or cubic centimeters (cc), oral suspension, or aqueous solution. The label may also indicate abbreviations or words that describe the form of the drug. Examples include CR (controlled-release), LA (long acting), DS (double strength), SR (sustained release), and XL (long acting). These abbreviations indicate that the drug has been prepared in a form that allows extended action, or slow release of a drug. Oftentimes these drugs are given less frequently. Examples are Procardia XL, Inderal LA, and Verapamil SR.

Route of Administration

This will tell how the medication is to be administered.

Example: Oral, I.M., I.V., topical

Total Volume

On solutions for injections or oral liquids total volume as well as dosage strength is stated.

Example: 30 mL may be the total volume on a medication label, but the solution or liquid contains 2 mg of medication per mL. On a bottle of Amoxicillin for oral use, the total volume would be 100 mL and the dosage strength would be 125 mg per 5 mL. **It's important to recognize the difference between the amount per mL and the total volume to avoid confusion and errors.**

Directions for Mixing or Reconstituting a Medication

When medication comes in a powdered form, the directions for how to mix or reconstitute it and with what solution are found on the label.

Precautions

Specific instructions related to safety, effectiveness, or administration that need to be adhered to are included on the label.

Medication labels also contain information such as the expiration date, storage information, lot numbers, the name of the drug manufacturer, and a National Drug Code (NDC) number. Some medication labels are more detailed than others; however, recognition of pertinent information on a medication label is an absolute requirement before calculation and administration.

Let's examine some medication labels.

1. On this label note the following:

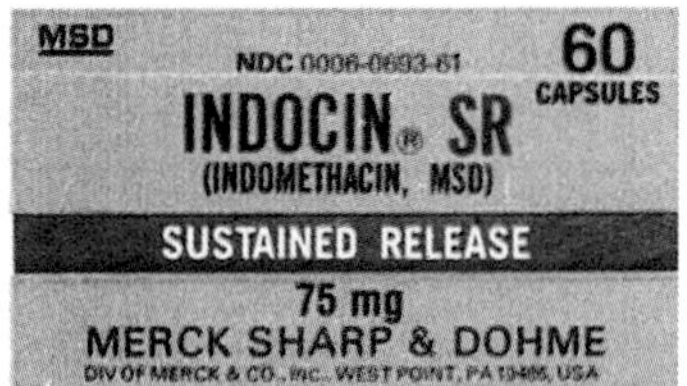

a) *Indocin* is the brand name.
b) *Indomethacin* is the generic name.
c) The drug form is capsule.
d) The dose strength is 75 mg per capsule.
e) The drug manufacturer is Merck Sharp & Dohme.

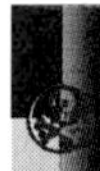

Think Critically to Avoid Drug Calculation Errors

Read labels carefully. Read the total volume on a medication container carefully. Confusion with dose strength can cause a serious medication error.

2. Note the following on this label:

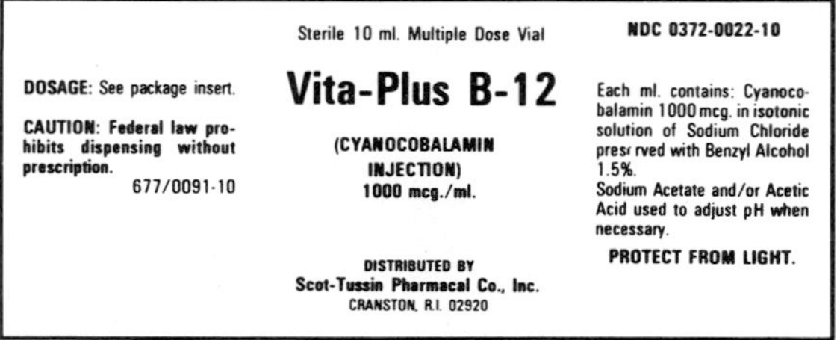

a) *Vita-Plus B-12* is the trade name.
b) *Cyanocobalamin* is the generic name.
c) Injection is the drug form or route.
d) 10 mL is the total volume of the vial.
e) 1000 mcg/mL is the dose strength.
f) Protect from light are the directions for storage.
g) Scot-Tussin Pharmacal Co, Inc. is the drug manufacturer.
h) The NDC is 0372-0022-10.

3. This label includes the following information:

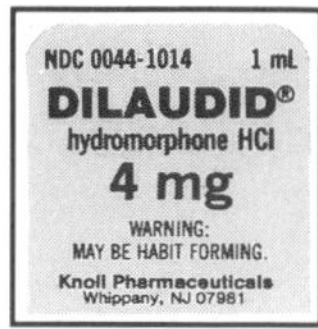

   a) *Dilaudid* is the trade name.
   b) *Hydromorphone HCl* is the generic name.
   c) The total volume of the ampule is 1 mL.
   d) The dose strength is 4 mg/mL.
   e) The NDC is 0044-1014.
   f) Knoll Pharmaceuticals is the drug manufacturer.
   g) May be habit forming is the warning.
4. The following information is indicated on this label:

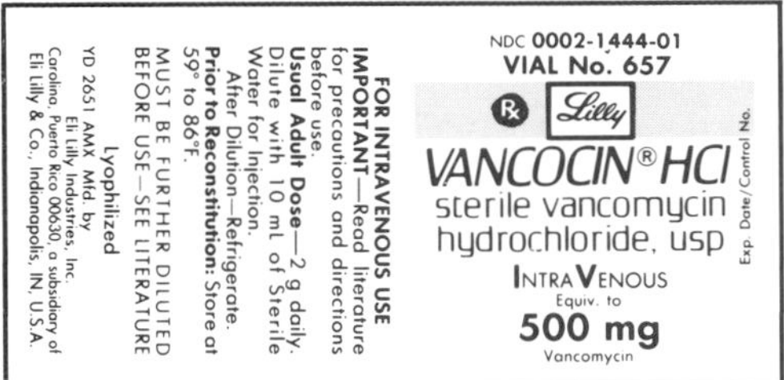

   a) *Vancocin HCl* is the trade name.
   b) *Vancomycin hydrochloride* is the generic name.
   c) Dilute with 10 mL of sterile water for injection are the directions for mixing.
   d) The dose strength (50 mg/mL) is 500 mg/10 mL.
   e) Injection is the form. The label specifies I.V. use.
   f) After dilution, refrigerate are the directions after reconstitution.
   g) Eli Lilly Industries, Inc. is the drug manufacturer.

In this chapter, a sample of medication labels is presented to assist you in the recognition of essential information on a drug label. It is important to note that some drugs may not give or indicate their strength but are ordered by the number of tablets (for example, multivitamin tablet 1 p.o. every day, Bactrim DS 1 tablet p.o. b.i.d., Percocet 1 tablet p.o. q4h p.r.n).

In hospitals that use unit dose, the medications will come to the unit in individually wrapped packets that are labeled. The label includes the generic name or trade name or sometimes both. The strength is indicated on the medication label. The nurse must read the label on unit-dose packages and note that sometimes even with this method calculation may be necessary. The pharmacy in some institutions provides the unit with a supply of medications that are available on units in multidose containers. These medications may be in unit-dose packaging but are used a great deal by the clients on the unit. Examples include Tylenol and aspirin. Some medications may also be dispensed in bottles for use—for example, 100 tablets of aspirin 325 mg.

Most hospital units have a combination of unit dose and multidose. Figure 12-1 shows examples of unit-dose packaging.

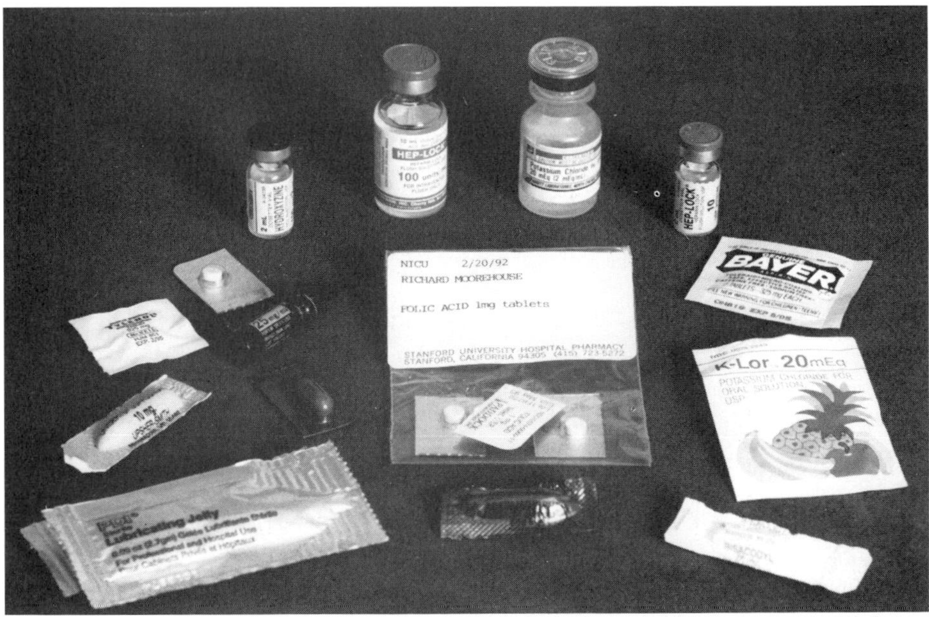

Figure 12-1. Unit-dose packages. (From Clayton B, Stock Y: *Basic pharmacology for nurses,* ed 10, St Louis, 1993, Mosby.)

Medication Labels That Show Combined Drugs

Some medication labels for certain drugs may indicate that a medication contains two drugs. These are usually indicated in the generic name of the drug, and the label specifies the dose strength for each next to the name.

Example 1: The label for Sinemet, which is the trade name for an antiparkinsonian drug, indicates the medication contains carbidopa and levodopa. The first number specifies the amount of carbidopa, and the second number represents the amount of levodopa. This is further indicated on the bottom of the label. (See sample labels.)

DU PONT PHARMA
DUPONT PHARMA
SINEMET®
(CARBIDOPA-LEVODOPA)
10-100
NDC 0056-0647-68
3346/7826602
7784/HC
100 TABLETS
Each tablet contains:
Carbidopa .... 10 mg*
*(Anhydrous equivalent)
Levodopa .... 100 mg
Marketed by:
DuPont Pharma
Wilmington, DE 19880
Manufactured by:
MERCK & CO., Inc.
WEST POINT, PA 19486, USA
USUAL ADULT DOSAGE: See accompanying circular.
PROTECT FROM LIGHT. Dispense in a well-closed, light-resistant container. This is a bulk package and not intended for dispensing.
CAUTION: Federal (USA) law prohibits dispensing without prescription.
SINEMET is a registered trademark of MERCK & CO., Inc.
Lot
Exp.

This label indicates the strength of carbidopa as 10 mg and levodopa as 100 mg.

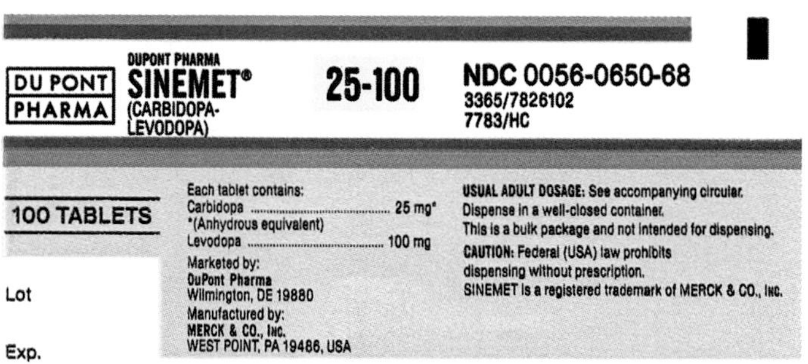

The dose strength of carbidopa is 25 mg and levodopa is 100 mg.

Example 2: Septra, (an antibiotic) that is also manufactured under the trade name Bactrim, is a combination of trimethoprim and sulfamethoxazole. For example, a Septra tablet contains 80 mg trimethoprim and 400 mg sulfamethoxazole. Septra DS is 160 mg trimethoprim and 800 mg sulfamethoxazole. (See labels for Septra.)

For indications, dosage, precautions, etc., see accompanying package insert.
Store at 15° to 25°C (59° to 77°F) in a dry place.
Dispense in a tight, light-resistant container as defined in the U.S.P.
Made in U.S.A. U.S. Patent No. 4,209,513 (tablet)
100 Tablets NDC 0173-0852-55
SEPTRA® TABLETS
(trimethoprim and sulfamethoxazole)
Each scored tablet contains
80 mg trimethoprim and
400 mg sulfamethoxazole.
CAUTION: Federal law prohibits dispensing without prescription.
Glaxo Wellcome Inc.
Research Triangle Park, NC 27709
Rev. 2/96
596154
LOT
EXP
N 3 0173-0852-55 7
6505-00-501-6452

Store at 15° to 25°C (59° to 77°F) in a dry place.
Dispense in tight, light-resistant container as defined in the U.S.P.
For indications, dosage, precautions, etc., see accompanying package insert.
6505-01-016-1470 Rev. 5/96 Made in U.S.A.
100 Tablets NDC 0173-0853-55
SEPTRA® DS
Double Strength
(trimethoprim and sulfamethoxazole)
Each scored tablet contains
160 mg trimethoprim and
800 mg sulfamethoxazole.
CAUTION: Federal law prohibits dispensing without prescription.
U.S. Patent No. 4,209,513 (Tablet)
Glaxo Wellcome Inc.
Research Triangle Park, NC 27709
595493
LOT
EXP
N 3 0173-0853-55 4

Note: Although frequently tablets and capsules that contain more than one drug are ordered by the brand name and number of tablets to be given (for example, Septra DS 1 tab p.o. b.i.d.), the doctor may order this medication by another route, for example, I.V. With the I.V. order, the nurse calculates the dose to be given based on the strength of the trimethoprim.

Example: Medication available: 10 mL multi-dose vial containing 160 mg trimethoprim (16 mg/mL) and 800 mg sulfamethoxazole (80 mg/mL)

Doctor's Order: Septra 320 mg IVPB q8h. (In calculating the dose, the nurse would calculate the amount to be given based on the trimethoprim [16 mg/mL]).

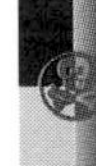

Think Critically to Avoid Drug Calculation Errors

Read the label carefully to validate you have the correct medication and dose for combined drugs.

Points to Remember

- Read medication labels 3 times.
- Read directions for mixing when indicated, and check expiration dates.
- Read labels carefully and don't confuse medication names; they are often deceptively similar. When in doubt, check appropriate resources such as a reference book or the hospital pharmacist.
- Read the label on combined drugs carefully to ascertain whether you're administering the correct medication dose.

Chapter Review (pp. 337-338)

Read the labels and fill in the following exercises.

RECOMMENDED STORAGE
STORE BELOW 86°F (30°C)
Dispense in tight, light resistant containers (USP).
†Each capsule contains prazosin hydrochloride equivalent to 1 mg of prazosin.
Manufactured by
Pfizer Pharmaceuticals, Inc., Barceloneta, P.R. 00617
4444
6505-01-039-6320
NDC0663-4310-71
250 Capsules
Minipress®
prazosin hydrochloride
1 mg†
CAUTION: Federal law prohibits dispensing without prescription.
Pfizer Distributed by LABORATORIES DIVISION New York, N.Y. 10017
READ ACCOMPANYING PROFESSIONAL INFORMATION
DOSAGE: See accompanying prescribing information.
IMPORTANT: This closure is not child-resistant.

1. Generic name __________ Form __________

   Trade name __________ Dose strength __________

LANOXIN® 2mL
(digoxin) Injection
500 µg (0.5 mg) in 2 mL
(250 µg [0.25 mg] per mL)
Store at 15° to 25°C (59° to 77°F).
PROTECT FROM LIGHT.
Glaxo Wellcome Inc.
Research Triangle Park, NC 27709
Rev. 1/96
542308

LOT
EXP

2. Generic name ______________ Form ______________

Trade name ______________ Dose strength ______________

Total volume ______________

USUAL ADULT DOSAGE:
See accompanying circular.
This is a bulk package and not intended for dispensing.
CAUTION: Federal (USA) law prohibits dispensing without prescription.
100 | No. 7592 7273206

MSD
NDC 0006-0020-68
100 TABLETS
Decadron
(Dexamethasone, MSD)
0.25 mg
MERCK SHARP & DOHME
DIVISION OF MERCK & CO., INC.
WEST POINT, PA 19486, USA

Lot

3. Generic name ______________ Form ______________

Trade name ______________ Dose strength ______________

Usual Adult Dose: See package insert.
Each ml of aqueous solution contains: gentamicin sulfate, USP equivalent to 40 mg gentamicin, 1.8 mg methylparaben and 0.2 mg propylparaben as preservatives, 3.2 mg sodium bisulfite, and 0.1 mg edetate disodium.
Store between 2° and 30°C (36° and 86°F).
GARAMYCIN Injectable should not be physically premixed with other drugs.

SCHERING
20 ml Multiple Dose Vial Sterile
For use in preparation of large volume parenterals
Garamycin® Injectable
brand of gentamicin sulfate injection, USP
40 mg/ml
20ml = 800mg
For Parenteral Administration
Caution: Federal law prohibits dispensing without prescription.
Schering Pharmaceutical Corporation (PR), Manati, Puerto Rico 00701
An Affiliate of Schering Corporation, Kenilworth, N.J. 07033

Read accompanying directions carefully.
Control No.
Exp. Date.
11788815 Rev. 1/81

4. Generic name ______________ Form ______________

Trade name ______________ Dose strength ______________

Total volume ______________ Instructions ______________

CAUTION—Federal (U.S.A.) law prohibits dispensing without prescription.
Keep Tightly Closed
Store at 59° to 86°F
WV 2160 AMX
ELI LILLY AND COMPANY
Indianapolis, IN 46285, U.S.A.
Exp. Date/Control No.

NDC 0002-1060-02
100 TABLETS No. 1703
℞ Lilly POISON
CRYSTODIGIN®
DIGITOXIN TABLETS
USP
0.1 mg

Usual Maintenance Dose—0.05 to 0.3 mg a day.
Each Tablet Contains: Crystalline Digitoxin, 0.1 mg
See accompanying literature.
Indiscriminate use may be dangerous.
Dispense in a tight, light-resistant container.

5. Generic name ______________ Form ______________

Trade name ______________ Dose strength ______________

NDC 0048-1040-03
NSN 6505-01-156-1807
Code 3P1043
SYNTHROID®
(Levothyroxine Sodium Tablets, USP)
50 mcg (0.05 mg)
100 TABLETS
Caution: Federal (USA) law prohibits dispensing without prescription.
BASF Pharma
knoll®

See full prescribing information for dosage and administration.
Dispense in a tight, light-resistant container as described in USP.
Store at controlled room temperature, 15°-30°C (59°-86°F).
Knoll Pharmaceutical Company
Mount Olive, NJ 07828
USA
7878-03

6. Generic name ______________ Form ______________

   Trade name ______________ Dose strength ______________

NDC **0002-2307-48**
100 mL (When Mixed) **M-126**
℞ Lilly
V-CILLIN K®
PENICILLIN V POTASSIUM FOR ORAL SOLUTION, USP
125 mg
(200,000 Units) **per 5 mL**
CAUTION—Federal (U.S.A.) law prohibits dispensing without prescription.
PULL

Usual Dose Range: One or two teaspoonfuls every 6 to 8 hours. See literature.
Contains Penicillin V Potassium equivalent to Penicillin V 2.5 g, in a dry, pleasantly flavored mixture, buffered with Sodium Citrate and Citric Acid.
Prior to Mixing. Store at Controlled Room Temperature 59° to 86°F (15° to 30°C)
Directions for Mixing—At the time of dispensing tap bottle lightly to loosen powder. Add 63 mL of water to the dry mixture in the bottle in **two** portions. Shake well after each addition.
Each 5 mL (approx. one teaspoonful) will then contain: Penicillin V Potassium equivalent to 125 mg (200,000 Units) Penicillin V
Slight color variation does not affect product efficacy.

YA 2546 AMX
Eli Lilly & Co., Indianapolis, IN 46285, U.S.A.
Expiration Date

To remove main label, cut or tear on perforation.

100 mL V-CILLIN K® PENICILLIN V POTASSIUM FOR ORAL SOLUTION, USP 125 mg (200,000 Units) per 5 mL. Oversize bottle provides extra space for shaking. Store in a refrigerator. May be kept for 14 days without significant loss of potency. Keep Tightly Closed. Discard unused portion after 14 days. **SHAKE WELL BEFORE USING**
Control No.

7. Generic name ______________ Dose strength ______________

   Trade name ______________ Directions for storage ______________

   Total volume ______________

LyphoMed®
POTASSIUM CHLORIDE
INJECTION, USP
(2 mEq/mL)
40 mEq
20 mL
Single Dose Vial

N 0469-6520-15 Sterile. Nonpyrogenic. 965-20
MUST BE DILUTED PRIOR TO IV ADMINISTRATION
Each mL contains: Potassium Chloride 149 mg; Water for Injection q.s. pH adjusted with HCl or KOH if necessary. 4000 mOsmol/L.
***Usual Dose:** See Package Insert.*
***LyphoMed, Inc.**, Rosemont, IL 60018* **B-87**

8. Generic name ______________ Form ______________

   Trade name ______________ Dose strength ______________

An aid in the treatment of temporary constipation.
Keep this and all medication out of the reach of children.
Warning: As with any drug, if you are pregnant or nursing a baby, seek the advice of a health professional before using this product.
Caution: If cramping pain occurs, discontinue the medication.
Manufactured by R.P. Scherer
Clearwater, Florida 33518
Expressly for:
HOECHST-ROUSSEL Pharmaceuticals Inc.
Somerville, New Jersey 08876
REG TM HOECHST AG
60210-2/85

NDC 0039-0002-10
Surfak®
docusate calcium USP
STOOL SOFTENER
Seal Under Cap
Printed Hoechst-Roussel
100 CAPSULES
50 MG EACH

Each capsule contains 50 mg docusate calcium USP and the following inactive ingredients: alcohol USP up to 1.3% (w/w), corn oil NF, FD&C Red #3, FD&C Red #40, gelatin NF, glycerin USP, parabens NF, sorbitol NF, soybean oil USP and other ingredients.
Usual Dosage: Adults—two or three capsules daily; children 6 to 12 and adults with minimal needs – one to three capsules daily. Continue for several days or until bowel movements are normal. For children under 6 consult a physician.
Preserve in a tight container. Store at controlled room temperature (59°-86°F) in a dry place.

9. Generic name ____________ Form ____________

Trade name ____________ Dose strength ____________

RECOMMENDED STORAGE IN DRY FORM
STORE BELOW 86° F (30° C)
Sterile reconstituted solutions should be protected from light and may be stored at room temperature for four weeks without significant loss of potency.
MADE IN U.S.A.

Sterile
Streptomycin Sulfate, USP
Equivalent to 5.0 g of Streptomycin Base
5.0 g
FOR INTRAMUSCULAR USE ONLY
CAUTION: Federal law prohibits dispensing without prescription
ROERIG Pfizer
A division of Pfizer Inc. N.Y., N.Y. 10017

Usual Daily Dosage
Adults: Varies with infection—consult package insert.
Adult average single injection: 0.5 to 1.0 g

ml Diluent added	mg/ml of Solution
9.0 ml	400 mg/ml

The dry powder is dissolved by adding Water for Injection, USP or Sodium Chloride Injection, USP in an amount to yield the desired concentration.

PATIENT ____________
ROOM NO. ____________
DATE DILUTED ____________

10. Generic name ____________ Directions for mixing ____________

Trade name ____________ Dose strength after reconstitution ______ ____

Form ____________ Storage instructions ____________

NDC 0173-0471-00
GlaxoWellcome
Epivir™ Oral Solution
(lamivudine oral solution)
10 mg/mL **240 mL**

Caution: Federal law prohibits dispensing without prescription.
See package insert for Dosage and Administration.
Store between 2° and 25°C (36° and 77°F) in tightly closed bottles. Contains 6% alcohol.

4 0 5 8 8 9 5
Glaxo Wellcome Inc.
Research Triangle Park, NC 27709
Manufactured in England under agreement from BioChem Pharma Inc.
Laval, Quebec, Canada
Rev. 10/95

11. Generic name ____________ Form ____________

Trade name ____________ Dose strength ____________

Total volume ____________

ZOVIRAX® STERILE POWDER 1000 mg NDC 0173-0952-01
(ACYCLOVIR SODIUM) equivalent to 1000 mg acyclovir
FOR INTRAVENOUS INFUSION ONLY
CAUTION: Federal law prohibits dispensing without prescription.
Preparation of Solution: Inject 20 mL Sterile Water for Injection into vial. Shake vial until a clear solution is achieved and use within 12 hours. DO NOT USE BACTERIOSTATIC WATER FOR INJECTION CONTAINING BENZYL ALCOHOL OR PARABENS.
Dilute to 7 mg/mL or lower prior to infusion. See package insert for additional reconstitution and dilution instructions.
For indications, dosage, precautions, etc., see accompanying package insert.
Store at 15° to 25°C (59° to 77°F).
Glaxo Wellcome Inc.
Research Triangle Park, NC 27709
U.S. Patent No. 4199574
Rev. 2/96
Made in U.S.A.
647627

12. Generic name __________ Form __________

Trade name __________ Dose strength __________

Directions for mixing ____________________

____

Storage ____________________

NDC 0173-0363-00
Glaxo Pharmaceuticals
Zantac®
(ranitidine hydrochloride) Injection
25 mg/mL*
40-mL Pharmacy Bulk Package—Not for Direct Infusion
Sterile
Caution: Federal law prohibits dispensing without prescription.

Contents should be used as soon as possible following initial closure puncture. Discard any unused portion within 24 hours of first entry.
* Each 1 mL of aqueous solution contains ranitidine 25 mg (as the hydrochloride); phenol 5 mg as preservative; monobasic potassium phosphate and dibasic sodium phosphate as buffers.
See package insert for Dosage and Administration and directions for use of Pharmacy Bulk Package.
Store between 4° and 30°C (39° and 86°F). Protect from light. Store vial in carton until time of use.
Zantac® Injection tends to exhibit a yellow color that may intensify over time without adversely affecting potency.
Glaxo Pharmaceuticals, Division of Glaxo Inc.
Research Triangle Park, NC 27709
Manufactured in England
4/93
4043014

13. Generic name __________ Form __________

Trade name __________ Dose strength __________

NDC number __________

DESCRIPTION: Each tablet contains ciprofloxacin hydrochloride equivalent to 750 mg of ciprofloxacin.
DOSAGE: See accompanying literature for complete information on dosage and administration.
RECOMMENDED STORAGE: Store below 86°F (30°C).
Batch: VOID
Expires:
Distributed by: Kaiser Foundation Hospitals
Manufactured by: Bayer Corporation Pharmaceutical Division
VOID

051438 NDC 0179-1226-50
CIPRO®
(ciprofloxacin hydrochloride)
Equivalent to
750 mg ciprofloxacin
50 Tablets
Caution: Federal (USA) law prohibits dispensing without a prescription.
Bayer
VOID
Bayer Corporation
Pharmaceutical Division
400 Morgan Lane
West Haven, CT 06516

N 3 0179-1226-50 2
PL500037 ©1995 Bayer Corporation 5402
Printed in USA

14. Generic name __________ Form __________

Trade name __________ Dose strength __________

Amount __________

1 vial NDC 0003-0437-30
NSN 6505-01-084-9453
50 mg
FUNGIZONE®
INTRAVENOUS
Amphotericin B
for Injection USP
FOR INTRAVENOUS INFUSION
IN HOSPITALS ONLY
Caution: Federal law prohibits
dispensing without prescription
Read all sides

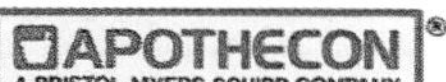

15. Generic name ____________ Form ____________

Trade name ____________ Drug manufacturer ____________

NDC 0009-7376-01
1 mL Single Dose Syringe
Depo-Provera®
Contraceptive Injection
sterile medroxyprogesterone
acetate suspension, USP
150 mg per mL
Intramuscular Use Only
Shake vigorously before use
81F 289 000 504711/1
The Upjohn Company
Lot:
EXP:

16. Generic name ____________ Form ____________

Trade name ____________ Dose strength ____________

Directions for use ____________

See package insert for complete product information.
Shake vigorously immediately before each use.
Store at controlled room temperature 15° to 30° C (59° to 86° F).
Each mL contains: Medroxyprogesterone acetate, 400 mg.
Also, polyethylene glycol 3350, 20.3 mg; sodium sulfate anhydrous, 11 mg; myristyl-gamma-picolinium chloride, 1.69 mg added as preservative. When necessary, pH was adjusted with sodium hydroxide and/or hydrochloric acid.
813 273 203
The Upjohn Company
Kalamazoo, Michigan 49001, USA

NDC 0009-0626-02
10 mL Vial
Depo-Provera®
Sterile Aqueous Suspension
sterile medroxyprogesterone
acetate suspension, USP
For intramuscular use only
400mg per mL
Caution: Federal law prohibits
dispensing without prescription.

17. Generic name ____________ Dose strength ____________

Trade name ____________ Directions for use ____________

NDC 0088-1792-47 6505-01-259-2914

120 mg Hoechst Marion Roussel

CARDIZEM®
(diltiazem HCl)

120 mg

100 Tablets

Each tablet contains: diltiazem hydrochloride. . . . . . 120 mg (equivalent to 110.3 mg as diltiazem). Dosage and Administration: Read package insert for prescribing information. CAUTION: Federal law prohibits dispensing without prescription. Warning: Keep out of reach of children. Pharmacist: Dispense in tight, light-resistant container as defined in USP. Important: This package is not child resistant. Store at controlled room temperature 59–86°F (15–30°C).

© 1996, Hoechst Marion Roussel, Inc.

Hoechst Marion Roussel, Inc. Kansas City, MO 64137 USA

EXP.: B6 50007212

3 0088-1792-47

18. Generic name ______________ Form ______________

Trade name ______________ Dose strength ______________

Amount ______________

Caution: Federal law prohibits dispensing without prescription. See package insert for complete product information. Store at controlled room temperature (20° to 25° C or 68° to 77° F) [see USP]. Each mL contains: Ibutilide fumarate, 0.1 mg; sodium chloride, 8.90 mg; sodium acetate trihydrate, 0.189 mg; water for injection. When necessary, pH was adjusted with sodium hydroxide and/or hydrochloric acid.

816 416 000

The Upjohn Company
Kalamazoo, MI 49001, USA

NDC 0009-3794-01 10 mL

Corvert™
Injection
ibutilide fumarate injection

0.1 mg per mL

For IV use only

19. Generic name ______________ Form ______________

Trade name ______________ Dose strength ______________

Directions for use ______________

See package insert for complete product information.

Store at controlled room temperature 15° to 30° C (59° to 86° F).

Each mL contains: Heparin sodium, 1,000 USP Units. Also sodium chloride, 9 mg; benzyl alcohol, 9.45 mg added as preservative.

811 326 403

The Upjohn Company
Kalamazoo, MI 49001, USA

Upjohn NDC 0009-0268-02
30 mL

Heparin Sodium Injection, USP
Sterile Solution
from beef lung
For subcutaneous or intravenous use

1,000 Units per mL

Caution: Federal law prohibits dispensing without prescription.

20. Generic name ______________ Dose strength ______________

Trade name ______________ Total volume ______________

Directions for use ______________

Chapter 13

Calculation of Doses Using Ratio-Proportion

Objectives

After reviewing this chapter the student will be able to do the following:

1. **State a ratio-proportion to solve a given dose calculation problem**
2. **Solve simple calculation problems using the ratio-proportion method**

Several methods are used for calculating doses. The most common methods are *ratio-proportion* and *use of a formula*. After presentation of the various methods, students can choose the method that they find easiest to use. First let's discuss calculating using ratio-proportion. If necessary, review Chapter 4 on ratio-proportion.

Use of Ratio-Proportion in Dose Calculation

Ratio-proportion is useful and easy to use in dose calculation, because frequently it is only necessary to find one unknown quantity.

For example, suppose you had a medication with a dose strength of 50 mg in 1 mL, and the doctor orders a dose of 25 mg. A ratio-proportion could be used to solve this. The known ratio is 50 mg : 1 mL, and x would be used to represent the unknown number of mL that would contain 25 mg. Therefore, to set this problem up in a ratio-proportion, the known ratio (50 mg : 1 mL) would be stated first, then the unknown ratio (25 mg : x mL). The known ratio is what you have **available,** or the information on the drug label.

It is important to remember when stating the ratios that the units of measure should be stated in the same sequence (in the example, mg : mL = mg : mL).

Example 1: 50 mg : 1 mL = 25 mg : x mL

(known) (unknown)

Solution: To solve for x use the principles presented in Chapter 4 on ratio-proportion.

50 mg : 1 mL = 25 mg : x mL

$50x$ = product of extremes

25 = product of means

$50x$ = 25 is the equation

$$\frac{50x}{50} = \frac{25}{50}$$ (Divide both sides by 50, the number in front of x.)

x = 0.5 mL

Note: As shown in Chapter 4 on ratio-proportion, this proportion could also be stated in fraction format.

Important Points When Calculating Doses Using Ratio-Proportion

1. Make sure that all terms are in the same unit and system of measure before calculating. If they are not, a conversion will be necessary before calculating the dose. Conversions can be made by changing what is ordered to the units in which the medication is available or by changing what is available to the units in which the medication is ordered. Try to be consistent as to how you make conversions. It is usual to convert what is ordered to the same unit and system of measure you have available.
2. Before calculating the dose, make a mental estimate of the approximate and reasonable answer.
3. Set up the proportion, labeling all of the terms in the proportion. This includes x. State the known ratio first (what is available or on the drug label).
4. Make sure the terms of the ratios are stated in the same sequence.
5. Label the value you obtain for x (for example, mL, tabs).

Let's use ratio-proportion to solve some more problems.

Example 2: Doctor's order: 40 mg p.o. of a drug.

Available: 20 mg tablets

Solution: 20 mg : 1 tab = 40 mg : x tab

(known) (unknown)

$$\frac{20x}{20} = \frac{40}{20}$$

x = 2 tabs

Note: When setting up the ratios, follow the sequence in stating the terms for both.

For example, mg : tab = mg : tab

This proportion could also be stated as a fraction and solved by cross multiplication.

Known Unknown

$$\frac{20 \text{ mg}}{1 \text{ tab}} = \frac{40 \text{ mg}}{x \text{ tab}}$$

Here the known is stated as the first fraction and the unknown as the second.

Example 3: Doctor's order: 1 g p.o. of an antibiotic

Available: 500 mg capsules. How many capsules will you give?

Solution: Notice the dose ordered is a different unit from what is available. Proceed first by changing the units of measure so they are the same. As shown in Chapter 8, ratio-proportion can be used for conversion.

After making the conversion, set up the problem and calculate the dose to be given. In this example the conversion required is within the same system (metric).

In this example the g are converted to mg by using the equivalent 1000 mg = 1 g. After making the conversion of 1 g to 1000 mg, the ratio is stated as follows:

500 mg : 1 caps = 1000 mg : x caps

(known) (unknown)

x = 2 caps

An alternate method of solving might be to convert mg to g. In doing this, 500 mg would be converted to g using the same equivalent: 1000 mg = 1 g. However, decimals are common when measures are changed from smaller to larger in the metric system: 500 mg = 0.5 g. Even though converting the mg to g would net the same final answer, *conversions that net decimals are frequently the source of calculation errors.* Therefore, if possible, avoid conversions that require their use. As a rule, it is best to convert to the measure stated on the drug label. Doing this consistently can prevent confusion. As with the other examples, this proportion could be stated as a fraction as well.

For the purpose of learning to calculate doses using ratio-proportion, this chapter emphasizes the mathematics of the answer. Determining whether an answer is logical will be discussed in later chapters covering the calculation of doses by various routes.

Points to Remember

- When stating the ratios, the known ratio is stated first. The known ratio is what is available, on hand, or the information obtained from the drug label.
- The unknown ratio is stated second. The unknown ratio is the dose desired, or what the doctor has ordered.
- The terms of the ratios in a proportion must be written in the same sequence of measurement.
- Label all terms of the ratios in the proportion including x.
- When conversion of units is required, it is usually easier to convert to the unit of measure on the drug label, or what the medication is available in.
- Estimate the answer.
- Label all answers obtained.
- A proportion may be stated in horizontal fashion or as a fraction.
- Double check all work.
- Be consistent in how ratios are stated and conversions are done.

Practice Problems (pp. 338-342)

Answer the following problems by indicating whether you need less than 1 tab or more than 1 tab.

1. A client is to receive gr 1/300 of a drug. The tablets available are gr 1/150. How many tablets do you need? ______________
2. A client is to receive gr 1/15 of a drug. The tablets available are gr 1/30. How many tablets do you need? ______________
3. A client is to receive gr 1/8 of a drug. The tablets available are gr 1/4. How many tablets do you need? ______________
4. A client is to receive gr 1/2 of a drug. The tablets available are gr 1/4. How many tablets do you need? ______________
5. A client is to receive gr 1/6 of a drug. The tablets available are gr 1/8. How many tablets do you need? ______________

Solve the following problems using ratio-proportion calculations. Express your answer to the nearest tenth where indicated, and include the units of measure in the answer.

6. The doctor orders 7.5 mg p.o. of a drug.

   Available: Tablets labeled 5 mg. ______________

7. The doctor orders gr 1/4 p.o. of a drug.

   Available: Tablets labeled 15 mg. ______________

8. The doctor orders gr $\overline{\text{iss}}$ p.o. of a drug.

   Available: Capsules labeled 100 mg. ______________

9. The doctor orders 0.25 mg I.M. of a drug.

   Available: 0.5 mg per cc. _______________

10. The doctor orders gr 1/4 I.M. of a drug.

    Available: gr 3/4 per cc. _______________

11. The doctor orders potassium chloride 20 mEq I.V.

    Available: Potassium chloride 40 mEq per 10 cc. _______________

12. The doctor orders 5,000 U s.c. of a drug.

    Available: 10,000 U per cc. _______________

13. The doctor orders 50 mg I.M. of a drug.

    Available: 80 mg per 2 cc. _______________

14. The doctor orders 0.5 g p.o. of an antibiotic.

    Available: Capsules labeled 250 mg. _______________

15. The doctor orders 400 mg p.o. of a liquid medication.

    Available: 125 mg per 5 cc. _______________

16. The doctor orders 50 mg I.M. of a drug.

    Available: 80 mg per mL. _______________

17. The doctor orders gr i of a drug.

    Available: gr$\overline{\text{ss}}$ per mL. _______________

18. The doctor orders gr xv of a drug.

    Available: Tablets labeled gr v. _______________

19. The doctor orders gr 1/300 of a drug.

    Available: Tablets labeled gr 1/150. _______________

20. The doctor orders gr 1/6 of a drug.

    Available: gr 1/4 per mL. _______________

21. The doctor orders 0.125 mg of a drug.

    Available: 0.5 mg per 2 mL. _______________

22. The doctor orders 0.75 mg of a drug.

    Available: 0.25 mg per mL. _______________

23. The doctor orders 375 mg of a drug.

    Available: 125 mg per 5 mL. __________

24. The doctor orders 10,000 U of a drug.

    Available: 7,500 U per mL. __________

25. The doctor orders 0.45 mg of a drug.

    Available: Tablets labeled 0.3 mg. __________

Chapter Review (p. 342)

Part I

Directions: Read the medication labels where available, and calculate the tablets or capsules necessary to provide the dose ordered. Include the unit of measure in your answer.

1. Doctor's Order: gr 1/4 p.o. of phenobarbital t.i.d.

   Available: Tablets labeled 15 mg. __________

2. Doctor's Order: Ampicillin 0.25 g p.o. q.i.d. __________

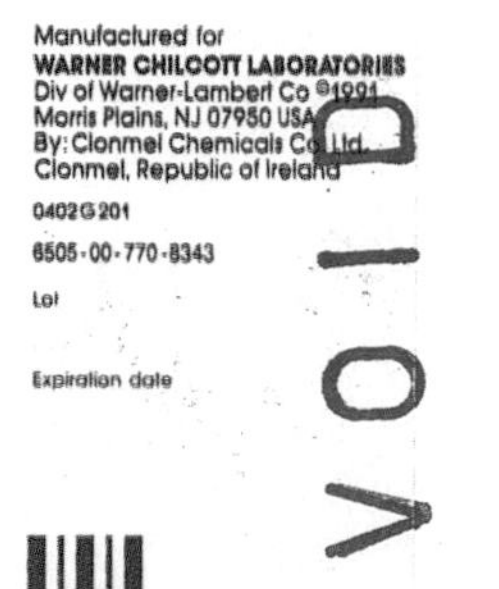

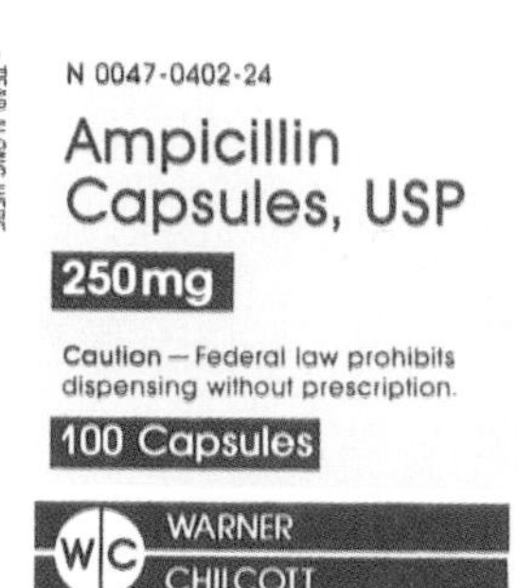

3. Doctor's Order: Ampicillin 1 g p.o. q6h. __________

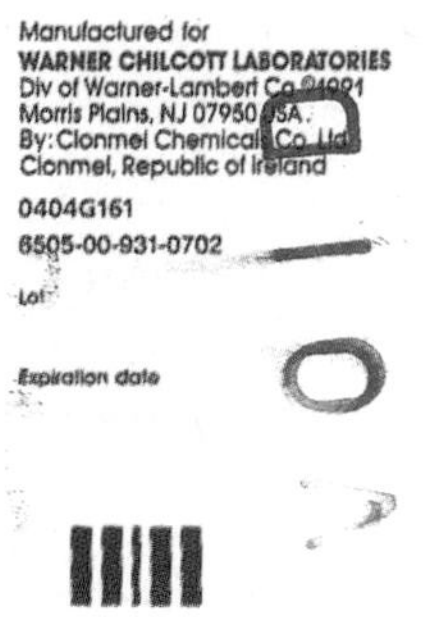

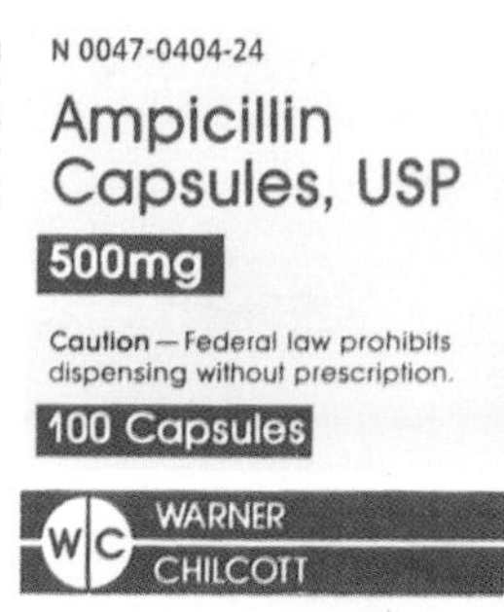

4. Doctor's Order: Phenobarbital 60 mg p.o. h.s.

   Available: Tablets labeled 30 mg. __________

5. Doctor's Order: Baclofen 20 mg p.o. t.i.d. ______________

NDC 0028-0023-61 FSC 2503
Lioresal® 10mg
baclofen
100 tablets–Unit Dose
Caution: Federal law prohibits dispensing without prescription.
Geigy

6. Doctor's Order: Isosorbide dinitrate 20 mg p.o. t.i.d.

   Available: Tablets labeled 40 mg. ______________

7. Doctor's Order: Dexamethasone 4 mg p.o. q6h. ______________

NDC 0054-8175-25
4 mg
10 x 10 Tablets
DEXAMETHASONE
Tablets USP

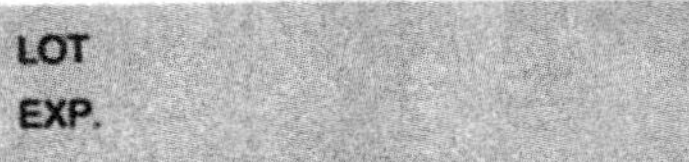

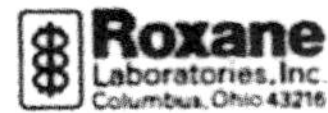

4238001 091

8. Doctor's Order: Diabinese 250 mg p.o. q.d. ______________

NDC 0663-3940-71
250 Tablets
Diabinese®
chlorpropamide
250 mg
CAUTION: Federal law prohibits dispensing without prescription.
6505-00-817-2279
Pfizer Distributed by LABORATORIES DIVISION
New York, N.Y. 10017

9. Doctor's Order: Digoxin 125 mcg p.o. q.d. ______________

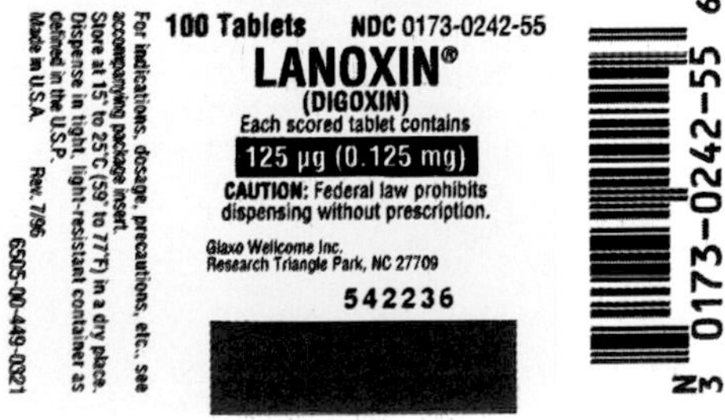

N 3 0173-0242-55 6

10. Doctor's Order: Synthroid 0.05 mg p.o. q.d. ______________

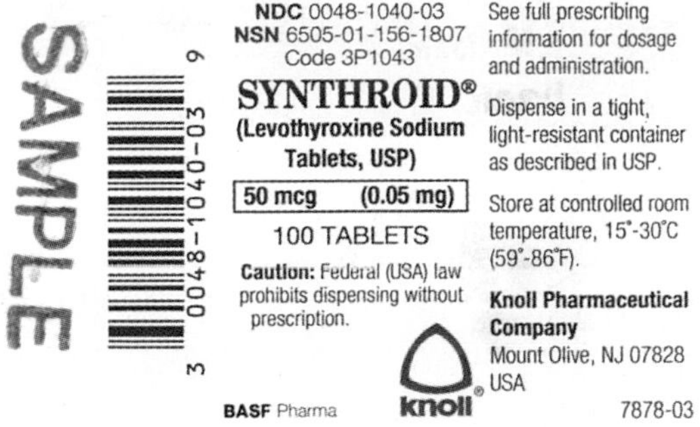

11. Doctor's Order: Restoril 30 mg p.o. h.s. p.r.n. ______________

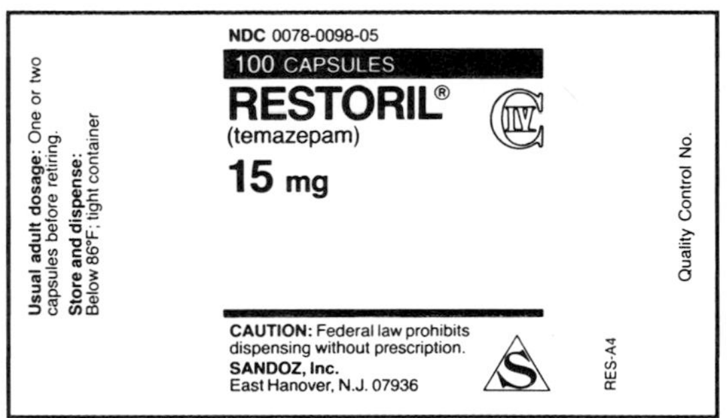

12. Doctor's Order: Phenobarbital gr i p.o. h.s. ______________

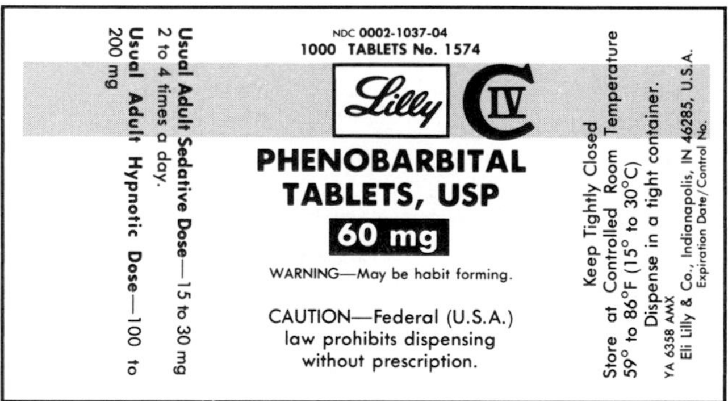

13. Doctor's Order: Macrodantin 100 mg p.o. t.i.d. ______________

Macrodantin
50 mg
100 capsules

14. Doctor's Order: Keflex 0.5 g p.o. q.i.d. ______________

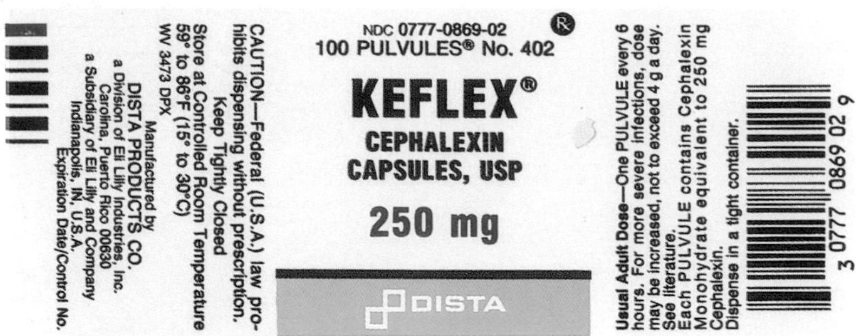

15. Doctor's Order: Cogentin 2 mg p.o. b.i.d. ______________

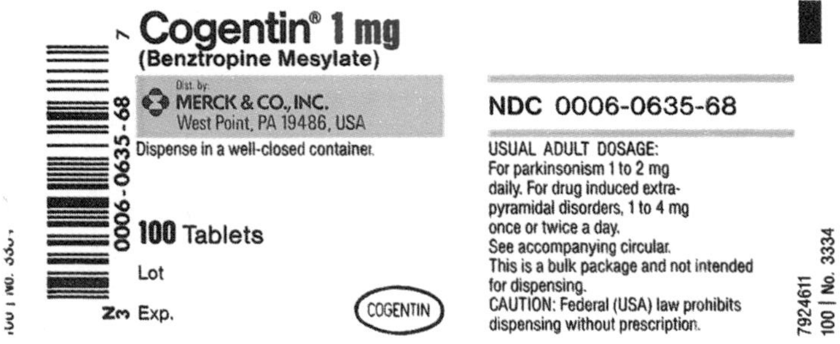

16. Doctor's Order: Augmentin 0.5 g p.o. q8h. ______________

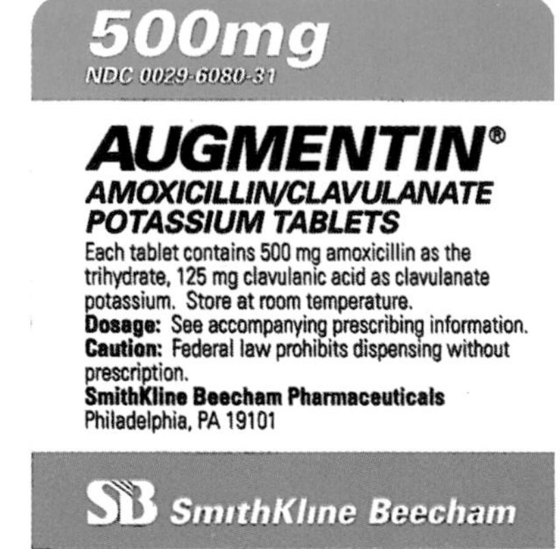

17. Doctor's Order: Zovirax 400 mg p.o. b.i.d. × 7 days. ______________

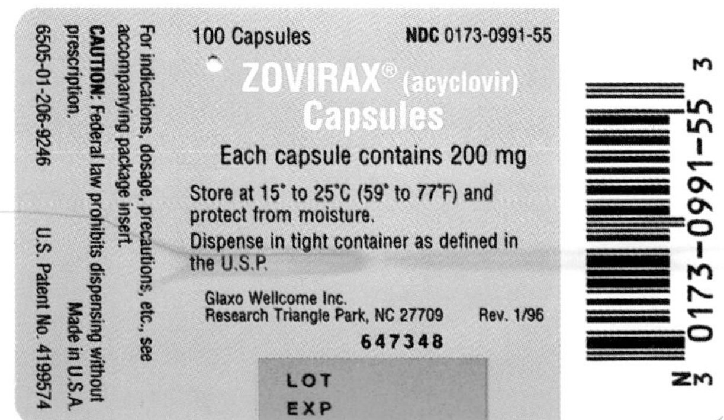

18. Doctor's Order: Rifampin 0.6 g p.o. o.d. _______________

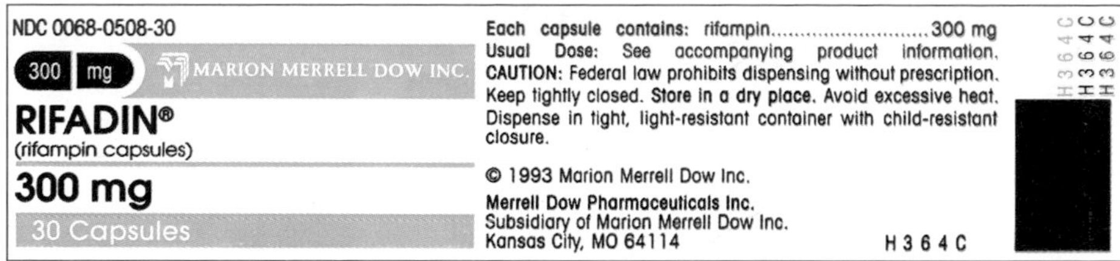

19. Doctor's Order: Carafate 1000 mg p.o. b.i.d. _______________

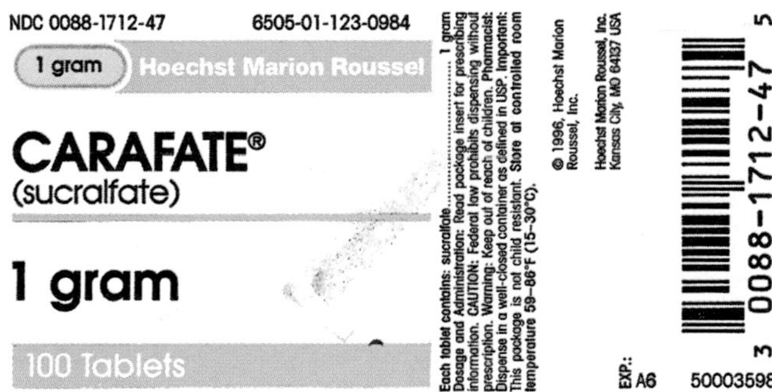

20. Doctor's Order: Cardizem 240 mg p.o. daily. _______________

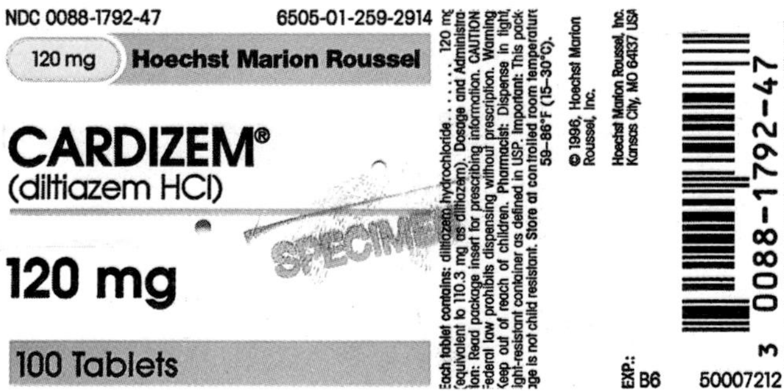

21. Doctor's Order: Xanax 0.25 mg p.o. b.i.d. _______________

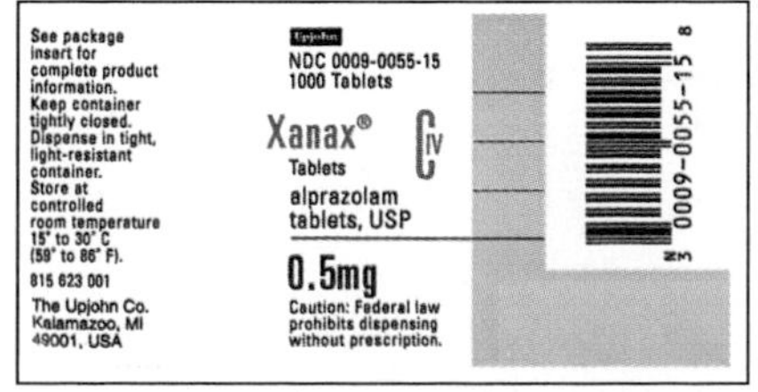

22. Doctor's Order: Septra DS 1 tab p.o. 3 × a week. ______________

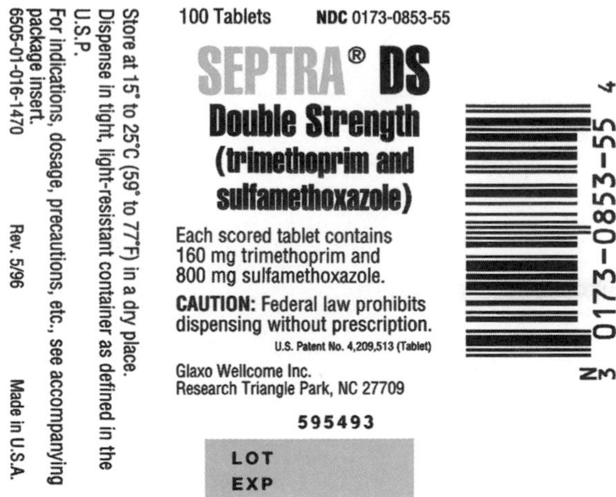

23. Doctor's Order: Sinemet 25-100 2 tabs p.o. t.i.d. ______________

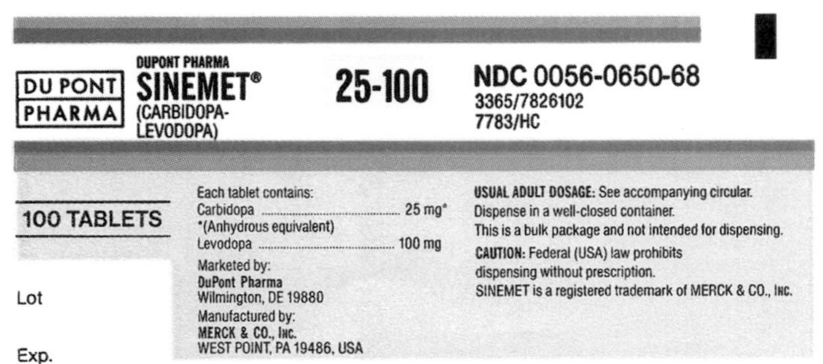

24. Doctor's Order: Retrovir 0.2 g p.o. t.i.d. ______________

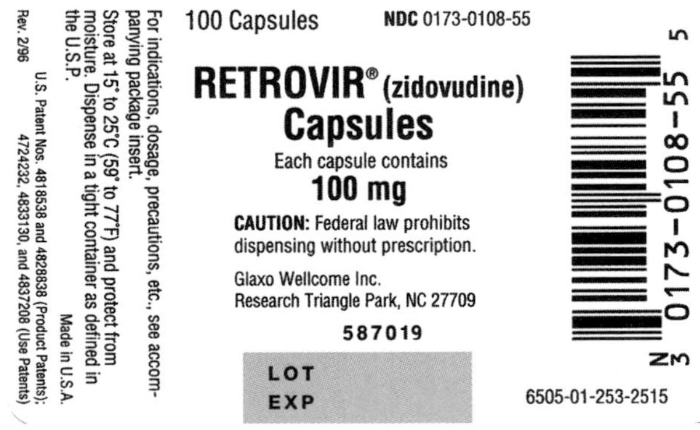

25. Doctor's Order: Lanoxicaps 0.05 mg p.o. q.o.d. ____________

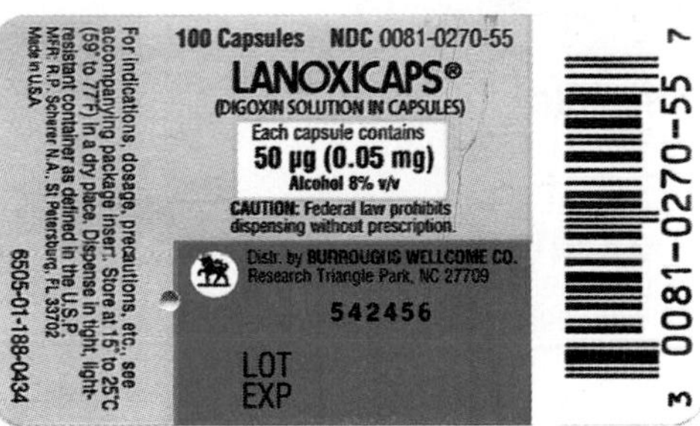

26. Doctor's Order: Risperdal 3 mg p.o. b.i.d.

    Available: Scored tablets labeled 1 mg. ____________

27. Doctor's Order: Flagyl 0.5g p.o. q8h.

    Available: Flagyl tablets labeled 500 mg. ____________

Part II

Directions: Read the medication labels where available, and calculate the volume necessary (in mL) to provide the dose ordered. Express your answer as a decimal fraction to the nearest tenth where indicated.

28. Doctor's Order: Dilantin 100 mg via gastrostomy tube t.i.d.

    Available: Dilantin 125 mg per 5 mL. ____________

29. Doctor's Order: Benadryl 50 mg p.o. h.s. ____________

Benadryl Elixir
4 Fluid Ounces
Available: 12.5 mg per 5 mL

30. Doctor's Order: Gentamicin 50 mg I.M. q8h. ____________

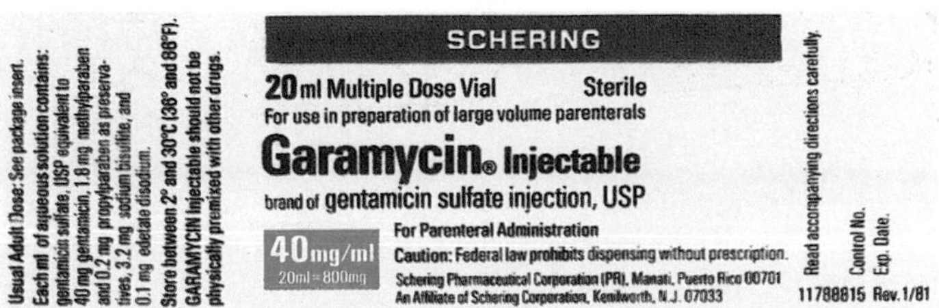

31. Doctor's Order: Vibramycin 100 mg p.o. q12h.

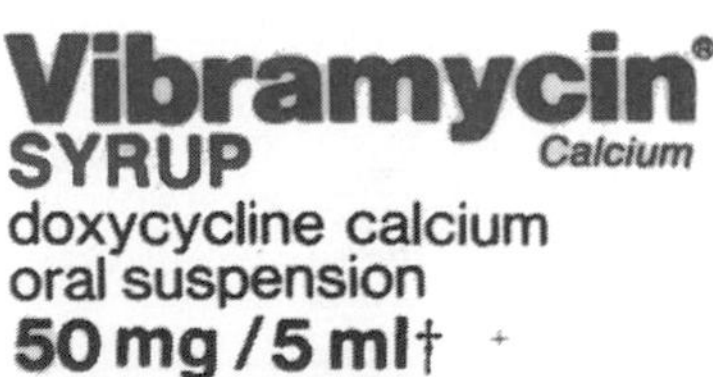

1 PINT (473 ml)
†Each teaspoonful (5 ml) contains doxycycline calcium equivalent to 50 mg of doxycycline.
USUAL DOSAGE:
Adults: 200 mg on the first day (100 mg every 12 hours) followed by a maintenance dose of 100 mg a day.
Children above eight years of age: Under 100 lbs.—2 mg/lb. of body weight daily divided in two doses on the first day, followed by 1 mg/lb. of body weight on subsequent days in one or two doses. Over 100 lbs.—See adult dosage.
doxycycline U.S. Pat. No. 3,200,149
READ ACCOMPANYING PROFESSIONAL INFORMATION
RECOMMENDED STORAGE
STORE BELOW 86°F. (30°C.)
Dispense in tight, light resistant containers (USP).
CAUTION: Federal law prohibits dispensing without prescription.
Pfizer LABORATORIES DIVISION
PFIZER INC.,
NEW YORK, N.Y. 10017
MADE IN U.S.A. 2

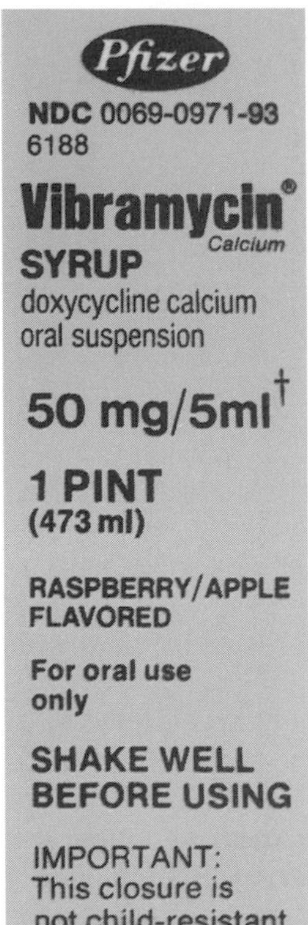

32. Doctor's Order: Meperidine hydrochloride 50 mg I.M. q4h p.r.n. for pain.

Available: Meperidine 75 mg/mL. __________

33. Doctor's Order: Gentamicin 90 mg I.V. q8h.

Available: Gentamicin 40 mg/mL. __________

34. Doctor's Order: Morphine gr 1/4 s.c. q4h p.r.n. __________

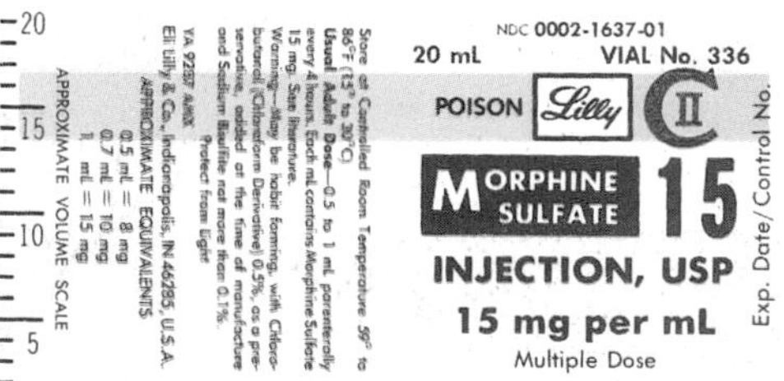

35. Doctor's Order: Vitamin B_{12} 1000 mcg I.M. once monthly. __________

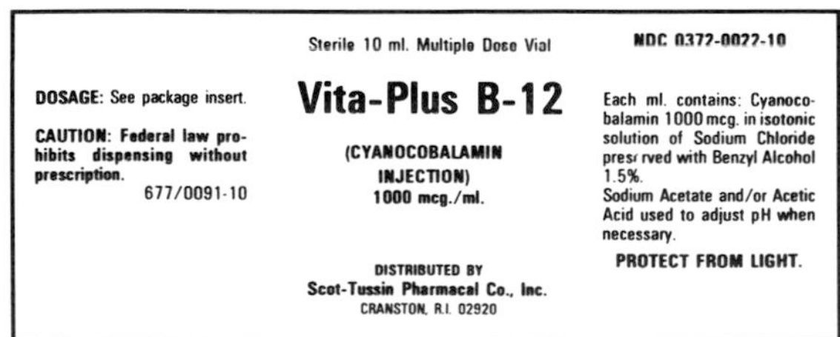

36. Doctor's Order: Morphine 10 mg s.c. stat. Express answer in hundredths.

    Available: Morphine 15 mg/mL. ______________

37. Doctor's Order: Kaon-Cl 20 mEq p.o. o.d.

    Available: Kaon-Cl 40 mEq/15 mL. ______________

38. Doctor's Order: Nystatin oral suspension 100,000 U swish and swallow q6h.

    Available: Nystatin oral suspension labeled 100,000 U per/mL. ______________

39. Doctor's Order: Heparin 5,000 U s.c. o.d. ______________

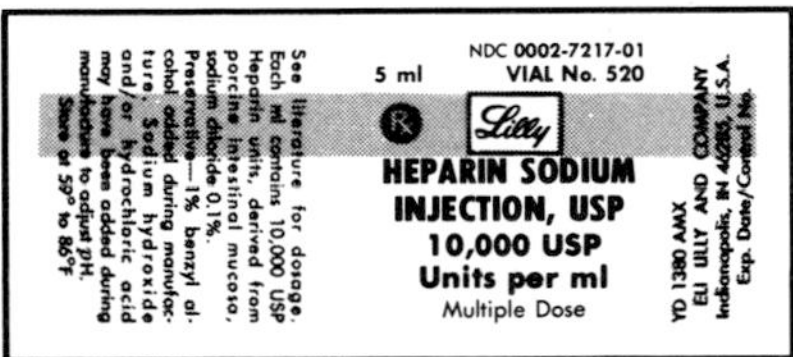

40. Doctor's Order: Atropine 0.2 mg s.c. stat. ______________

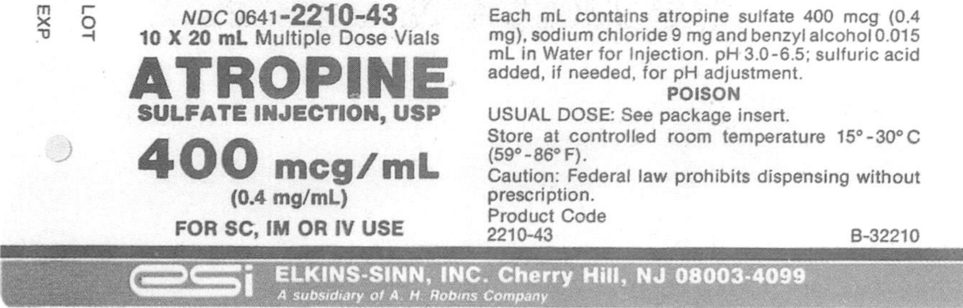

41. Doctor's Order: Amoxicillin 500 mg p.o. q6h × 7 days. ______________

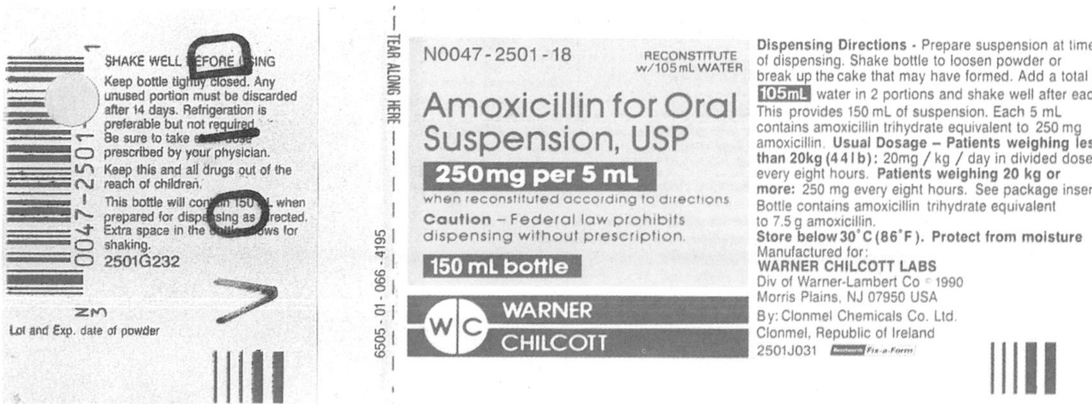

42. Doctor's Order: Heparin 7,500 U s.c. o.d. Express answer in hundredths.

    Available: Heparin 10,000 U/mL. ______________

43. Doctor's Order: Solu-Medrol 70 mg I.V. o.d. ______________

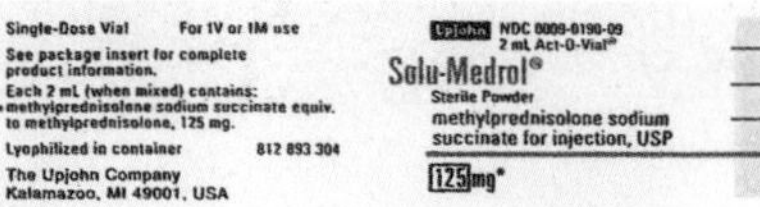

44. Doctor's Order: Ativan 2 mg I.M. q4h p.r.n. agitation. ______________

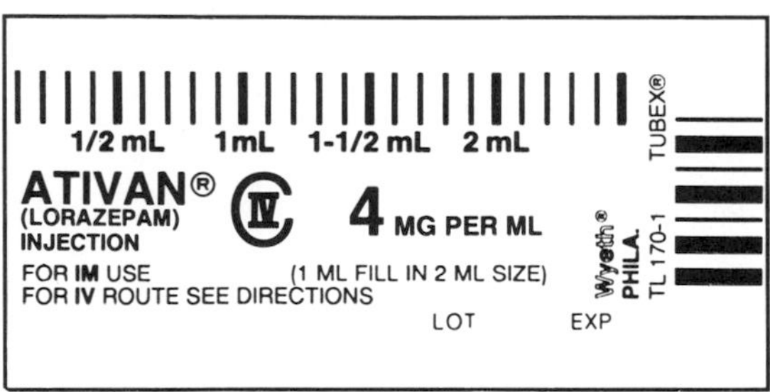

45. Doctor's Order: Vistaril 25 mg I.M. on call to operating room (OR). ______________

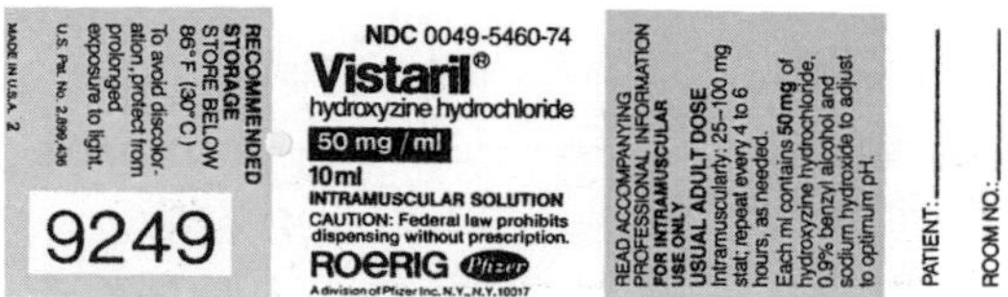

46. Doctor's Order: Phenobarbital gr $\overline{\text{iss}}$ I.M. stat. ______________

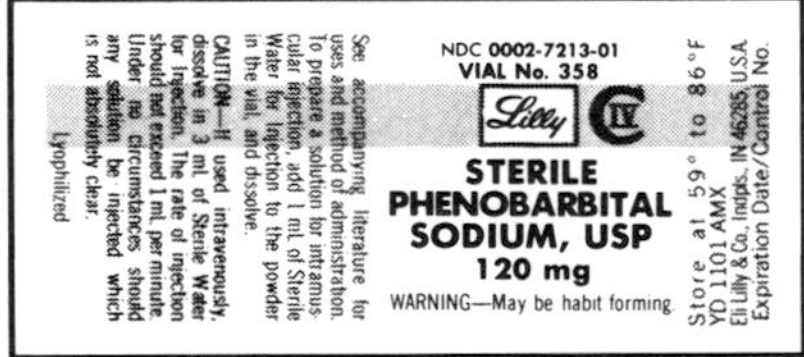

47. Doctor's Order: Aminophylline 100 mg I.V. q6h. ______________

Aminophylline Injection, USP
500 mg/20 mL
(25 mg/mL)

48. Doctor's Order: Zantac 150 mg I.V. q.d. ______________

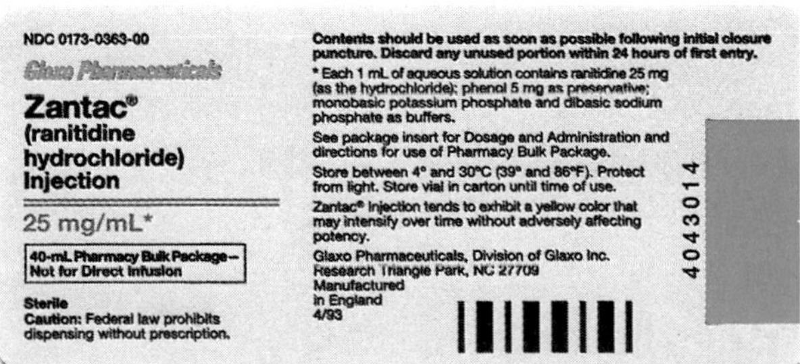

49. Doctor's Order: Augmentin 0.5 g p.o. q8h. ______________

AUGMENTIN®

400mg/5mL
NDC 0029-6092-39

Tear along perforation

Directions for mixing: Tap bottle until all powder flows freely. Add approximately 2/3 of total water for reconstitution (total = 66 mL); shake vigorously to wet powder. Add remaining water; again shake vigorously.
Dosage: Administer every 12 hours. See accompanying prescribing information.
Phenylketonurics: Contains phenylalanine 7 mg per 5 mL.

Tear along perforation

Keep tightly closed.
Shake well before using.
Must be refrigerated.
Discard after 10 days.

AUGMENTIN®
AMOXICILLIN/
CLAVULANATE
POTASSIUM
FOR ORAL SUSPENSION

When reconstituted, each 5 mL contains:
AMOXICILLIN, 400 MG,
as the trihydrate
CLAVULANIC ACID, 57 MG,
as clavulanate potassium

75mL (when reconstituted)

SB SmithKline Beecham

Use only if inner seal is intact.
Net contents: Equivalent to 6 g amoxicillin and 0.855 g clavulanic acid.
Store dry powder at or below 25°C (77°F).
Caution: Federal law prohibits dispensing without prescription.
SmithKline Beecham Pharmaceuticals
Philadelphia, PA 19101

EXP.

LOT

3 0029-6092-39 1

9405817-A

50. Doctor's Order: Thorazine concentrate 75 mg p.o. q.d. ______________

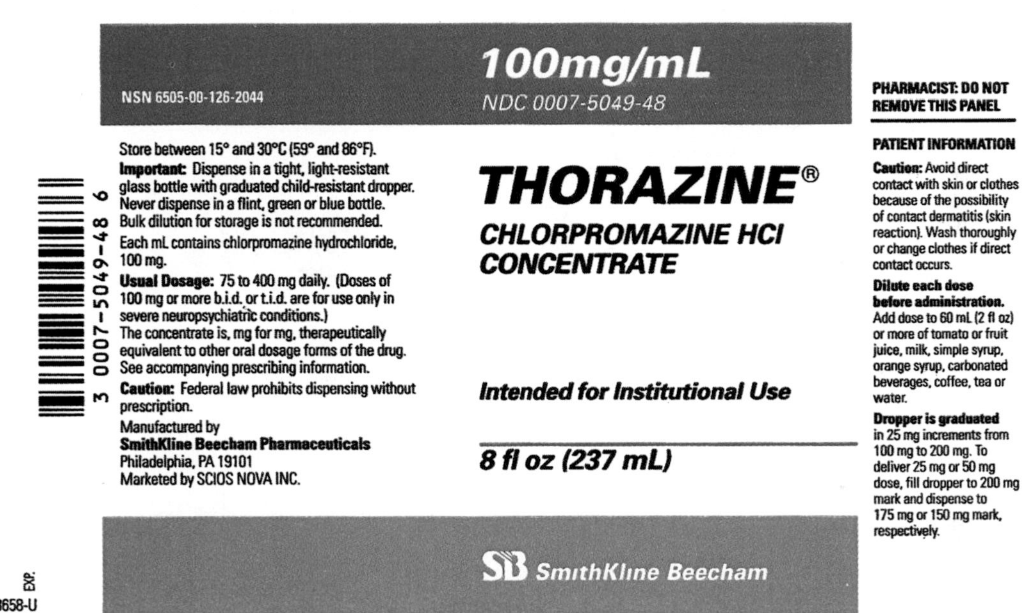

51. Doctor's Order: Retrovir 200 mg via nasogastric tube t.i.d. ______________

240 mL **NDC** 0173-0113-18

RETROVIR®
(zidovudine)
Syrup

Each 5 mL (1 teaspoonful) contains zidovudine 50 mg and sodium benzoate 0.2% added as a preservative.

CAUTION: Federal law prohibits dispensing without prescription.

U.S. Patent Nos. 4818538 (Product Patent); 4724232, 4833130, and 4837208 (Use Patents)

For indications, dosage, precautions, etc., see accompanying package insert.
Store at 15° to 25°C (59° to 77°F).

Made in U.S.A. Rev. 5/96 587023

GlaxoWellcome
Glaxo Wellcome Inc.
Research Triangle Park, NC 27709

LOT
EXP

52. Doctor's Order: Epivir 0.3 g p.o. b.i.d. ____________

NDC 0173-0471-00

GlaxoWellcome

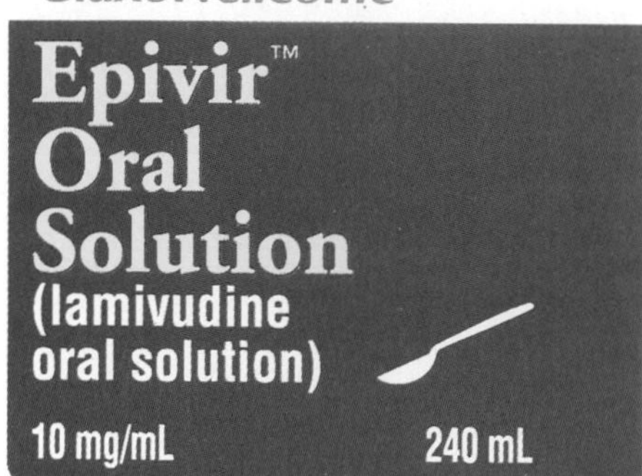

Caution: Federal law prohibits dispensing without prescription.

See package insert for Dosage and Administration.

Store between 2° and 25°C (36° and 77°F) in tightly closed bottles. Contains 6% alcohol.

4 05889 5

Glaxo Wellcome Inc.
Research Triangle Park,
NC 27709
Manufactured in England
under agreement from
BioChem Pharma Inc.
Laval, Quebec, Canada
Rev. 10/95

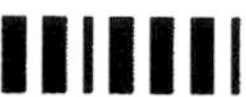

53. Doctor's Order: Cipro 0.4 g I.V. q12h. ____________

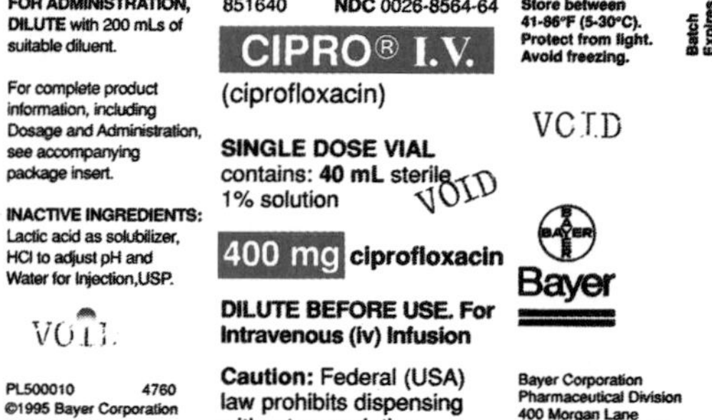

54. Doctor's Order: Prozac 40 mg p.o. q.d. ____________

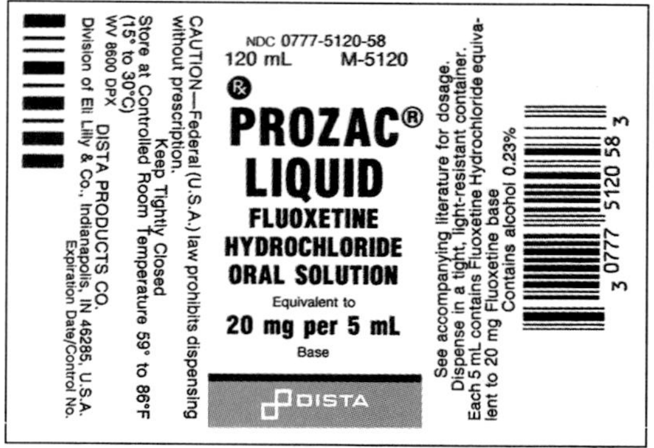

55. Doctor's Order: Depo-Provera 0.4 g I.M. once a week. ____________

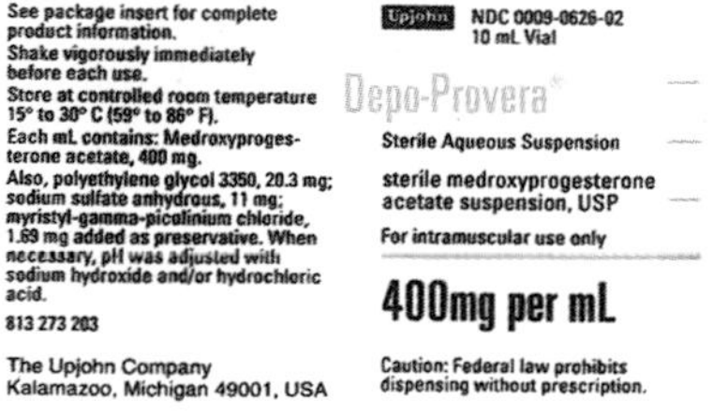

Chapter 14

Dose Calculation Using the Formula Method

Objectives

After reviewing this chapter the student will be able to do the following:

1. Identify the information from a calculation problem to place into the formulas given
2. Solve problems using the stated formula

This chapter shows how to use a formula for dose calculation, which requires substituting information from the problem into the formula. There are two formulas that may be used to calculate doses. **The nurse should choose a formula and consistently use it in its entirety to avoid calculation errors.**

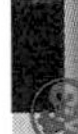

Think Critically to Avoid Drug Calculation Errors

Do not rely solely on formulas when calculating doses to be administered. Use critical thinking skills such as considering what the answer should be, reasoning, problem solving, and finding rational justification for your answer. Formulas should be used as a tool for validating the dose you THINK should be given.

Formulas for Calculating Doses

The formulas presented in this chapter can be used when calculating doses in the same system or after converting when the dose desired and the dose on hand are in different systems. We can write the first formula as

$$\frac{D}{H} \times Q = x$$

where

D = The dose desired, or what the doctor has ordered, including the weights—for example, 5 mg, gr 1/2, 1 g.

H = The dose strength that is available, what is on hand, or the weight of the drug on the label, including the weights—for example, 25 mg, gr 1, 10 g.

Q = The quantity or the unit of measure that contains the dose that is available. When solving problems that involve solid forms of medication (tabs, caps), Q is always 1 and can be eliminated from the equation. **For consistency and to avoid chances of error when Q is not 1, always include Q even with tablet and capsule problems.** When solving problems for medications in solution, the amount for Q varies and must always be included.

x = The unknown, the dose you are looking for, the dosage you are going to administer, how many mL, tab, etc. you will give.

The second formula (Copyright Research Foundation, New York) is a ratio-proportion; the terms in the proportion are labeled differently and set up as a fraction. We can write it as

$$\frac{DW}{SW} = \frac{DV}{SV}$$

where:

DW = Dose weight—The dose desired, or what the doctor has ordered, including the weights—for example, 5 mg, 0.5 g.

SW = Stock weight—The dose strength that is available, what is on hand, or the weight of the drug on the label, including the weights—for example, gr 5, 1 g.

DV = Dose volume—The unknown, the dose you are looking for, the dose you are going to administer—x is used to represent this value. The number of mL, tab, caps, etc. of x is always labeled.

SV = Stock volume—The quantity or unit of measure that contains the dose that is available. For solid forms of medication (tabs, caps) the SV is always 1 (for example, 1 tab, 1 caps). For medications in solution the amount for SV varies. To avoid errors in calculation always include the SV even if the value is 1.

Steps for Use of the Formulas

Either of the formulas presented may be used to calculate a dose to administer. The nurse should choose a formula and use it consistently. Regardless of which formula is used, remember the steps for using the formula (see box below).

Now we will look at sample problems illustrating the use of the formulas for calculation that have been presented.

Example 1: The doctor orders 0.375 mg p.o. of a drug. The tablets available are 0.25 mg.

Solution: The dose 0.375 mg is desired, the dose strength available is 0.25 mg per tablet. No conversion is necessary. What is desired is in the same system and unit of measure as what you have on hand.

Formula Setup

$$\frac{D}{H} \times Q = x$$

The desired (D) is 0.375 mg. You have on hand (H) 0.25 mg per (Q) 1 tablet. The label on x is tablet. Notice the label on x is always the same as Q.

$$\frac{(D)\ 0.375\ mg}{(H)\ 0.25\ mg} \times (Q)\ 1\ tab = x\ tab$$

$$\frac{0.375}{0.25} \times 1 = x$$

OR

$$\frac{DW}{SW} = \frac{DV}{SV}$$

The desired (DW) is 0.375 mg. You have on hand (SW) 0.25 mg per (SV) 1 tablet. The label on x is tablet (DV). Notice the label on x is always the same as SV.

$$\frac{(DW)\ 0.375\ mg}{(SW)\ 0.25\ mg} = \frac{(DV)\ x\ tab}{(SV)\ 1\ tab}$$

$$0.25 \times (x) = 0.375 \times 1$$

$$\frac{0.25\ x}{0.25} = \frac{0.375}{0.25} \qquad \frac{0.375}{0.25} = x$$

Therefore, x = 1.5 tabs, or 1 1/2 tabs. (Because 0.375 mg is larger than 0.25 mg, you will need more than 1 tab to administer 0.375 mg.) Note: Although 1.5 tabs is the same as 1 1/2 tabs, in terms of administration it would be best to state it as 1 1/2 tabs.

Steps for Using a Formula

1. Memorize the formula.
2. Place the information from the problem into the formula in the correct position.
3. Make sure all measures are in the same units and system of measure or a conversion must be done *before* calculating the dose.
4. Think logically and consider what a reasonable amount would be to administer.
5. Calculate your answer.
6. Label all answers—tabs, caps, mL, etc.

Example 2: The doctor orders 7,000 U s.c. of a drug. The drug is available 10,000 U in 2 mL.

Solution:

$$\frac{\text{(D) } 7{,}000 \text{ U}}{\text{(H) } 10{,}000 \text{ U}} \times \text{(Q) } 2 \text{ mL} = x \text{ mL}$$

$$\frac{7{,}000}{10{,}000} \times 2 = x$$

$$\frac{14{,}000}{10{,}000} = x$$

Note: Omitting Q here could result in an error. A liquid medication is involved; Q must be included.

OR

$$\frac{\text{(DW) } 7{,}000 \text{ U}}{\text{(SW) } 10{,}000 \text{ U}} = \frac{\text{(DV) } x \text{ mL}}{\text{(SV) } 2 \text{ mL}}$$

$$10{,}000 \times (x) = 7{,}000 \times 2$$

$$\frac{10{,}000}{10{,}000}x = \frac{14{,}000}{10{,}000} \qquad \frac{14{,}000}{10{,}000} = x$$

Note: SV here is 2 mL and is important to include since with liquid medications this can vary.

Therefore, $x = 1.4$ mL. (Because 7,000 U × 2 is more than 10,000 U, it will take more than 1 mL to administer the dose.)

Example 3: The doctor orders gr 1/2 p.o. Available are tablets labeled 15 mg. Note: What is desired and what is available must be in the *same units and system of measure*. Remember it is usual to convert what is desired to what is available. Therefore change gr to mg; this will also eliminate the fraction and decrease the chance of error in calculation.

Rule for Different Units or Systems of Measure

Whenever the desired amount and the dose on hand are in different units or systems of measure, follow these steps:

1. Choose the identified equivalent.
2. Convert what is ordered to the same units or system of measure as what is available on hand by using one of the methods presented in the chapter on converting.
3. Use the formula $\frac{D}{H} \times Q = x$ or $\frac{DW}{SW} = \frac{DV}{SV}$ to calculate the dose to administer.

Solution: Convert gr 1/2 to mg. The equivalent to use is 60 mg = gr 1. Therefore gr 1/2 = 30 mg.

Now that you have everything in the same system and units of measure, use either formula presented to calculate the dose to be administered.

Solution:

$$\frac{\text{(D) } 30 \text{ mg}}{\text{(H) } 15 \text{ mg}} \times \text{(Q) } 1 \text{ tab} = x \text{ tab}$$

$$\frac{30}{15} \times 1 = x \qquad \frac{30}{15} = x$$

OR

$$\frac{\text{(DW) } 30 \text{ mg}}{\text{(SW) } 15 \text{ mg}} = \frac{\text{(DV) } x \text{ tab}}{\text{(SV) } 1 \text{ tab}}$$

$$15 \times (x) = 30 \times 1$$

$$\frac{15x}{15} = \frac{30}{15} \qquad \frac{30}{15} = x$$

Therefore, $x = 2$ tabs. (Because 30 mg is a larger dose than 15 mg, it will take more than 1 tab to administer the desired dose.)

Example 4: The doctor orders gr 1/6 of a drug. The drug is available gr 1/2 per mL.

Solution:

$$\frac{\text{(D) gr } \frac{1}{6}}{\text{(H) gr } \frac{1}{2}} \times \text{(Q) } 1 \text{ mL} = x \text{ mL}$$

$$\frac{1}{6} \div \frac{1}{2} = x \qquad \frac{1}{6} \times \frac{2}{1} = \frac{2}{6} = \frac{1}{3} \qquad \frac{1}{3} = x$$

OR

$$\frac{\text{(DW) gr } \frac{1}{6}}{\text{(SW) gr } \frac{1}{2}} = \frac{\text{(DV) } x \text{ mL}}{\text{(SV) } 1 \text{ mL}}$$

$$\frac{1}{2} \times (x) = \frac{1}{6} \times 1 \qquad \frac{\frac{1}{2}}{\frac{1}{2}}x = \frac{\frac{1}{6}}{\frac{1}{2}} \qquad \frac{1}{6} \div \frac{1}{2} = x$$

$$\frac{1}{6} \times \frac{2}{1} = \frac{2}{6} = \frac{1}{3} \qquad \frac{1}{3} = x$$

Therefore, $x = 0.33$ mL = 0.3 mL, 0.3 cc. (Because 1/2 is a larger dose than 1/6, it will take less than 1 cc to administer the required dose.)

Points to Remember

- The formula $\frac{D}{H} \times Q = x$ or $\frac{DW}{SW} = \frac{DV}{SV}$ can be used to calculate the dose to be administered.
- The Q and SV are always 1 for solid forms of medications (tabs, caps, etc.) but vary when a solution is being used.
- Always set up the formula with the units of measure included.
- Before the dose to be given is calculated, the dose desired must be in the same units and system of measure as the dose available or a conversion is necessary.
- Double check all of your math and think logically about the answer obtained.
- Label all answers obtained.

Chapter Review (pp. 343-345)

Calculate the following problems using one of the formulas presented in this chapter.

1. The doctor orders gr 1/150 p.o.

   Available: Tablets labeled gr 1/300. ____________

2. The doctor orders 0.75 g p.o.

   Available: Capsules labeled 250 mg. ____________

3. The doctor orders 90 mg p.o.

   Available: Tablets labeled 60 mg. ____________

4. The doctor orders 7.5 mg p.o.

   Available: Tablets labeled 2.5 mg. ____________

5. The doctor orders 0.05 mg p.o.

   Available: Tablets labeled 25 mcg. ____________

Calculate the following problems in mL; round to the nearest tenth where indicated.

6. The doctor orders 40 mg I.M.

   Available: 80 mg per 2 mL. ____________

7. The doctor orders 4,500 U s.c.

   Available: 5,000 U per mL. ____________

8. The doctor orders gr 1/200 I.M.

   Available: 0.3 mg per mL. ____________

9. The doctor orders 0.75 mg I.M.

   Available: 0.25 mg per mL. ____________

10. The doctor orders gr 1/6 s.c.

    Available: 15 mg per mL. ______________

Calculate the following doses, using the medication label or information provided. Express answers in mL; round to the nearest tenth where indicated.

11. Doctor's Order: Phenobarbital gr ss p.o. t.i.d. ______________

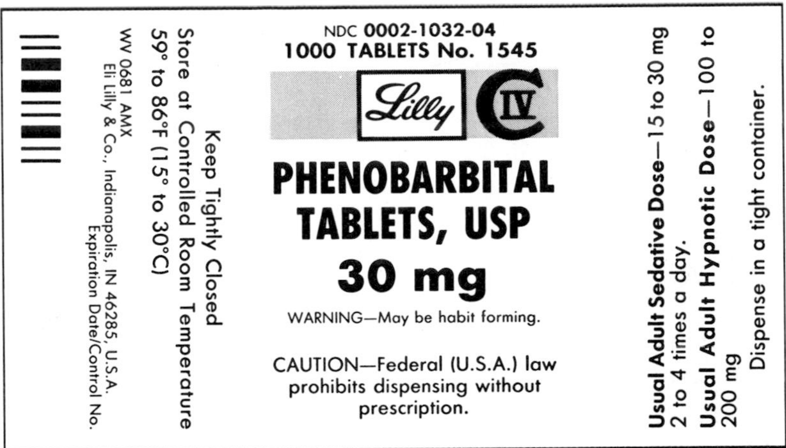

12. Doctor's Order: Gantrisin 500 mg p.o. q.i.d. ______________

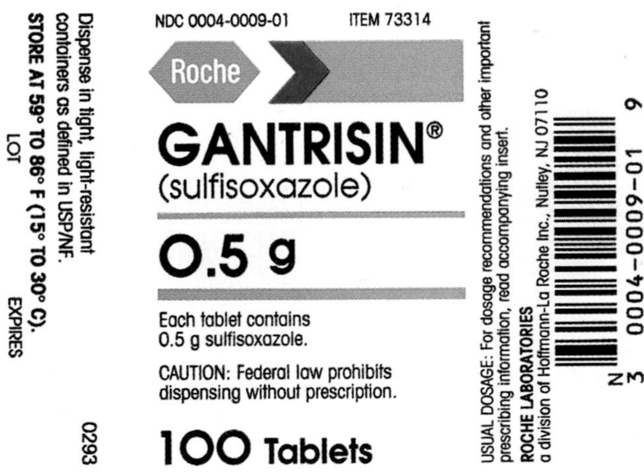

13. Doctor's Order: Indocin 50 mg p.o. t.i.d. ______________

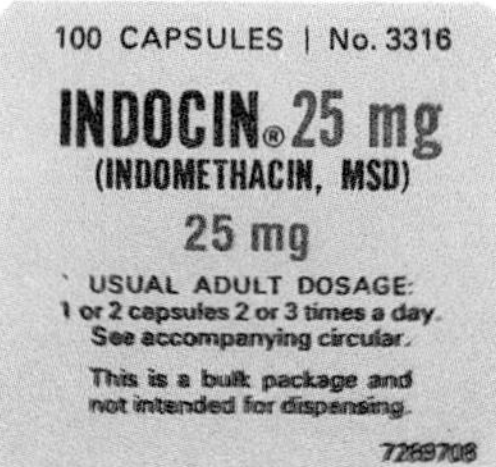

14. Doctor's Order: Hydrochlorothiazide 50 mg p.o. b.i.d. ______________

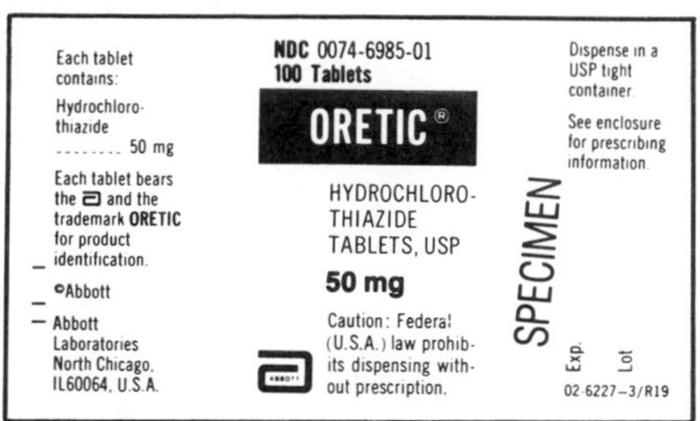

15. Doctor's Order: Aspirin gr x p.o. q4h p.r.n. for pain. ______________

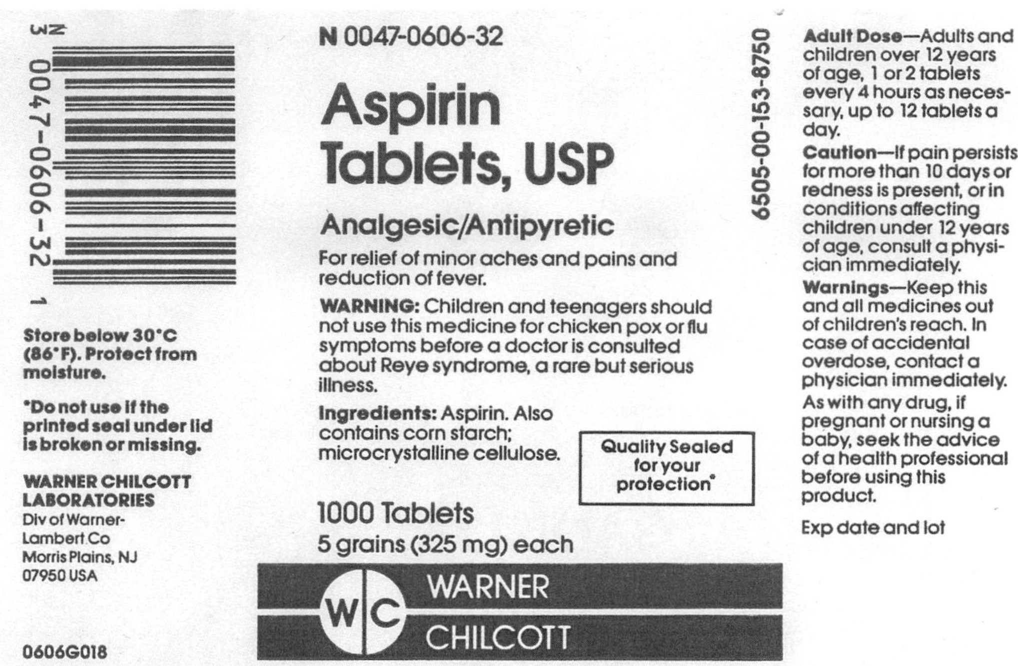

16. Doctor's Order: Digoxin 0.375 mg p.o. o.d.

Available: Lanoxin 250 mcg (0.25 mg) per tab. ______________

17. Doctor's Order: Keflex 0.25 g p.o. q6h. ______________

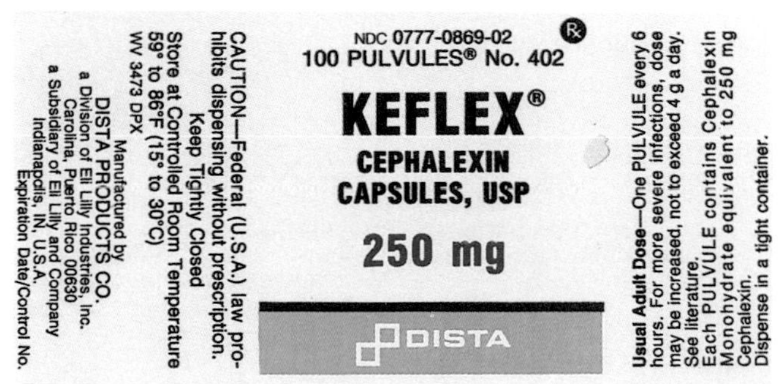

18. Doctor's Order: Seconal 100 mg p.o. h.s. __________

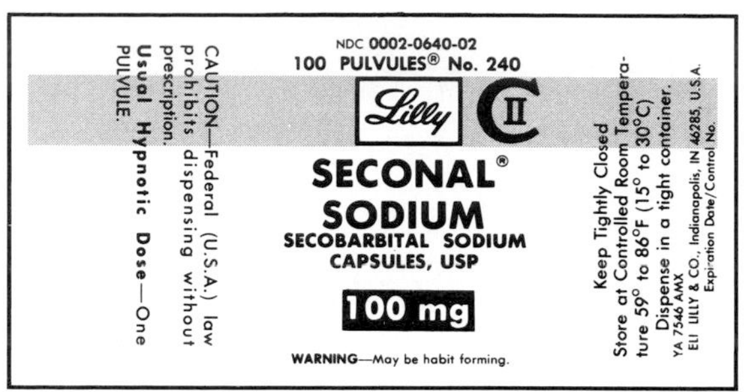

19. Doctor's Order: Minipress 2 mg p.o. b.i.d. × 2 days.

    Available: Minipress 1 mg caps. __________

20. Doctor's Order: Crystodigin 0.2 mg p.o. o.d. __________

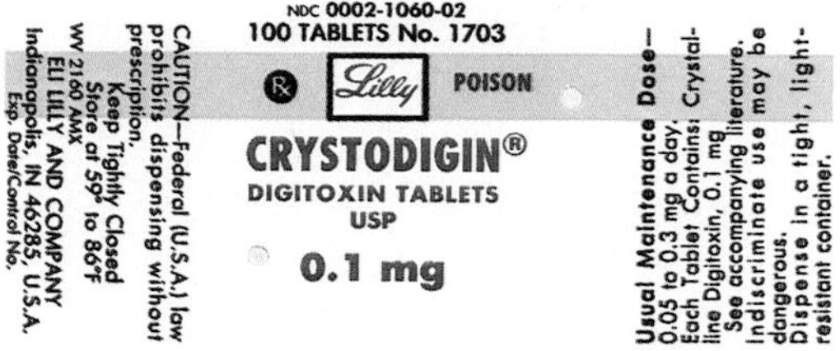

21. Doctor's Order: Codeine gr 3/4 p.o. q4h p.r.n. for pain.

    Available: Codeine 30 mg (gr 1/2) tab. __________

22. Doctor's Order: Cephradine 0.5 g p.o. q6h.

    Available: Cephradine 250 mg caps. __________

23. Doctor's Order: Cogentin 0.5 mg p.o. h.s. __________

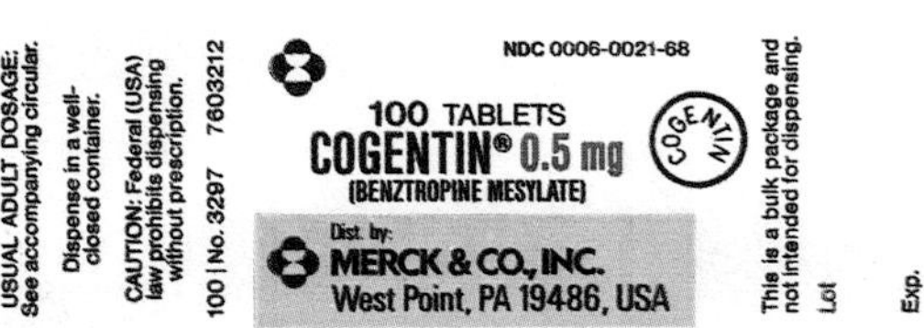

24. Doctor's Order: Thorazine 75 mg p.o. b.i.d. __________

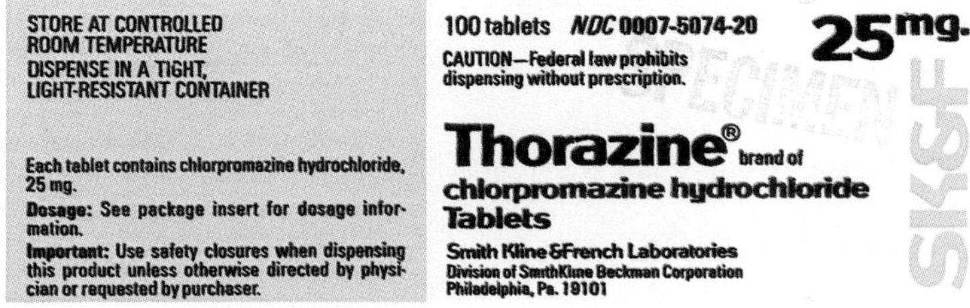

25. Doctor's Order: Dilantin 60 mg p.o. b.i.d. ____________

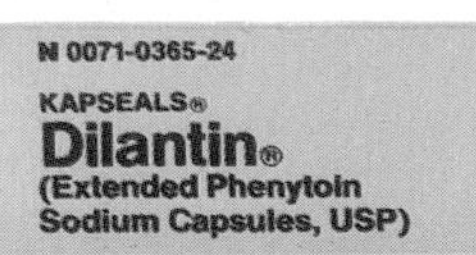

26. Doctor's Order: Meperidine hydrochloride 50 mg I.M. q4h p.r.n. for pain.

    Available: Meperidine 75 mg/mL. ____________

27. Doctor's Order: Solu-Medrol 60 mg I.V. o.d. ____________

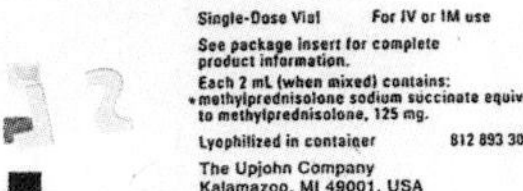

28. Doctor's Order: Amikacin 90 mg I.M. q12h. ____________

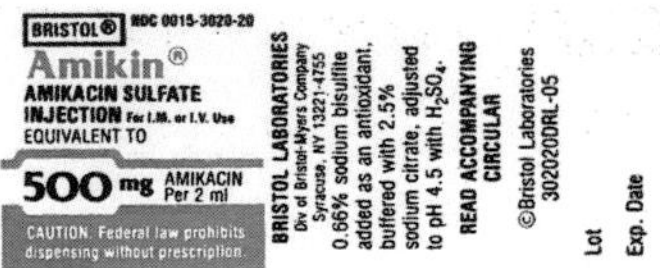

29. Doctor's Order: Amoxicillin 300 mg p.o. q8h.

    Available: Amoxicillin 125 mg/5 mL. ____________

30. Doctor's Order: V-cillin K 300,000 U p.o. q6h. ____________

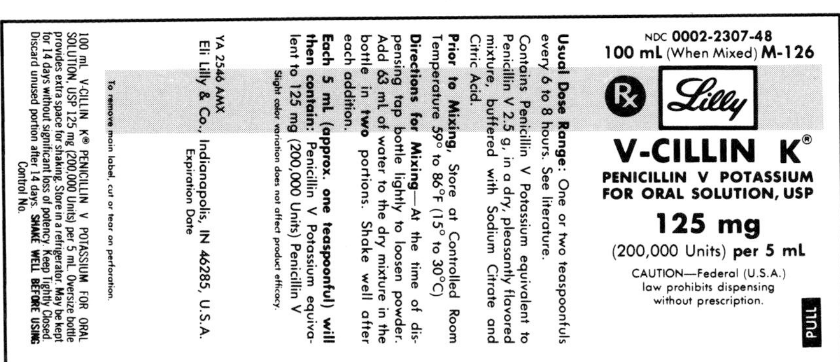

31. Doctor's Order: Phenobarbital elixir 45 mg p.o. b.i.d.

    Available: Phenobarbital elixir 20 mg/5 mL. ____________

32. Doctor's Order: Heparin 3,000 U s.c. b.i.d. ____________

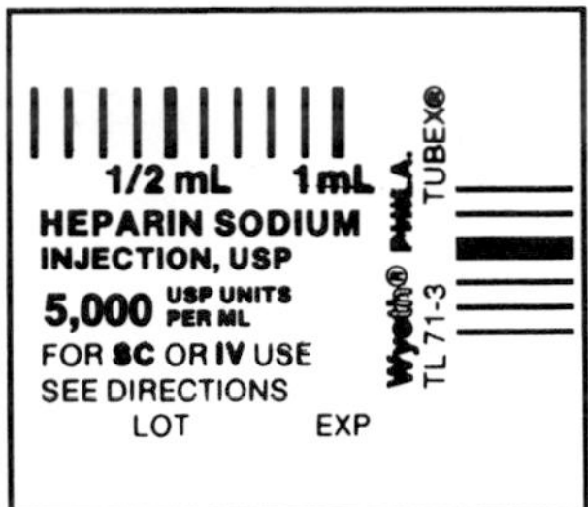

33. Doctor's Order: Procaine penicillin 600,000 U I.M. q12h. ____________

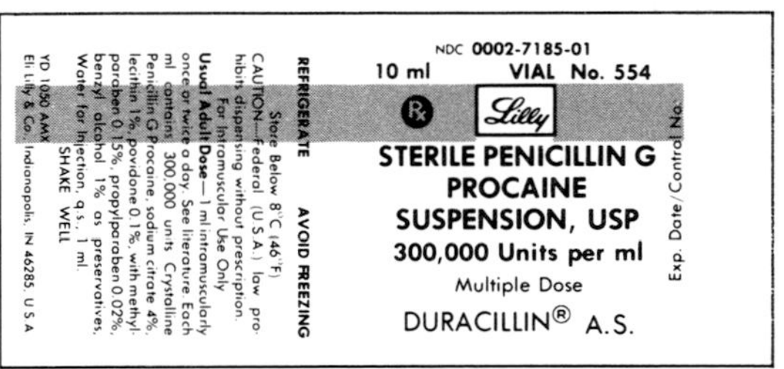

34. Doctor's Order: Gentamicin 70 mg I.V. q8h.

    Available: Gentamicin 40 mg/mL. ____________

35. Doctor's Order: Add potassium chloride 20 mEq to each I.V. bag.

    Available: Potassium chloride 2 mEq/mL. ____________

36. Doctor's Order: Depo-Medrol 60 mg I.M. q. Monday × 2 weeks. ____________

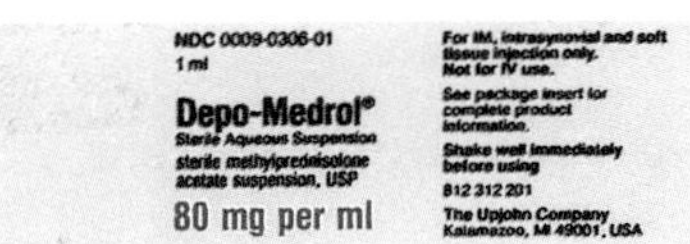

37. Doctor's Order: Vistaril 100 mg I.M. stat.

    Available: Vistaril 50 mg/mL. ____________

38. Doctor's Order: Morphine sulfate 6 mg s.c. q4h p.r.n. for pain.

    Available: Morphine 10 mg/mL. ____________

39. Doctor's Order: Atropine 0.3 mg I.M. stat. ____________

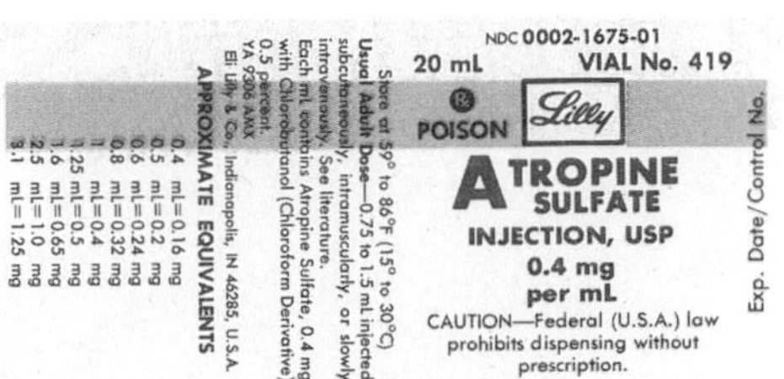

40. Doctor's Order: Stadol 1 mg I.M. q4h p.r.n. for pain. ______________

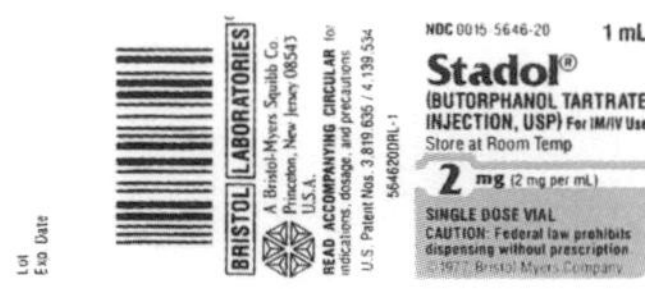

41. Doctor's Order: Ativan 1 mg I.M. stat.

Available: Ativan 4 mg/mL. ______________

42. Doctor's Order: Kanamycin 250 mg I.M. q6h. ______________

Kantrex Injection Label
Available 500 mg/ 2mL

43. Doctor's Order: Robinul 0.4 mg I.M. stat on call to OR. ______________

5 mL Multiple Dose Vial NDC 0031-7890-93
Robinul® Injectable
(Glycopyrrolate Injection, USP)
0.2 mg/mL
Water for Injection, USP q.s./Benzyl Alcohol, NF (preservative) 0.9%.
NOT FOR USE IN NEWBORNS
pH adjusted, when necessary, with hydrochloric acid and/or sodium hydroxide.

CAUTION: Federal law prohibits dispensing without prescription.
For I.M. or I.V. administration.
For dosage and other directions for use, consult accompanying product literature.
Store at Controlled Room Temperature, Between 15°C and 30°C (59°F and 86°F).
MANUFACTURED FOR PHARMACEUTICAL DIVISION
A.H. ROBINS COMPANY, RICHMOND, VA. 23220
by ELKINS-SINN, INC., CHERRY HILL, N.J. 08003
a subsidiary of A.H. Robins 10.87
LOT
EXP.

44. Doctor's Order: Aminophylline 80 mg I.V. q6h.

Available: Aminophylline 25 mg/mL. ______________

45. Doctor's Order: Lithium citrate oral solution 300 mg t.i.d.

Available: Lithium citrate 300 mg/5 mL. ______________

46. Doctor's Order: Sinemet 25/100 p.o. q.i.d. ______________

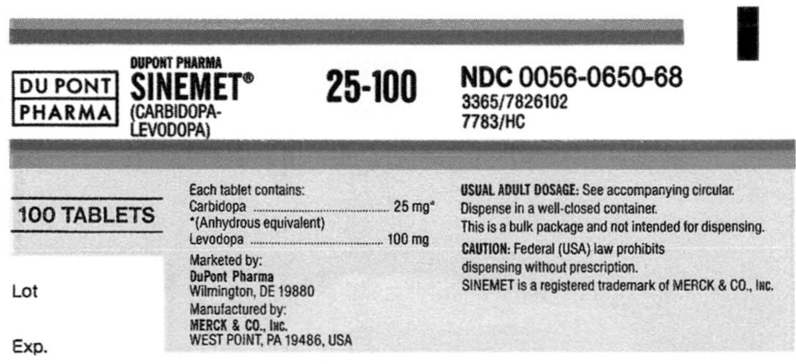

47. Doctor's Order: Lopid 0.6 g p.o. b.i.d. 30 minutes before meals. ____________

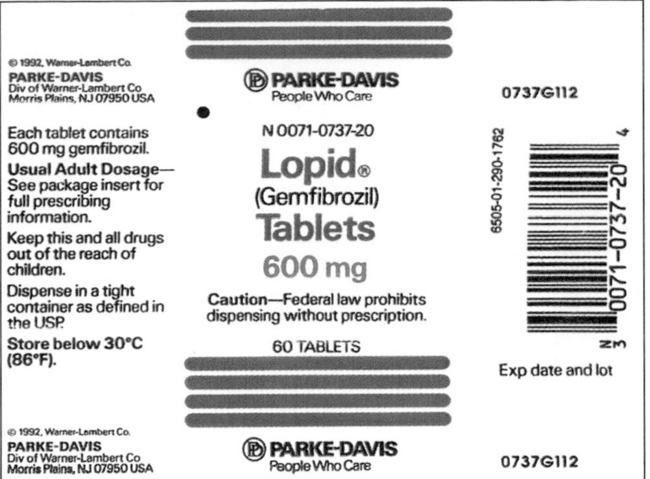

48. Doctor's Order: Prozac 20 mg p.o. q.d. ____________

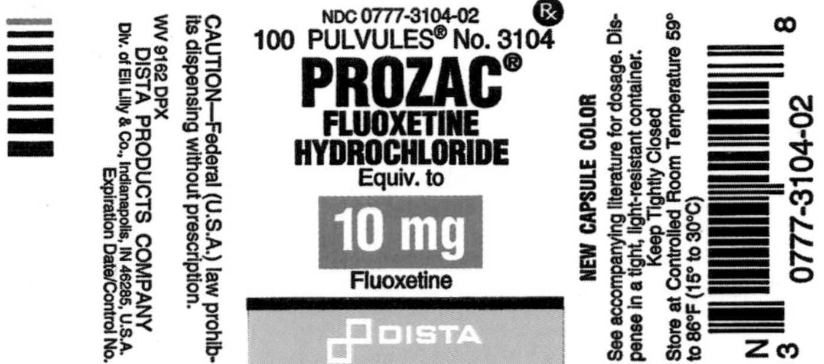

49. Doctor's Order: Potassium chloride 10 mEq I.V. × 2 L. ____________

Potassium Chloride Label
40 mEq/20 mL
(2 mEq/mL)

50. Doctor's Order: Augmentin 0.875 g p.o. q12h. ____________

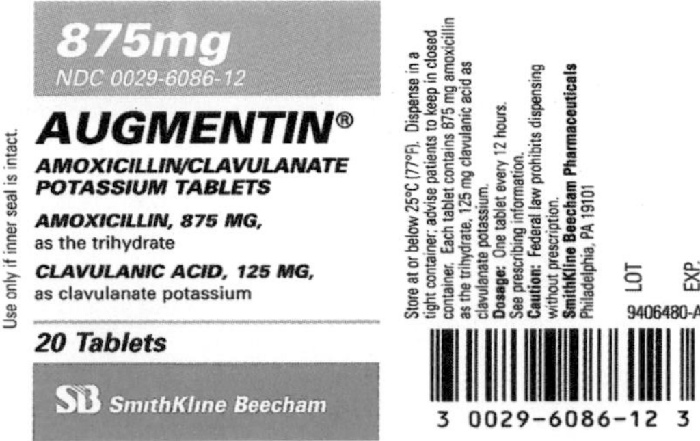

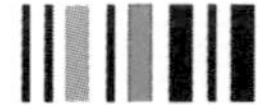

51. Doctor's Order: Tagamet 800 mg p.o. h.s. ______________

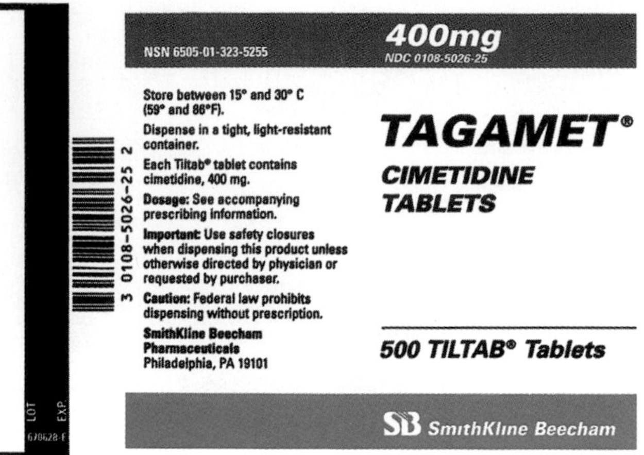

52. Doctor's Order: Depo-Provera 500 mg I.M. once a week. ______________

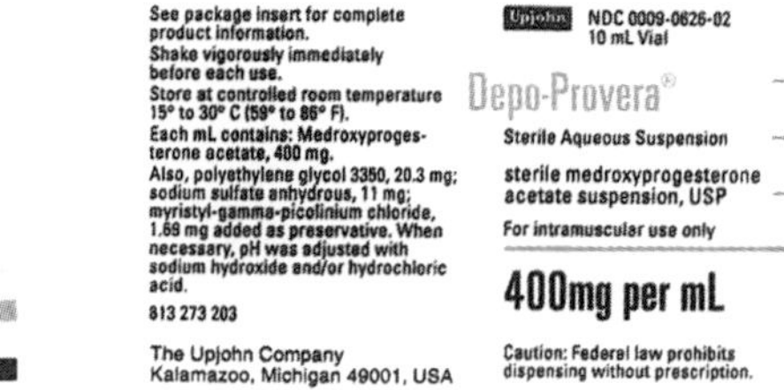

53. Doctor's Order: Tagamet 300 mg I.V. q8h. ______________

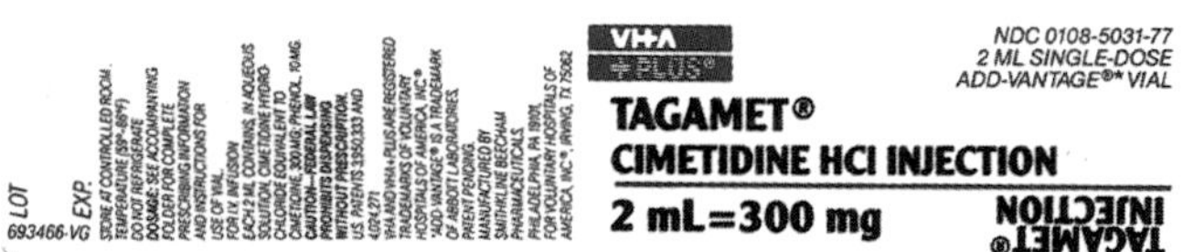

54. Doctor's Order: Nembutal 150 mg I.M. h.s. p.r.n. ______________

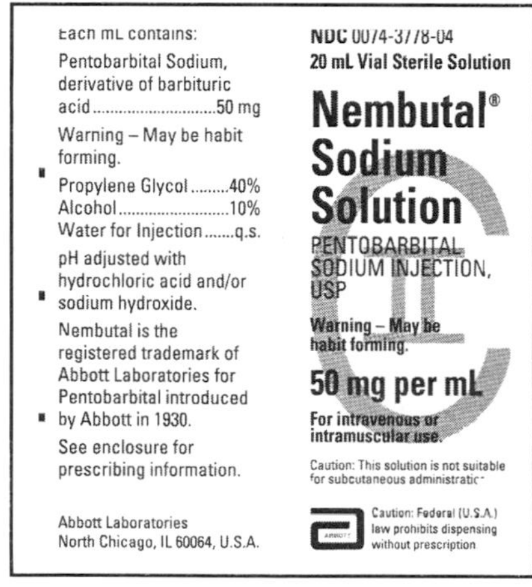

55. Doctor's Order: Cipro 1.5 g p.o. q12h. ______________

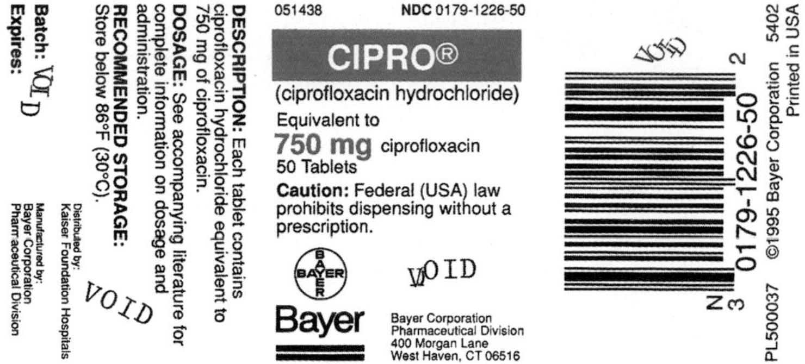

UNIT FOUR

Oral and Parenteral Doseforms, Insulin, and Pediatric Dose Calculations

Oral medications are the easiest, most economical, and most frequently used medications, but sometimes parenteral (non–gastrointestinal tract) dosage routes are necessary. Both oral and parenteral drugs can be administered in liquid or powder form. In addition to oral and parenteral doseforms, this unit examines the varying types of insulin, as well as pediatric dose calculations.

Chapter 15

Calculation of Oral Medications

Objectives

After reviewing this chapter the student will be able to do the following:

1. **Identify the forms of oral medication**
2. **Identify the terms on the medication label to be used in calculation of doses**
3. **Calculate doses for oral and liquid medications using ratio-proportion or the formula method**
4. **Apply principles learned concerning tablet and liquid preparations to obtain a rational answer**

The easiest, most economical, and most frequently used method of medication administration is p.o. Drugs for oral administration are available in solid forms such as tablets and capsules or as liquid preparations. To calculate doses appropriately the nurse needs to understand the principles that apply to administration of medications by this route.

Forms of Solid Medications

Tablets

Tablets are preparations of powdered drugs that have been molded into various sizes and shapes. Tablets come in a variety of doses that can be expressed in apothecaries' or metric measure—for example, milligrams and grains. There are different types of tablets.

Caplets. Caplet is a tablet that has an elongated shape like a capsule and is coated for ease of swallowing. Tylenol is available in caplet form.

Scored tablets. These are tablets that are designed to administer a dose that is less than what is available in a single tablet. In other words, scored tablets have indentations or markings that allow you to break the tablet into halves or quarters. Only scored tablets may be broken. Examples of scored tablets are Lanoxin and Capoten (Figure 15-1).

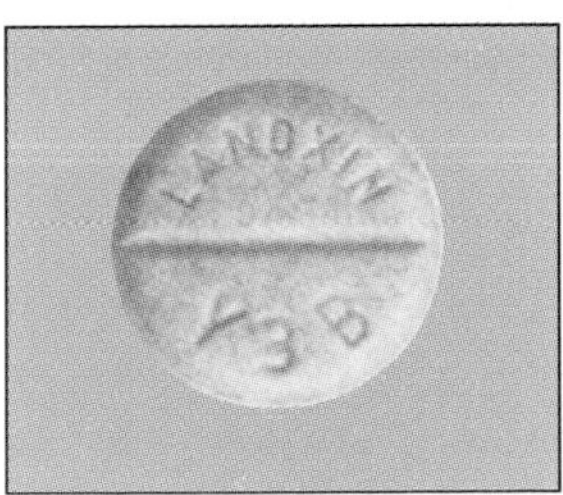

Figure 15-1. Lanoxin tablet scored in half. (From Brown M, Mulholland J: *Drug calculations: process and problems for clinical practice,* ed 5, St Louis, 1996, Mosby.)

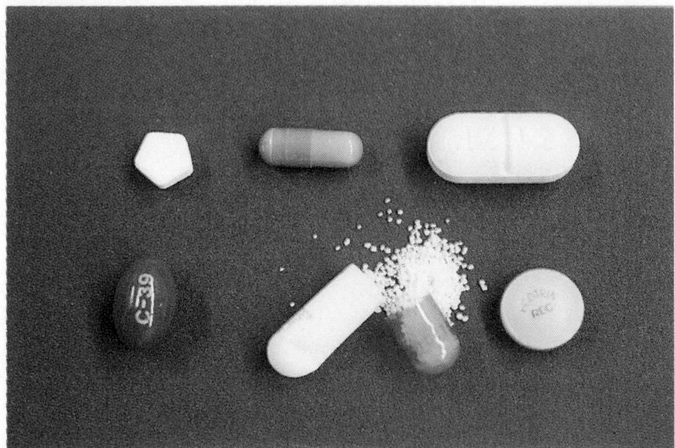

Figure 15-2. Forms of solid oral medications. *Top row,* Unique shape tablet, capsule, scored tablet; *bottom row,* gelatin-coated liquid capsule, extended-release capsule, enteric-coated tablet. (From Elkin M, Perry A, Potter P: *Nursing interventions and clinical skills,* St Louis, 1996, Mosby.)

Enteric-coated tablets. These are tablets with a special coating that protects them from the effects of gastric secretions and prevents them from dissolving in the stomach. They are dissolved and absorbed in the intestines.

The enteric coating also prevents the drug from becoming a source of irritation to the gastric mucosa, thereby preventing gastrointestinal upset. Examples include enteric-coated aspirin and iron tablets such as ferrous gluconate. Enteric-coated tablets should never be crushed, since crushing them would destroy the special coating on them and defeat its purpose.

Sublingual tablets. These tablets are designed to be placed under the tongue, where they dissolve in saliva and the medication is absorbed. Sublingual tablets should never be swallowed because this will prevent them from achieving their desired effect. Nitroglycerine, which is used for the relief of acute chest pain, is usually administered sublingually.

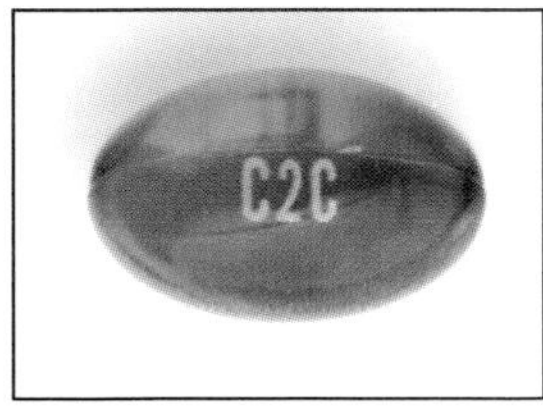

Figure 15-3. Lanoxin capsule (liquid medication contained in gelatin capsule). (From Brown M, Mulholland J: *Drug calculations: process and problems for clinical practice,* ed 5, St Louis, 1996, Mosby.)

In addition to the types of tablets mentioned, "timed release" and extended release tablets are available. Medication from these tablets is released over a period of time, at specific time intervals.

Capsules

A capsule is a form of medication that contains a powder, liquid, or oil enclosed in a hard or soft gelatin. Capsules come in a variety of colors, sizes, and doses. Some capsules have special shapes and colorings to identify which company produced them. Capsules are also available as "timed release," sustained release, and spansules and work over a period of time. Capsules cannot be divided or crushed. Capsules should only be administered as a whole. Examples of medications that come in capsule form are ampicillin, tetracycline, Colace, and Lanoxicaps (Figures 15-2 to 15-4).

Although there are other forms of solid preparations for oral administration—such as lozenges and troches—tablets, capsules, and pulvules are the most frequent forms of solids encountered by the nurse that require calculation. Figure 15-2 shows forms of solid oral medications.

Calculating Doses Involving Tablets and Capsules

When administering medications, you will have to calculate the number of tablets or capsules needed to administer the dose ordered. To help you determine if your calculated dose is sensible, accurate, and safe, remember the following points:

Points to Remember

- Converting drug measures from one system to another and one unit to another to determine the dose to be administered can result in discrepancies, depending on the conversion factor used.
- Example: Aspirin may indicate on the label 5 grains (325 mg). This is based on the equivalent 65 mg = gr 1. On the other hand, another label on aspirin may indicate 5 grains (300 mg). Here the equivalent 60 mg = gr 1 was used. Both of the equivalents are correct. **Remember, equivalents are not exact.** Use the common equivalents when making conversions—for example, 60 mg = gr 1.
- When the precise number of tablets or capsules is determined and you find that administering the amount calculated is unrealistic or impossible, always use the following rule to avoid an error in administration: *No more than 10% variation should exist between the dose ordered and the dose administered.* For example, you may determine a client should receive 0.9 tablet or 0.9 capsule. Administration of such an amount accurately would be impossible. Following the stated rule, if you determined that 0.9 tablet or 0.9 capsule should be given, you could safely administer 1 tab or 1 caps.
- Capsules are not scored and cannot be divided. They are administered in whole amounts only. If a client has difficulty swallowing a capsule, check to see if a liquid preparation of the same drug is available. Never crush or open a timed-release capsule or empty its contents into a liquid or food; this may cause release of all the medication at once. There are, however, some instances in which a soft gelatin capsule that is filled with liquid may be pierced with a small sterile needle and the medication squeezed out for sublingual use. For example, Procardia (nifedipine) has been used in this way. However, the action is erratic and short-term and is not approved by the FDA for use in this manner.
- Pulvules are proprietary capsules containing a dose of a drug in powder form. For example, the popular and new antidepressant, Prozac, comes in pulvule form.
- Tablets and capsules may be available in different strengths for administration, and you may have a choice when giving a dose. For example, 75 mg of a drug may be ordered. When you check what is available, it may be in tablet or capsule form as 10, 25, or 50 mg. In deciding the best combination of tablets or capsules to give, the nurse should always choose the strength that would allow the least number of tablets or capsules to be administered without breaking a tablet if possible, since breaking is found to result in variations in dosage. In the example given, the best combination to use to administer 75 mg would be one of the 50-mg tablets or capsules and one of the 25-mg tablets or capsules.
- The maximum number of tablets or capsules given to a client to achieve a certain dose is usually three. Any more than this is unusual and may indicate an error in the interpretation of the order or in calculation.
- When using the formula or ratio-proportion method to calculate tablet and capsule problems, remember that each tablet and capsule contains a certain weight of the drug. The weight indicated on a label is per tablet or per capsule. This is particularly important when reading a medication label on bottles or single packages such as unit dose.
- In calculating oral doses you may encounter measures other than apothecaries' or metric measure. For example, electrolytes such as potassium will indicate the number of milliequivalents (mEq) per tablet. Units is another measure you may see for oral antibiotics or vitamins. For example, a vitamin E capsule will indicate 400 U per capsule. Units and milliequivalents are measurements that are specific to the drug they are being used for. There is no conversion that exists between these and apothecaries' or metric measure.

Figure 15-4. Various sizes and numbers of gelatin capsules. (From Clayton B, Stock Y: *Basic pharmacology for nurses,* ed 10, St Louis, 1993, Mosby.)

Remembering the points mentioned will be helpful when starting to calculate doses. Any of the methods presented in Chapters 13 and 14 can be used to determine the dose to be administered.

To compute doses accurately it is necessary to review a few reminders that were presented in previous chapters.

Reminders

1. Read the problem carefully and
   a) Identify known factors in the problem
   b) Identify unknown factors in the problem
   c) Eliminate unnecessary information that is not relevant
2. Make sure that what is ordered and what is available are in the same system of measurement and units, or a conversion will be necessary. When a conversion is necessary, it is usual to convert what the doctor has ordered into what you have available or what is indicated on the drug label. You can, however, convert the measure in which the drug is available into the same units and system of measure as the dose ordered. The choice is usually based upon whichever is easier to solve. Using any of the methods presented in Chapter 8, make conversions consistently one way to avoid confusion. If necessary, go back and review that chapter.
3. Consider what would be a reasonable answer based on what is ordered.
4. Set up the problem using ratio-proportion or the formula method.
5. Label the final answer (tablet, capsule).
6. For administration purposes, state answers to problems in fractions. Example: 1/2 tab, 1 1/2 tabs, instead of 0.5 tabs, 1.5 tabs.

Let's look at some sample problems calculating the number of tablets or capsules to administer.

Example 1: Doctor's order: Digoxin 0.375 mg p.o. o.d.

Available: Scored tablets labeled 0.25 mg.

Problem Setup

1. No conversion is necessary; the units are in the same system of measure.
   Order: 0.375 mg
   Available: 0.25 mg
2. Think critically: Tablets are scored; 0.375 mg is larger than 0.25 mg; therefore you will need more than 1 tab to administer the correct dose.
3. Solve using ratio-proportion or the formula method.

Solution Using Ratio-Proportion Method

$$0.25 \text{ mg} : 1 \text{ tab} = 0.375 \text{ mg} : x \text{ tab}$$

(Known) (Unknown)

(What's available) (What's ordered)

$$0.25x = 0.375$$

$$x = \frac{0.375}{0.25}$$

Therefore, $x = 1.5$ tabs or 1 1/2 tabs. (It is best to state it as 1 1/2 tabs for administration purposes.)

Note: You can administer 1 1/2 tabs because the tablets are scored. The above ratio-proportion could have been written as a fraction as well. (If necessary, review Chapter 4 on ratio-proportion.)

Solution Using the Formula Method

$$\frac{\text{(D)}0.375 \text{ mg}}{\text{(H)}0.25 \text{ mg}} \times \text{(Q) } 1 \text{ tab} = x \text{ tab}$$

$$\frac{0.375}{0.25} \times 1 = x = 1\frac{1}{2} \text{ tabs}$$

OR

$$\frac{\text{(DW) } 0.375 \text{ mg}}{\text{(SW) } 0.25 \text{ mg}} = \frac{\text{(DV)}x \text{ tab}}{\text{(SV) } 1 \text{ tab}}$$

$$x = \frac{0.375}{0.25} = 1\frac{1}{2} \text{ tabs}$$

Example 2: Doctor's order: Ampicillin 0.5 g p.o. q6h.

Available: Capsules labeled 250 mg per capsule.

1. Note: A conversion is necessary. The ordered dose and the available dose are in the same system of measurement (metric), but the units are different (g and mg). Before calculating the dose to be administered, you must have the ordered dose and the available dose in the same units.
   Order: 0.5 g
   Available: 250-mg capsules
2. After making the necessary conversion, think, what is a reasonable amount to administer?
3. Calculate the dose to be administered using ratio-proportion or the formula method.
4. Label your final answer (tablets, capsules).

Problem Setup

1. Convert g to mg. Equivalent: 1000 mg = 1 g

$$1000 \text{ mg} : 1 \text{ g} = x \text{ mg} : 0.5 \text{ g}$$

$$x = 1000 \times 0.5$$

$$x = 500 \text{ mg}$$

   Therefore 0.5 g is equal to 500 mg. Converting the g to mg eliminated a decimal, which is often the source of calculation errors. Converting mg to g would necessitate a decimal. Whenever possible, conversions that result in a decimal should be avoided to decrease the chance of error in calculating. Remember, a ratio-proportion could also be stated as a fraction. If necessary, review Chapter 4 on ratio-proportion. Since the measures are metric in this problem (g, mg), the other method that can be used is to move the decimal the desired number of places (0.5 g = 500 mg).
2. After making the conversion, you are now ready to calculate the dose to be given, using ratio-proportion or the formula method. In this problem we will use the answer obtained from converting what was ordered to what's available (0.5 g = 500 mg).

Solution Using Ratio-Proportion Method

$$250 \text{ mg} : 1 \text{ caps} = 500 \text{ mg} : x \text{ caps}$$

$$250x = 500$$

$$x = \frac{500}{250}$$

$$x = 2 \text{ caps}$$

Note: 2 caps is a logical answer. Capsules are administered in whole amounts; they are not dividable. Using the conversion obtained from converting mg to g in this problem would also net a final answer of 2 caps.

Solution Using the Formula Method

$$\frac{(\text{D})500 \text{ mg}}{(\text{H})250 \text{ mg}} \times (\text{Q})\ 1 \text{ caps} = x \text{ caps}$$

$$\frac{500}{250} \times 1 = x = 2 \text{ caps}$$

OR

$$\frac{(\text{DW})500 \text{ mg}}{(\text{SW})250 \text{ mg}} = \frac{(\text{DV})x \text{ caps}}{(\text{SV})1 \text{ caps}}$$

$$x = \frac{500}{250} = 2 \text{ caps}$$

Example 3: Doctor's order: Nitroglycerine gr 1/150 sublingual p.r.n. for chest pain.

Available: Sublingual tablets labeled 0.4 mg.

Problem Setup

1. Conversion is required.
   Doctor's order: gr 1/150
   Available: 0.4 mg
   Equivalent 60 mg = gr 1. Convert what is ordered to the same system and units of what is available (gr is apothecaries', mg is metric).

$$60 \text{ mg} : \text{gr } 1 = x \text{ mg} : \text{gr } \frac{1}{150}$$

$$x = 60 \times \frac{1}{150}$$

$$x = \frac{60}{150}$$

$$x = 0.4 \text{ mg}$$

   Note: In this problem it was easier to change gr to mg; gr 1/150 is equal to 0.4 mg.
2. Think critically—It's obvious after making the conversion that you will give 1 tab.
3. Solve to obtain the desired dose.

Solution Using Ratio-Proportion Method

$$0.4 \text{ mg} : 1 \text{ tab} = 0.4 \text{ mg} = x \text{ tab}$$

$$0.4x = 0.4$$

$$x = \frac{0.4}{0.4}$$

$$x = 1 \text{ tab}$$

Solution Using the Formula Method

$$\frac{\text{(D) } 0.4 \text{ mg}}{\text{(H) } 0.4 \text{ mg}} \times \text{Q (1 tab)} = x \text{ tab}$$

$$\frac{0.4}{0.4} \times 1 = x = 1 \text{ tab}$$

OR

$$\frac{\text{(DW)}0.4 \text{ mg}}{\text{(SW)}0.4 \text{ mg}} = \frac{\text{(DV)}x \text{ tab}}{\text{(SV)}1 \text{ tab}}$$

$$x = \frac{0.4}{0.4} = 1 \text{ tab}$$

Note: This involved the division of decimals. Remember the rule for dividing decimals. If necessary, review Chapter 3 on decimals.

Alternate Method of Doing Example 3

An alternate way of solving the problem in Example 3 would be to eliminate the decimal and therefore convert 0.4 mg to gr. In doing this, more mathematical steps are involved. The same equivalent would be used.

$$60 \text{ mg} : \text{gr } 1 = 0.4 \text{ mg} : x \text{ gr}$$

$$60x = 0.4$$

$$x = \frac{0.4}{60}$$

Remember: Apothecaries' measures are expressed using fractions. Therefore 0.4 must be divided by 60. To divide 0.4 by 60, the decimal point in the numerator is eliminated by moving the decimal point one place to the right to make it 4. For every place the decimal point is moved to make the numerator a whole number, a zero is added to the denominator; therefore it would be as follows:

$$\frac{0.4}{60} = \frac{4}{600}$$

$$\frac{4}{600} = \frac{1}{150}$$

Converting this way will net the same answer when calculating the dose to be given.

Alternate Solution Using Ratio-Proportion Method

$$\text{gr } \frac{1}{150} : 1 \text{ tab} = \text{gr } \frac{1}{150} : x \text{ tab}$$

$$\frac{\frac{1}{150}x}{\frac{1}{150}} = \frac{\frac{1}{150}}{\frac{1}{150}}$$

$$x = \frac{1}{150} \div \frac{1}{150}$$

$$x = \frac{1}{150} \times \frac{150}{1}$$

$$x = \frac{150}{150}$$

$$x = 1 \text{ tab}$$

Alternate Solution Using the Formula Method

$$\frac{\text{(D) gr } \frac{1}{150}}{\text{(H) gr } \frac{1}{150}} \times \text{Q (1 tab)} = x \text{ tab}$$

$$\frac{\frac{1}{150}}{\frac{1}{150}} \times 1 = x = 1 \text{ tab}$$

OR

$$\frac{\text{(DW) gr } \frac{1}{150}}{\text{(SW) gr } \frac{1}{150}} = \frac{\text{(DV)}x \text{ tab}}{\text{(SV)}1 \text{ tab}}$$

$$x = \frac{\frac{1}{150}}{\frac{1}{150}} = 1 \text{ tab}$$

Example 4: Doctor's order: Nembutal gr 1 1/2 p.o. h.s. p.r.n.

Available: Capsules labeled 100 mg

Problem Setup

1. Convert gr 1 1/2 to mg. Equivalent: 60 mg = gr 1

$$60 \text{ mg} : \text{gr } 1 = x \text{ mg} : \text{gr } 1\frac{1}{2}$$

$$60 \text{ mg} : \text{gr } 1 = x \text{ mg} : \text{gr } \frac{3}{2}$$

$$x = 60 \times \frac{3}{2} = \frac{180}{2}$$

$$x = 90 \text{ mg}$$

2. Solve for the dose to be administered.

Solution Using Ratio-Proportion Method

$$100 \text{ mg} : 1 \text{ caps} = 90 \text{ mg} : x \text{ caps.}$$

$$100x = 90$$

$$x = \frac{90}{100}$$

$$x = 0.9 \text{ caps} = 1 \text{ caps}$$

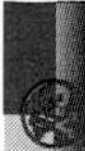

Think Critically to Avoid Drug Calculation Errors

Capsules are not dividable; 0.9 is closer to 1 caps. It is safe to administer 1 caps; 1 caps falls within the 10% variation allowed between the dose ordered and the dose given.

Solution Using the Formula Method

$$\frac{(D)100\text{ mg}}{(H)\ 90\text{ mg}} \times Q\ (1\text{ caps}) = x\text{ caps}$$

$$\frac{100}{90} \times 1 = x = 0.9\text{ caps} = 1\text{ caps}$$

OR

$$\frac{(DW)100\text{ mg}}{(SW)90\text{ mg}} = \frac{(DV)x\text{ caps}}{(SV)1\text{ caps}}$$

$$x = \frac{100}{90} = 0.9\text{ caps} = 1\text{ caps}$$

As already discussed, alternate equivalents may be used to achieve the same answer in terms of the dose to be administered. For example, if the equivalent 65 mg = gr 1 is used to convert gr 1 1/2 to mg, the answer for the conversion is 97.5 mg.

Therefore, in calculating the dose to administer, the precise answer would have been 0.975 caps. This would still require that 1 caps be administered. Remember, there is a 10% margin because of approximate equivalents.

Another alternative to the conversion for this problem might be to think 1000 mg = 1 g. Therefore, since gr 15 = 1 g, 100 mg could be converted to gr as follows:

$$1000\text{ mg} : \text{gr } 15 = 100\text{ mg} : x\text{ gr}$$

$$1000x = 1500$$

$$x = \frac{1500}{1000}$$

$$x = \text{gr } 1\frac{1}{2}$$

Converting in this manner will give the same answer of 1 caps as illustrated using the ratio-proportion method to calculate the dose to be given.

$$\text{gr } 1\frac{1}{2} : 1\text{ caps} = \text{gr } 1\frac{1}{2} : x\text{ caps}$$

Note: gr 1 1/2 can be changed to an improper fraction for the purpose of calculating.

$$\text{gr } \frac{3}{2} : 1\text{ cap} = \text{gr } \frac{3}{2} : x\text{ caps}$$

$$\frac{3}{2}x = \frac{3}{2}$$

$$x = \frac{3}{2} \div \frac{3}{2}$$

$$x = \frac{3}{2} \times \frac{2}{3}$$

$$x = \frac{6}{6}$$

$$x = 1\text{ caps}$$

Example 5: Doctor's order: Thorazine 100 mg p.o. t.i.d.

Available: Tablets labeled 25 mg and 50 mg

Problem Setup

1. No conversion is necessary.
2. Thinking critically: 100 mg is larger than 25 or 50 mg. Therefore more than 1 tab is needed to administer the dose. The client should always be given the strength of tablets or capsules that would require the least number to be taken.
3. In this problem, selection of the 50-mg tablets would require the client to receive 2 tabs, while using 25-mg tablets would require 4 tabs to be administered.

Solution Using Ratio-Proportion Method

$$50\text{ mg} : 1\text{ tab} = 100\text{ mg} : x\text{ tab}$$

$$50x = 100$$

$$x = 2\text{ tabs } (50\text{ mg each})$$

Solution Using the Formula Method

$$\frac{(D)100\text{ mg}}{(H)50\text{ mg}} \times Q\ (1\text{ tab}) = x\text{ tab}$$

$$\frac{100}{50} \times 1 = x = 2\text{ tabs of } 50\text{ mg each}$$

OR

$$\frac{(DW)100\text{ mg}}{(SW)50\text{ mg}} = \frac{(DV)x\text{ tab}}{(SV)1\text{ tab}}$$

$$x = \frac{100}{50} = 2\text{ tabs of } 50\text{ mg each}$$

Note: In Example 5 not only is the number of tablets specified, but the strength of tablets chosen is specified as well.

Variation of Tablet and Capsule Problems

Frequently, to decide how many tablets or capsules are needed requires knowing the dosage and frequency.

Example 1: Doctor's order: Valium 10 mg p.o. q.i.d.

How many 5-mg tablets would be needed for 7 days?

Solution: To obtain 10 mg the client requires two 5-mg tablets each time. Therefore eight 5-mg tablets are necessary to administer the dose q.i.d. (four times a day).
(Number of days ordered for) × (Number of tablets needed per day) = Total number of tablets needed

$8 \times 7 = 56$

Answer: Total number of tablets needed for 7 days would be 56 tabs

Determining the Dose to be Given Each Time

Example 2: A client is to receive 1 g of a drug p.o. daily. The drug should be given in four equally divided doses.

How many mg should the client receive each time the medication is administered?

Solution:
$$\frac{\text{Total daily allowance}}{\text{Number of doses per day}} = \text{Dose to be administered}$$

Answer:
$$\frac{1\text{ g }(1000\text{ mg})}{4} = 250\text{ mg}$$

Points to Remember

- The maximum number of tablets and capsules to administer to achieve a desired dose is usually three.
- Before calculating a dose, make sure that the dose ordered and what's available are in the same system of measurement and units. When a conversion is required, it is usually best to convert the dose ordered to what's available.
- No more than a 10% variation should exist between the dose ordered and the dose administered.
- Regardless of the method used to calculate a dose, it is important to develop the ability to think critically about what is a reasonable amount.
- State doses as you are actually going to administer them. Example: 0.5 tab = 1/2 tab.

Practice Problems on Tablets and Capsules (pp. 345-349)

Directions: Calculate the correct number of tablets or capsules to be administered in the following problems using the labels or information provided. Use any of the methods presented to calculate the dose.

Remember to label your answers.

1. Doctor's Order: Synthroid 0.025 mg p.o. o.d.

   Available: Scored tablets. ______________

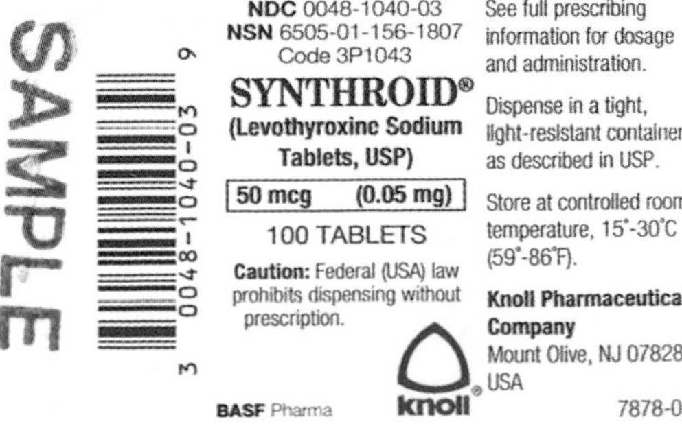

2. Doctor's Order: Capoten 6.25 mg p.o. b.i.d.

   Available: Tablets scored in fourths. ____________

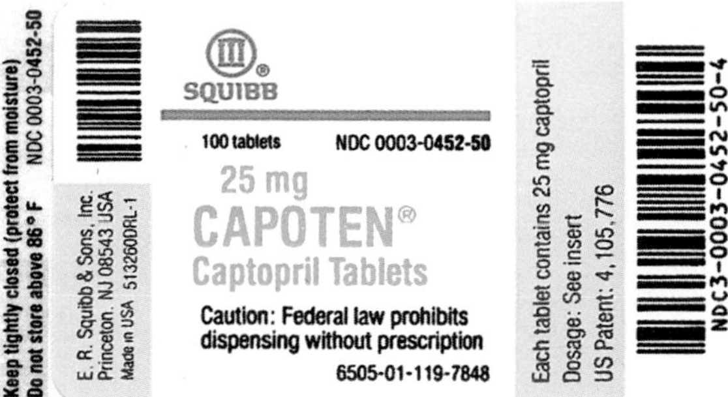

3. Doctor's Order: Ethambutol 1.2 g p.o. o.d.

   Available: ____________

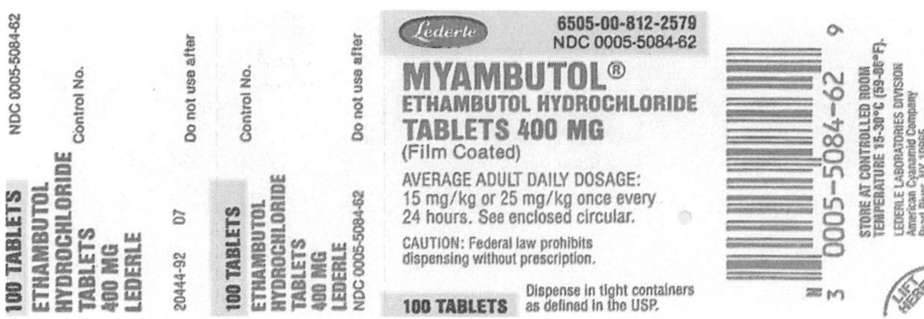

4. Doctor's Order: Coumadin 7.5 mg p.o. h.s.

   Available: Scored tablets. ____________

   a) What would be the appropriate strength tablet to use? ____________

COUMADIN® 2½ mg	COUMADIN® 5 mg
(Warfarin Sodium Tablets, USP)	(Warfarin Sodium Tablets, USP)
Crystalline	Crystalline
DuPont Pharma	DuPont Pharma
Wilmington, Delaware 19880	Wilmington, Delaware 19880
LOT JJ275A	LOT KA009A
EXP 8/98	EXP 1/99

5. Doctor's Order: Lanoxin 0.125 mg p.o. o.d.

   Available: Scored tablets. ____________

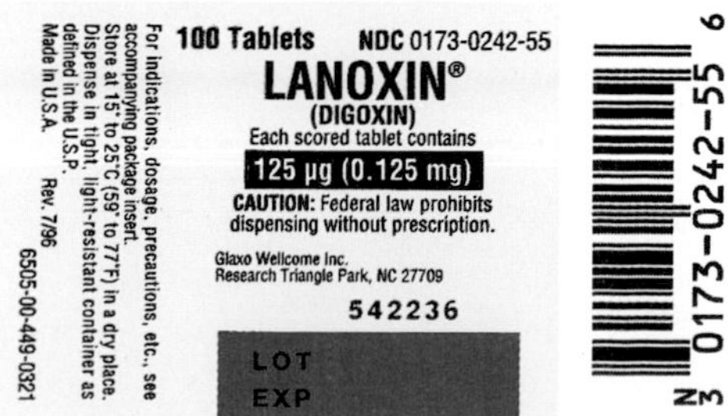

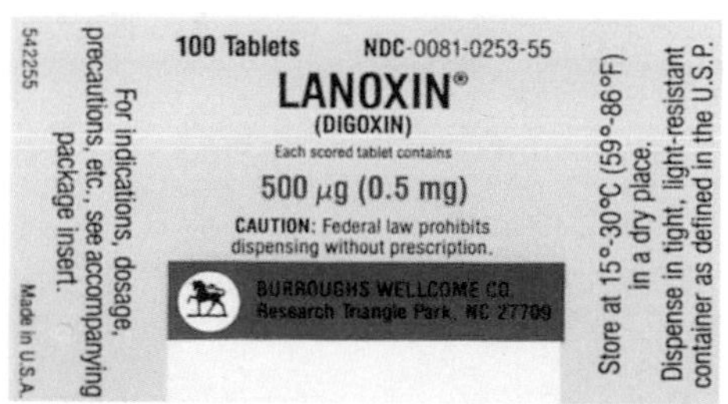

   a) What would be the appropriate strength tablet to use? ____________

   b) What will you prepare to administer? ____________

6. Doctor's Order: Ampicillin 1 g p.o. q6h.

   Available: Capsules labeled 500 mg and 250 mg. ____________

   a) Which strength of capsules would be appropriate to use? ____________

   b) How many capsules are needed for one dose? ____________

   c) What is the total number of capsules needed if the medication is ordered for 7 days? ____________

7. Doctor's Order: Reglan 10 mg p.o. t.i.d. 1/2 hr a.c.

   Available: Tablets labeled 5 mg. ____________

8. Doctor's Order: Baclofen 15 mg p.o. t.i.d. × 3 days.

   Available: Scored tablets.

   NDC **0028-0023-61** FSC **2503**
   Lioresal® 10mg
   baclofen

   100 tablets–Unit Dose

   Caution: Federal law prohibits dispensing without prescription.

   Geigy

   a) How many tablets are needed for one dose? ____________

   b) What is the total number of mg the client will receive in 3 days? ____________

9. Doctor's Order: Synthroid 0.075 mg p.o. q.d.

   Available: Scored tablets labeled 50 mcg. ____________

10. Doctor's Order: Calcium carbonate 1.3 g p.o. o.d.

    Available: Tablets labeled 650 mg. ____________

11. Doctor's Order: Dilantin 90 mg p.o. t.i.d.

    Available: Capsules labeled 30 mg. ____________

12. Doctor's Order: Tegretol 200 mg p.o. t.i.d.

    Available:

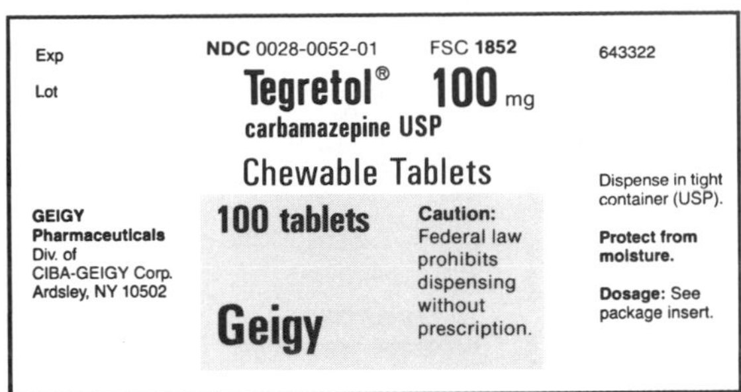

    a) How many tablets will you administer for each dose? ______________

13. Doctor's Order: Dicloxacillin 1 g p.o. as an initial dose and 0.5 g p.o. q6h thereafter.

    Available:

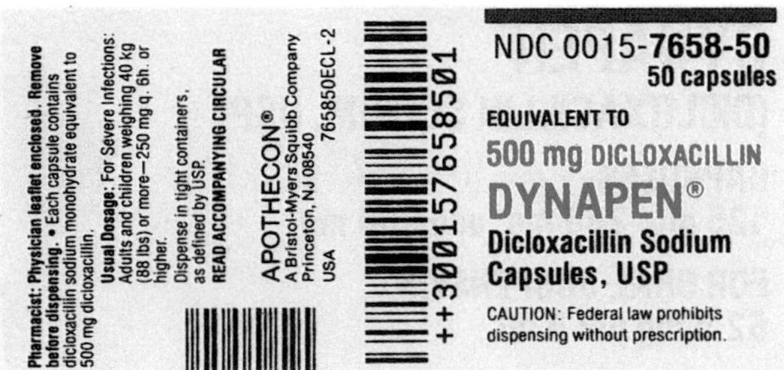

    a) How many capsules will you need for the initial dose? ______________

    b) How many capsules are needed for each subsequent dose? ______________

14. Doctor's Order: Aldomet 250 mg p.o. b.i.d.

    Available: ______________

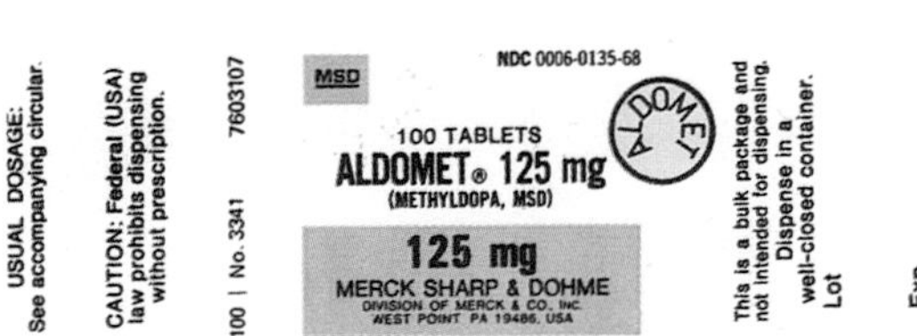

    a) How many tablets will you administer for each dose? ______________

15. Doctor's Order: Phenobarbital gr iss p.o. h.s.

    Available: Phenobarbital 15-mg tabs and 30-mg tabs. ______________

    a) Which strength of tablets would be the best to administer? ______________

    b) How many tablets of which strength will you prepare to administer? ______________

16. Doctor's Order: Decadron 3 mg p.o. b.i.d. × 2 days.

Available:

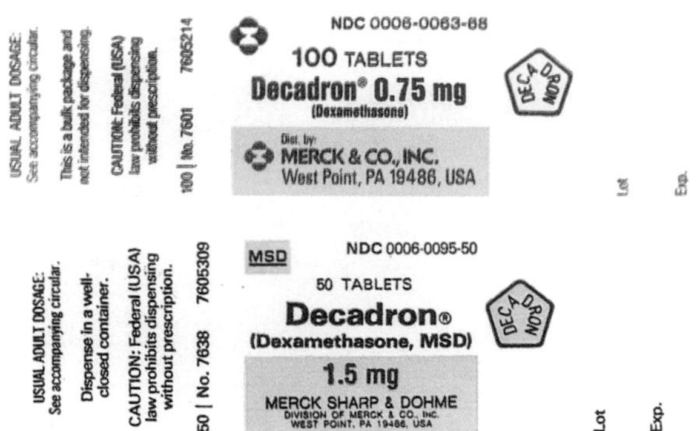

a) Which would be the best strength to administer?

17. Doctor's Order: Thorazine 100 mg p.o. t.i.d.

Available: __________

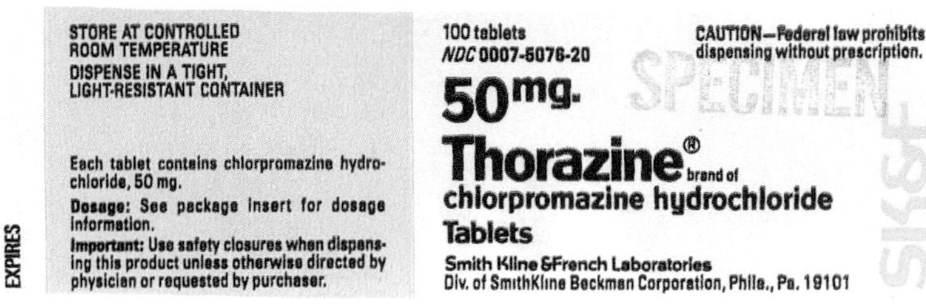

a) How many tablets are needed for 3 days? __________

18. Doctor's Order: Verapamil 120 mg p.o. t.i.d. Hold for systolic blood pressure <100, heart rate <55.

Available: Scored tablets labeled 80 mg and 40 mg. __________

a) Which would be the best strength tablets to use? __________

b) How many of which strength tablet will you administer? __________

19. Doctor's Order: Acetaminophen gr x p.o. q4h p.r.n. for a temp >101° F.

Available: __________

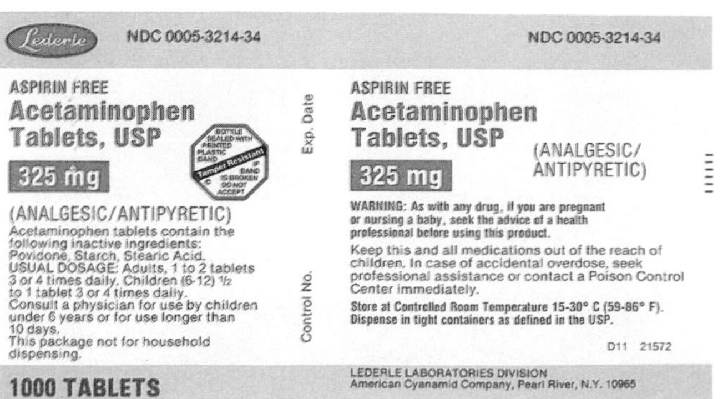

20. Doctor's Order: Cogentin 1 mg p.o. t.i.d.

    Available: ________________

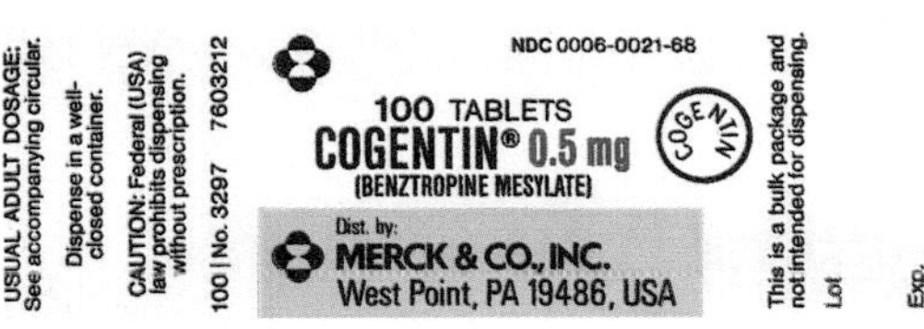

21. Doctor's Order: Prazosin hydrochloride 3 mg p.o. b.i.d.

    Available: Capsules labeled 1 mg. ________________

22. Doctor's Order: Nitroglycerine gr 1/150 SL p.r.n.

    Available: ________________

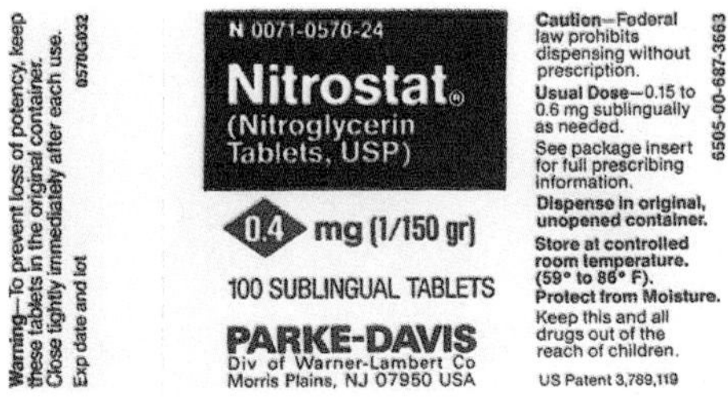

23. Doctor's Order: Dexamethasone 6 mg p.o. o.d.

    Available: Tablets (scored).

    a) How many of which strength tablets will you give? ________________

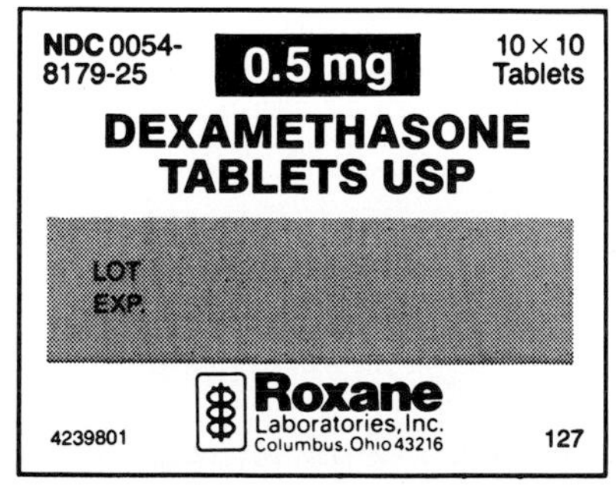

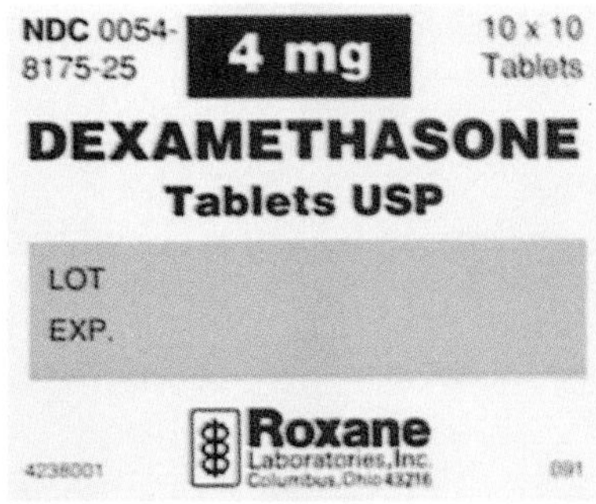

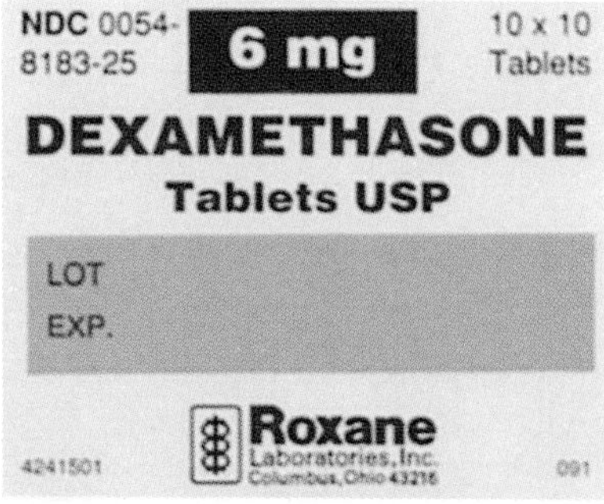

24. Doctor's Order: Pyridium 0.2 g p.o. q8h.

    Available: ________________

Pyridium
100 mg/100 tablets

25. Doctor's Order: Lasix 60 mg p.o. stat.

    Available: Scored tablets. ______________

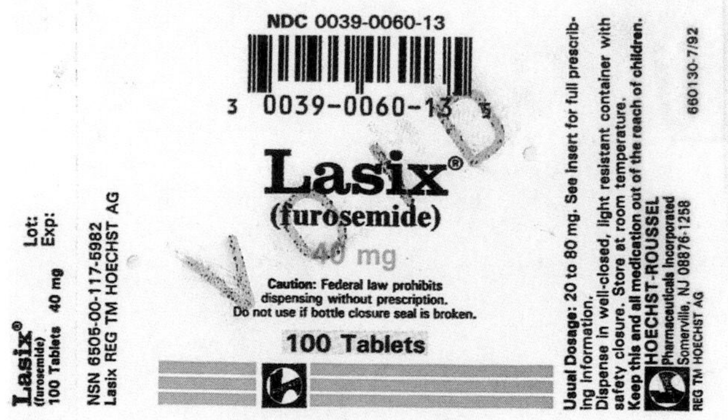

26. Doctor's Order: Glyburide 2.5 mg p.o. o.d.

    Available: Scored tablets labeled 5 mg.

    a) How many tablets will you administer for each dose? ______________

27. Doctor's Order: Tagamet 400 mg p.o. b.i.d.

    Available: Tablets labeled 200 mg.

    a) How many tablets will you administer for each dose? ______________

28. Doctor's Order: Indocin 150 mg p.o. b.i.d.

    Available:

MSD
NDC 0006-0693-61
60 CAPSULES
INDOCIN® SR
(INDOMETHACIN, MSD)
SUSTAINED RELEASE
75 mg
MERCK SHARP & DOHME
DIV OF MERCK & CO., INC., WEST POINT, PA 19486, USA
← Remove and place left edge of pharmacy label here ←
Lot
Exp.
USUAL ADULT DOSAGE: See accompanying circular.
CAUTION: Federal (USA) law prohibits dispensing without prescription.
60 | No.3370 7516902
LIFT HERE

    a) How many capsules will you administer for each dose? ______________

29. Doctor's Order: Sulfasalazine 1 g p.o. q6h.

    Available:

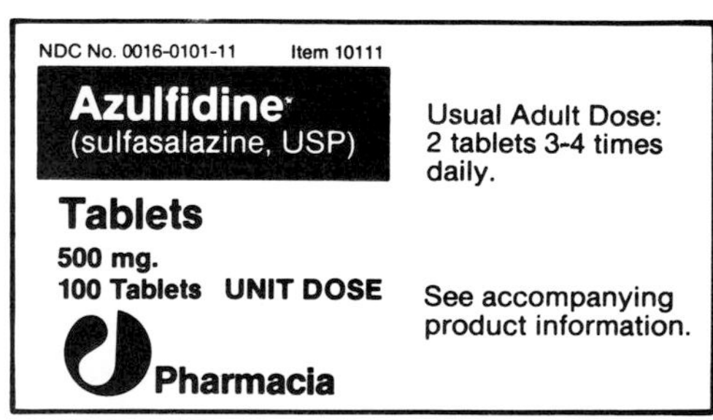

    a) How many tablets will you administer for each dose? ______________

30. Doctor's Order: Capoten 12.5 mg p.o. b.i.d.

    Available: Scored tablets (quarters) labeled 25 mg.

    a) How many tablets will you administer for each dose? ____________

31. Doctor's Order: Synthroid 100 mcg p.o. o.d.

    Available: Tablets labeled 75 mcg and 25 mcg.

    a) How many tablets of which strength will you use to administer the dose? ____________

32. Doctor's Order: Capoten 6.25 mg p.o. q8h.

    Available: Scored tablets (quarters). ____________

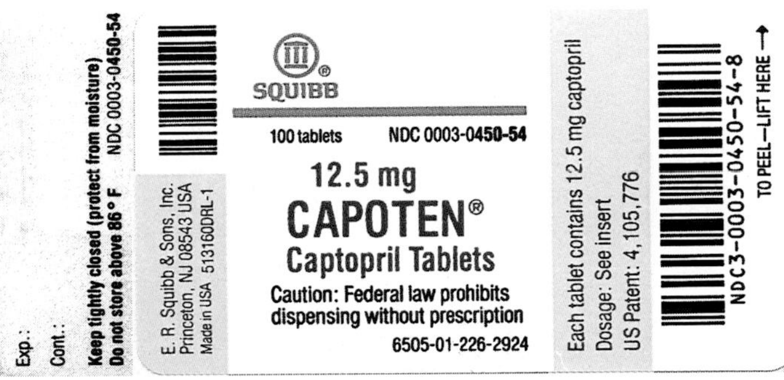

33. Doctor's Order: Clonazepam 0.25 mg p.o. b.i.d. and h.s.

    Available: Scored tablets labeled 0.5 mg. ____________

34. Doctor's Order: Augmentin 0.25 g p.o. q8h.

    Available: ____________

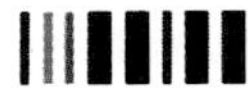
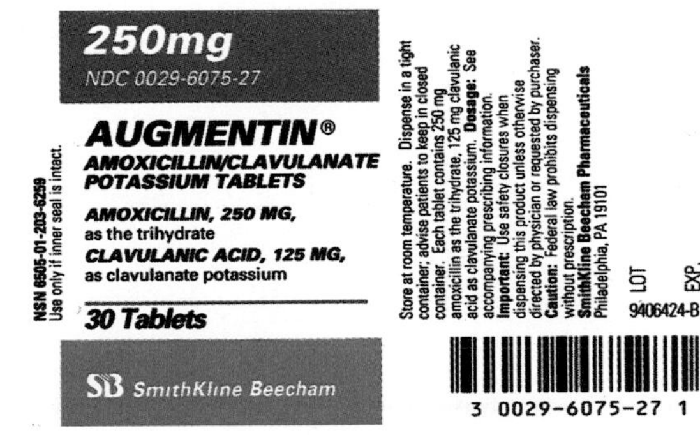

35. Doctor's Order: Synthroid 25 mcg p.o. o.d.

    Available: Tablets labeled 0.025 mg (25 mcg). ____________

36. Doctor's Order: Aspirin 650 mg p.o. q4h p.r.n.

 Available: ____________

37. Doctor's Order: Dilantin extended capsules 0.2 g p.o. t.i.d.

 Available: ____________

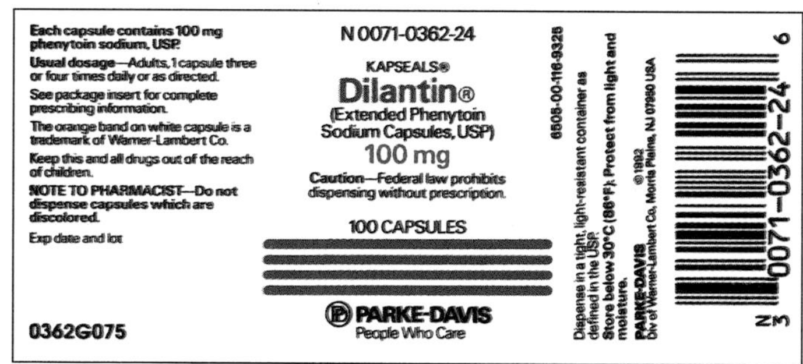

38. Doctor's Order: Motrin 800 mg p.o. q6h p.r.n.

 Available: ____________

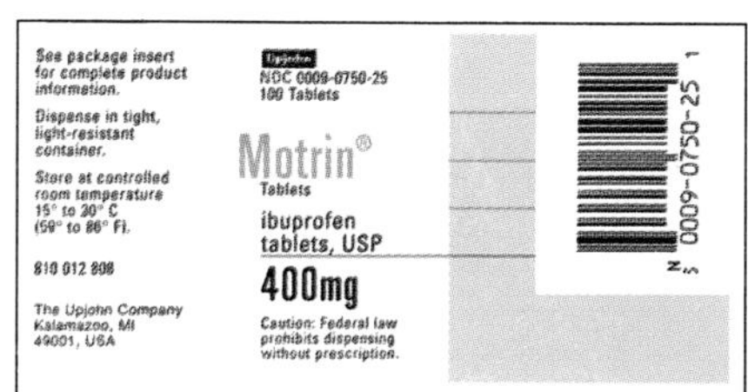

39. Doctor's Order: Procardia XL 60 mg p.o. q.d.

 Available: Procardia XL labeled 30 mg per tablet. ____________

40. Doctor's Order: Isoniazid 0.3 g p.o. q.d.

Available: ____________

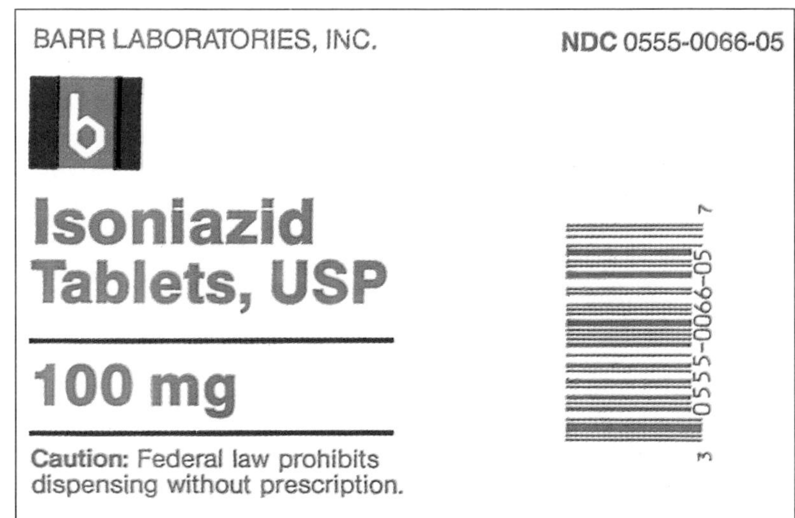

41. Doctor's Order: Inderal LA 160 mg p.o. q.d.

Available: Inderal LA capsules labeled 80 mg. ____________

Calculating Oral Liquids

Medications are also available in liquid form for oral administration. Liquid medications are desirable to use for clients who have dysphagia (difficulty swallowing) or who are receiving medications by tubes such as nasogastric (tube in nose to stomach), gastrostomy (tube placed directly into stomach), or jejunostomy (tube directly into intestines). Liquid medications are also desired for use in young children and infants. When medications are ordered that cannot be crushed for administration, the availability of the medication in liquid form should be investigated. Medications in liquid form contain a specific amount or weight of a drug in a given amount of solution that is indicated on the label. Liquid medications are prepared in different forms, as follows:

1. Elixir—Alcohol solution that is sweet and aromatic.
   Example: Phenobarbital elixir.
2. Suspension—One or more drugs finely divided into a liquid such as water.
   Example: Penicillin suspension.
3. Syrup—Medication dissolved in concentrated solution of sugar and water.
   Example: Colace.

Liquid medications also come as tincture and extract preparations for oral use. Even though oral liquids may be administered by means other than p.o., as already discussed, they should **never** be given by any other route, such as I.V. or by injection.

In solving problems that involve oral liquids, the methods presented in Chapters 13 and 14 can be used; however, you must calculate the volume or amount of liquid that contains the dose of the medication. This information is usually indicated on the medication label and can be expressed per milliliter, cubic centimeter, ounce, etc.—for example, 25 mg per mL. The amount may also be expressed in terms of multiple milliliters or cubic centimeters. Example: 80 mg per 2 mL, 125 mg per 5 mL.

When calculating liquid medications, the stock or what you have available is in liquid form; therefore the label on your answer will always be expressed in liquid measures such as mL, cc, m, etc.

Measuring Oral Liquids

The measurement of liquid medications can be done in several ways:

1. The standard measuring cup (plastic), which is calibrated in metric, apothecaries', and household measures, can be used. When pouring liquid medications, pour them at eye level and read at the meniscus (a curvature made by the solution) (Figure 15-5).

2. Calibrated droppers are also used for the measurement of liquid medications (Figure 15-6).
3. Syringes may also be used to measure medications. The medication is poured in a medication cup and drawn up in the syringe without the use of a needle. This is often done when the amount desired cannot be measured accurately in a cup. *Oral syringes* are designed for this purpose (Figure 15-7).

Before we proceed to calculate liquid medications, let's review some helpful pointers.

1. The label on the medication container must be read carefully to determine the dose strength in the volume of solution, since it varies. Do not confuse dose strength with the total volume. Example: the label on a medication may indicate a total volume of 100 cc, but the dose strength may be 125 mg per 5 cc. Figure 15-8 illustrates sample labels on oral medications.
2. Answers are labeled using liquid measures. Example: cc, mL.
3. Calculations can be done using the same methods (formula, ratio-proportion) and the same steps as for solid forms of oral medications.

Now let's look at some sample problems that involve the calculation of oral liquids.

Example 1: Doctor's order: Dilantin 200 mg p.o. t.i.d.

Available: Dilantin suspension labeled 125 mg per 5 mL.

Problem Setup

1. No conversion is required. Everything is in the same units of measure and the same system.
   Doctor's Order: 200 mg.
   Available: 125 mg per 5 mL.
2. Think critically: What would be a logical answer? Looking at Example 1, you can assume the answer will be greater than 5 mL.
3. Set up the problem using ratio-proportion or formula method.
4. Label the final answer with the correct unit of measure. In this case the label will be mL. Remember: The answer has no meaning without the appropriate label.

Solution Using Ratio-Proportion Method

$$125 \text{ mg} : 5 \text{ mL} = 200 \text{ mg} : x \text{ mL}$$

(Known) (Unknown)

$$125x = 200 \times 5$$

$$125x = 1000$$

$$x = \frac{1000}{125} = 8 \text{ mL}$$

Solution Using the Formula Method

$$\frac{(D)200 \text{ mg}}{(H)125 \text{ mg}} \times (Q)\ 5 \text{ mL} = x \text{ mL}$$

$$\frac{200}{125} \times 5 = \frac{1000}{125} = x = 8 \text{ mL}$$

OR

$$\frac{(DW)200 \text{ mg}}{(SW)125 \text{ mg}} = \frac{(DV)x \text{ mL}}{(SV)5 \text{ mL}}$$

$$x = \frac{1000}{125} = 8 \text{ mL}$$

Note: When possible, reduction of the numbers can be done to make them smaller and easier to deal with.

Figure 15-5. Measuring container. (From Clayton B, Stock Y: *Basic pharmacology for nurses,* ed 10, St Louis, 1993, Mosby.)

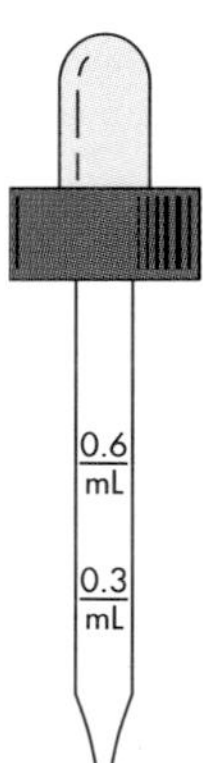

Figure 15-6. Medicine dropper. (From Brown M, Mulholland J: *Drug calculations: process and problems for clinical practice,* ed 5, St Louis, 1996, Mosby.)

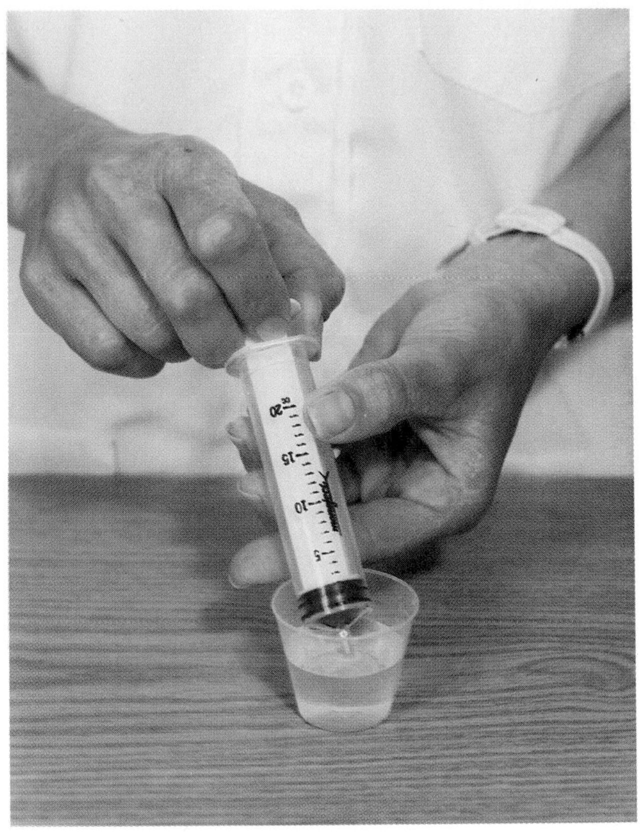

Figure 15-7. Filling syringe directly from medicine cup. (From Lilley L, Aucker R, Albanese J: *Pharmacology and the nursing process,* St Louis, 1996, Mosby.)

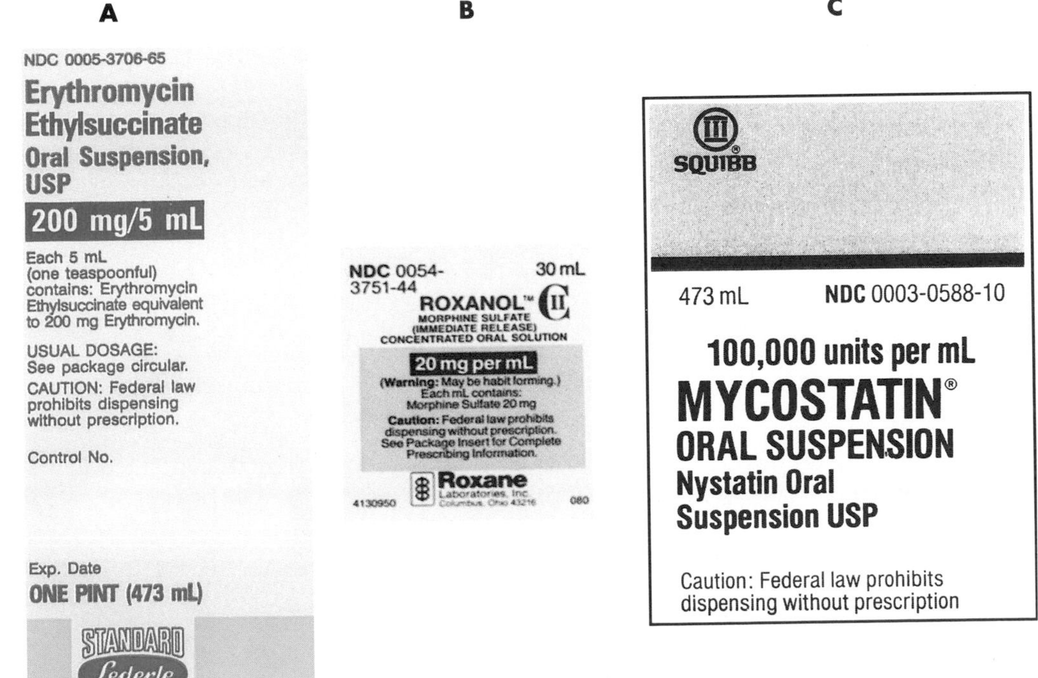

Figure 15-8. Drug labels. **A,** Erythromycin 200 mg. **B,** Roxanol 20 mg. **C,** Mycostatin 100,000 U. (From Dison N: *Simplified drugs and solutions for nurses,* ed 10, St Louis, 1992, Mosby.)

Example 2: Doctor's order: Lactulose 30 g p.o. b.i.d.

Available: Lactulose labeled 10 g = 15 mL.

➢Solution Using Ratio-Proportion Method

$$10 \text{ g} : 15 \text{ mL} = 30 \text{ g} : x \text{ mL}$$
$$10x = 450$$
$$x = 45 \text{ mL}$$

➢Solution Using the Formula Method

$$\frac{(D)30 \text{ g}}{(H)10 \text{ g}} \times (Q)\ 15 \text{ mL} = x \text{ mL}$$

$$\frac{30}{10} \times 15 = x = \frac{450}{10} = 45 \text{ mL}$$

OR

$$\frac{(DW)30 \text{ g}}{(SW)10 \text{ g}} = \frac{(DV)x \text{ mL}}{(SV)15 \text{ mL}}$$

$$x = \frac{450}{10} = 45 \text{ mL}$$

Example 3: Doctor's order: Elixir of phenobarbital gr iss p.o. o.d.

Available: Elixir of phenobarbital labeled 20 mg per 5 mL.

Note: A conversion is necessary before calculating the dose. What the doctor has ordered is different from what's available.

Doctor's order: gr iss

Available: 20 mg per 5 mL.

Equivalent: 60 mg = gr 1

$$60 \text{ mg} : \text{gr } 1 = x \text{ mg} : \text{gr } 1\frac{1}{2}\left(\frac{3}{2}\right)$$

$$60 \text{ mg} : \text{gr } 1 = x \text{ mg} : \text{gr } \frac{3}{2}$$

$$x = \frac{180}{2} = 90 \text{ mg}$$

➢Solution Using Ratio-Proportion Method

$$20 \text{ mg} : 5 \text{ mL} = 90 \text{ mg} : x \text{ mL}$$
$$20x = 450$$
$$x = \frac{450}{20}$$
$$x = 22.5 \text{ mL} \quad \text{or} \quad 22\frac{1}{2} \text{ mL}$$

➢Solution Using the Formula Method

$$\frac{(D)90 \text{ mg}}{(H)20 \text{ mg}} \times (Q)\ 5 \text{ mL} = x \text{ mL}$$

$$\frac{90}{20} \times 5 = x = \frac{450}{20} = 22.5 \text{ mL or } 22\frac{1}{2} \text{ mL}$$

OR

$$\frac{(DW)90 \text{ mg}}{(SW)20 \text{ mg}} = \frac{(DV)x \text{ mL}}{(SV)5 \text{ mL}}$$

$$x = \frac{450}{20} = 22.5 \text{ mL or } 22\frac{1}{2} \text{ mL}$$

Some medication orders that may be written by the doctor state the specific amount to be given and therefore require no calculation. Example: milk of magnesia ℥ i p.o. h.s., Robitussin 15 mL p.o. q4h p.r.n., multivitamin 1 tab p.o. o.d., Fer-In-Sol 0.2 cc p.o. o.d.

Points to Remember

- Liquid medications can be calculated using the same methods as those used for solid forms (tabs, caps).
- Read labels carefully on medication containers; identify the dose strength contained in a certain amount of solution.
- Administration of accurate doses of liquid medications may require the use of calibrated droppers or syringes.
- The use of ratio-proportion or a formula is a means of validating an answer; however, it still requires thinking in terms of the dose you will administer and applying principles learned to calculate doses that are sensible and safe.

Practice Problems on Oral Liquids (pp. 349-352)

Calculate the following doses for oral liquids in mL. Don't forget to label your answer. Labels have been included where possible. Round answers to the nearest tenth where indicated.

42. Doctor's Order: Colace syrup 100 mg by jejunostomy tube t.i.d.

    Available: ____________

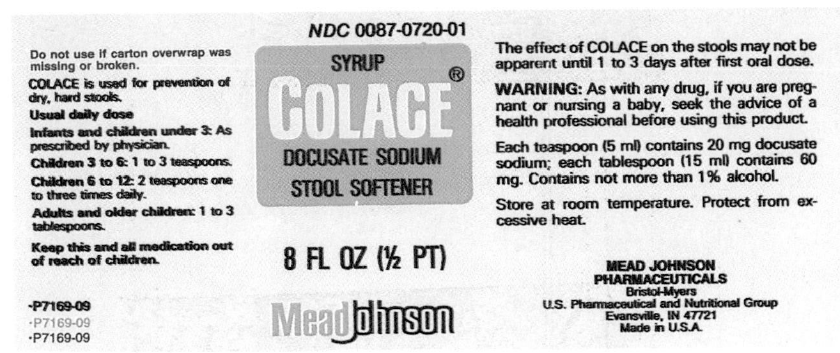

43. Doctor's Order: Ascorbic acid 1 g by nasogastric tube b.i.d.

    Available: Ascorbic acid solution 500 mg = 10 mL. ____________

44. Doctor's Order: Kaon-Cl 40 mEq p.o. o.d.

    Available: Potassium oral solution 40 mEq = 15 mL. ____________

45. Doctor's Order: Theophylline elixir 120 mg p.o. b.i.d.

    Available: Theophylline elixir 80 mg/5 mL. ____________

46. Doctor's Order: Erythromycin oral suspension 250 mg po q6h.

    Available: Erythromycin suspension 200 mg/5 mL.

    a) Determine how much solution is needed to administer the dose. ____________

47. Doctor's Order: Dilantin 100 mg p.o. t.i.d.

    Available: Dilantin suspension 125 mg/5 mL.

    a) Determine how much solution is needed to administer the dose. ____________

48. Doctor's Order: Digoxin 125 mcg p.o. o.d.

Available: ____________

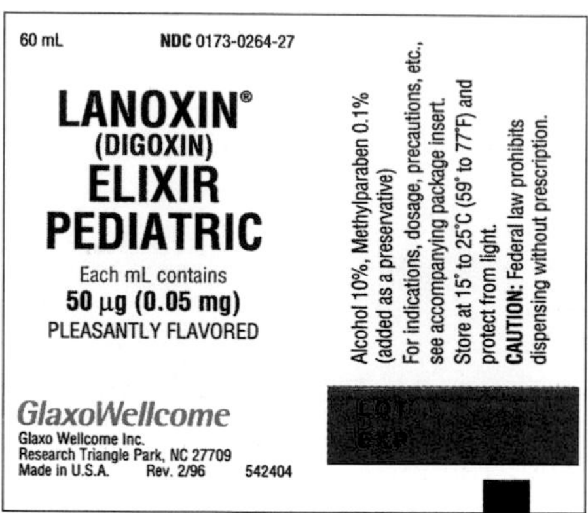

49. Doctor's Order: Keflex 250 mg p.o. q6h.

Available: ____________

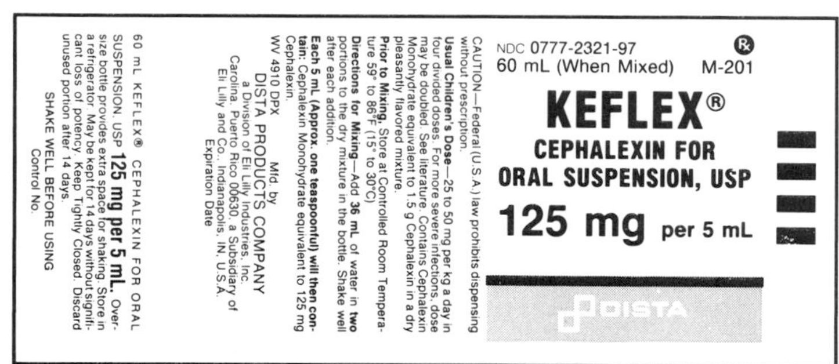

50. Doctor's Order: Amoxicillin 0.5 g p.o. q6h.

Available: Amoxicillin oral suspension 125 mg/5 mL.

a) Calculate the dose you will administer. ____________

51. Doctor's Order: Phenobarbital 60 mg p.o. h.s.

Available: Phenobarbital elixir 20 mg/5 mL.

a) Calculate the dose you will administer. ____________

52. Doctor's Order: Mellaril 150 mg p.o. b.i.d.

Available: Mellaril 30 mg/mL. ____________

53. Doctor's Order: Diphenhydramine HCl 25 mg p.o. b.i.d. p.r.n. for agitation.

Available: Diphenhydramine hydrochloride elixir 12.5 mg/5 mL.

a) Calculate the amount of medication you will administer. ____________

54. Doctor's Order: Lithium carbonate 600 mg p.o. h.s.

    Available: Lithium citrate syrup. Each 5 mL container contains lithium carbonate 300 mg.

    a) How many mL are needed to administer the required dose? ____________

    b) How many containers of the drug will you need to prepare the dose? ____________

55. Doctor's Order: Haldol 10 mg p.o. b.i.d.

    Available: Haldol concentrate labeled 2 mg/mL. ____________

56. Doctor's Order: Dicloxacillin sodium 0.5 g by gastrostomy tube q6h.

    Available: Dicloxacillin suspension 100 mL, labeled 62.5 mg per 5 mL. ____________

57. Doctor's Order: V-Cillin K suspension 500,000 U p.o. q.i.d.

    Available: V-Cillin K oral solution 200,000 Units per 5 mL.

    a) Calculate the dose you will administer. ____________

58. Doctor's Order: Keflex 1 g by nasogastric tube q6h.

    Available: Keflex oral suspension 125 mg/5 mL.

    a) Calculate the dose you will administer. ____________

59. Doctor's Order: Trilafon 24 mg p.o. b.i.d.

    Available: Trilafon concentrate labeled 16 mg/5 mL. ____________

60. Doctor's Order: Acetaminophen elixir 650 mg by nasogastric tube q4h p.r.n. for temperature greater than 101° F.

    Available: ____________

NDC 0054-8006

DELIVERS 10.15 ml

ACETAMINOPHEN
(Cherry)
325 mg per 10.15 ml

Elixir USP

ANALGESIC
Alcohol 7%
See Package Insert

Roxane Laboratories, Inc.
Columbus, Ohio 43216

PEEL
083

61. Doctor's Order: Tagamet 400 mg p.o. q6h.

    Available: Tagamet labeled 300 mg/5 mL. ____________

62. Doctor's Order: Epivir 150 mg p.o. b.i.d.

    Available: ______________

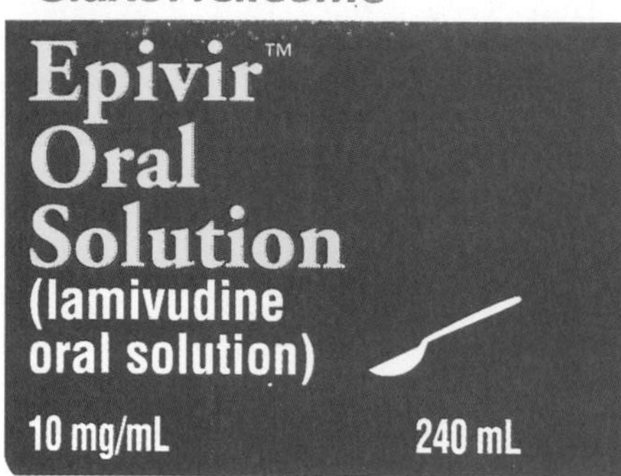

See package insert for Dosage and Administration.

Store between 2° and 25°C (36° and 77°F) in tightly closed bottles. Contains 6% alcohol.

4 0 5 8 8 9 5

Glaxo Wellcome Inc.
Research Triangle Park,
NC 27709
Manufactured in England
under agreement from
BioChem Pharma Inc.
Laval, Quebec, Canada
Rev. 10/95

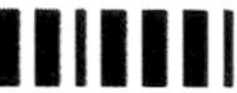

63. Doctor's Order: Retrovir 0.3 g p.o. b.i.d.

    Available: ______________

240 mL NDC 0173-0113-18

RETROVIR®
(zidovudine)
Syrup

Each 5 mL (1 teaspoonful) contains zidovudine 50 mg and sodium benzoate 0.2% added as a preservative.

CAUTION: Federal law prohibits dispensing without prescription.

U.S. Patent Nos. 4818538 (Product Patent); 4724232, 4833130, and 4837208 (Use Patents)

For indications, dosage, precautions, etc., see accompanying package insert.
Store at 15° to 25°C (59° to 77°F).

Made in U.S.A. Rev. 5/96 587023

GlaxoWellcome
Glaxo Wellcome Inc.
Research Triangle Park, NC 27709

LOT
EXP

64. Doctor's Order: Mycostatin suspension 200,000 U p.o. b.i.d.

    Available: ____________

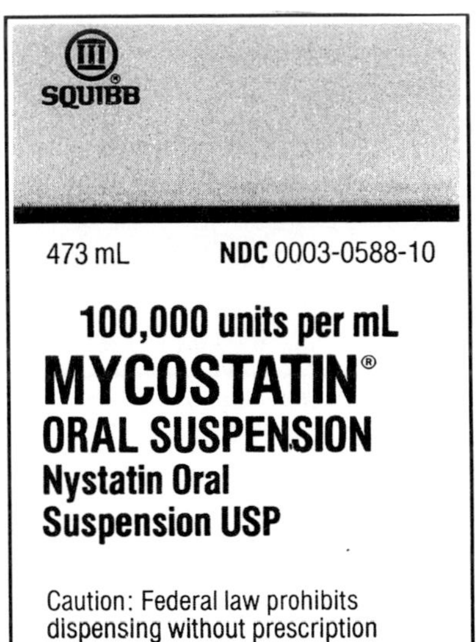

65. Doctor's Order: Thorazine concentrate 150 mg p.o. b.i.d.

    Available: ____________

Thorazine HCl Concentrate
100 mg/mL

66. Doctor's Order: Augmentin 0.25 g p.o. q8h.

    Available:

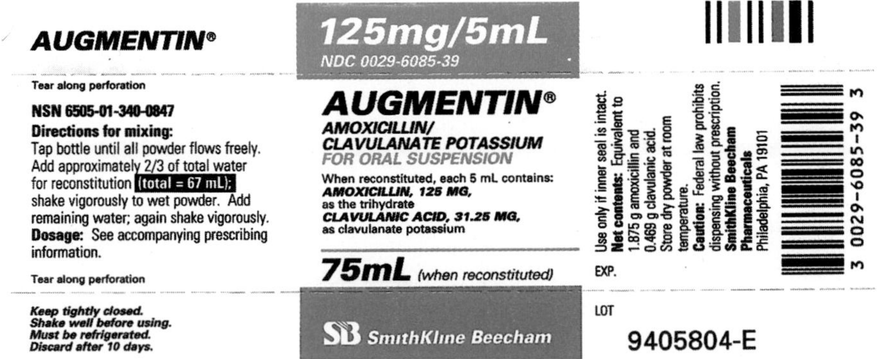

67. Doctor's Order: Zovirax 200 mg p.o. q4h 5×/day while awake × 5 days.

    Available: ______________

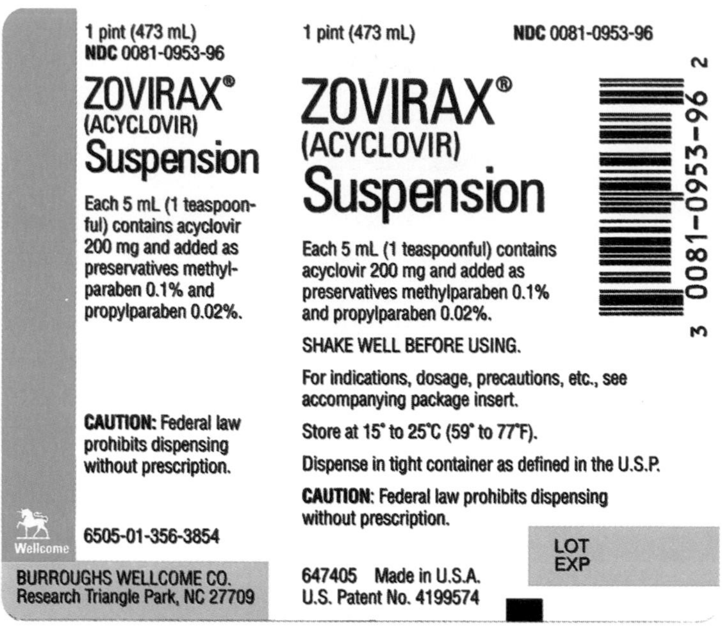

68. Doctor's Order: Prozac 30 mg p.o. q.d. in am & h.s.

    Available: ______________

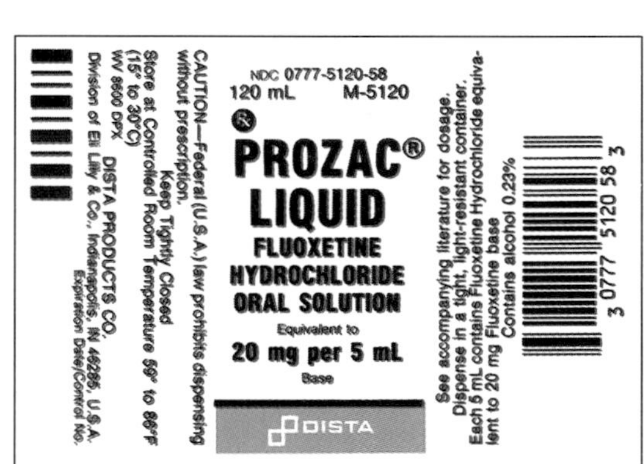

69. Doctor's Order: Zantac 150 mg b.i.d. via nasogastric tube.

Available: ____________

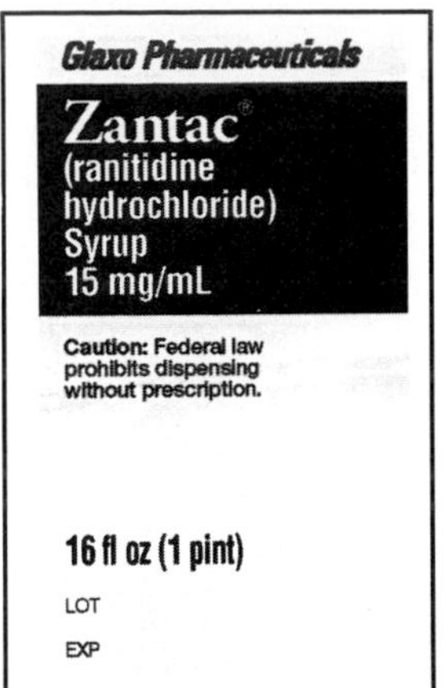

70. Doctor's Order: Milk of Magnesia ℥ i p.o. h.s.

Available: ____________

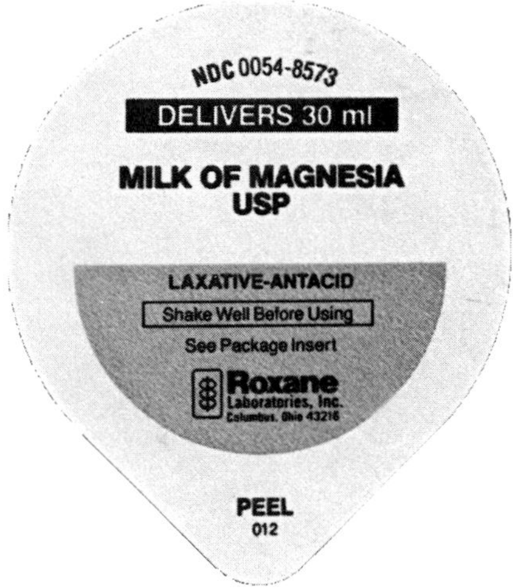

71. Doctor's Order: Mellaril 50 mg p.o. t.i.d.

Available: ______________

Dosage: See package insert for dosage information.
It is recommended that the Concentrate be used only for severe neuropsychiatric conditions.
Immediately before administration, dilute the dose of Concentrate with distilled water, acidified tap water, or suitable juices.
Suggested Dilution: 25 mg dose in 2 teaspoonfuls of diluent-liquid. For higher doses increase the volume of diluent.

2891-41 MEL-A19

NDC 0078-0001-31

4 fl. oz. (118 ml)

CONCENTRATE

MELLARIL®

(thioridazine) HCl
oral solution, USP

30 mg/ml

Each ml contains:
thioridazine HCl, USP .... 30 mg
alcohol, USP .... 3.0% by volume

CAUTION: Federal law prohibits dispensing without prescription.

6505-00-059-3497

Store and dispense: Below 86°F; tight, amber glass bottle

SANDOZ
PHARMACEUTICALS
CORPORATION
EAST HANOVER, NJ 07936

SPECIMEN

Quality Control No.
Exp.

Chapter 16

Parenteral Medications

Objectives

After reviewing this chapter the student will be able to do the following:

1. **Identify the various types of syringes used for parenteral administration**
2. **Read and measure doses on a syringe**
3. **Read medication labels on parenteral medications**
4. **Calculate doses of parenteral medications already in solution**
5. **Identify appropriate syringes to administer doses calculated**

The term *parenteral* is used to indicate medications that are administered by any route other than through the digestive system. However, the term parenteral is commonly used to refer to the administration of medications by injection with the use of a needle and syringe. Examples of common parenteral routes are I.M., s.c., intradermal, and I.V. Medications that are administered by the parenteral route act more quickly than oral medications because they are absorbed more rapidly into the bloodstream. The parenteral route may be desired when a rapid action of a drug is necessary, for a client who is unable to take a medication orally due to emesis (vomiting), or if a client is in an unconscious state. This route may also be desired for the client who is displaying irrational behavior and refuses medications by the oral route. Medications for parenteral use are available in liquid (solution) or powder. When medications are available in powder form, they must be diluted with a liquid or solvent (reconstituted) before they can be used. Reconstitution of drugs in powder form will be covered in Chapter 17.

Packaging of Parenteral Medications

Parenteral medications are packaged in various forms:

1. Ampule—This is a sealed glass container usually designed to hold a single dose of medication. Ampules have a particular shape with a constricted neck. They are designed to snap open. The neck of the ampule may be scored or have a darkened line or ring around it to

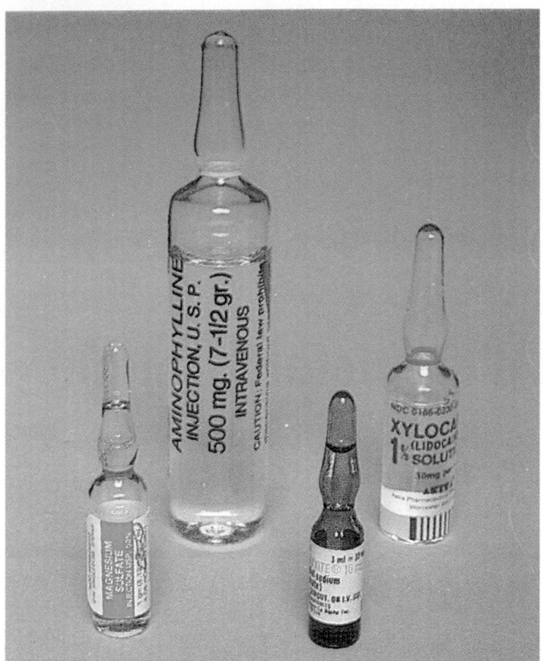

Figure 16-1. Medication in ampules. (From Elkin M, Perry A, Potter P: *Nursing interventions and clinical skills,* St Louis, 1996, Mosby.)

indicate where it should be broken to withdraw medication (Figure 16-1).

To withdraw the medication from an ampule the neck is snapped off by grasping the neck with an alcohol wipe or sterile gauze and breaking it off. An aspiration (filter) needle is inserted to withdraw the medication.

2. Vial—This is a plastic or glass container that has a rubber stopper (diaphragm) on the top. The rubber stopper is covered with a metal lid to maintain sterility until the vial is used for the first time (Figure 16-2). Vials are available in different sizes. Multidose vials contain more than one dose of the medication. The label on the vial will specify the amount of medication in a certain amount of solution, for example, 60 mg per mL, 0.2 mg per 0.5 mL. Single-dose vials contain a single dose of medication for injection. Most of the vials are multidose size. The medication in a vial may be in liquid (solution) form, or it may contain a powder that has to be reconstituted before administration.

   To withdraw medication from a vial, the top is wiped with alcohol, air equal to the amount of solution being withdrawn is injected into the vial through the rubber stopper, the vial is inverted, and the desired volume of medication is withdrawn. Withdrawal of large amounts of medication may require less air to be injected.
3. Mix-o-vial—Some medications come in mix-o-vials, for example, Solu-Medrol, Solu-Cortef. The vial usually contains a single dose of medication. The mix-o-vial has two compartments that are separated by a rubber stopper. The top compartment contains the sterile liquid (diluent), and the bottom compartment contains the powdered medication. When pressure is placed on the top of the vial, the rubber stopper that separates the medication and liquid is released. This allows the liquid and medication to be mixed, thereby dissolving the drug (Figure 16-3). A needle is inserted to withdraw the medication.
4. Cartridge—Some medications are packaged in a prefilled glass or plastic container. The cartridge is clearly marked, indicating the amount of medication in it. Certain cartridges require a special holder called a *Tubex* or *Carpujet* to release the medication from the cartridge. The cartridge usually contains a single dose of medication. The unused portion of medication is discarded (Figure 16-4).
5. Prepackaged syringe—The medication comes prepared for administration in a syringe with the needle attached. A specific amount of

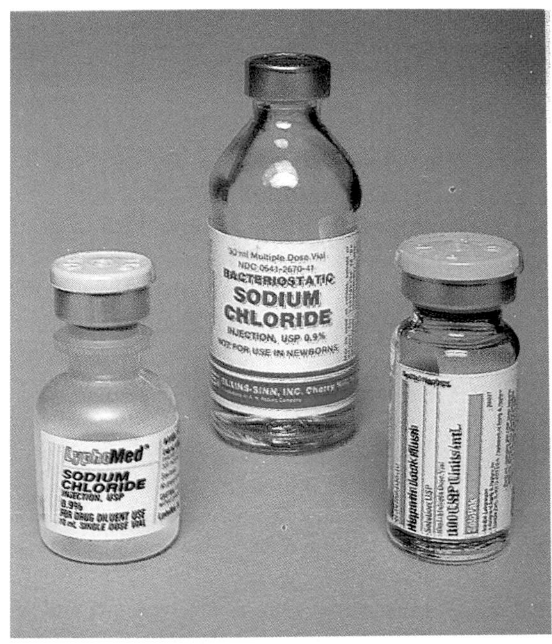

Figure 16-2. Medication in vials. (From Elkin M, Perry A, Potter P: *Nursing interventions and clinical skills,* St Louis, 1996, Mosby.)

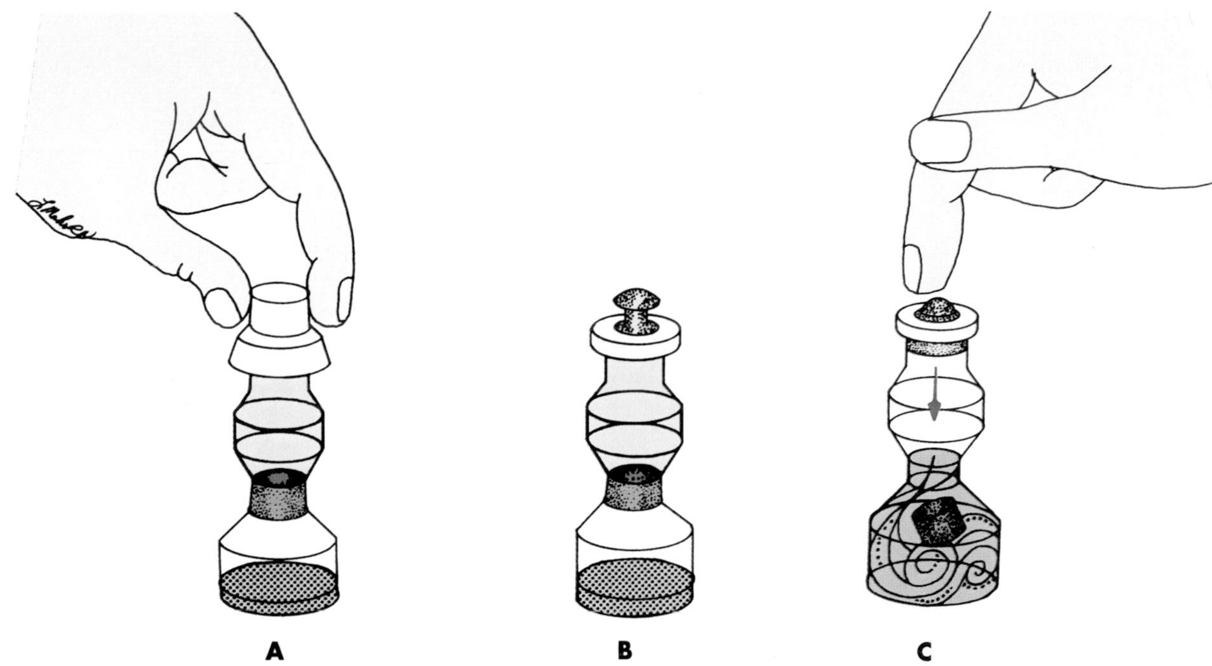

Figure 16-3. Mix-o-vial directions. (From Clayton B, Stock Y: *Basic pharmacology of nurses,* ed 10, St Louis, 1993, Mosby.)

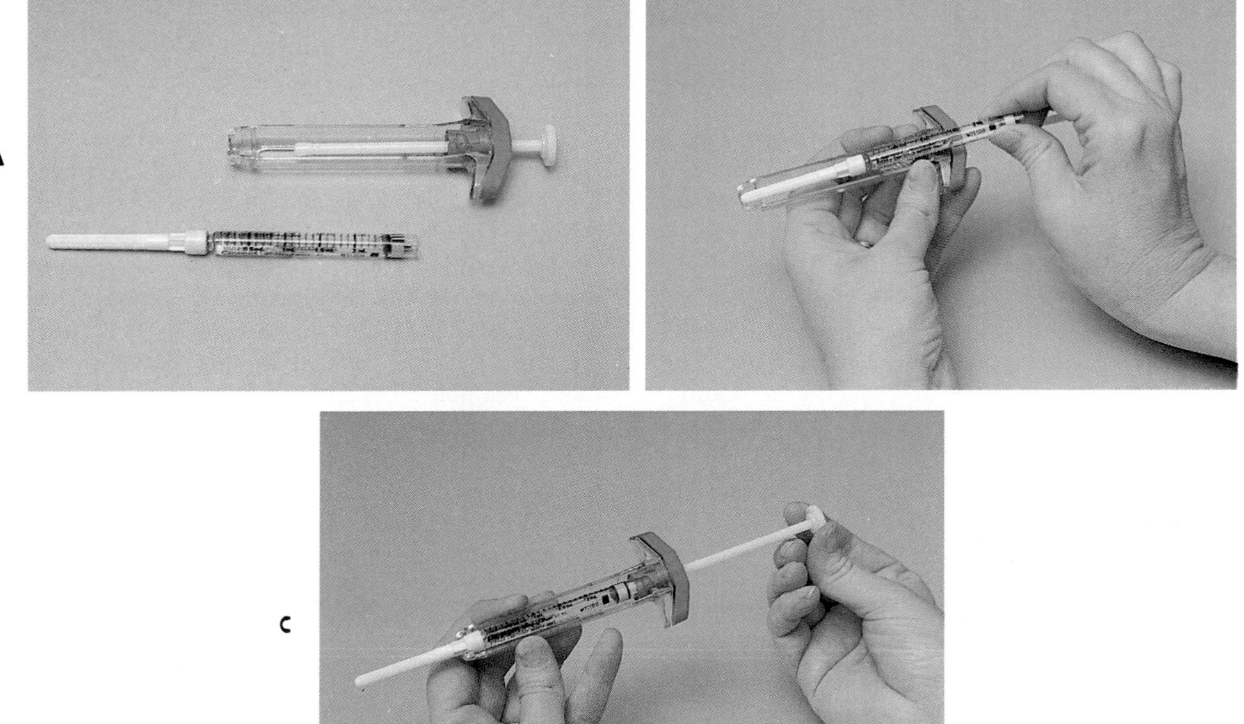

Figure 16-4. **A,** Carpujet syringe and prefilled sterile cartridge with needle. **B,** Assembling the Carpujet. **C,** Cartridge locks at needle end; plunger screws into opposite end. (From Elkin M, Perry A, Potter P: *Nursing interventions and clinical skills,* St Louis, 1996, Mosby.)

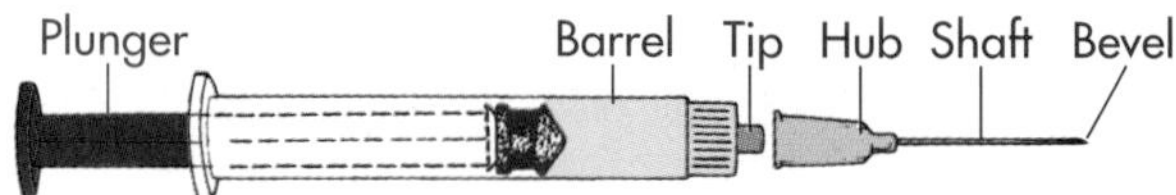

Figure 16-5. Parts of syringe. (From Elkin M, Perry A, Potter P: *Nursing interventions and clinical skills,* St Louis, 1996, Mosby.)

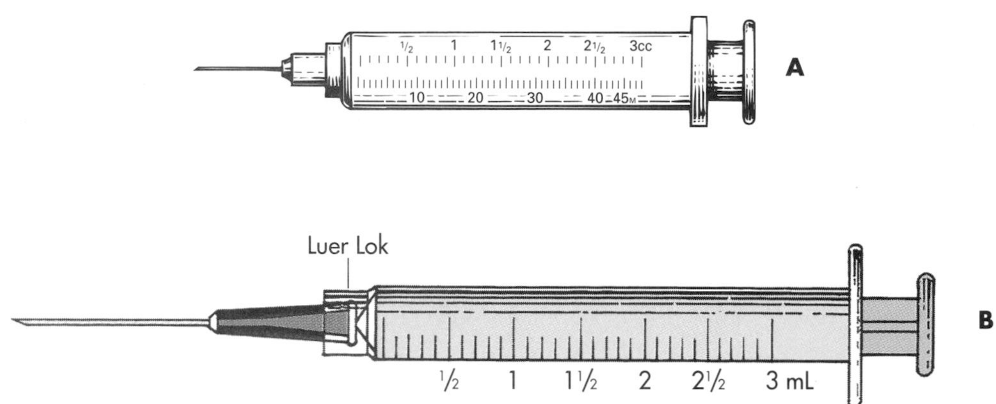

Figure 16-6. **A** and **B,** Small hypodermics. (**A,** From Brown M, Mulholland J: *Drug calculations: process and problems for clinical practice,* ed 5, St Louis, 1996, Mosby; **B,** from Elkin M, Perry A, Potter P: *Nursing interventions and clinical skills,* St Louis, 1996, Mosby.)

medication is contained in the syringe. The amount desired is administered, and the remainder is disposed of. These syringes are for single use only. Example: Valium comes in prepackaged syringes.

Syringes

Various size syringes are available for use. They have different capacities and specific calibrations. Syringes are made of plastic and glass. The plastic syringes are used more frequently. They are disposable and designed for one-time use only. Syringes have three parts:

1. The barrel—The outer portion that has the calibrations of the syringe on it
2. The plunger—The inner device that is pushed to eject the medication from the syringe
3. The tip—The end of the syringe that holds the needle (Figure 16-5). The tip can be plain or Luer-Lok (Figure 16-6)

Types of Syringes

The three types of syringes are hypodermic, tuberculin, and insulin.

Hypodermic syringes. Hypodermic syringes come in a variety of sizes. All the syringes are calibrated or marked in cc but hold varying capacities. The smaller-capacity syringes (2, 2 1/2, 3 cc) are used more often for the administration of medication; however, hypodermic syringes are also available in larger sizes (10, 20, 50 cc). There are some syringes labeled in mL, however, the most common labeling seen is cc. The smaller-capacity syringes (2, 2 1/2, 3 cc) are also calibrated in minims (m) (Figure 16-6).

For small hypodermics decimal numbers are used to express doses. (Example: 1.2 mL, 0.3 mL) Notice that the small hypodermics up to 3-cc size also have fractions on them. Therefore to state doses involving the decimal 0.5 it is realistic to state the answer as a fraction for administrative purposes. Example: state 0.5 mL as 1/2 mL.

Notice the side that indicates cc or mL. There are 10 spaces between the largest markings. This indicates the syringe is marked in tenths of a cc. Each of the lines is 0.1 cc. The longer lines indicate 1/2 (0.5) and full cc measures. On the other side of the syringe there are minim markings. Each small line counts as 1 minim, and the longer lines represent 5-minim increments—5, 10, etc.

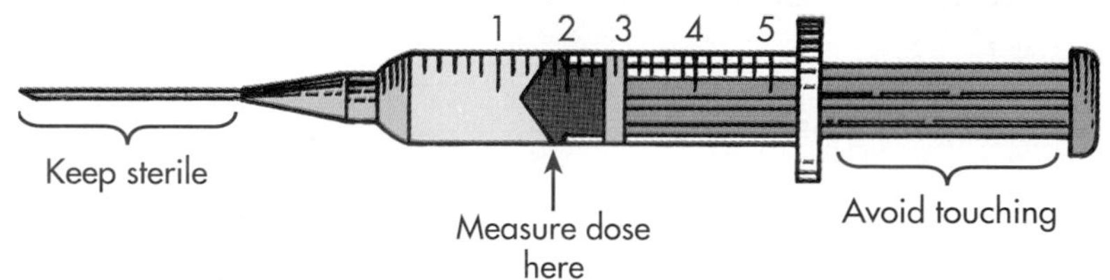

Figure 16-7. Reading measured amount of medication in a syringe. (From Elkin M, Perry A, Potter P: *Nursing interventions and clinical skills,* St Louis, 1996, Mosby.)

When looking at the syringe shown in Figure 16-7, notice the rubber ring. When measuring medication and reading the medication withdrawn, the forward edge of the plunger head indicates the amount of medication withdrawn. The point where the rubber plunger tip makes contact with the barrel is the spot that should be lined up with the amount desired.

Let's examine the syringes below to illustrate specific amounts in a syringe.

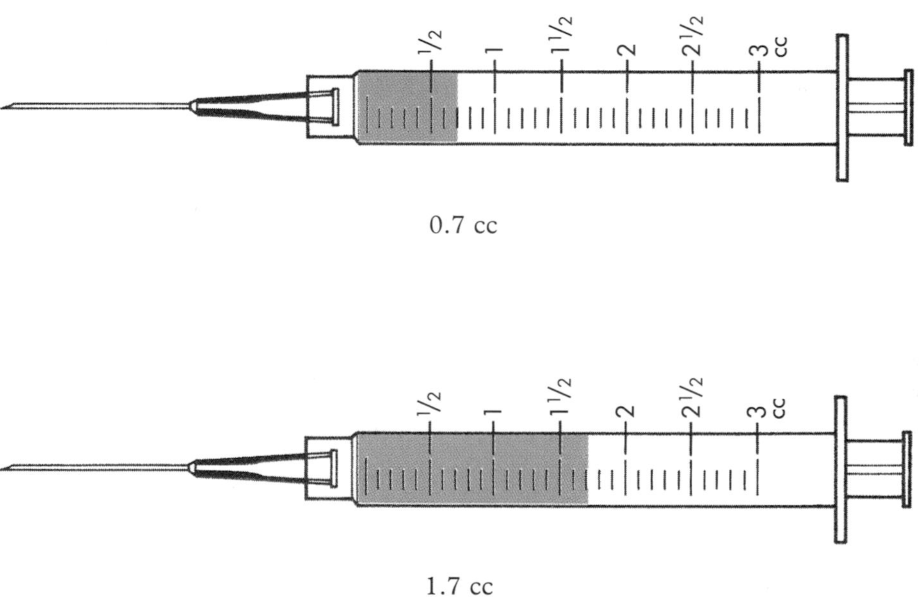

Since the smaller-capacity syringes are used most often for the administration of medications, it is very important to know how to read them to draw up amounts accurately.

Points to Remember

- Small-capacity hypodermics (2, 2 1/2, 3 cc) are calibrated in 0.1 cc and minims. Doses administered with them must correlate to the calibration.
- Remember cc and mL are equivalent, and syringes are labeled using both abbreviations. However, the abbreviation or measurement seen most often is cc.

Practice Problems (p. 353)

Shade in the indicated amounts on the syringes.

1. 0.8 cc
2. 1.2 cc
3. m 10
4. 1.5 cc
5. 2.4 cc

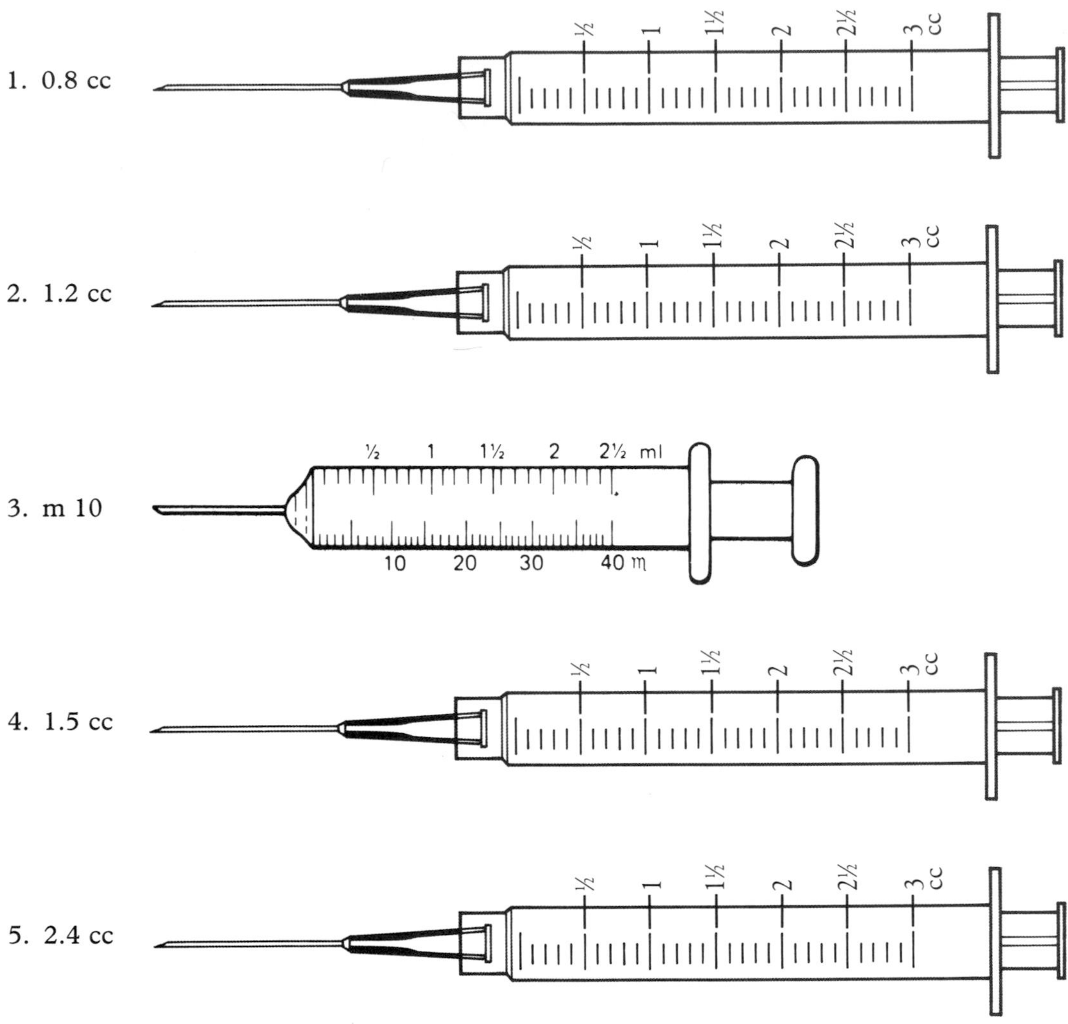

Identify the number of m shaded in on the syringe in Problem 6 and the number of cc shaded in on the syringes in Problems 7-10.

6. __________

7. __________

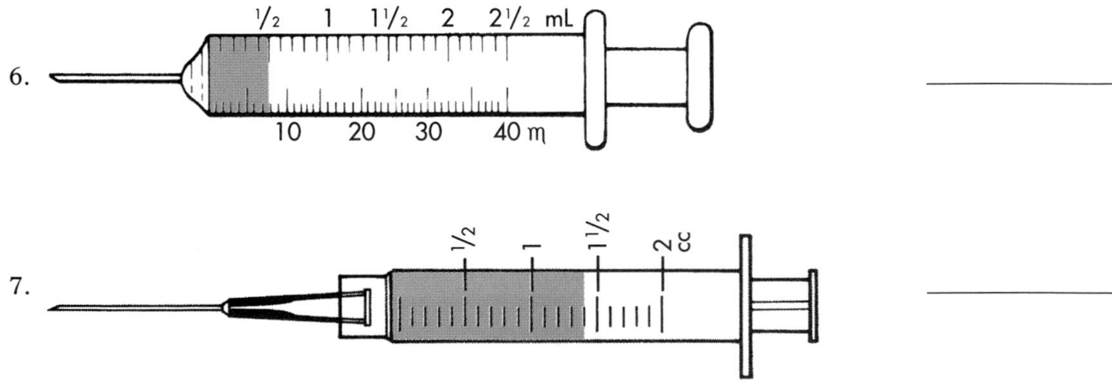

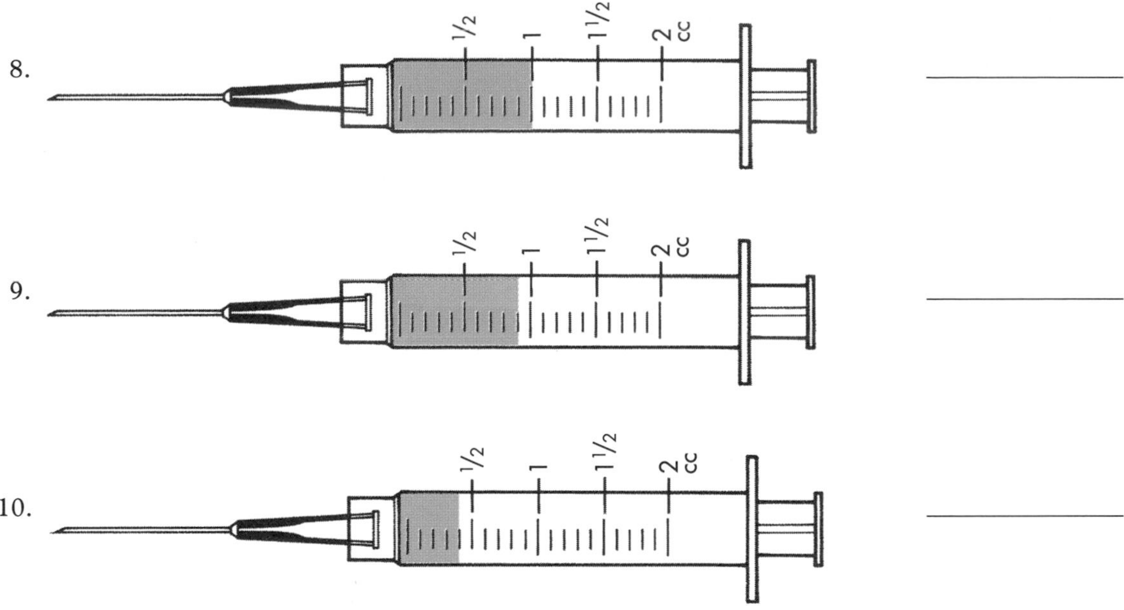

The larger hypodermics (5, 6, 10, 12 cc) are used when volumes larger than 3 cc are desired. These syringes are used to measure whole numbers of cc as opposed to smaller units such as a tenth of a cc. There are no minim markings on the larger syringes. Syringes 5, 6, 10, and 12 cc in size are calibrated in increments of fifths of a cc (0.2 cc), with whole number indicated by the long lines. Figure 16-8, *A*, shows 0.8 cc of medication drawn up, and Figure 16-8, *B*, shows 4.8 cc drawn up. Syringes that are 20 cc and larger are calibrated in full cc measures and can have other measures, such as ounces, on them.

Remember: The larger the syringe, the larger the calibration.

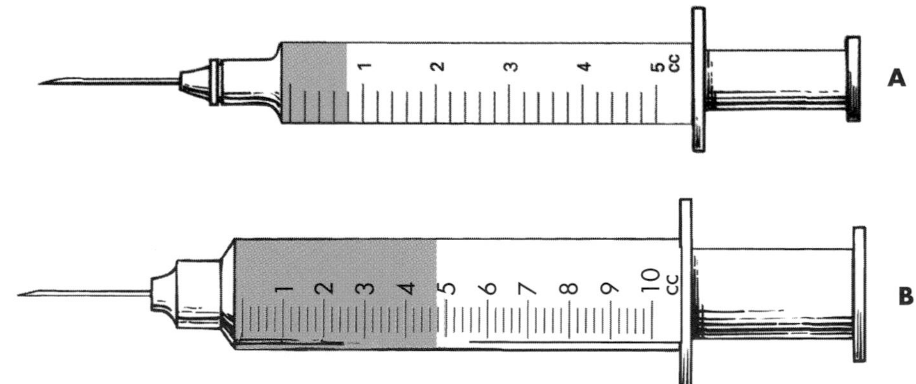

Figure 16-8. Large hypodermic. **A,** 5-cc syringe filled with 0.8 cc. **B,** 10-cc syringe filled with 4.8 cc. (From Brown M, Mulholland J: *Drug calculations: process and problems for clinical practice,* ed 5, St Louis, 1996, Mosby.)

Practice Problems (p. 353)

Indicate the number of ccs shaded in on the following syringes.

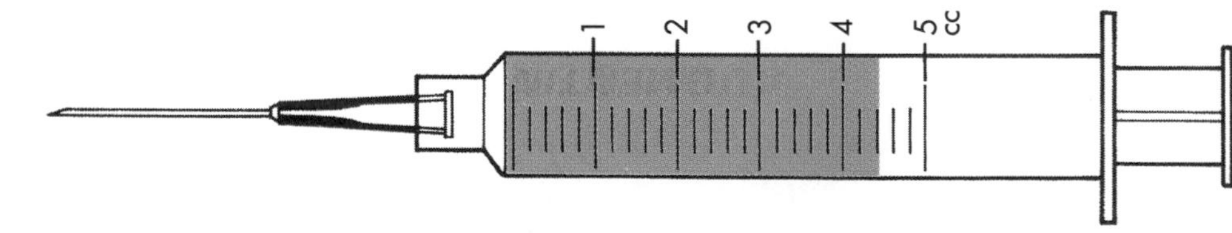

11. ____________

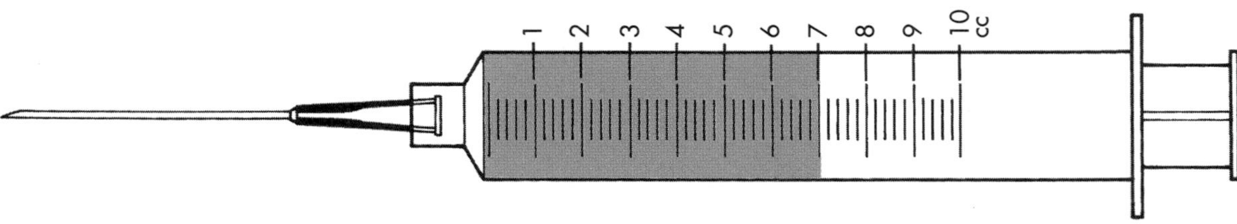

12. ____________

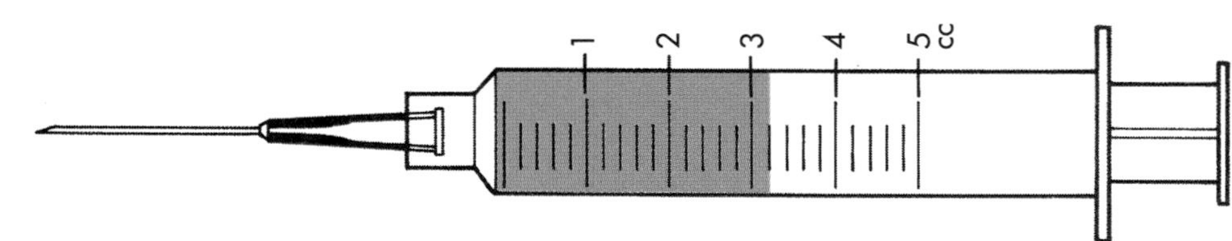

13. ____________

Tuberculin syringe. This is a narrow syringe that has a total capacity of 1 cc. The volume of a tuberculin syringe can be measured on the cc or the minim scale. On the minim side of the syringe, the lines represent 1 minim. On the cc side of the syringe the syringe is calibrated in hundredths of a cc. The markings on the syringe (lines) are closer together to indicate how small the calibrations are (Figure 16-9).

Tuberculin syringes are used to accurately measure medications that are given in very small volumes (for example, heparin). This syringe is also frequently used in pediatrics and for diagnostic purposes (for example skin testing, test for tuberculosis). It is recommended that doses less than 0.5 mL be measured using a tuberculin syringe to make certain that the correct dose is administered to a client. Doses such as 0.42 cc and 0.37 cc can be measured accurately using a tuberculin syringe. When using a tuberculin syringe, it is important to read it carefully to avoid error.

Insulin syringes. These syringes are designed for the administration of insulin. Insulin doses are measured in units (U). Insulin syringes are calibrated to match the dose strength of the insulin being used. They are marked U-100 and are designed to be used with insulin that is marked U-100. There are two types of insulin syringes.

The *Lo-Dose syringe* is used to measure small doses and is 0.5 mL in size. It may be used for clients receiving 50 U or less of U-100 insulin. It has a capacity of 50 U. The scale on the Lo-Dose syringe is easy to read. Each calibration (shorter lines) measures 1 U, and each 5-U increment is numbered (long lines) (Figure 16-10).

A 30 U syringe is also available for use with U-100 insulin only and is designed for small doses of 30 U or less. Each increment on the syringe represents 1 U (Figure 16-11).

The *1-mL size syringe* is designed to hold 100 U. There are currently two types on the market. One type of 1 CC (100 U) capacity has each 10-U increment numbered. This syringe is calibrated in 2-U increments. Odd-numbered units are therefore measured between the even calibrations (Figure 16-12). Use of this syringe should be avoided if possible since accuracy of the dose is questionable. The second type of 1 cc-capacity syringe has two scales on it. The odd numbers are on the left of the syringe and the even are on the right. The calibrations are in 1 U increments. The best method for using this type of syringe is the following: Measure uneven doses on the left, and measure even doses using the scale on the right (Figure 16-13). The calculation of insulin doses and reading of the calibrations are discussed in more detail in Chapter 18.

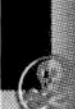

Think Critically to Avoid Drug Calculation Errors

- Doses must be measurable and appropriate for the syringe used.
- When reading syringes with both minim (m) and cubic centimeter calibration (cc), remember they are not the same measurement. It is critical to avoid making errors with m and cc.
- The insulin syringe and the tuberculin syringe are different. Confusion of the two can cause a medication error.
- If the dose cannot be accurately measured, don't give it.

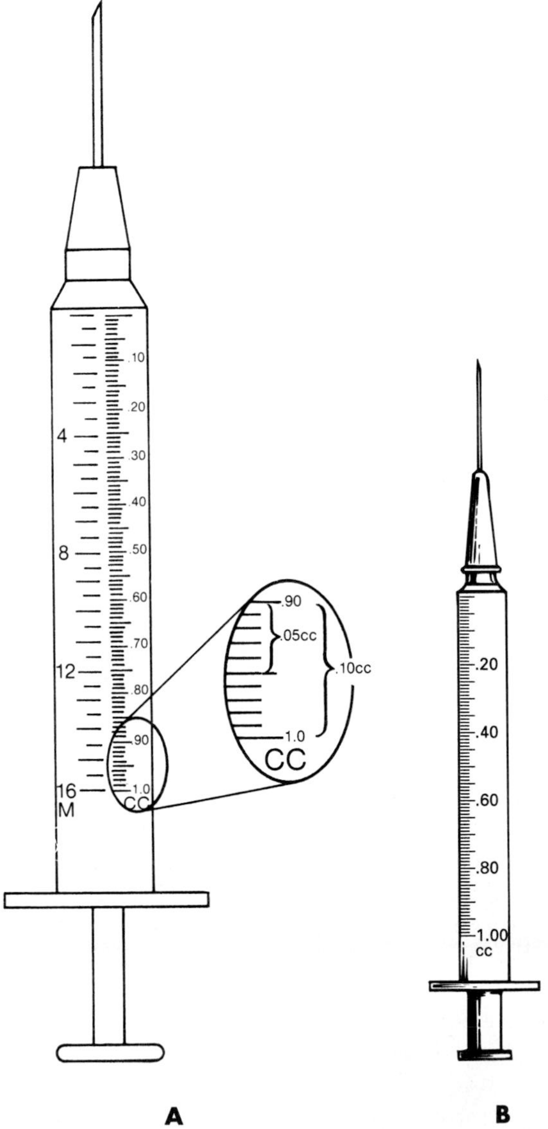

Figure 16-9. Tuberculin syringes. **A,** Marked in 0.01 cc increments. **B,** 1 cc syringe. (From Brown M, Mulholland J: *Drug calculations: process and problems for clinical practice,* ed 5, St Louis, 1996, Mosby.)

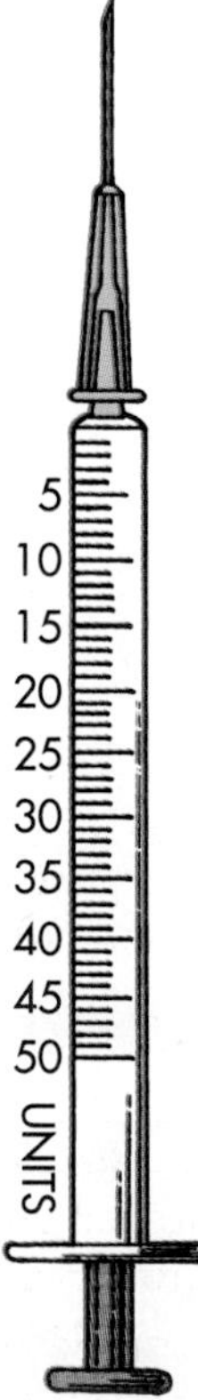

Figure 16-10. Lo-Dose syringe 1/2 mL in size (50 U). (From Elkin M, Perry A, Potter P: *Nursing interventions and clinical skills,* St Louis, 1996, Mosby.)

Points to Remember

- Hypodermic syringes—2, 2 1/2, and 3 cc—are marked in minims and 0.1 cc. These small-capacity syringes are most often used for medication administration.
- Hypodermic syringes—5, 6, 10, and 12 cc—are marked in increments of 0.2 cc and 1 cc.
- Hypodermic syringes—20 cc and larger—are marked in 1-cc increments and may have other markings, such as ounces.
- Tuberculin syringes—small syringes that are marked in minims and hundredths of a cc. They are used for the administration of small doses and are recommended for use with a dose less than 0.5 cc.
- Insulin syringes—marked U-100 for administration with U-100 Insulin only. Insulin is measured in units.
- The larger the syringe, the larger the calibration.
- For small hypodermics, doses involving the decimal 0.5 should be expressed as a fraction up to 3 cc in size. Other values are expressed as decimal numbers.

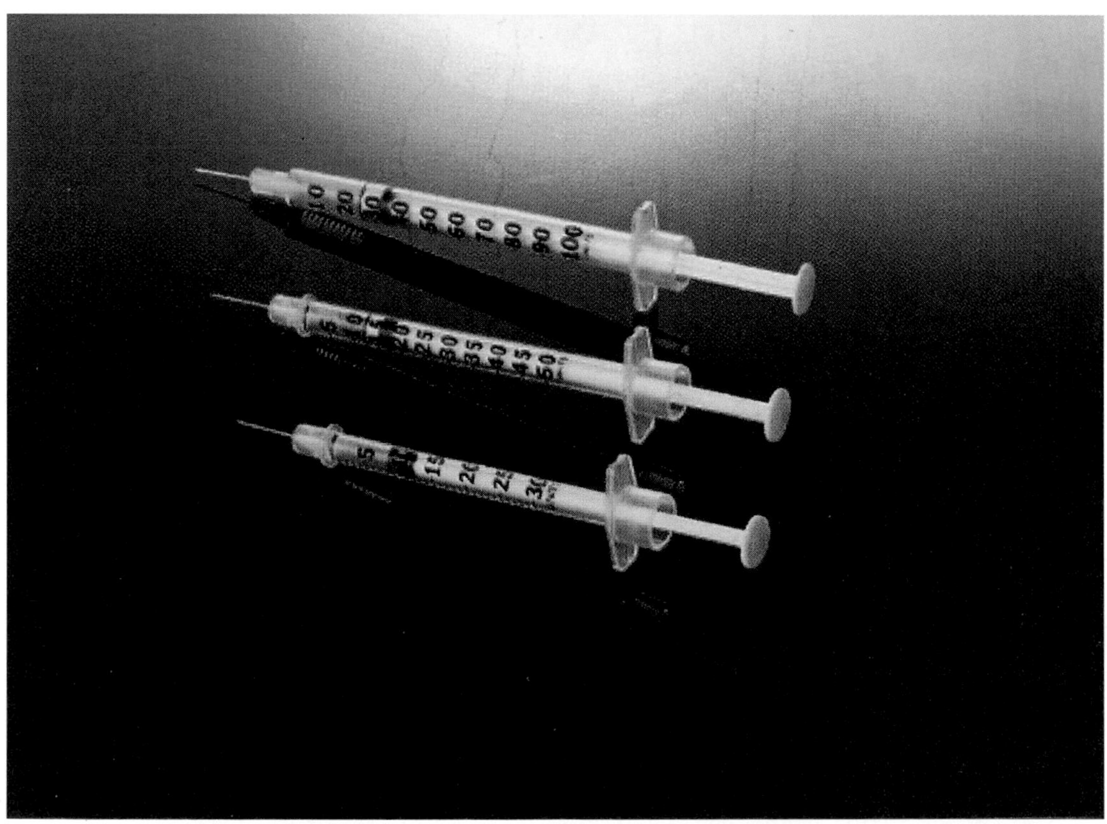

Figure 16-11. Insulin syringes of 30, 50, and 100 U. (From Brown M, Mulholland J: *Drug calculations: process and problems for clinical practice,* ed 5, St Louis, 1996, Mosby.)

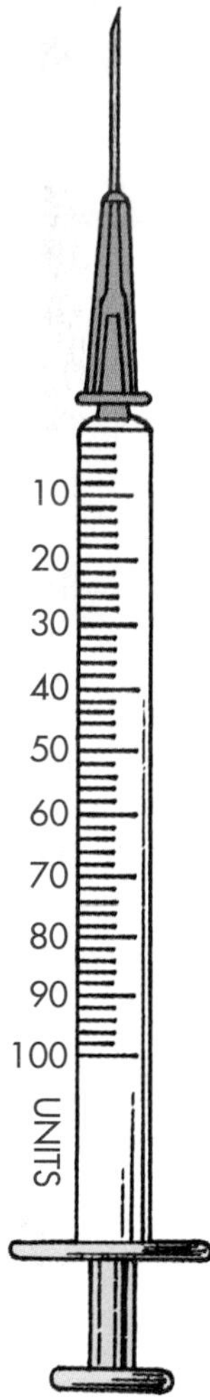

Figure 16-12. 1-cc capacity syringe (holds 100 units). (From Elkin M, Perry A, Potter P: *Nursing interventions and clinical skills,* St Louis, 1996, Mosby.)

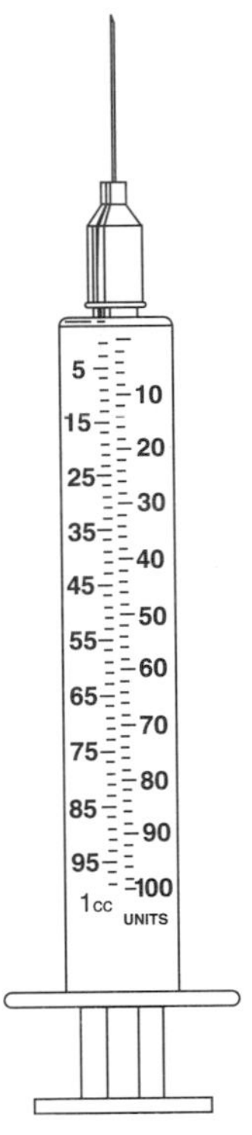

Figure 16-13. 1-cc capacity syringe—insulin syringe with two scales. (From Brown M, Mulholland J: *Drug calculations: process and problems for clinical practice,* ed 5, St Louis, 1996, Mosby.)

Before proceeding to discuss calculation of parenteral doses, it is necessary to review some specifics in terms of reading labels. Reading the label and understanding what information is essential is important in determining the correct dose to administer.

Reading Parenteral Labels

The information contained on the parenteral label is similar to the information on an oral liquid label. It contains the total volume of the container and the dose strength (amount of medication in solution) expressed in cc or mL. It is important to read the label carefully to determine the dose strength and volume. Example: 25 mg per mL

Let's examine some labels. In examining the Vistaril label on p. 120 in Chapter 13, notice the total size of the vial is 10 mL. The dose strength is 50 mg per mL.

The atropine label following shows that the total vial size is 20 mL; however, there are 0.4 mg per mL. It is important to realize that although there is a total of 20 mL, each mL contains 0.4 mg.

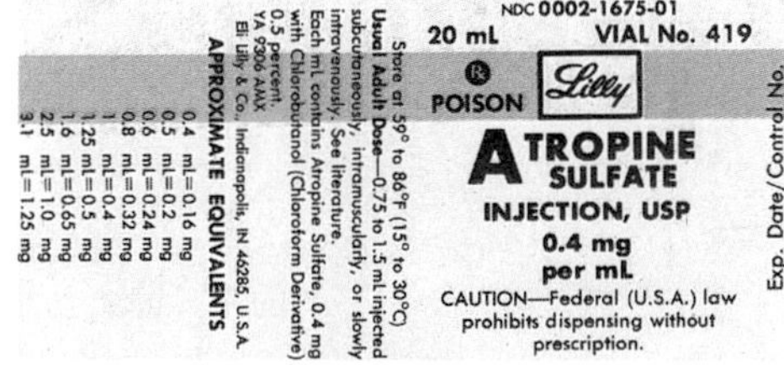

The codeine label has a combination of two systems of measurement: grains, which is apothecaries', and mg and mL, which are metric. The vial size is 20 mL. Notice it states 30 mg (1/2 gr) per mL. If 60 mg = gr 1, then gr 1/2, which is 30 mg, is contained in 1 mL.

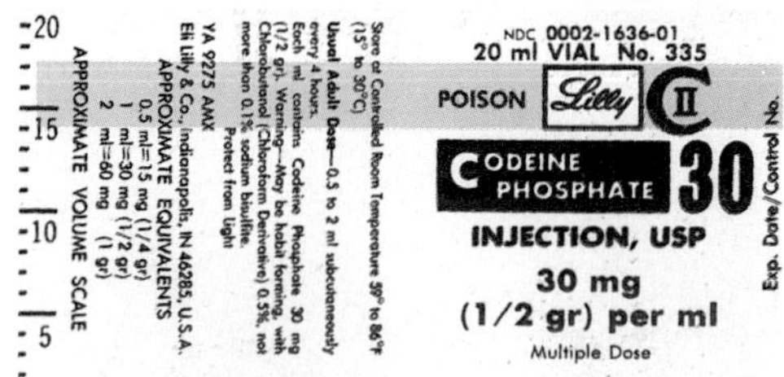

As you can see, the dose strength on parenteral labels can be expressed in metric, apothecaries', or a combination of both.

Practice Problems: Reading Parenteral Labels (p. 353)

Use the labels provided to answer the questions.

Aminophylline Injection, USP
500 mg/20 mL
(25 mg/mL)

14. What is the total volume of the ampule? __________

15. What is the dose strength? __________

16. If 250 mg were ordered, how many mL would this be? __________

Caution: Federal law prohibits dispensing without prescription. See package insert for complete product information. Store at controlled room temperature (20° to 25° C or 68° to 77° F) [see USP]. Each mL contains: Ibutilide fumarate, 0.1 mg; sodium chloride, 8.90 mg; sodium acetate trihydrate, 0.189 mg; water for injection. When necessary, pH was adjusted with sodium hydroxide and/or hydrochloric acid.
816 416 000
The Upjohn Company
Kalamazoo, MI 49001, USA

NDC 0009-3794-01 10 mL
Corvert™
Injection
ibutilide fumarate injection
0.1 mg per mL
For IV use only

17. What is the total volume of the vial? __________

18. What is the dose strength? __________

19. What is the route of administration? __________

NSN 6505-01-156-1981
Dilute before I.V. use. Store below 86°F
Do not freeze. Protect from light.
Each mL contains, in aqueous solution, chlorpromazine hydrochloride, 25 mg; ascorbic acid, 2 mg; sodium bisulfite, 1 mg; sodium sulfite, 1 mg; sodium chloride, 1 mg. Contains benzyl alcohol, 2%, as preservative. See accompanying prescribing information. For deep I.M. injection.
Caution: Federal law prohibits dispensing without prescription.
Manufactured by **SmithKline Beecham Pharmaceuticals**, Philadelphia, PA 19101
Marketed by SCIOS NOVA INC.
LOT EXP.
683897-AE

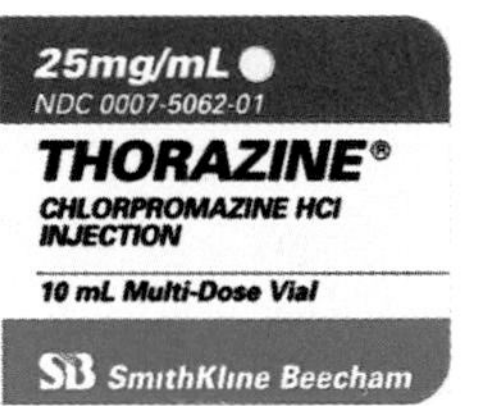

20. What is the total volume of the vial? __________

21. What is the dose strength? __________

22. If 50 mg were ordered, how many mL would this be? __________

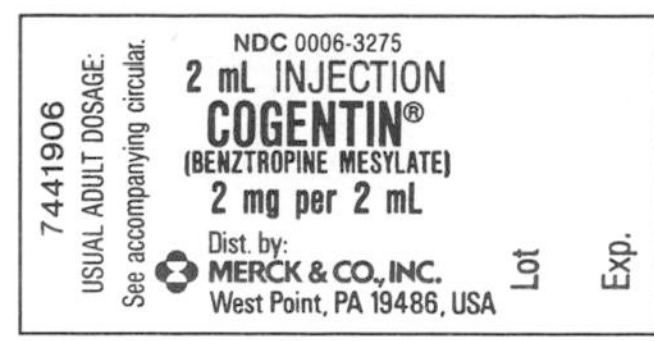

23. What is the total volume of the ampule? ____________

24. What is the dose strength? ____________

25. If 1 mg were ordered, how many mL would this be? ____________

Parenteral labels can express medications in percentage strengths, as well as units and milliequivalents.

Drugs Labeled in Percentage Strengths

Drugs that are labeled as percentage solutions give information such as the percentage of the solution and the total volume of the vial or ampule. Although percentage is used, metric measures are used as well. Example: The figure below, which shows a label of Lidocaine 1%. Notice there are 10 mg/mL.

5 mL NDC 0074-4713-02
1% Lidocaine
HCl Inj., USP
50 mg (10 mg/mL)
06-5915-2/R5-6/86
Abbott Laboratories
N. Chicago, IL60064, USA

Often no calculation is necessary when giving medications expressed in percentage strength. The doctor usually states the number of cc or mL to prepare or may state it in the number of ampules or vials. Example: Calcium gluconate 10% may be ordered as "Administer one vial of 10% calcium gluconate or 10 cc of 10% calcium gluconate" (see figure below).

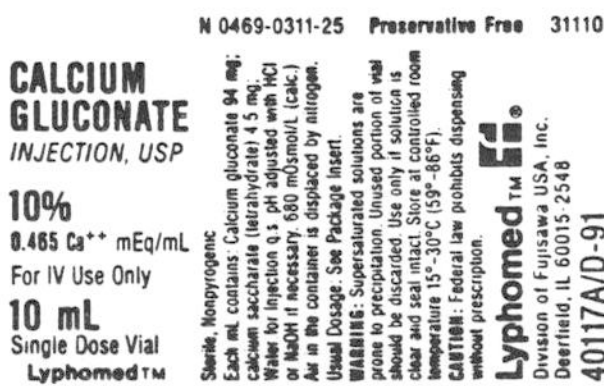

Solutions Expressed in Ratio Strength

A medication commonly expressed in terms of ratio strength is epinephrine. Drugs expressed this way include metric measures as well and are often ordered by the number of cc and mL. Example: Epinephrine may state 1:1000 and indicate 1 mg/mL.

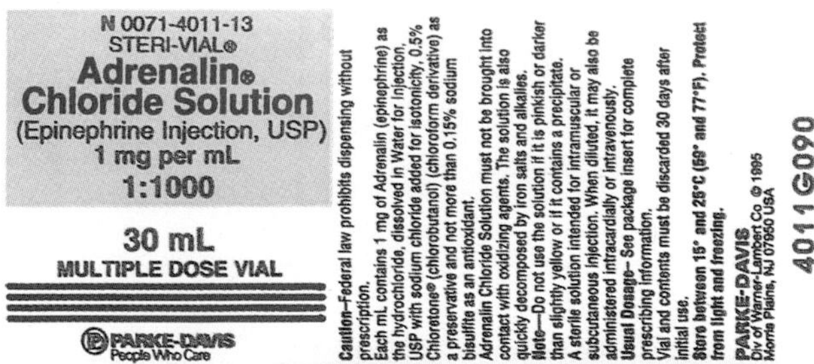

Parenteral Medications Measured in Units

Some medications measured in units for parenteral administration are heparin, pitocin, insulin, and penicillin. Notice the labels indicate how many units per mL. Example: Pitocin 10 U/mL, Heparin 1000 U/mL. Units express the amount of drug present in 1 mL of solution, and they are specific to the drug for which they are used.

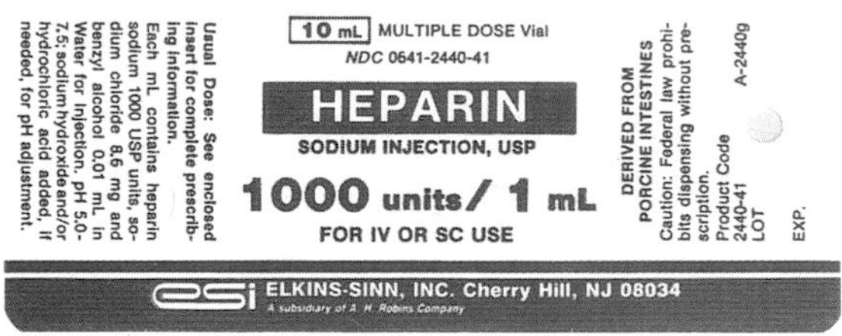

Parenteral Medications in Milliequivalents

Potassium and sodium bicarbonate are drugs that are expressed in milliequivalents. Like units, milliequivalents are specific measurements that have no conversion to another system and are specific to the medication used. Milliequivalent (mEq) is used to measure electrolytes (for example, potassium) and the ionic activity of a drug.

Practice Problems (p. 353)

Use the labels provided to answer the questions.

Potassium Chloride Label
40 mEq/20 mL
(2 mEq/mL)

26. What is the total volume of the vial? ____________

27. What is the dose in mEq/mL? ____________

Sodium Bicarbonate Injection Label
84 mg/mL
50 mL Single dose vial

28. What is the total volume of the vial? ____________

29. What is the dose strength? ____________

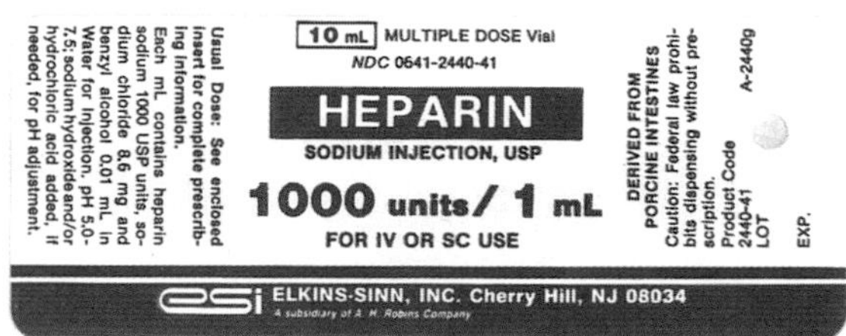

30. What is the total volume of the vial? ____________

31. What is the dose strength? ____________

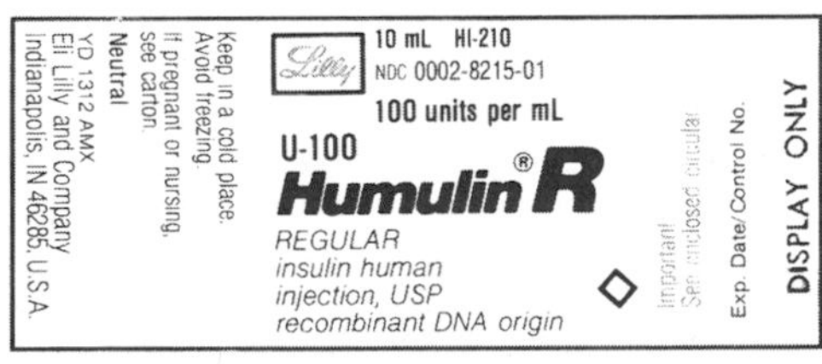

32. What is the total volume of the vial? ____________

33. What is the dose strength? ____________

NDC 0002-2307-48
100 mL (When Mixed) M-126

Rx Lilly

V-CILLIN K®

PENICILLIN V POTASSIUM
FOR ORAL SOLUTION, USP

125 mg
(200,000 Units) per 5 mL

CAUTION—Federal (U.S.A.) law prohibits dispensing without prescription.

PULL

Usual Dose Range: One or two teaspoonfuls every 6 to 8 hours. See literature.
Contains Penicillin V Potassium equivalent to Penicillin V 2.5 g, in a dry, pleasantly flavored mixture, buffered with Sodium Citrate and Citric Acid.
Prior to Mixing, Store at Controlled Room Temperature 59° to 86°F (15° to 30°C)
Directions for Mixing—At the time of dispensing tap bottle lightly to loosen powder. Add 63 mL of water to the dry mixture in the bottle in **two** portions. Shake well after each addition.
Each 5 mL (approx. one teaspoonful) will then contain: Penicillin V Potassium equivalent to 125 mg (200,000 Units) Penicillin V
Slight color variation does not affect product efficacy.

YA 2546 AMX
Eli Lilly & Co., Indianapolis, IN 46285, U.S.A.
Expiration Date

To remove main label, cut or tear on perforation.

100 mL V-CILLIN K® PENICILLIN V POTASSIUM FOR ORAL SOLUTION, USP 125 mg (200,000 Units) per 5 mL. Oversize bottle provides extra space for shaking. Store in a refrigerator. May be kept for 14 days without significant loss of potency. Keep Tightly Closed. Discard unused portion after 14 days. **SHAKE WELL BEFORE USING.**
Control No.

34. What is the total volume of the oral container? ______________

35. What is the dose strength? ______________

Remember: It is important to read the label on parenteral medications carefully. Labels on parenteral medications include a variety of units to express dose strengths. To calculate doses to administer it is important to know the strength of the medication in solution per mL or cc. Confusing dose strength with total volume can lead to medication error.

Calculating Parenteral Dosages

The calculation of parenteral doses can be done using the same rules and methods that were used in computing oral doses. The ratio-proportion and formula methods have been presented in earlier chapters. There are guidelines that will help you calculate a dose that is logical, reasonable, and accurate.

Guidelines for Calculating Parenteral Dosages

1. Use ratio-proportion or formula method to calculate the dose to be administered.
2. The rules and the steps for calculating parenteral doses are the same as those used for computing oral doses.
3. Remember, the stock volume varies and is not always per 1 mL or cc. Read the label carefully to determine the dose strength contained in a certain volume of solution.
4. Although cc and mL are used interchangeably, labels to answers should be based on whether one strength is available in cc or mL.
5. Accuracy in calculating parenteral doses depends on the syringe used. Therefore it is important to be able to understand syringes.
6. Small-capacity syringes—2, 2 1/2, 3 cc (mL)—are marked in minims and tenths (0.1) of a mL (cc). These syringes are used most often for the administration of I.M. medications. Doses are stated using decimal numbers. Doses involving decimal 0.5 are stated as fractions. The syringe has fraction markings.
7. Tuberculin syringes are used for small doses and are calibrated in hundredths (0.01) of a mL. Tuberculin syringes have a total capacity of 1 mL; they are designed to administer small doses and potent medications. They frequently are used in pediatrics.
8. **Insulin syringes are designed for insulin only.** Measurement of insulin in an insulin syringe requires no calculation or conversion. In an emergency situation or when insulin syringes are not available, the tuberculin syringe may be used to administer insulin. This is possible because 100 units of insulin equals 1 mL. It is safest to measure insulin with an insulin syringe! Insulin will be discussed in more detail in Chapter 18.

Calculating Injectable Medications According to the Syringe

Now that you have an understanding of syringes, let's discuss obtaining an answer that is measurable according to the syringe being used.

Points to Remember

- cc (mL) are never rounded off to a whole unit.
- Minims are expressed only as whole numbers.
- mL and cc are used interchangeably. Label problems (answers) accordingly.
- When using a 2, 2 1/2, 3 cc syringe, round answers in mL (cc) to the nearest tenth or express them in minims.

  a) For an answer in mL (cc), math is carried two decimal places and rounded to the nearest tenth.

  Example: 1.75 mL (cc) = 1.8 mL (cc)

  b) To calculate minims, the math is carried out to the tenths place and rounded to the nearest whole number.

  Example: 16.9 = m 17
- Using the equivalent m 16 = 1 cc (mL) is preferred and gives a more accurate answer. The maximum number of minims on a syringe is 40. A dose greater than 40 minims can't be measured.
- Remember: Minims is an apothecaries' measure and is not exact. It is better to express answers in metric measures such as mL or cc.
- When using a tuberculin syringe to calculate a dose in mL (cc), math is carried to the thousandth place and rounded to the nearest hundredth because the syringe is marked in hundredths (0.01) of a mL (cc).

  Example: 0.876 mL (cc) = 0.88 mL (cc)

  a) When a calculation comes to the hundredth place evenly, rounding off is not necessary.

  Example: A dose of 0.53 mL (cc) can be drawn up accurately without rounding off.

  b) To calculate minims on this syringe, math is carried to the nearest hundredth and rounded to the nearest whole minim.

  Example: 9.28 = m 9. (A dose of 9.28 rounds off to 9.3; because 0.3 is less than 0.5, it is dropped.)
- For injectable medications there are guidelines as to the amount of medication that can be administered. When the dose exceeds these guidelines, the dose should be questioned and the calculation double checked.

  a) I.M.—The range for an average adult dose is between 1 and 3 mL (cc). According to "Back to basics: administering IM injections the right way" by Beyea and Nicoll in *American Journal of Nursing,* Vol 96, No. 1, January 1996, a developed adult client can tolerate as much as 4 mL (cc) in large muscles. For children and persons with less developed muscles, the recommendation is 1 to 2 mL (cc). Whaley and Wong *Essentials of Pediatric Nursing* (1997) recommends giving no more than 1 mL (cc) to small children and older infants. The maximum dose that can be given to an adult is 4 mL (cc) in a large muscle.

  b) Subcutaneous—The volume that can be administered safely is 1 mL (cc) or less.
- In administering medications by injection, the absorption and consistency of the medication is also considered. For example, a dose of 3 mL (cc) of a thick oily substance may be divided into two injections of 1.5 mL (cc) each.
- Doses administered are measured in mL, cc, and minims; therefore the answer is labeled accordingly.
- Proceed with calculations in a logical and reasonable manner.
- Injectables that are added to an I.V. solution may have a volume greater than 5 mL (cc).

Now, with the guidelines in mind, let's look at some sample problems. Regardless of what method you use to calculate, the following steps are used.

1. Check to make sure everything is in the same system and unit of measure.
2. Think critically about what the answer should logically be.
3. Consider the type of syringe that is being used. **The cardinal rule should always be any dose given must be able to be measured accurately in the syringe you are using.**
4. Use the ratio-proportion or formula method to calculate the dose.

Let's look at some sample problems calculating parenteral doses.

Example 1: Doctor's Order: Gentamicin 75 mg I.M. q8h.

Available: Gentamicin labeled 40 mg = 1 mL.

Note: No conversion is necessary here. Think—the dose ordered is going to be more than 1 mL but less than 2 mL. Set up and solve.

Solution Using Ratio-Proportion Method

$$40 \text{ mg} : 1 \text{ mL} = 75 \text{ mg} : x \text{ mL}$$

$$40x = 75$$

$$x = 1.87 \text{ mL}$$

Answer: 1.9 mL

The answer here is rounded to the nearest tenth of a mL (cc). Remember, the syringe you are using is marked in tenths of a mL and minims.

Solution Using the Formula Method

$$\frac{(D)75 \text{ mg}}{(H)40 \text{ mg}} \times (Q)\ 1 \text{ mL} = x \text{ mL} \qquad \textbf{OR} \qquad \frac{(DW)75 \text{ mg}}{(SW)40 \text{ mg}} = \frac{(DV)x \text{ mL}}{(SV)1 \text{ mL}}$$

$$\frac{75}{40} = x \qquad\qquad \frac{40\,x}{40} = \frac{75}{40}$$

$$x = 1.87 \text{ mL} \qquad\qquad \frac{75}{40} = x$$

$$x = 1.87 \text{ mL}$$

Answer: 1.9 mL

The answer to Example 1 could also be expressed as minims. When changing to minims, do not round off the number of cc to the nearest tenth. Change the answer to minims by multiplying the value obtained for cc before it is rounded off. Use m 16 = 1 mL. Remember, however, it is always preferable to express the answer in metric measures, since apothecaries' measures are not exact. **Minims are rarely used; however, remember small hypodermics have minim calibrations. It is crucial that you use a syringe with minim calibrations when the amount of medication you are going to administer is calculated in minims.** To convert to minims use any of the methods presented in Chapter 8. In Example 1, we would change to minims as follows:

$$\text{m } 16 : 1 \text{ mL} = x \text{ m} : 1.87 \text{ mL}$$

$$x = 1.87 \times 16$$

$$x = \text{m } 29.92 \quad \text{(Answer: m 30)}$$

Remember: Minims are expressed as whole numbers; therefore the answer to the nearest whole number is m 30.

Look at the syringes below, illustrating the amounts shaded in on a syringe.

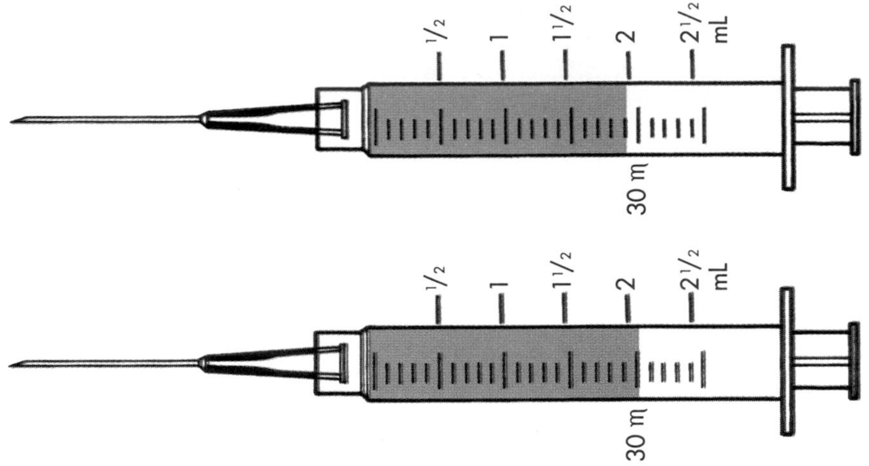

Example 2: Doctor's Order: Kantrex 500 mg I.M. q12h.

Available: Kanamycin (Kantrex) labeled 0.5 g per 2 mL.

In this problem a conversion is necessary. Equivalent: 1000 mg = 1 g. Convert what is ordered to what is available: 500 mg = 0.5 g. To get rid of the decimal point, convert what's available to what's ordered: 0.5 g = 500 mg. Remember, either way will net the same final answer.

Think—The dose you will need to give is greater than 1 mL, and it's being given I.M. The dose therefore should fall within the range that is safe for I.M. The solution after making conversion is as follows:

Solution Using Ratio-Proportion Method

$$0.5 \text{ g} : 2 \text{ mL} = 05. \text{ g} : x \text{ mL}$$

$$0.5x = 1.0$$

$$x = \frac{1.0}{0.5}$$

$$x = 2 \text{ mL}$$

Solution Using the Formula Method

$$\frac{(\text{D})0.5 \text{ g}}{(\text{H})0.5 \text{ g}} \times (\text{Q})2 \text{ mL} = x \text{ (mL)}$$

$$\frac{0.5 \times 2}{0.5 \times 1} = x$$

$$\frac{1.0}{0.5} = x$$

$$x = 2 \text{ mL}$$

OR

$$\frac{(\text{DW})500 \text{ mg}}{(\text{SW})500 \text{ mg}} = \frac{(\text{DV})x \text{ mL}}{(\text{SV})2 \text{ mL}}$$

$$\frac{500x}{500} = \frac{1000}{500}$$

$$\frac{1000}{500} = x$$

$$x = 2 \text{ mL}$$

Look at the syringe illustrating 2 mL drawn up.

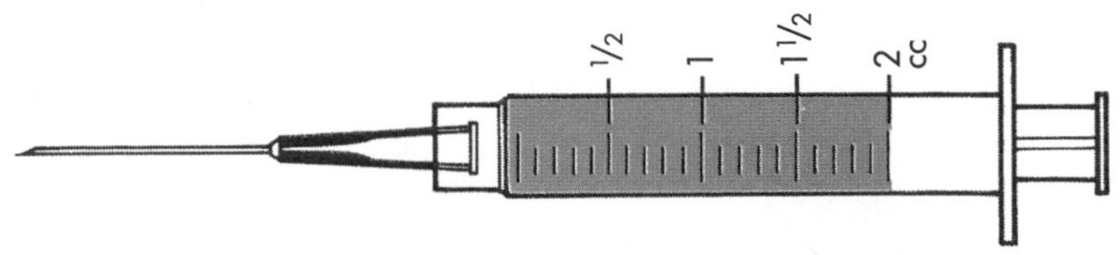

Example 3: Doctor's Order: Morphine sulfate gr 1/2 I.M. stat.

Available: Morphine sulfate in a 20-mL vial, labeled 15 mg per mL.

Problem Setup

1. A conversion is necessary. Convert gr 1/2 to mg using the equivalent 60 mg = gr 1, gr 1/2 therefore is 30 mg.
2. Think—You will need more than 1 mL to administer the dose.
3. Set up the problem, and calculate the dose to be administered.

Solution Using Ratio-Proportion Method

$$15 \text{ mg} : 1 \text{ mL} = 30 \text{ mg} : x \text{ mL}$$

$$15x = 30$$

$$x = 2 \text{ mL}$$

Solution Using the Formula Method

$$\frac{(\text{D})30 \text{ mg}}{(\text{H})15 \text{ mg}} \times (\text{Q})1 \text{ mL} = x \text{ (mL)} \quad \textbf{OR} \quad \frac{(\text{DW})30 \text{ mg}}{(\text{SW})15 \text{ mg}} = \frac{(\text{DV})\ x \text{ mL}}{(\text{SV})1 \text{ mL}}$$

$$\frac{30}{15} = x \qquad\qquad \frac{15x}{15} = \frac{30}{15}$$

$$x = 2 \text{ mL} \qquad\qquad \frac{30}{15} = x$$

$$x = 2 \text{ mL}$$

Note: Refer to the Example 2 to visualize 2 mL in a syringe.

Example 4: Doctor's Order: Atropine sulfate gr 1/100 I.M. stat.

Available: Atropine sulfate in 20-mL vial labeled 0.4 mg per mL.

Problem Setup

1. Conversion is necessary. Use the equivalent 60 mg = gr 1. gr 1/100 = 0.6 mg
2. Think—The dose will be greater than 1 mL to administer the required dose.
3. Set up the problem to solve for the dose to administer.

Solution Using Ratio-Proportion Method

$$0.4 \text{ mg} : 1 \text{ mL} = 0.6 \text{ mg} : x \text{ mL}$$

$$0.4x = 0.6$$

$$x = \frac{0.6}{0.4}$$

x = 1.5 mL or 1 1/2 mL (For administrative purposes it is best to state this answer as 1 1/2 mL. Note that the small hypodermics have fraction markings.)

Solution Using the Formula Method

$$\frac{(\text{D})0.6 \text{ mg}}{(\text{H})0.4 \text{ mg}} \times (\text{Q})1 \text{ mL} = x \text{ (mL)} \quad \textbf{OR} \quad \frac{(\text{DW})0.6 \text{ mg}}{(\text{SW})0.4 \text{ mg}} = \frac{(\text{DV})\ x \text{ mL}}{(\text{SV})1 \text{ mL}}$$

$$\frac{0.6}{0.4} = x \qquad\qquad \frac{0.4x}{0.4} = \frac{0.6}{0.4}$$

$$x = 1.5 \text{ mL, } 1\ 1/2 \text{ mL} \qquad\qquad \frac{0.6}{0.4} = x$$

$$x = 1.5 \text{ mL, } 1\ 1/2 \text{ mL}$$

Let's look at this amount shaded in on a syringe.

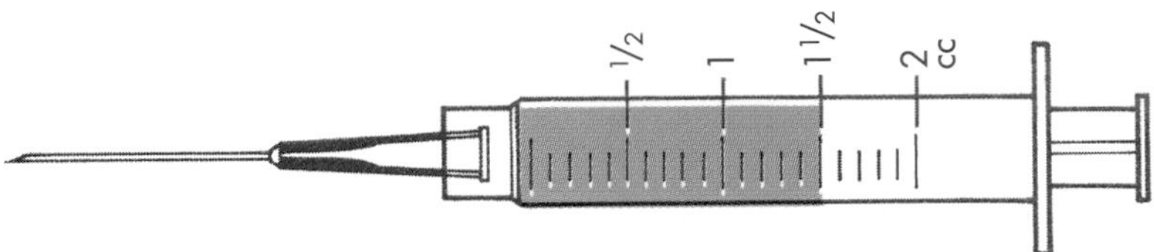

Calculating Doses for Medications in Units

Certain drugs are measured in units. Some medications measured in units include vitamins, antibiotics, insulin, and heparin. The calculation of insulin will be discussed in Chapter 18. In determining the dose to administer when medications are measured in units, use the same steps as with other parenteral medications. Doses of certain medications such as heparin are administered with a tuberculin syringe, as opposed to a hypodermic (2, 2 1/2, 3 cc). Because of its effects, heparin is never rounded off, but rather exact doses are given. Heparin will also be discussed in more detail in Chapter 21. Let's look at sample problems with units.

Example 1: Doctor's Order: Heparin 750 U. s.c. o.d.

Available: Heparin 1000 U per mL

Using a 1-cc (tuberculin) syringe, calculate the dose to be administered.

Problem Setup

1. No conversion is required. No conversion exists for units.
2. Think—The dosage to be given is less than 1 cc. This dose can be accurately measured in a 1-cc tuberculin syringe. To administer in a hypodermic (2, 2 1/2, 3 cc) the dose would have to be expressed to the nearest tenth of a mL or expressed as minims.
3. Set up the problem, and calculate the dose to be given.

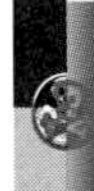

Think Critically to Avoid Drug Calculation Errors

Due to the action of heparin, an exact dose is crucial; the dose would not be rounded off.

Solution Using Ratio-Proportion Method

$$1000 \text{ U} : 1 \text{ mL} = 750 \text{ U} : x \text{ mL}$$

$$1000x = 750$$

$$x = \frac{75}{1000}$$

$$x = 0.75 \text{ mL}$$

Solution Using the Formula Method

$$\frac{\text{(D) } 750 \text{ U}}{\text{(H) } 1000 \text{ U}} \times \text{(Q)} 1 \text{ mL} = x \text{ (mL)} \quad \textbf{OR} \quad \frac{\text{(DW)} 750 \text{ U}}{\text{(SW)} 1000 \text{ U}} = \frac{\text{(DV) } x \text{ mL}}{\text{(SV) } 1 \text{ mL}}$$

$$\frac{750}{1000} = x \qquad \frac{1000x}{1000} = \frac{750}{1000}$$

$$x = 0.75 \text{ mL} \qquad \frac{750}{1000} = x$$

$$x = 0.75 \text{ mL}$$

Let's look at the 1-cc (1-mL) syringe illustrating 0.75 mL shaded in.

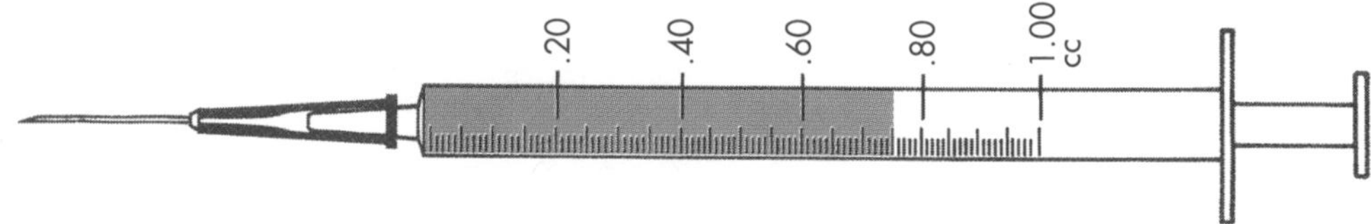

Example 2: Doctor's Order: Penicillin G 500,000 U I.M. b.i.d.

Available: Penicillin G labeled 300,000 U per mL.

Problem Setup

1. No conversion is required.
2. Think—The dose ordered is more than what is available. Therefore more than 1 cc would be required to administer the dose.
3. Set up the problem in ratio-proportion or formula to calculate the dose.

Solution Using the Ratio-Proportion Method

$$300{,}000 \text{ U} : 1 \text{ mL} = 500{,}000 \text{ U} : x \text{ mL}$$

$$300{,}000x = 500{,}000$$

$$x = \frac{500{,}000}{300{,}000}$$

$$x = 1.66 \text{ mL}$$

Note: The division here is carried two decimal places. This answer is then rounded off to 1.7 mL. Remember the hypodermic syringe (2, 2 1/2, 3 cc) is marked in tenths of a mL.

Solution Using the Formula Method

$$\frac{\text{(D) } 500{,}000 \text{ U}}{\text{(H) } 300{,}000 \text{ U}} \times \text{(Q)}1 \text{ mL} = x \text{ (mL)} \quad \textbf{OR} \quad \frac{\text{(DW) } 500{,}000 \text{ U}}{\text{(SW) } 300{,}000 \text{ U}} = \frac{\text{(DV) } x \text{ mL}}{\text{(SV)}1 \text{ mL}}$$

$$\frac{500{,}000}{300{,}000} = x \qquad\qquad \frac{300{,}000x}{300{,}000} = \frac{500{,}000}{300{,}000}$$

$$x = 1.66 \text{ mL} \qquad\qquad x = 1.66 \text{ mL}$$

$$x = 1.7 \text{ mL} \qquad\qquad x = 1.7 \text{ mL}$$

Illustration of the dose calculated in a hypodermic syringe.

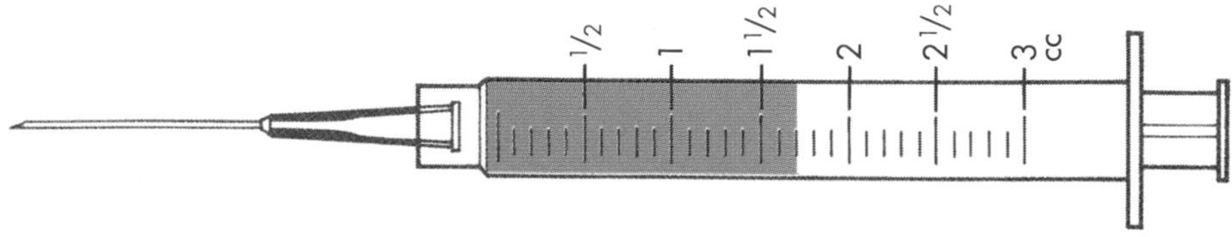

> **Caution**
>
> Read orders carefully when the order is expressed in units. Do not confuse the "U" when written in an order with an "0." To avoid confusion some institutions require doctors to write out the word *units* to avoid misinterpretation of an order—for example, "50 U" as 500 units.

Chapter Review (pp. 354-364)

Calculate the doses for the problems below and shade in the dose on the syringe provided. Use labels where provided to calculate the volume necessary to administer the dose ordered. Express your answers to the nearest tenth except where indicated.

1. Doctor's Order: Sandostatin 0.05 mg s.c. o.d.
   Available: Sandostatin labeled 1 mL = 100 mcg.

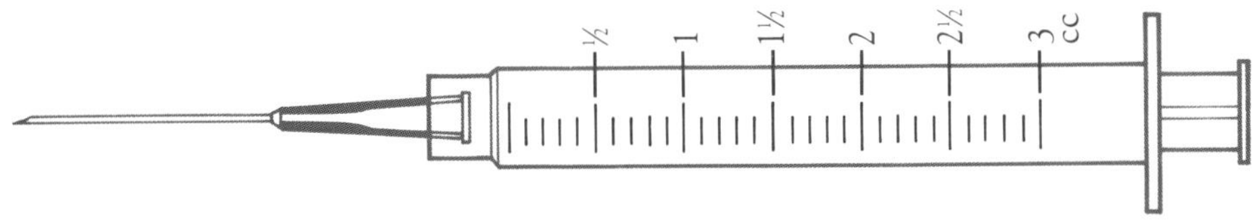

2. Doctor's Order: Demerol 50 mg I.M. and Vistaril 25 mg I.M. q4h p.r.n. for pain.
   Available: Demerol labeled 75 mg/mL.
   Vistaril labeled 50 mg/mL.

   What is the total amount of mL you will administer? ____________

   Shade the total number of cc (mL) on the syringe provided.

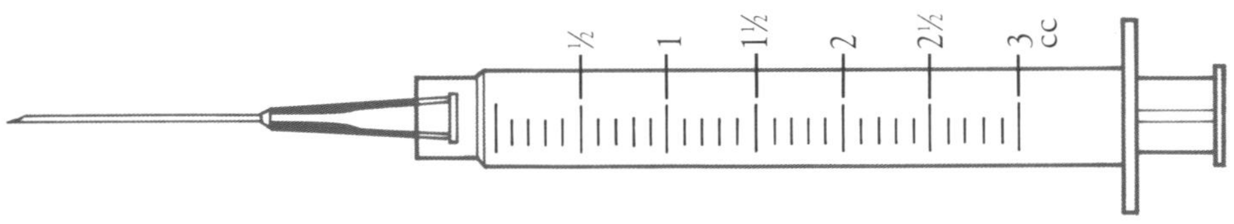

3. Doctor's Order: Reglan 5 mg I.M. b.i.d. 1/2 hour a.c.
   Available: Reglan labeled 10 mg per 2 mL.

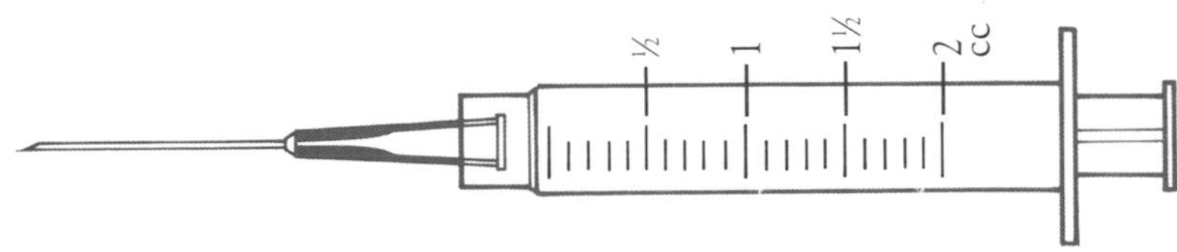

4. Doctor's Order: Heparin 5,000 U s.c. b.i.d.
   Available:

   Heparin Sodium Injection Label
   20,000 USP Units/mL
   1 mL Vial

   Express your answer in hundredths.

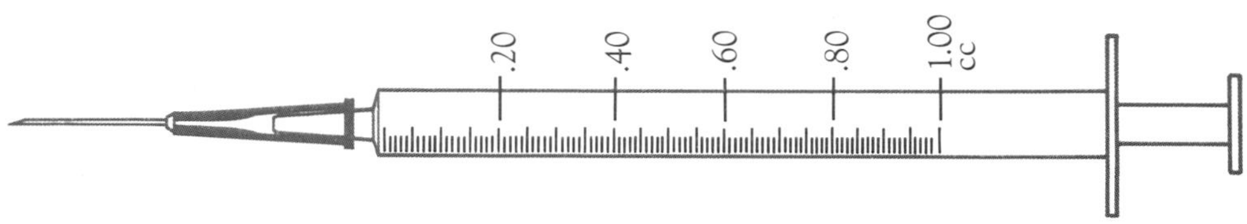

5. Doctor's Order: Morphine sulfate gr 1/4 I.M. q4h p.r.n.
   Available:

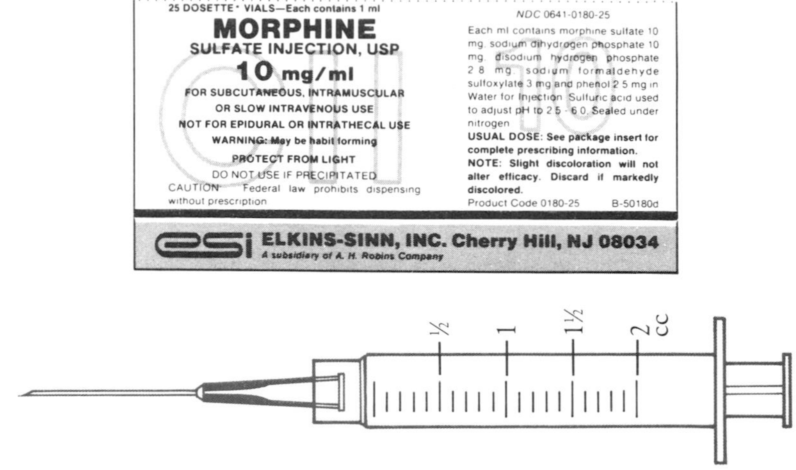

6. Doctor's Order: Lasix (furosemide) 20 mg I.M. stat.
   Available:

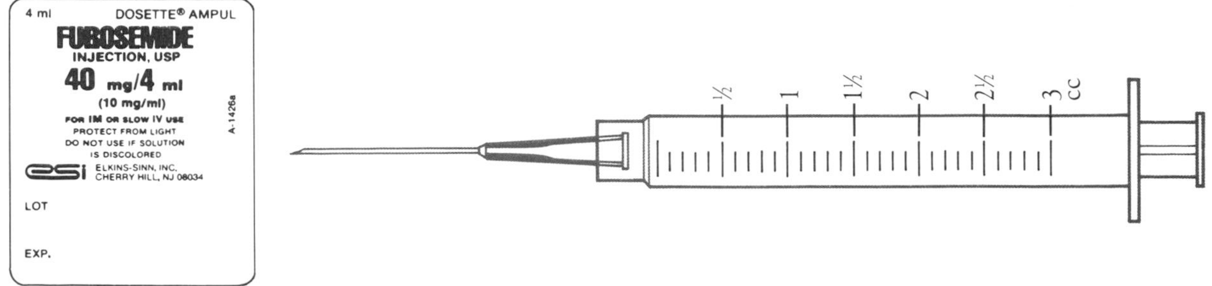

7. Doctor's Order: Clindamycin 0.3 g I.M. q6h.
   Available:

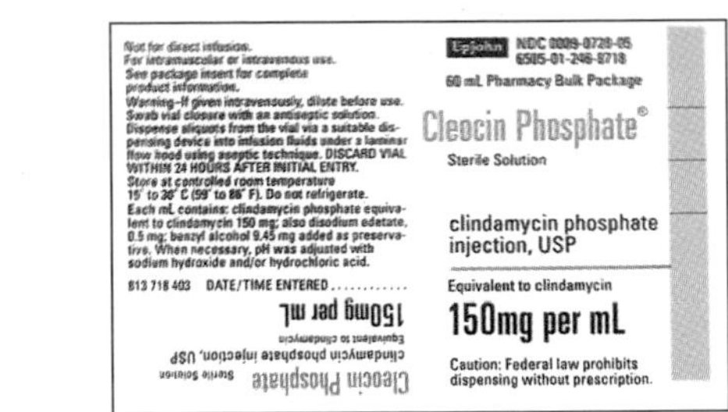

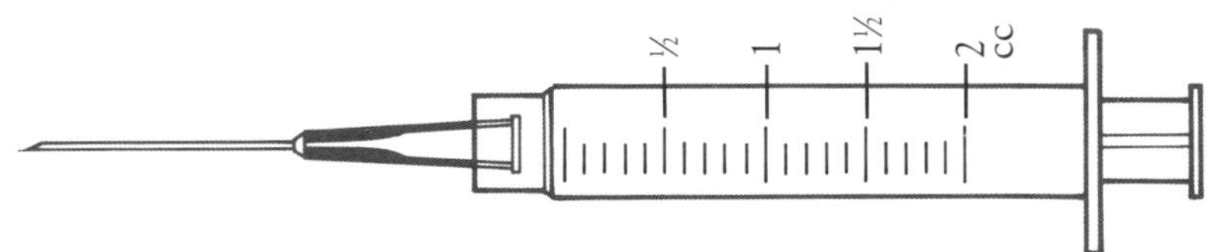

8. Doctor's Order: Atropine gr 1/150 I.M. stat.
   Available: Atropine 0.4 mg per mL.

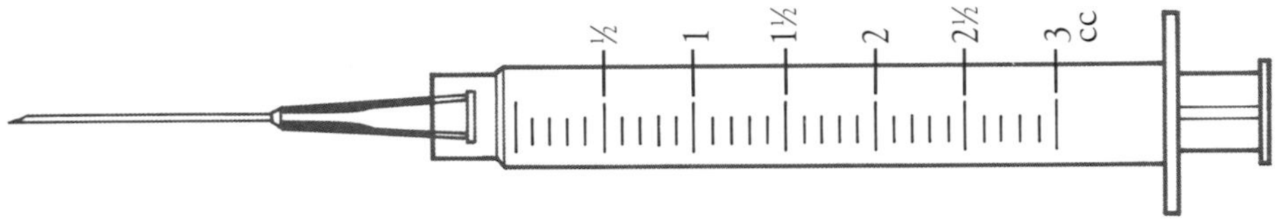

9. Doctor's Order: Kefzol 0.5 g I.M. q6h.
   Available: After reconstitution 225 mg per mL.

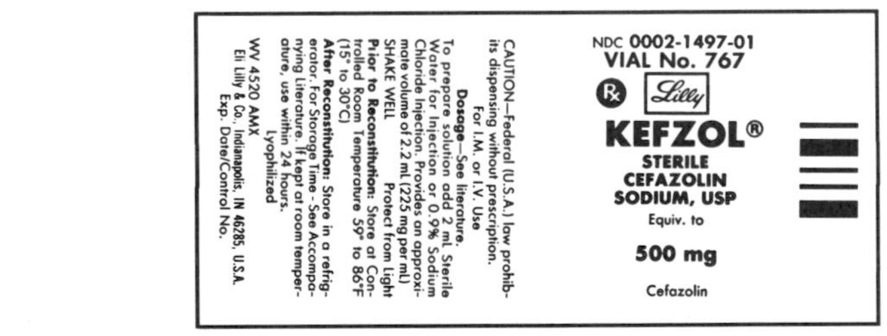

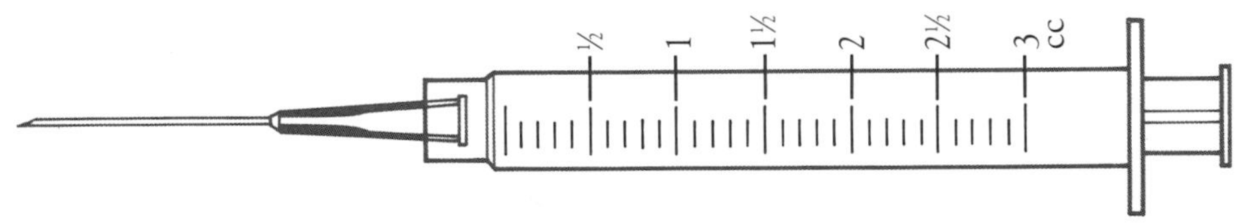

10. Doctor's Order: Digoxin 100 mcg I.M. q.d.
    Available: Digoxin injection 0.5 mg/2 mL.

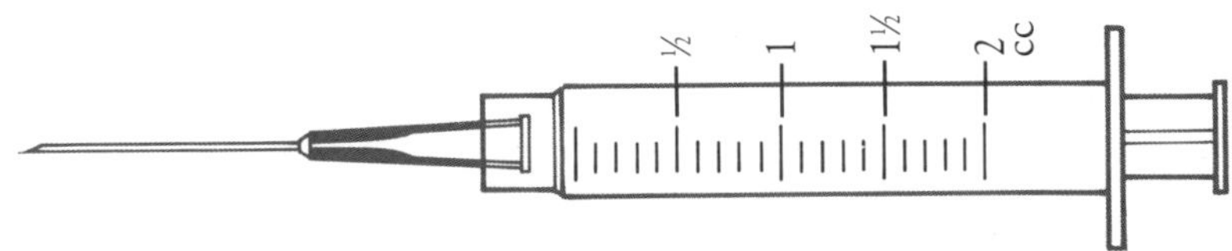

11. Doctor's Order: Phenobarbital gr 1/2 I.M. b.i.d.
    Available: Phenobarbital labeled 120 mg per mL.

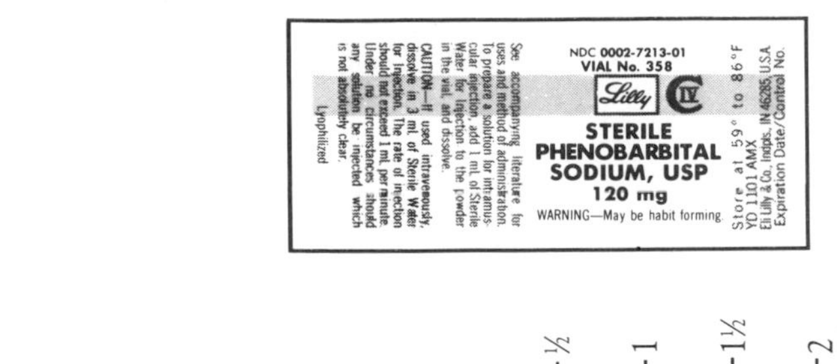

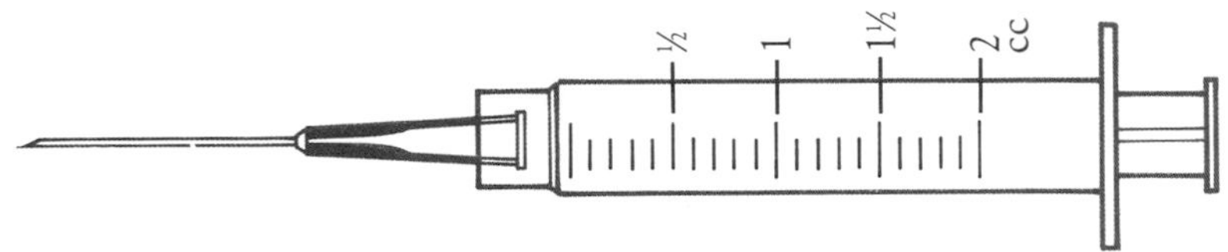

12. Doctor's Order: Dilaudid 2 mg s.c. q4h p.r.n. for pain.
    Available:

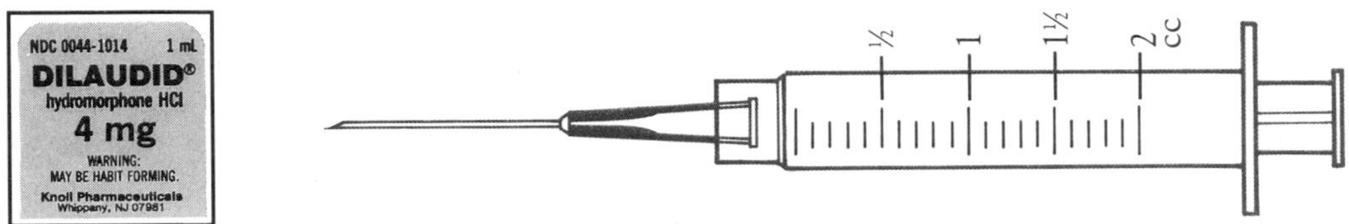

13. Doctor's Order: Penicillin G 250,000 U I.M. q6h.
    Available:

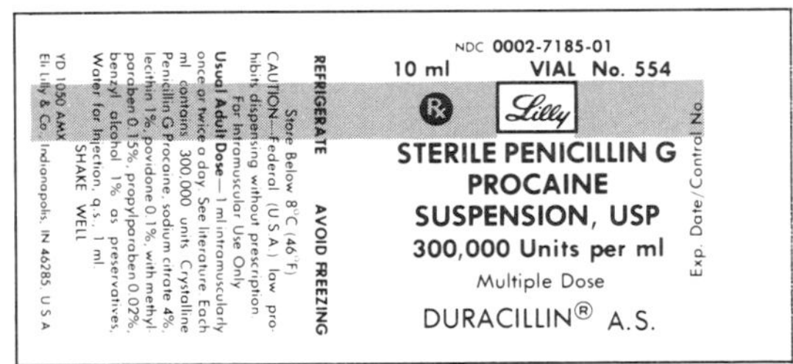

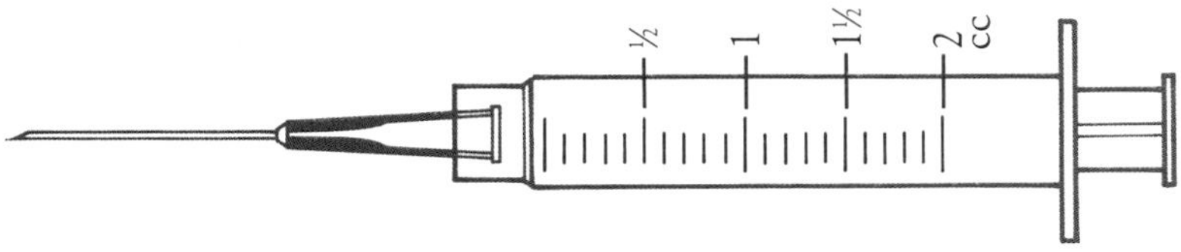

14. Doctor's Order: Solu-Medrol 100 mg I.M. q8h × 2 doses.
    Available:

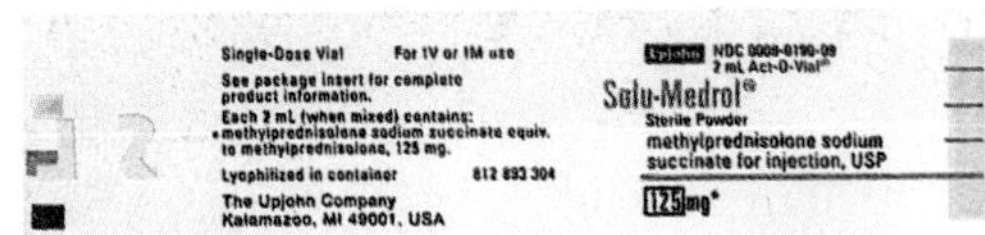

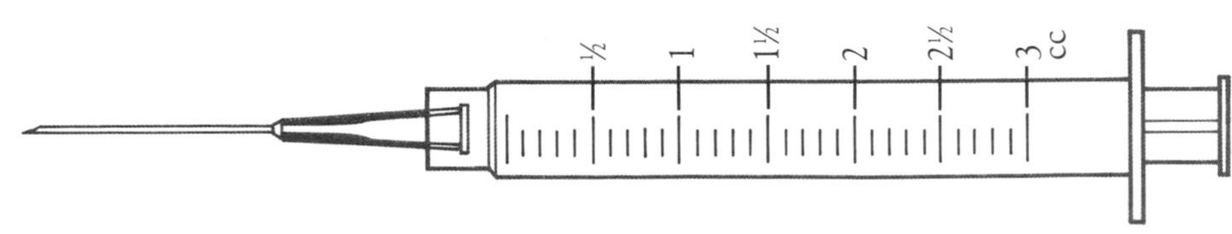

15. Doctor's Order: Methergine 0.4 mg I.M. q4h × 3 doses.
    Available: Methergine labeled 0.2 mg/mL.

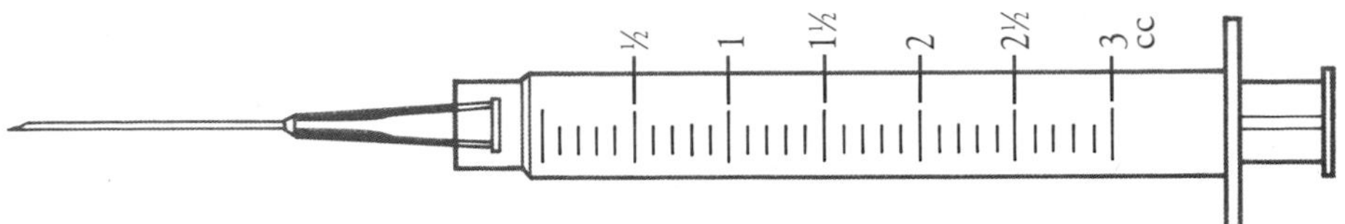

16. Doctor's Order: Heparin 8,000 U s.c. q12h.
    Available:

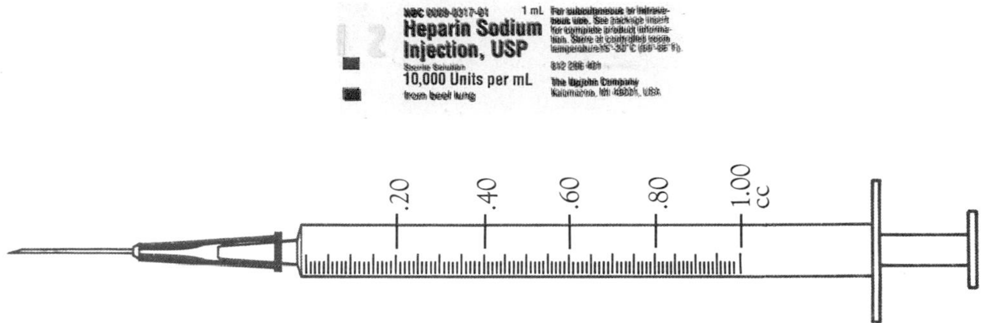

17. Doctor's Order: Morphine sulfate 4 mg I.M. q4h p.r.n.
    Available: Morphine 10 mg per mL.

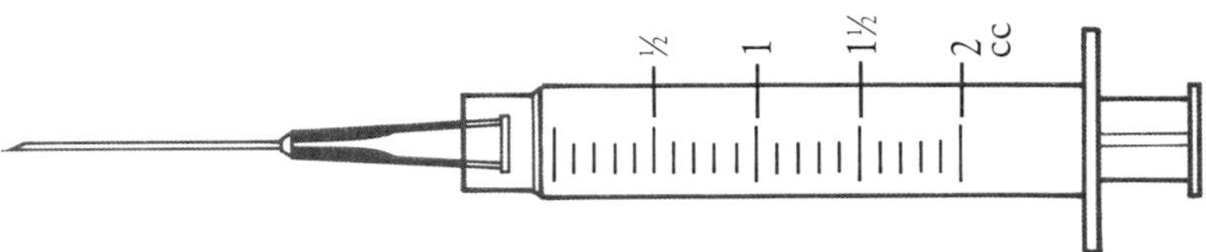

18. Doctor's Order: Vitamin K 10 mg I.M. q.d. × 3 days.
    Available: Vitamin K labeled 5 mg per mL.

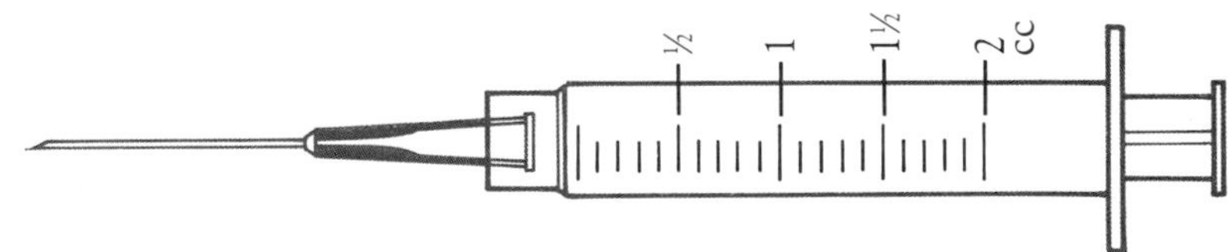

19. Doctor's Order: Codeine gr 1/4 I.M. q4h p.r.n. for pain.
    Available: Codeine phosphate 30 mg (gr 1/2) per mL.

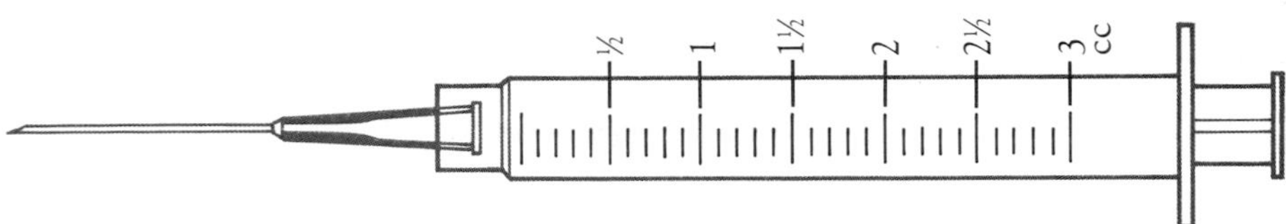

20. Doctor's Order: Phenergan 25 mg I.M. q4h p.r.n. for nausea.
    Available: Phenergan labeled 50 mg per mL.

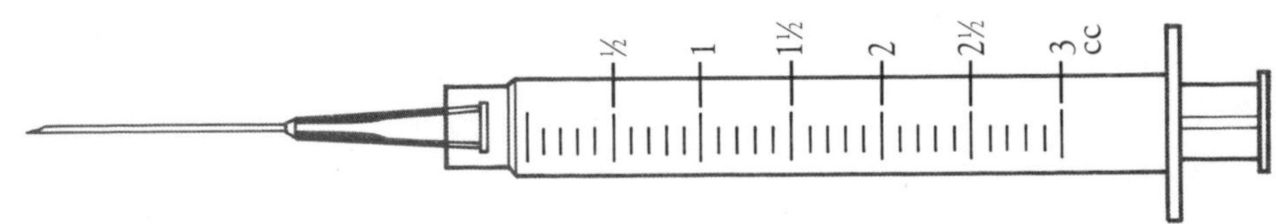

21. Doctor's Order: Stadol 1.5 mg I.M. q3-4h for pain.
    Available: Stadol labeled 2 mg per mL.

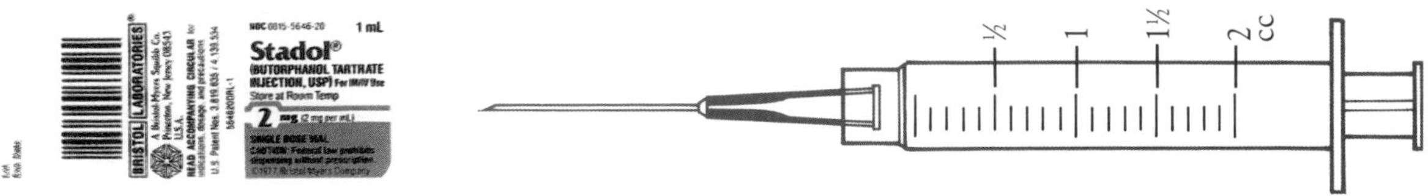

22. Doctor's Order: Dilaudid 3 mg I.M. q4h prn.
    Available: Dilaudid 4 mg per mL.

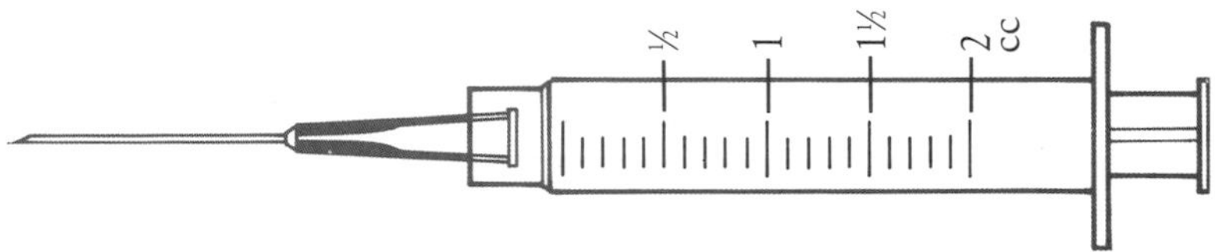

23. Doctor's Order: Scopolamine gr 1/300 s.c. stat.
    Available:

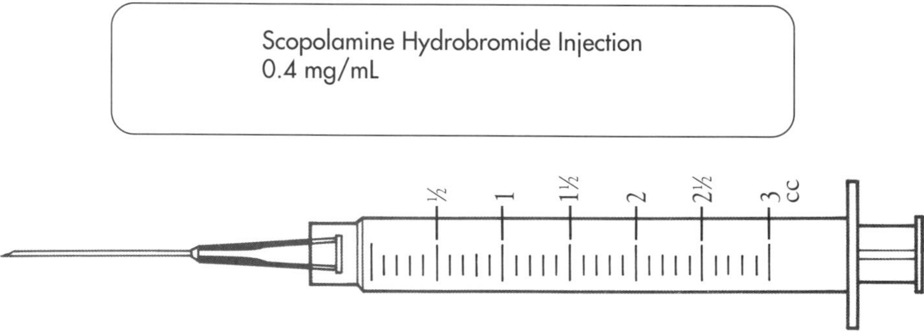

24. Doctor's Order: Haldol 3 mg I.M. q6h p.r.n.
    Available:

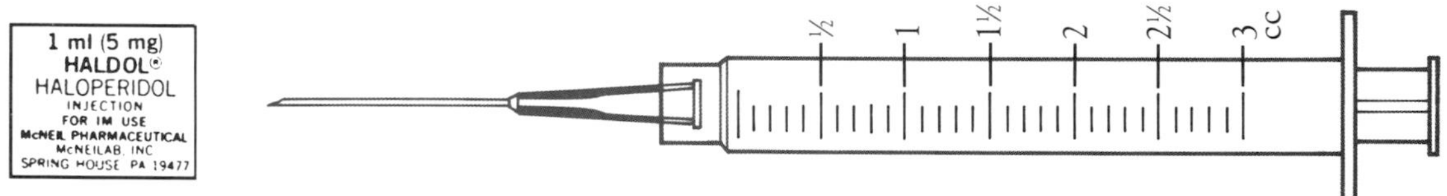

25. Doctor's Order: Seconal Sodium 90 mg I.M. h.s. p.r.n.
    Available:

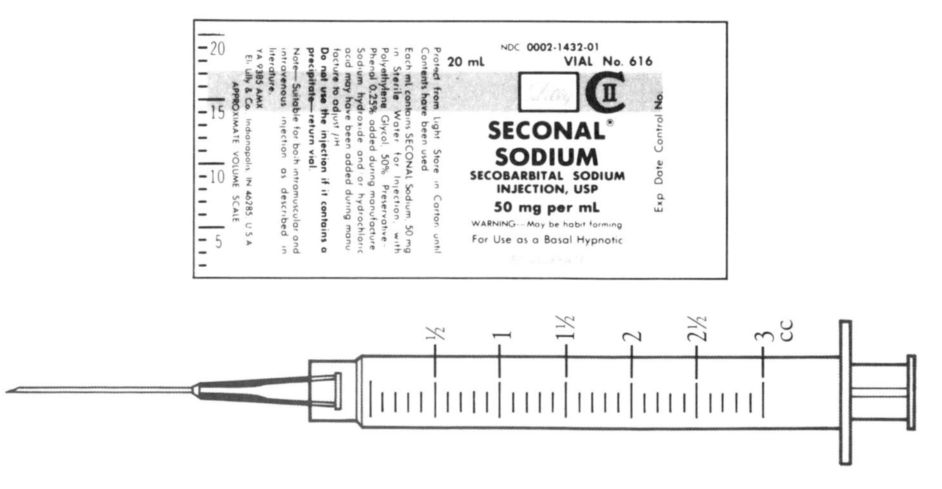

26. Doctor's Order: Solu-Cortef 400 mg I.V. o.d. for a severe inflammation.
    Available:

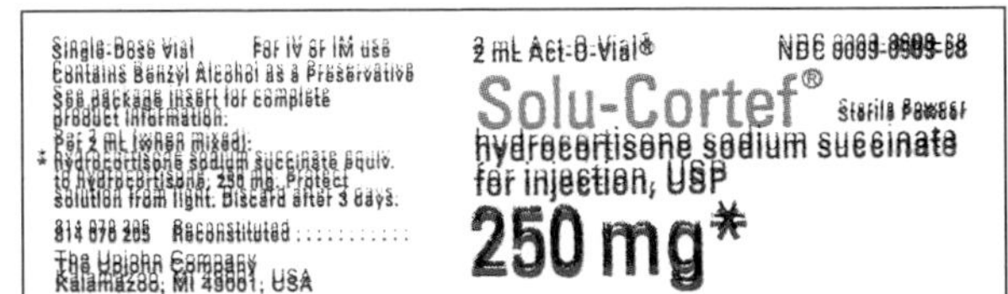

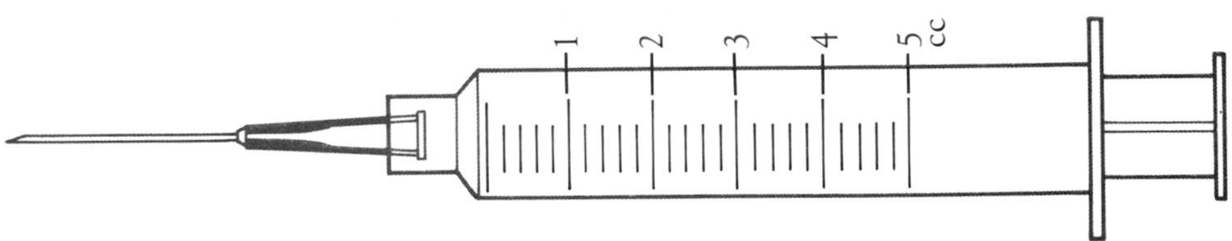

27. Doctor's Order: Solu-Medrol 40 mg I.V. q6h × 3 days.
    Available: Solu-Medrol 125 mg per 2 mL.

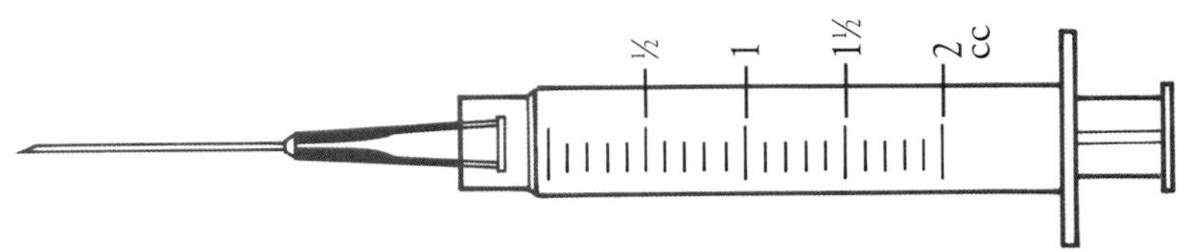

28. Doctor's Order: Robinul 200 mcg I.M. on call to the O.R.
    Available:

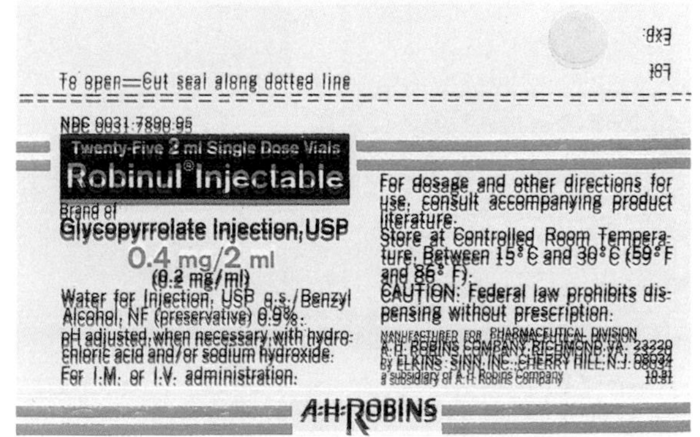

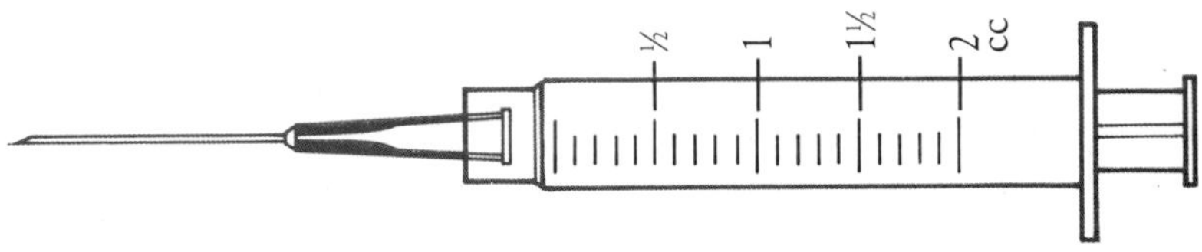

29. Doctor's Order: Heparin 2,500 U s.c. o.d.
    Available:

Heparin Sodium Injection Label
5000 USP Units/mL
1 mL Vial

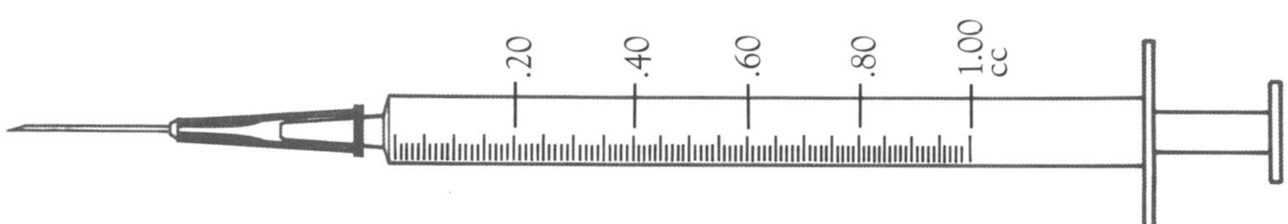

30. Doctor's Order: Vistaril 35 mg I.M. stat.
    Available:

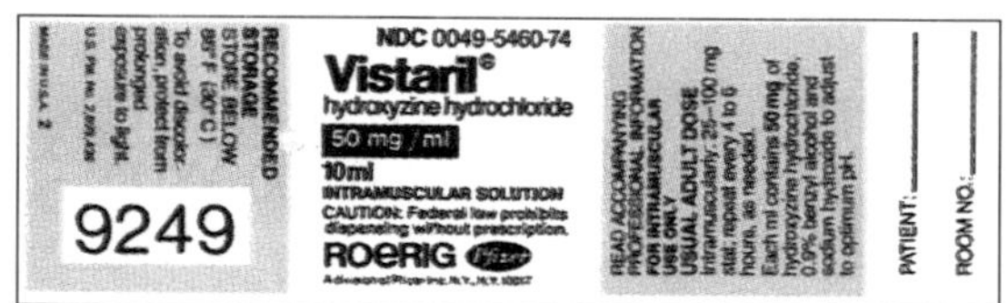

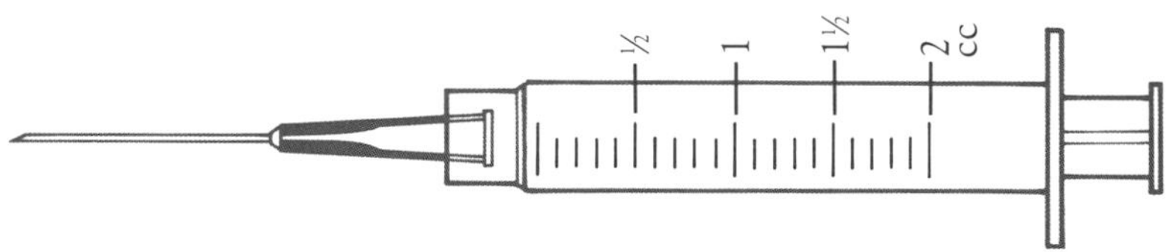

31. Doctor's Order: Meperidine 60 mg I.M. q3-4h p.r.n. for pain.
    Available: Meperidine 75 mg per mL.

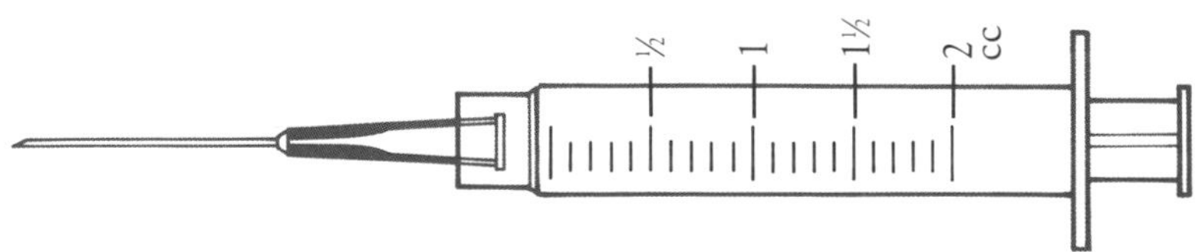

32. Doctor's Order: Bicillin 400,000 U I.M. q4h.
    Available:

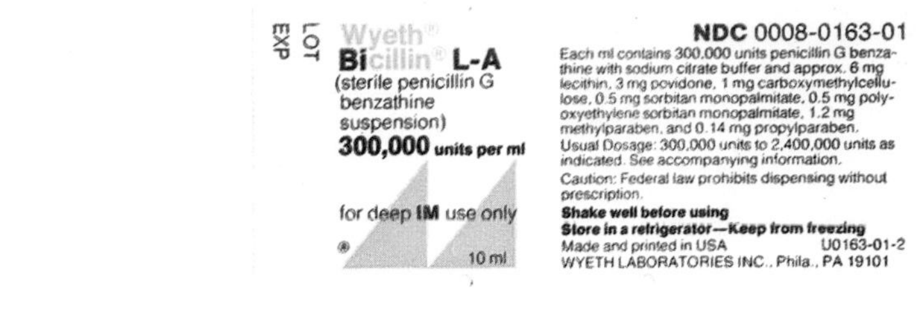

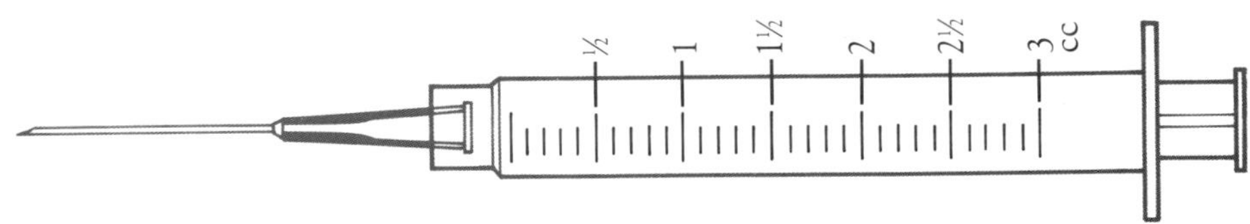

33. Doctor's Order: Lanoxin 0.4 mg I.M. stat.
    Available:

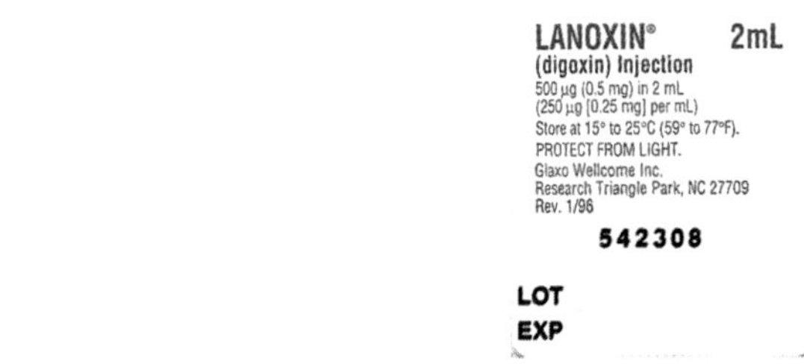

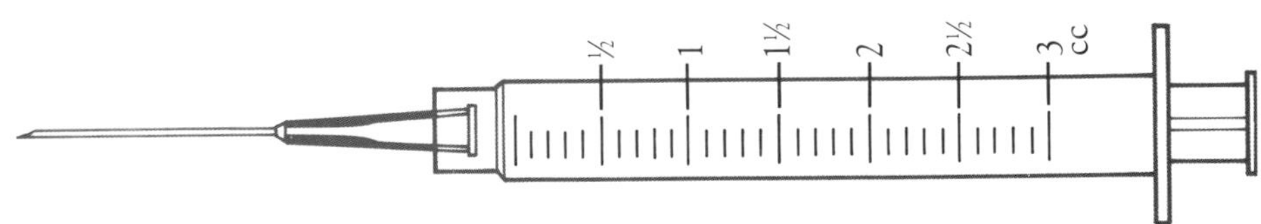

34. Doctor's Order: Amikin 100 mg I.M. q8h.
    Available:

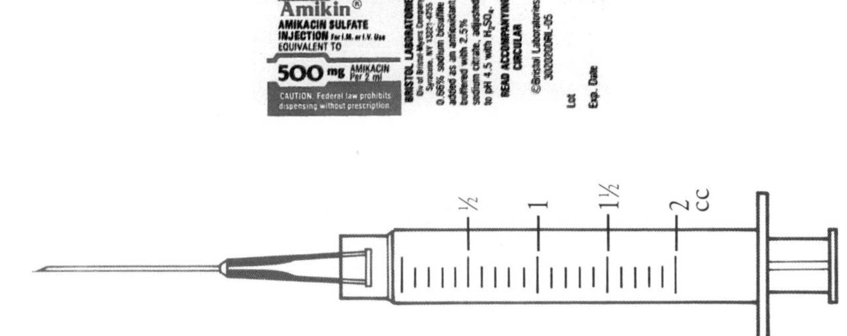

35. Doctor's Order: Depo-Medrol 60 mg I.M. b.i.d. × 3 days.
    Available:

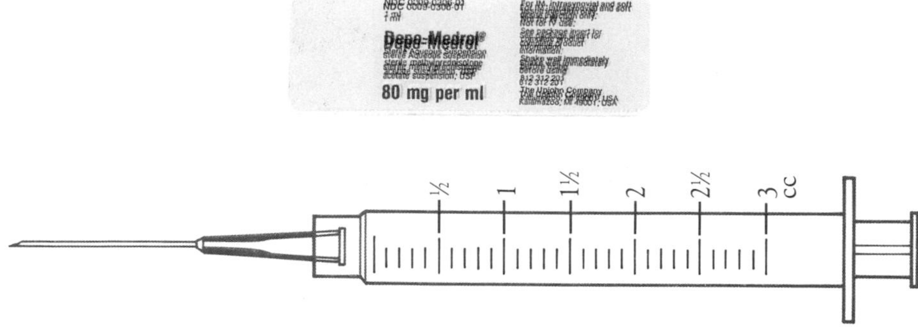

36. Doctor's Order: Ativan 2 mg I.M. b.i.d. p.r.n. for agitation.
    Available:

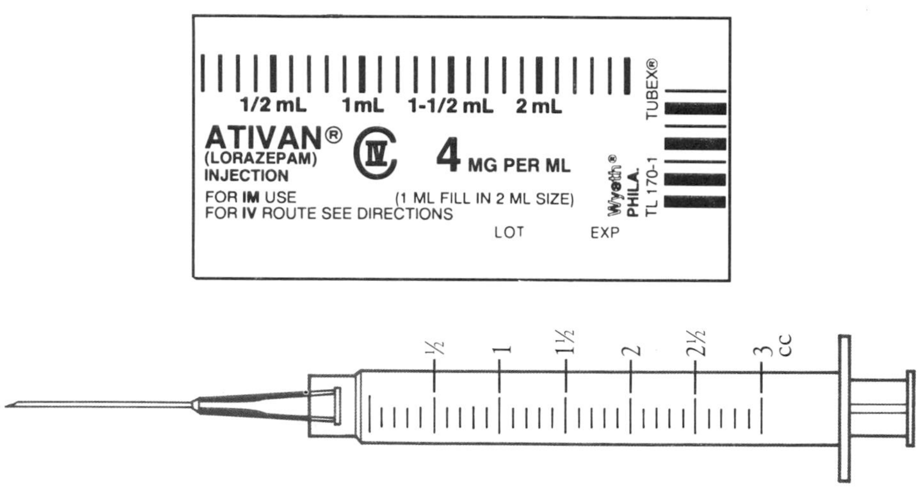

37. Doctor's Order: Thorazine 75 mg I.M. q4h p.r.n.
    Available:

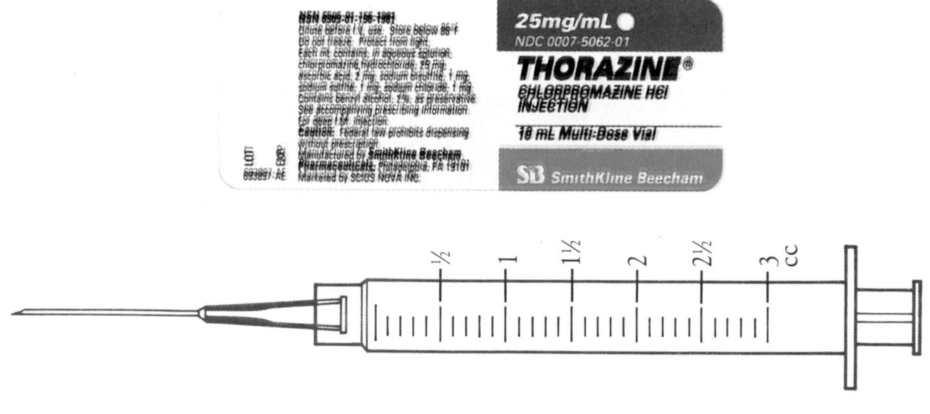

38. Doctor's Order: Nembutal sodium 120 mg I.M. h.s. p.r.n.
    Available:

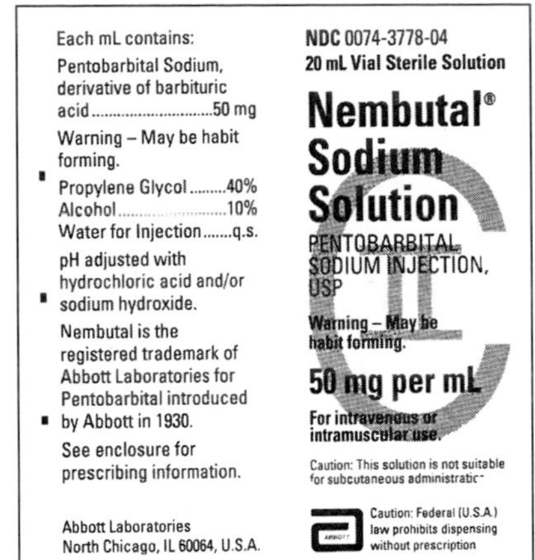

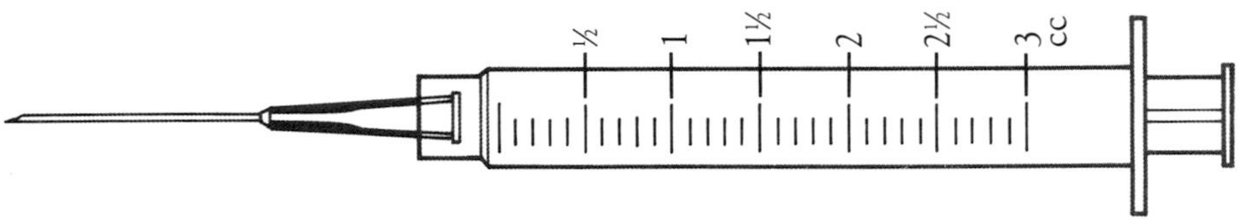

39. Doctor's Order: Epogen 3,000 U s.c. o.d. every Monday, Wednesday, and Friday.
    Available: Epogen labeled 2,000 U per mL.

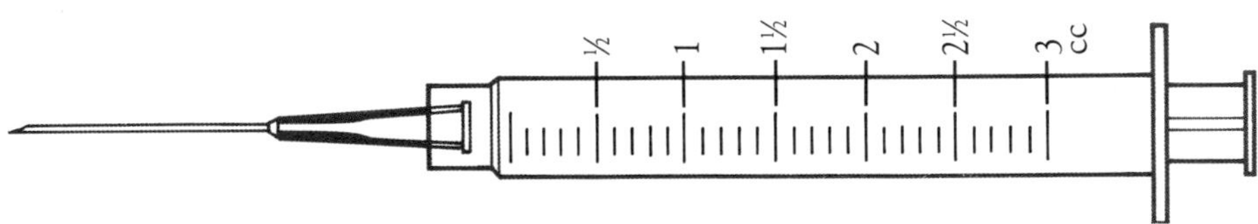

40. Doctor's Order: Zantac 50 mg I.M. q8h.
    Available:

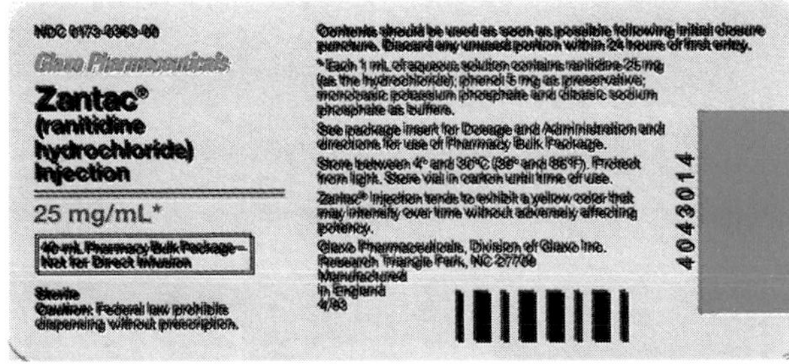

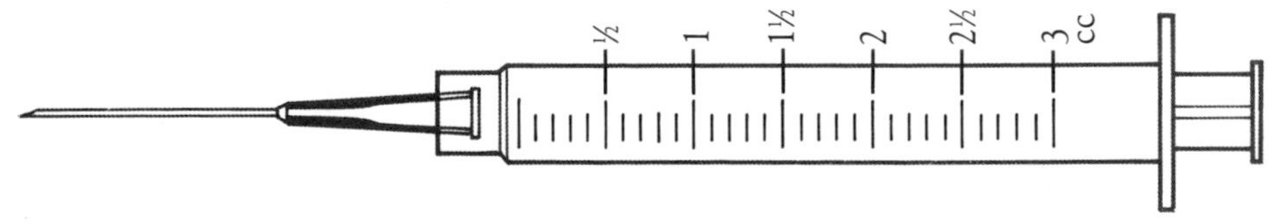

41. Doctor's Order: Lovenox 30 mg s.c. q12h.
    Available:

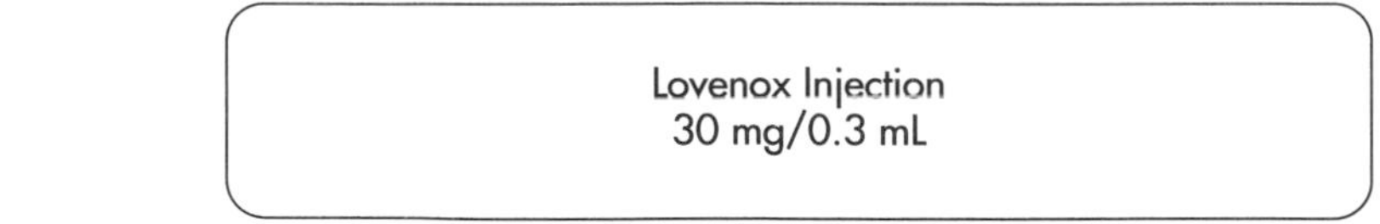

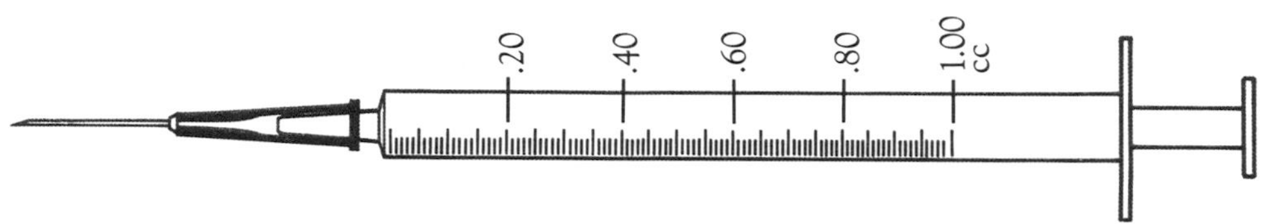

42. Doctor's Order: Cimetidine 0.3 g I.V. t.i.d.
    Available:

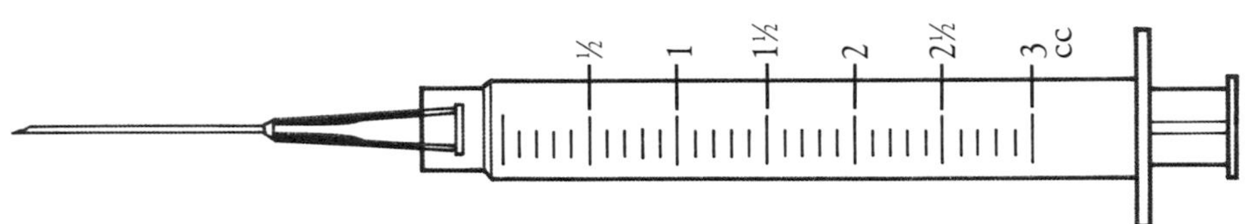

43. Doctor's Order: Valium 7.5 mg I.M. stat.
    Available: Valium 5 mg per mL.

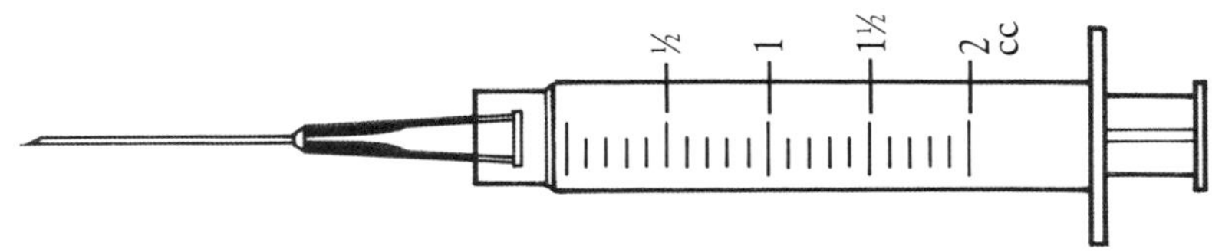

44. Doctor's Order: Numorphan 1 mg s.c. q4h p.r.n.
    Available:

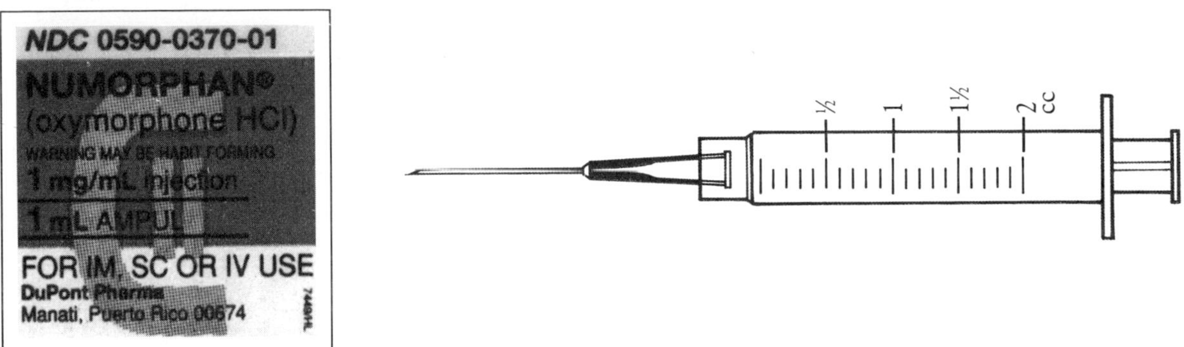

45. Doctor's Order: Lasix 30 mg I.V. stat.
    Available: Lasix 20 mg per 2 mL.

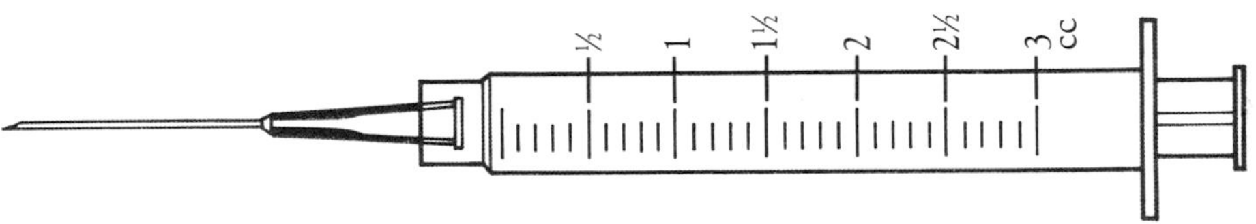

46. Doctor's Order: Betamethasone 12 mg I.M. q24h × 2 doses.
    Available: Betamethasone 4 mg per mL

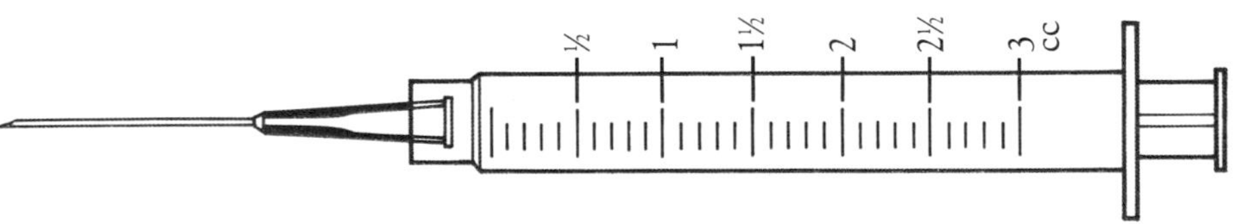

47. Doctor's Order: Aminophylline 0.25 g I.V. q6h.
    Available: Aminophylline 500 mg per 20 mL.

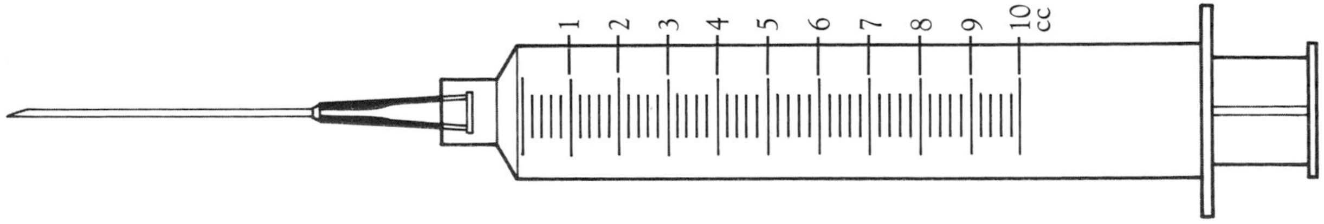

48. Doctor's Order: Pronestyl 0.5 g I.V. stat.
    Available: Pronestyl 500 mg per mL.

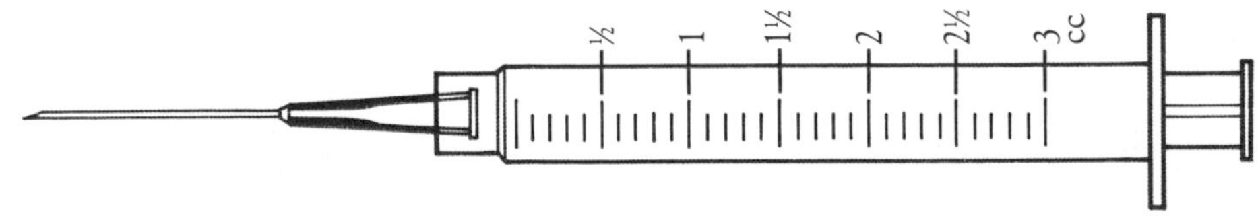

Chapter 17

Powdered Drugs

Objectives

After reviewing this chapter the student will be able to do the following:

1. **Prepare a solution from a powdered medication according to directions on the vial or other resources**
2. **Identify essential information to be placed on the vial of a medication after it is reconstituted**
3. **Determine the best concentration strength for medications ordered, when there are several directions for mixing**
4. **Calculate doses from reconstituted medications**

Some drugs are unstable in liquid form for long periods of time and therefore are packaged in powdered form. When medications come in powdered form, they must be diluted with a liquid referred to as a *diluent* or *solvent* before they can be administered to a client. Once a liquid is added to a powdered drug, the solution may be used for only 1 to 14 days, depending on the type of medication.

The process of adding a solvent or liquid to a medication that is in the form of a powder is called *reconstitution.* If you think about it, this process is something you do in everyday situations. For example, when you make Kool-Aid or iced tea (powdered form), what you're doing in essence is reconstituting. The Kool-Aid, for example, is the powder, and the water you add to it is considered the diluent, or solvent. Medications requiring reconstitution can be for oral or parenteral use (Figure 17-1).

Basic Principles for Reconstitution

The initial step in preparing a powdered medication is to carefully read the information on the vial or the package insert since directions for reconstituting are indicated there.

1. The drug manufacturer provides directions for reconstitution, including information regarding the number of mL of diluent or solvent that should be added, as well as the type of solution that should be used to reconstitute the medication. The concentration (or strength) of the medication after it has been

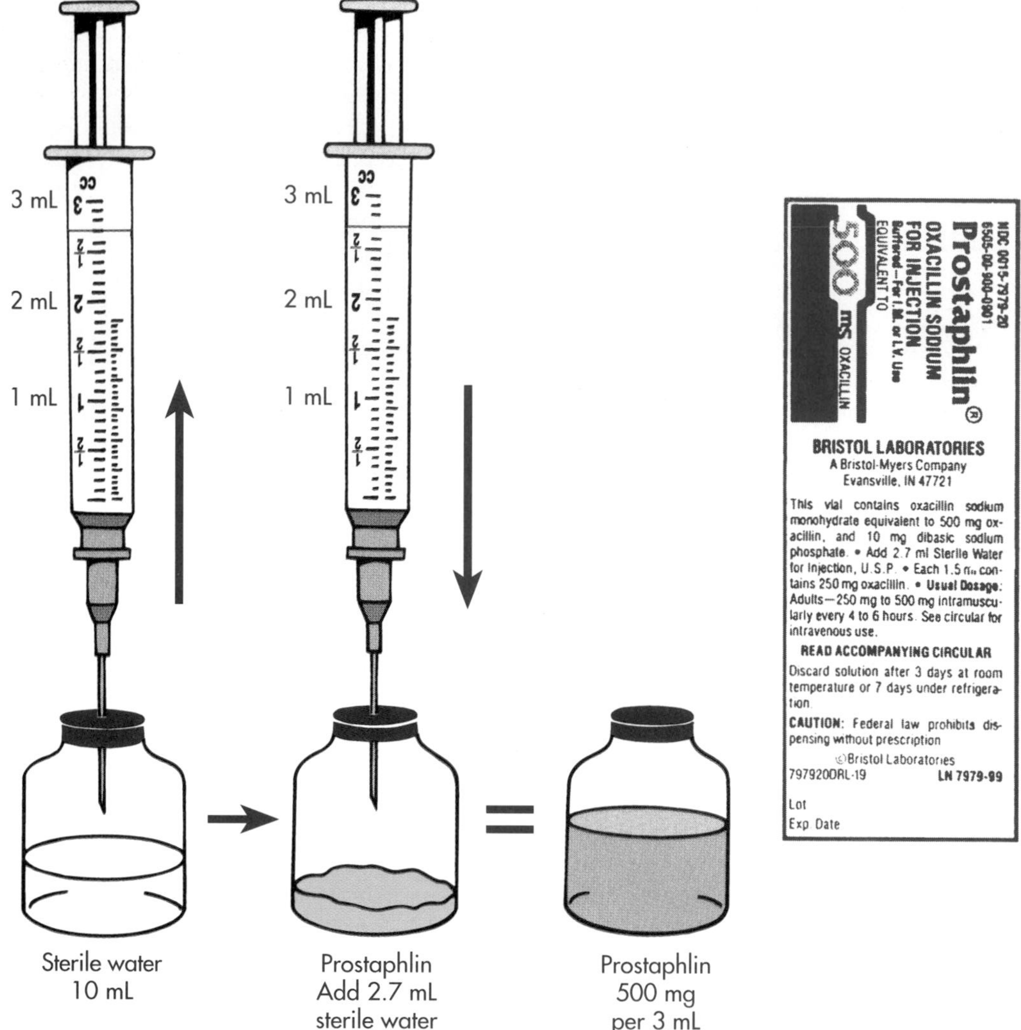

Figure 17-1. Example showing reconstitution. (From Brown M, Mulholland J: *Drug calculations: process and problems for clinical practice*, ed 5, St Louis, 1996, Mosby.)

reconstituted according to the directions is also indicated on some medications. The directions for reconstituting must be read carefully and followed.

2. The diluent (solvent, liquid) commonly used for reconstitution is sterile water or sterile normal saline, prepared for injection. Other solutions that may be used are 5% dextrose and water and bacteriostatic water. Some powdered medications for oral use may be reconstituted with tap water. The manufacturer's directions will tell you which solution to use. If the medication requires a special solution for reconstitution, it is usually supplied by the drug manufacturer and packaged with the medication. When the solution for reconstitution is not indicated, most solutions can be safely mixed with sterile water.
3. Once you have located the directions on the label for reconstitution of the medication, you need to identify the following information:
   a) The type of diluent to use for reconstitution
   b) The amount of diluent to add
   c) The length of time the medication is good once it is reconstituted
   d) Directions for storing the medication after mixing
   e) The strength or concentration of the medication after it's reconstituted
4. If there are no directions for reconstitution on the label or on a package insert, or if any of the information (listed in number 3) is missing, consult appropriate resources such as the *Physician's Desk Reference* (PDR), a pharmacology text, the hospital drug formulary, or the pharmacy.

5. After mixing the powdered drug, you must place the following information on the medication vial.
   a) **Your initials.**
   b) **The date and time prepared and the expiration date and time.** Note: If all of the solution is used that is mixed, this information is not necessary. Information regarding the date and time of preparation and date and time for expiration is crucial when all of the medication is not used. Powdered medications once reconstituted must be used within a certain time period. For example, ampicillin once reconstituted must be used within an hour.
6. When reconstituting medications that are in multiple-dose vials or have several directions as to how they can be prepared, information regarding the dose strength or final concentration **(what the medication's strength or concentration is after you mixed it) must be on the label, for example, 500 mg/mL. This is important since others using the medication after you need to know this in determining the dose to administer.**
7. After adding the diluent to the powdered medication, the total reconstituted volume will be greater than the amount of diluent. The reconstituted material represents the diluent plus the powder. For example, you may add 1.5 mL of diluent to a powder and have a total volume of 2.5 mL. **(The total volume of the prepared solution will always yield a greater volume than the diluent you add.)**

Let's examine some labels of powdered medications by looking first at the reconstitution instructions for a single-strength solution. Examine the label for ampicillin 1 g.

Practice Problems (pp. 364-366)

Using the label for Polycillin- N, answer the following questions.

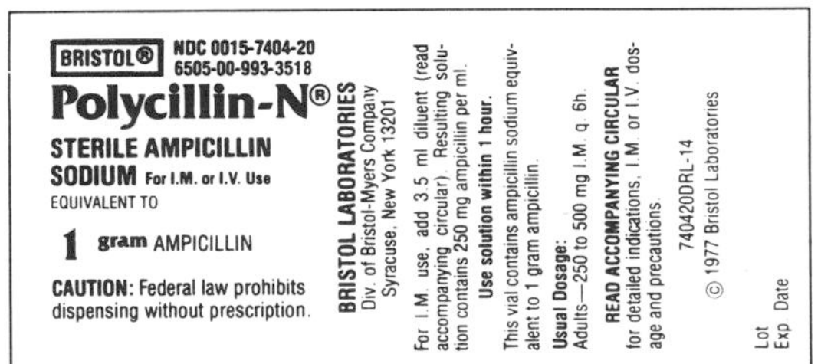

1. How much diluent is added to the vial to prepare the drug for I.M. use? ____________
2. What kind of solution can be used for the diluent? ____________
3. What is the final concentration of the prepared solution for I.M. administration? ____________
4. How long will reconstituted material retain its potency? ____________
5. The doctor ordered 500 mg I.M. q6h. How many mL will you give? Shade the amount on the syringe provided.

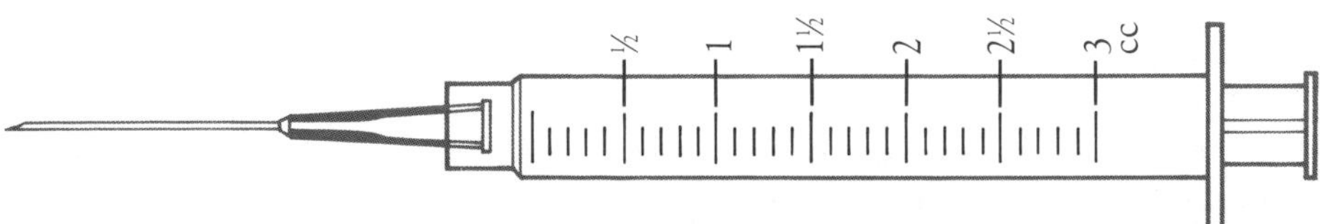

Using the label for Prostaphlin, answer the following questions.

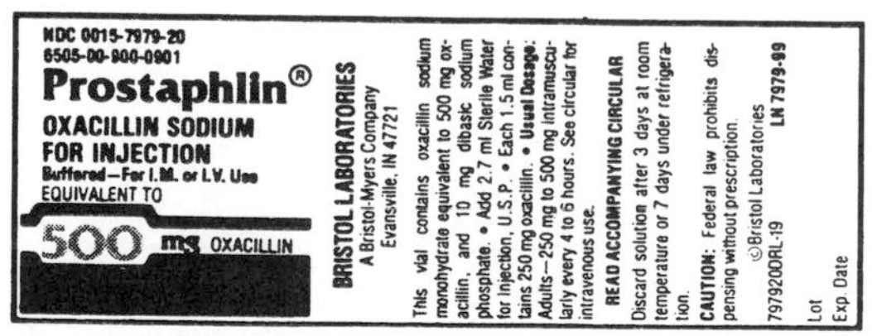

6. How many mL of diluent are needed to prepare the solution? ____________

7. What kind of solution is used as the diluent? ____________

8. What is the dose strength of the prepared solution? ____________

9. How long does the medication retain its potency at room temperature? ____________

10. How long does the medication retain its potency if it is refrigerated? ____________

11. The doctor ordered 400 mg I.M. q6h. How many mL will you give? Shade in the amount on the syringe provided.

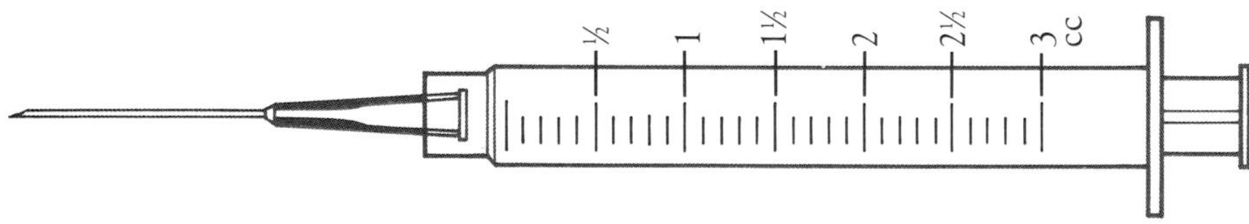

Using the label for Kefzol, answer the following questions.

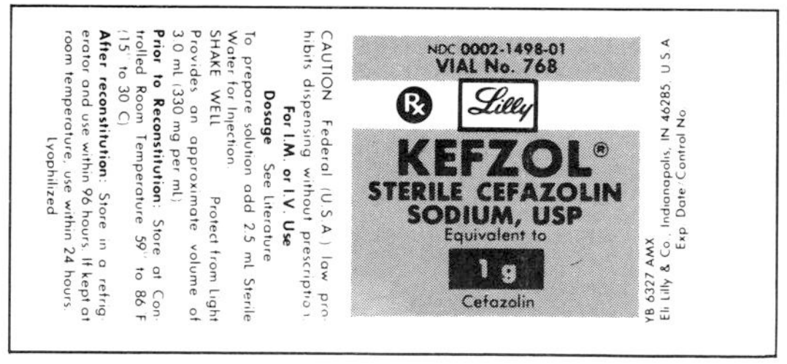

12. How much diluent must be added to the vial to prepare an I.M. dose? ____________

13. What kind of solution is used as the diluent? ____________

14. What is the dose strength of the prepared solution? ____________

15. How long will the reconstituted solution maintain its potency if refrigerated? ____________

16. The doctor ordered Kefzol 500 mg I.M. q6h. How many mL will you give? Shade in the amount on the syringe provided.

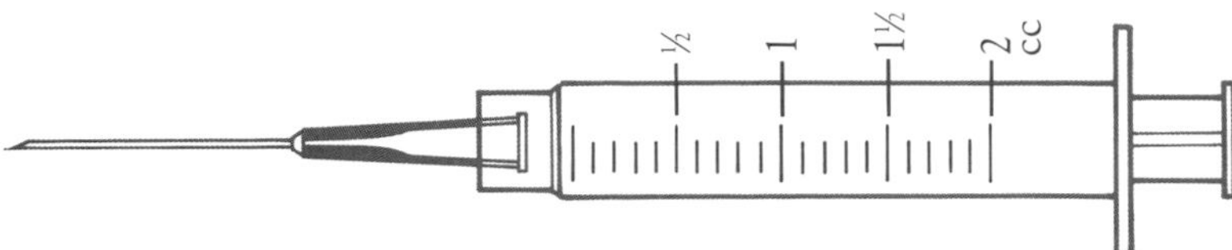

Using the label for Cefobid, answer the following questions.

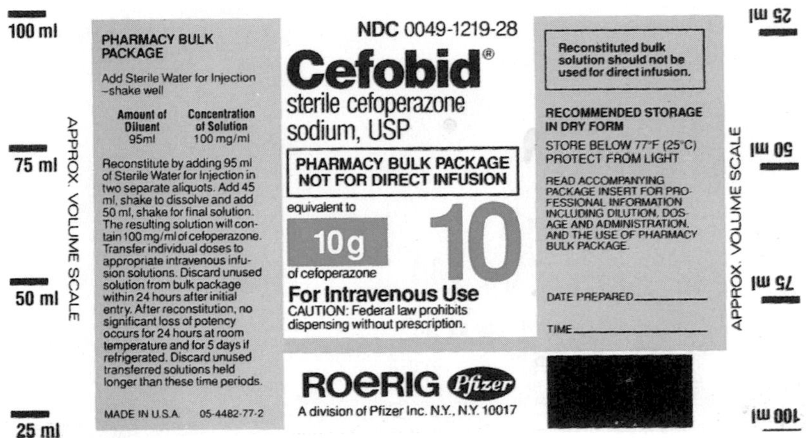

17. What route of administration is the medication indicated for? __________

18. How much diluent must be added to prepare the solution? __________

19. Whay type of solution is used for the diluent? __________

20. What is the dose strength of the prepared solution? __________

21. How long does the medication maintain its potency at room temperature? __________

22. How long does the medication maintain its potency if refrigerated? __________

23. The doctor ordered 1 g I.V. q6h. How many mL will you give? Shade in the amount on the syringe provided.

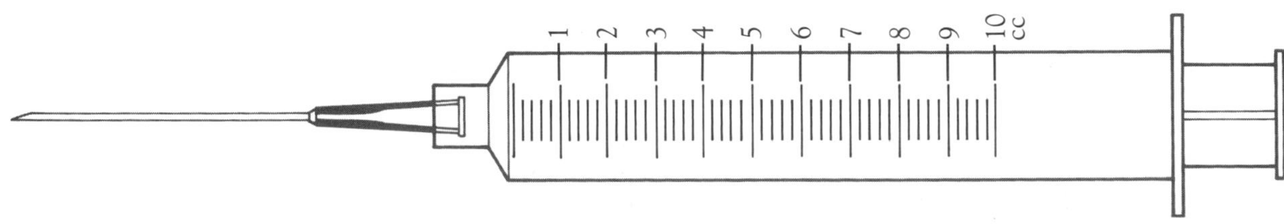

Using the label for Augmentin, answer the following questions.

Product No. 609064 NOT FOR SALE
Store dry powder at or below 25°C (77°F). After mixing, refrigerate, keep tightly closed and use within 24 hours. Shake well before using.
Directions for mixing: Tap bottle until all powder flows freely. Add approximately 1 teaspoonful (5 mL) of water; shake vigorously. When reconstituted, each 5 mL will contain 250 mg amoxicillin as the trihydrate and 62.5 mg clavulanic acid as clavulanate potassium. 9406441-E
250mg/5mL Patient Starter Package
AUGMENTIN®
AMOXICILLIN/CLAVULANATE POTASSIUM
FOR ORAL SUSPENSION
1 x 5mL (when reconstituted)
SB SmithKline Beecham
Use only if inner seal is intact.
Caution: Federal law prohibits dispensing without prescription.
SmithKline Beecham Pharmaceuticals
Philadelphia, PA 19101
LOT
EXP.

24. How much diluent must be added to prepare the solution? ____________

25. What type of solution is used for the diluent? ____________

26. What is the dose strength of the prepared solution? ____________

27. How should the medication be stored after it is mixed? ____________

Using the label for Zovirax and a portion of the package insert, answer the following questions.

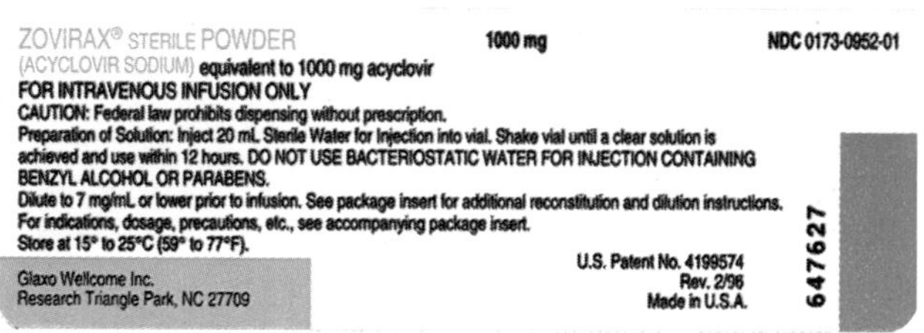

Method of Preparation: Each 10 mL vial contains acyclovir sodium equivalent to 500 mg of acyclovir. Each 20 mL vial contains acyclovir sodium equivalent to 1000 mg of acyclovir. The contents of the vial should be dissolved in Sterile Water for Injection as follows:

Contents of Vial	Amount of Diluent
500 mg	10 mL
1000 mg	20 mL

The resulting solution in each case contains 50 mg acyclovir per mL (pH approximately 11). Shake the vial well to assure complete dissolution before measuring and transferring each individual dose. DO NOT USE BACTERIOSTATIC WATER FOR INJECTION CONTAINING BENZYL ALCOHOL OR PARABENS.

28. How much diluent must be added to prepare the solution? ____________

29. What type of solution is used for the diluent? ____________

30. What is the dose strength of the prepared solution? ____________

31. What is the route of administration? ____________

Using the label for Erythromycin, answer the following questions.

TO PATIENT:
Shake well before using.
Keep tightly closed. Store in refrigerator and discard unused portion after ten days. Oversize bottle provides shake space.
TO THE PHARMACIST:
When prepared as directed, each 5 mL teaspoonful contains erythromycin ethylsuccinate equivalent to 200 mg of erythromycin in a cherry-flavored suspension.
Bottle contains erythromycin ethylsuccinate equivalent to 8 g of erythromycin.
Usual Dose: See package outsert.
Store at room temperature in dry form.
Child-Resistant closure not required; Reference: Federal Register Vol.39 No.29.
DIRECTIONS FOR PREPARATION: Slowly add 140 mL of water and shake vigorously to make 200 mL of suspension.
BARR LABORATORIES, INC.
Pomona, NY 10970
R11-90

BARR LABORATORIES, INC.

Erythromycin Ethylsuccinate for Oral Suspension, USP

200 mg of erythromycin activity per 5 mL reconstituted

Caution: Federal law prohibits dispensing without prescription.

200 mL (when mixed)

NDC 0555-0215-23
NSN 6505-00-080-0653

3 0555-0215-23 3

SAMPLE

Exp. Date:

Lot No.:

32. How much diluent must be added to prepare the solution? __________

33. What is the volume of the solution after it is mixed? __________

34. What is the dose strength of the prepared solution? __________

35. How long is the reconstituted solution good? __________

Reconstituting Medications with More than One Direction for Mixing

Some medications come with a choice of how to reconstitute them, thereby providing a choice of dose strengths. In this case the nurse must choose the concentration or dose strength appropriate for the dose ordered. A common medication that has a choice of dose strengths is penicillin. When a medication comes with several directions for preparation or offers a choice of dose strengths, the following guidelines may be used.

Guidelines for Choosing Appropriate Concentrations

1. Consider the route of administration.
   a) I.M.—You are concerned that the amount does not exceed the maximum allowed I.M. However you don't want to choose a concentration that will result in irritation when injected into a muscle. When a choice of strengths can be made, do not choose an amount that would exceed the amount allowed I.M. or that is very concentrated.
   b) I.V.—Keep in mind that this medication is usually further diluted because once reconstituted, the reconstituted material is then placed in additional fluid of 50 to 100 cc, depending on the medication being administered. Example: Erythromycin requires the reconstituted solution be placed in 250 cc of fluid before administration to a client. In pediatrics a medication may be given in a smaller volume of fluid depending on the age, the child's size, and the medication.
2. Choose the concentration or dose strength that comes closest to what the doctor has ordered. The dose strengths are given for the amount of diluent used.
   Example: If the doctor orders 300,000 U of a particular medication I.M., and the choices of strength are 200,000 U/ml, 250,000 U/mL, and 500,000 U/mL, the strength that is closest to 300,000 U/mL is 250,000U/mL. It allows you to administer a dose within the range for I.M., and it is not the most concentrated.
3. The word respectively may be used sometimes on a medication label for directions on reconstitution. For example, reconstitute with 23 mL, 18 mL, 8 mL of diluent to provide concentrations of 200,000 U, 250,000 U,

500,000 U per mL, respectively. The word *respectively* means in the order given. In terms of the directions for reconstitution, this means if you add 23 mL diluent, it will provide 200,000 U per mL; 18 mL diluent will provide 250,000 U per mL, etc. In other words, the amounts of diluent correspond to the order in which the concentrations are written. Remember: **When you are mixing a medication that is a multiple-strength solution, the dose strength that you prepare must be written on the vial.**

Let's look at a sample label that shows a multiple-strength solution.

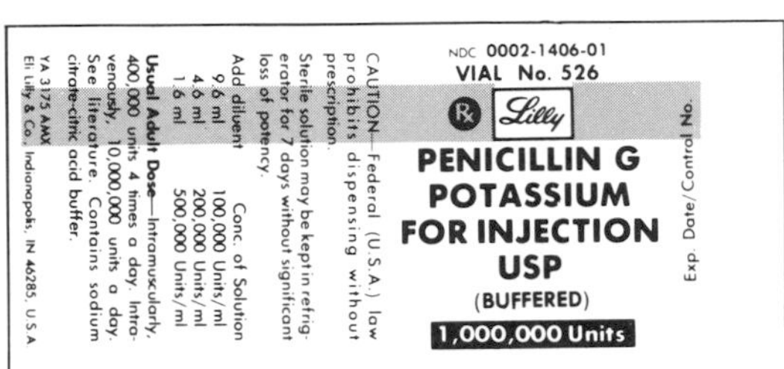

When looking at the penicillin label, notice it states 1,000,000 U. This means there is a total of 1,000,000 U of Penicillin in the vial. The directions for reconstitution and the dose strengths that can be obtained are listed on the left side of the label. If the dosage ordered for the client was, for example, 200,000 U q6h, the most appropriate strength to mix would be 200,000 U per mL. When reading the directions, if you look across next to the dose strength, you will notice that 4.6 mL of diluent must be added to obtain a concentration of solution 200,000 U per mL. Since this is a multiple-strength solution, the dose strength you choose must be indicated on the vial after you reconstitute it. Since the type of diluent is not indicated on the label, other resources such as those recommended previously in our discussion must be consulted.

Practice Problems (p. 366)

Using the label for penicillin G potassium, answer the following questions.

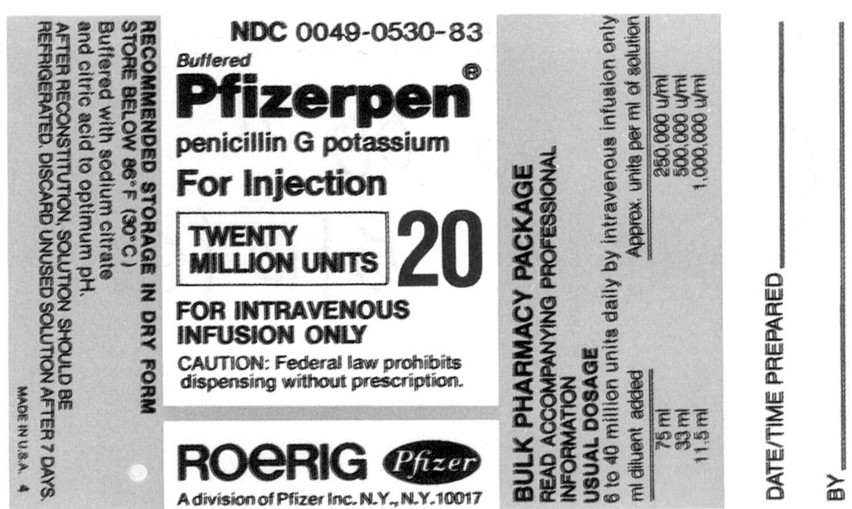

36. What is the total number of units of penicillin contained in the vial? __________

37. If you add 33 mL of diluent to the vial, what dose strength will you print on the label? __________

38. If the doctor ordered 2,000,000 U I.V., which dose strength would be appropriate to use? __________

39. How long will the medication maintain its potency if refrigerated? __________

Using the label for penicillin G potassium, answer the following questions.

NDC 0002-1406-01
VIAL No. 526
℞ Lilly
PENICILLIN G
POTASSIUM
FOR INJECTION
USP
(BUFFERED)
1,000,000 Units
Exp. Date/Control No.

CAUTION—Federal (U.S.A.) law prohibits dispensing without prescription.
Sterile solution may be kept in refrigerator for 7 days without significant loss of potency.

Add diluent	Conc. of Solution
9.6 ml	100,000 Units/ml
4.6 ml	200,000 Units/ml
1.6 ml	500,000 Units/ml

Usual Adult Dose—Intramuscularly, 400,000 units 4 times a day. Intravenously, 10,000,000 units a day. See literature. Contains sodium citrate-citric acid buffer.
YA 3175 AMX
Eli Lilly & Co., Indianapolis, IN 46285, U.S.A.

40. What is the total number of units of penicillin contained in the vial? __________

41. If the doctor ordered 700,000 U I.M., which dose strength would be appropriate to use? __________

42. Where will you store any unused medication? __________

43. How long will the medication maintain its potency? __________

44. What concentration strength would be obtained if you added 1.6 mL of diluent? __________

45. How long can the potency of the medication be obtained if it is refrigerated? __________

Calculation of Medications When the Final Concentration (Dosage Strength) Is Not Stated

Sometimes medications come with directions for only one way to reconstitute them, and the label does not indicate the final dose strength after it is mixed, such as "becomes 250 mg per cc." Example: A particular medication is available in 1 g in powder. Directions tell you that adding 2.5 cc of sterile water yields 3 cc of solution. When you add 2.5 cc of sterile water, the solution expands to 3 cc. The concentration is not changing; you will get 3 cc of solution; however, it will be equal to 1 g.

The problem is therefore calculated using 1 g = 3 cc.

Before we proceed to calculate doses, let's review the steps to use with medications that have been reconstituted.

1. The formula or the ratio-proportion method may be used to calculate the dose. What's available becomes the dose strength you obtain after mixing the medication according to the directions.
2. Powdered medications expand when a liquid is added (diluent + powder).
3. The volume the medication expands to must be considered when calculating the problem.
4. When the final concentration is not stated, the total weight of the medication in powdered form is used, and the number of ccs produced is indicated after the solvent or liquid has been added.
5. As with all calculation problems, check to make sure that the ordered and the available medications are in the same system of measurement and the same units.
6. Don't forget to label your answer.

Calculation of Doses to Administer

To calculate the dose to administer after reconstituting a medication, the ratio-proportion or formula method may be used, as with other forms of medication. However, the H (have or what's available) is the dose strength you obtain when you mix the medication according to the directions. If using ratio-proportion, therefore the known ratio is also the dose strength obtained when you mix the medication.

In $\frac{D}{H} \times Q = x$, Q is the volume of solution that contains the dose strength.

In $\frac{DW}{SW} = \frac{DV}{SV}$, SV is the volume of solution that contains the dose strength.

To illustrate, let's calculate the dose you would administer if you mixed the penicillin and made a solution containing 1,000,000 U/mL. The doctor has ordered 2,000,000 U I.M.

Solution Using the Ratio-Proportion Method

1,000,000 U : 1 mL = 2,000,000 U : x mL

(Known) (Unknown)

$$\frac{1{,}000{,}000}{1{,}000{,}000}x = \frac{2{,}000{,}000}{1{,}000{,}000}$$

$$x = \frac{2{,}000{,}000}{1{,}000{,}000}$$

$$x = 2 \text{ mL}$$

Solution Using the Formula Method

$$\frac{D}{H} \times Q = x$$

$$\frac{2{,}000{,}000 \text{ U}}{1{,}000{,}000 \text{ U}} \times 1 \text{ mL} = x \text{ mL}$$

$$\frac{2{,}000{,}000}{1{,}000{,}000} = x$$

$$x = 2 \text{ mL}$$

OR

$$\frac{DW}{SW} = \frac{DV}{SV}$$

$$\frac{2{,}000{,}000 \text{ U}}{1{,}000{,}000 \text{ U}} = \frac{x \text{ mL}}{1 \text{ mL}}$$

$$\frac{2{,}000{,}000}{1{,}000{,}000} = x$$

$$x = 2 \text{ mL}$$

Sample Problem: Doctor orders 0.5 g of an antibiotic I.M. q4h.

Available: 1 g of the drug in powdered form; the label reads: Add 1.7 mL of sterile water; each mL will then contain 500 mg.

Problem Setup

1. A conversion is necessary. Equivalent 1000 mg = 1 g. Convert what's ordered into the available units. This will eliminate a decimal point.
2. Think: What would a logical answer be?

Solution Using the Ratio-Proportion Method

500 mg : 1 mL = 500 mg : x mL

(Known) (Unknown)

$$\frac{500}{500}x = \frac{500}{500}$$

$$x = \frac{500}{500}$$

$$x = 1 \text{ mL}$$

Solution Using the Formula Method

$$\frac{D}{H} \times Q = x$$

$$\frac{500 \text{ mg}}{500 \text{ mg}} \times 1 \text{ mL} = x \text{ mL}$$

$$\frac{500}{500} = x$$

$$x = 1 \text{ mL}$$

OR

$$\frac{DW}{SW} = \frac{DV}{SV}$$

$$\frac{500 \text{ mg}}{500 \text{ mg}} = \frac{x \text{ mL}}{1 \text{ mL}}$$

$$\frac{500}{500} = x$$

$$x = 1 \text{ mL}$$

Points to Remember

- If the medication is not used entirely after it is mixed, any medication remaining for use must have the following information clearly written on the label.

  a) Initials of the preparer

  b) The dose strength (final concentration) per volume of solution (cc, mL)

  c) Date and time of preparation and the date and time of expiration

  Note: If there is no area on the label for this information to be indicated, the information can be written directly on the vial in an area that can be read clearly.

- Read all directions carefully; if there are no instructions on the vial, the package insert, the pharmacy, or other reliable resources may be used to find the necessary information for reconstitution.

- When directions on the label are for I.M. and I.V. reconstitution, read the label carefully for the solution you are preparing.

- Read directions relating to storage and the time period for maintaining potency relating to how the medication is stored (room temperature, refrigeration).

Chapter Review (pp. 366-372)

In the following problems, calculate the amount of mL you will prepare to administer. Use the labels where provided to obtain the necessary information and shade in the dose you calculated on the syringe when provided. Round answers to the nearest tenth where indicated.

1. Doctor's Order: Ampicillin 400 mg I.M. q4h.

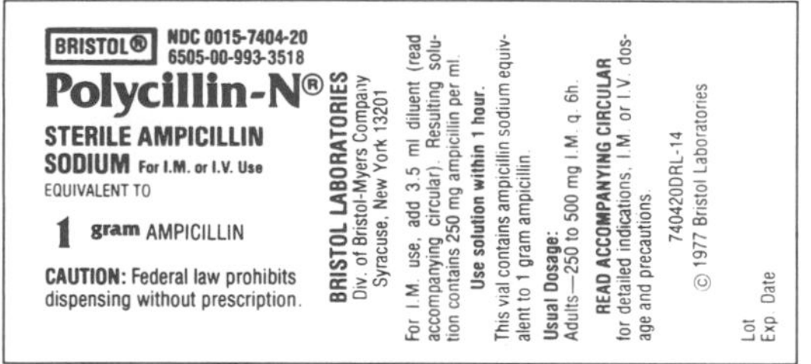

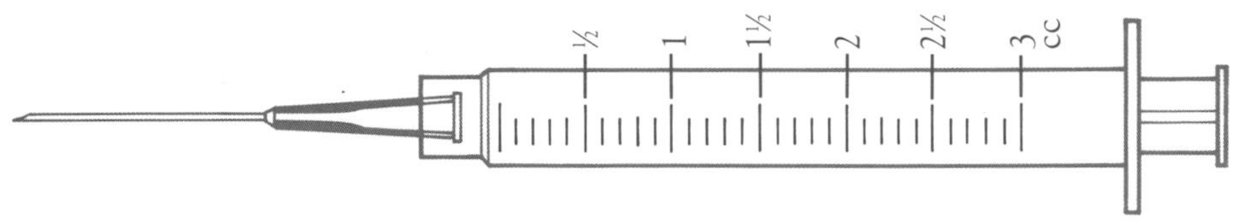

2. Doctor's Order: Ampicillin 1 g I.V. q6h.

   Directions state the following for I.V. administration: Reconstitute with 10 mL of diluent. The vial contains ampicillin 1 g.

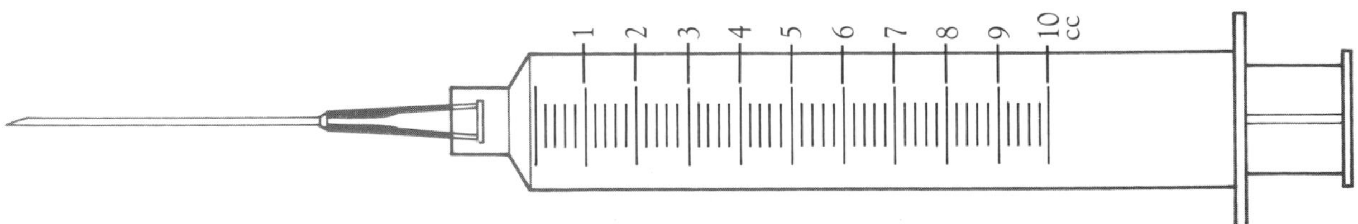

3. Doctor's Order: Oxacillin 300 mg I.M. q6h.

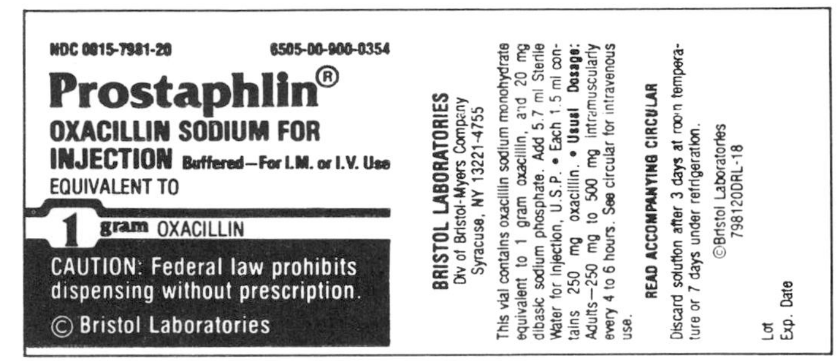

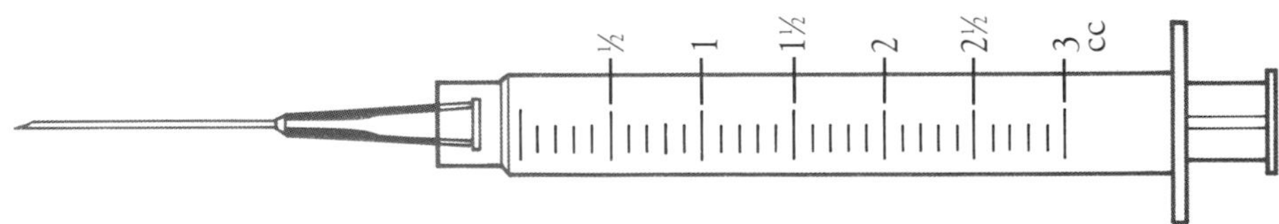

4. Doctor's Order: Mezlocillin 1.5 g I.V. q6h.
   Label states: For I.V. use reconstitute with 30 mL sterile water for injection.
   Each 30 mL of reconstituted solution will contain 3 g mezlocillin.
   How many will you administer? __________

5. Doctor's Order: Ticar 1 g I.M. q6h.
   a) How many mL of diluent must be added? __________
   b) What type of diluent is used? __________
   c) What is the dose strength of the reconstituted solution? __________

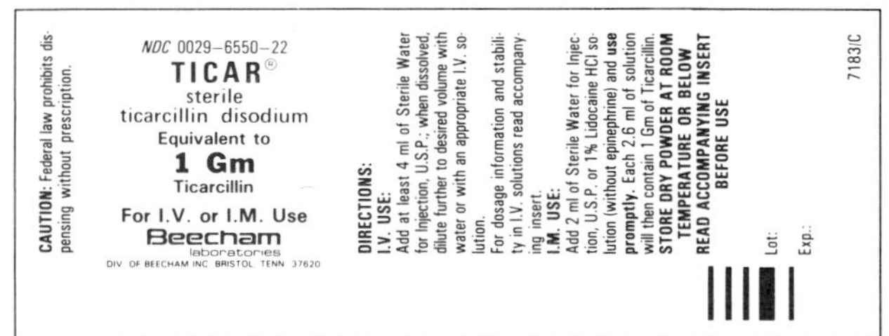

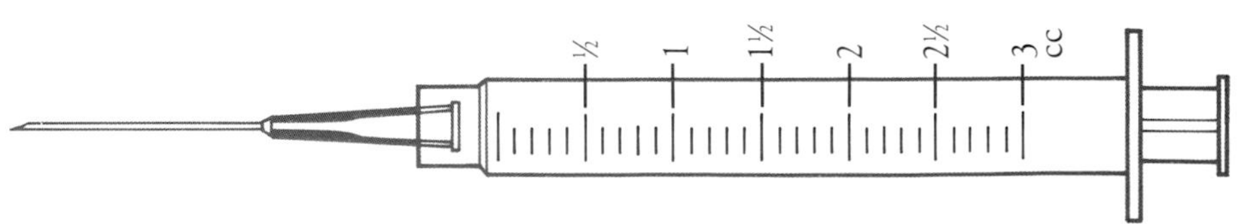

6. Doctor's Order: Penicillin G 600,000 U I.V. q4h.
   a) Which dosage strength would be best to choose? __________
   b) How many mL of diluent would be needed to make the dose strength? __________

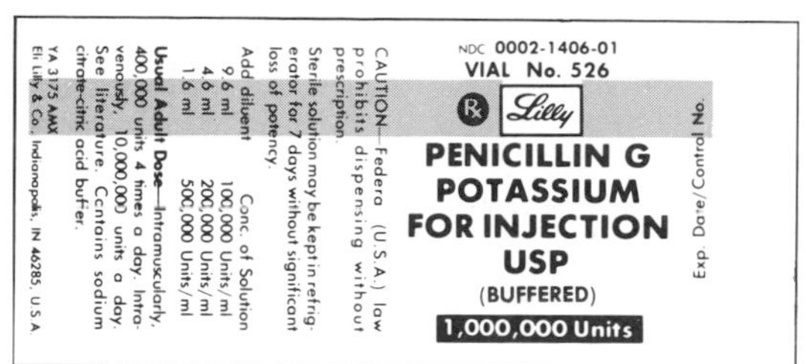

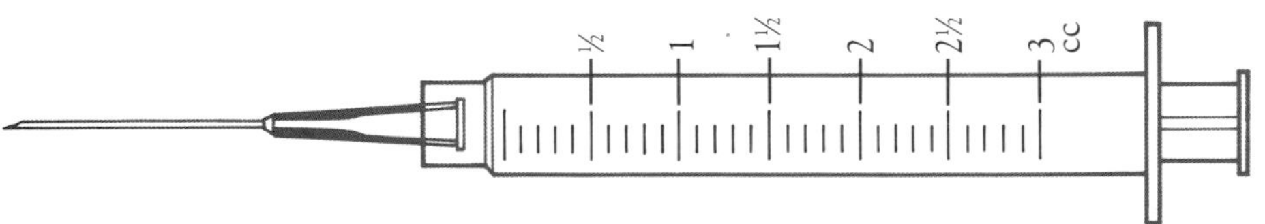

7. Doctor's Order: Solu-Cortef 200 mg I.V. q6h × 1 week.
   a) How many mg per mL is the reconstituted material? __________

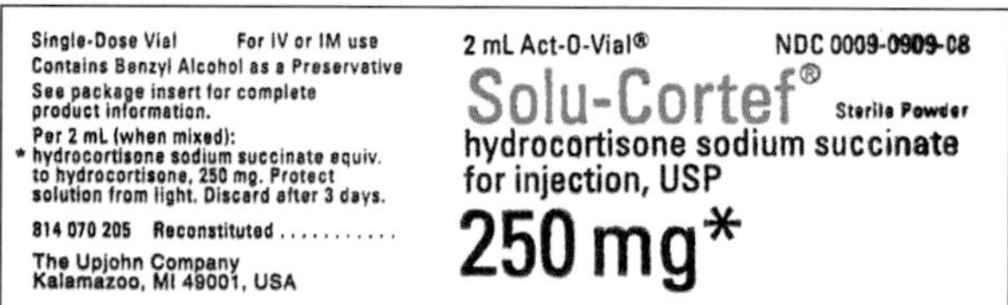

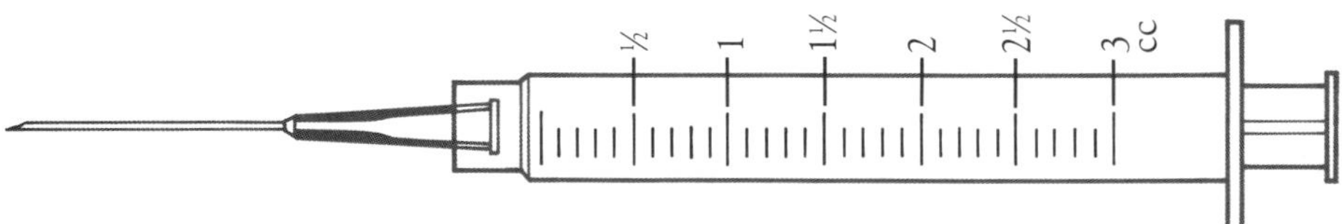

8. Doctor's Order: Carbenicillin 1 g I.M. q6h.
   a) What type of diluent is used? __________
   b) If you reconstitute with 9.5 mL of diluent, how many mL will you administer? __________

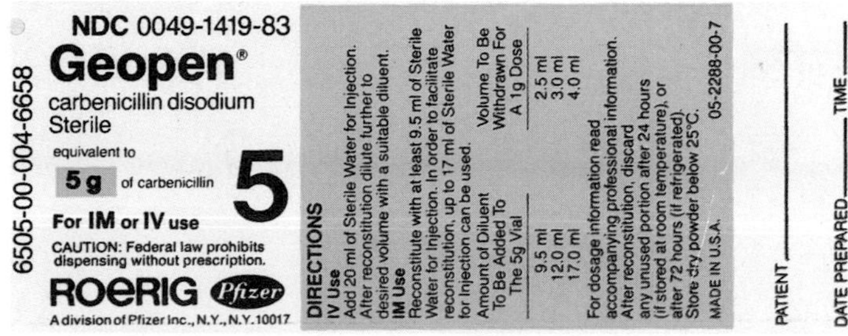

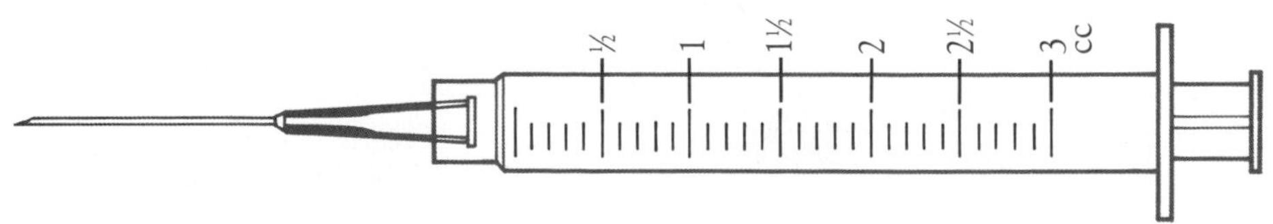

9. Doctor's Order: Amoxicillin 500 mg p.o. q6h.
   a) How many mL of diluent must be added? ________
   b) What is the dose strength after reconstitution? ________
   c) How many mL are needed to administer the required dose? ________

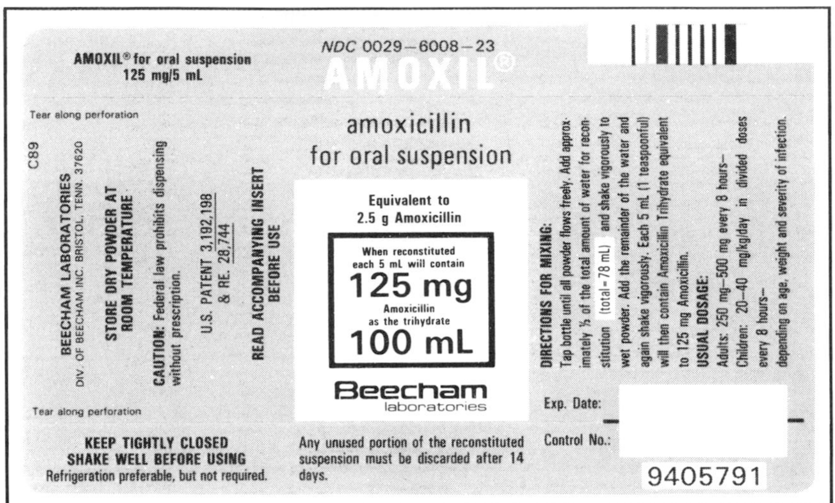

10. Doctor's Order: Staphcillin 1 g I.M.
    a) How much diluent must be added for I.M.? ________

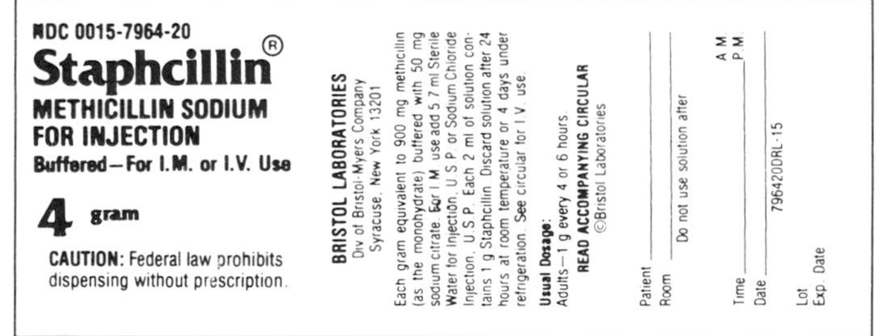

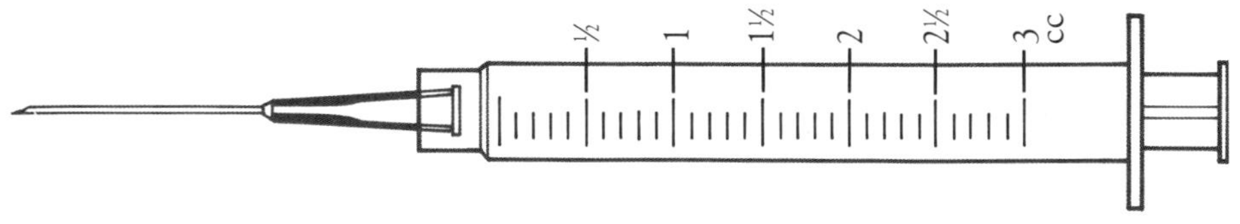

11. Doctor's Order: Ancef 500 mg I.M. q8h.
    a) How many mL of diluent should be used to reconstitute? ________
    b) What will be the dose strength of the reconstituted Ancef? ________

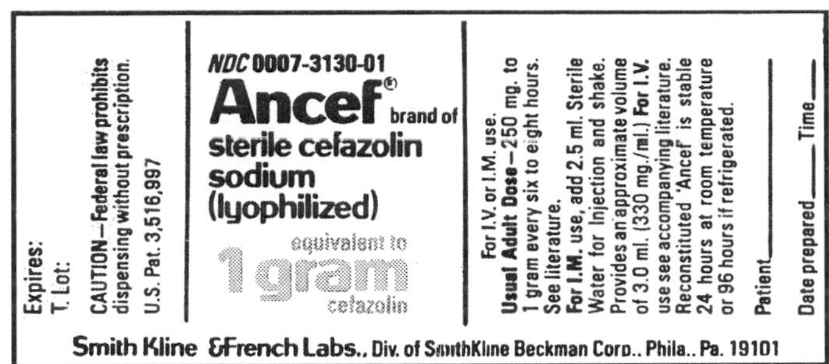

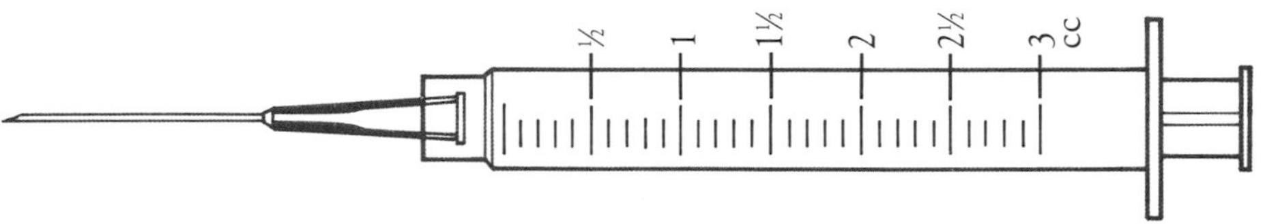

12. Doctor's Order: Nafcillin 1 g I.M. q6h.
    a) What is the dose strength of the reconstituted nafcillin? ________

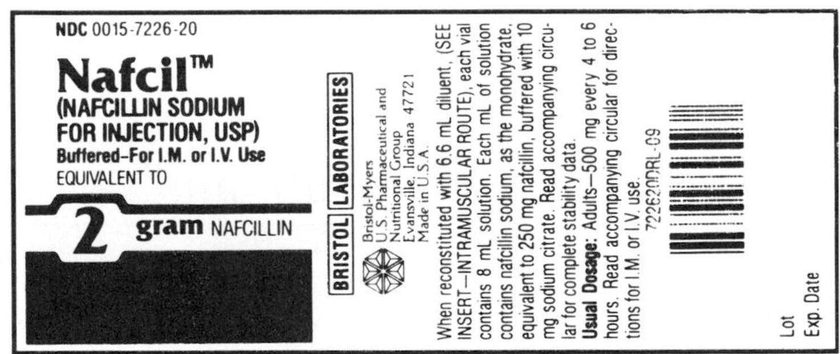

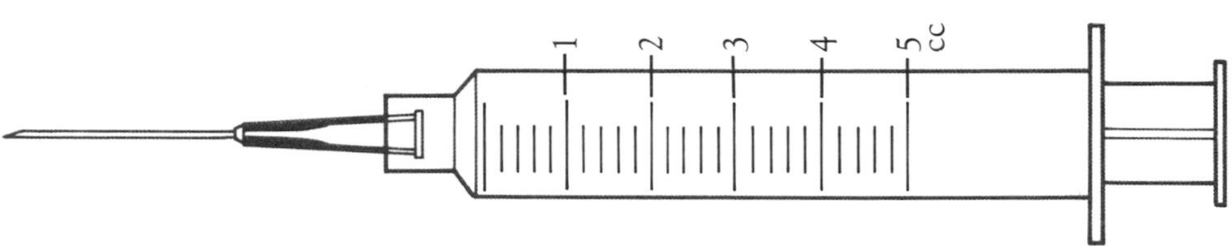

13. Doctor's Order: Cefotaxime 750 mg I.M. q8h.
    Available: Cefotaxime with the package insert below.
    a) What is the total grams of cefotaxime in the vial? ________
    b) According to the package insert, what volume of diluent is used for I.M. reconstitution? ________
    c) What is the dose strength of the reconstituted cefotaxime? ________

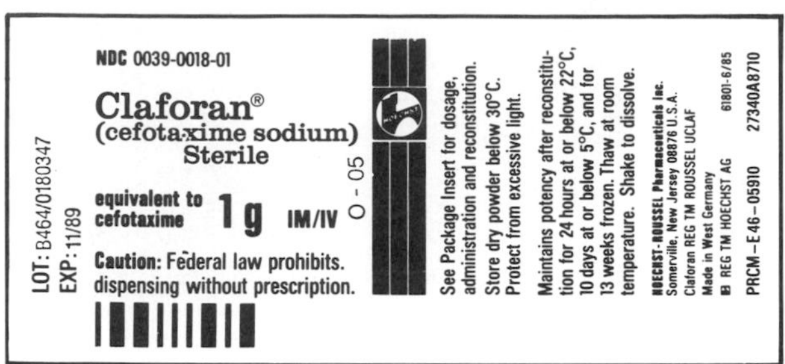

PREPARATION OF CLAFORAN STERILE

Claforan for IM or IV administration should be reconstituted as follows:

Strength	Diluent (mL)	Withdrawable Volume (mL)	Approximate Concentration (mg/mL)
1g vial (IM)*	3	3.4	300
2g vial (IM)*	5	6.0	330
1g vial (IV)*	10	10.4	95
2g vial (IV)*	10	11.0	180
1g infusion	50-100	50-100	20-10
2g infusion	50-100	50-100	40-20
10g bottle	47	52.0	200
10g bottle	97	102.0	100

*in conventional vials

Shake to dissolve; inspect for particulate matter and discoloration prior to use. Solutions of Claforan range from very pale yellow to light amber, depending on concentration, diluent used, and length and condition of storage.

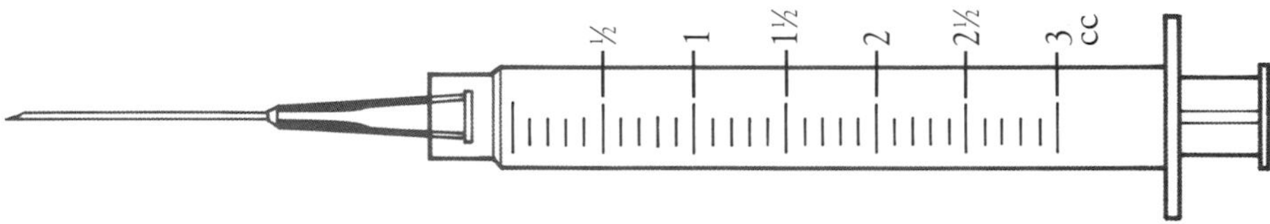

14. Doctor's Order: Streptomycin 0.5 g I.M. q6h.
    a) What is the total grams of streptomycin in the vial? ________
    b) What is the volume of diluent used for reconstitution? ________
    c) What is the dose strength of the reconstituted streptomycin? ________

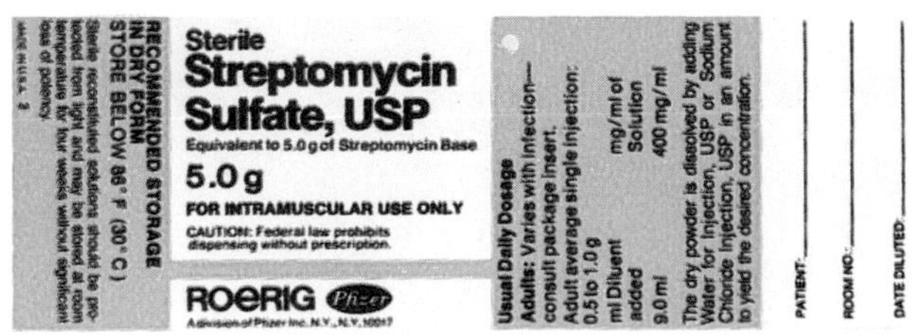

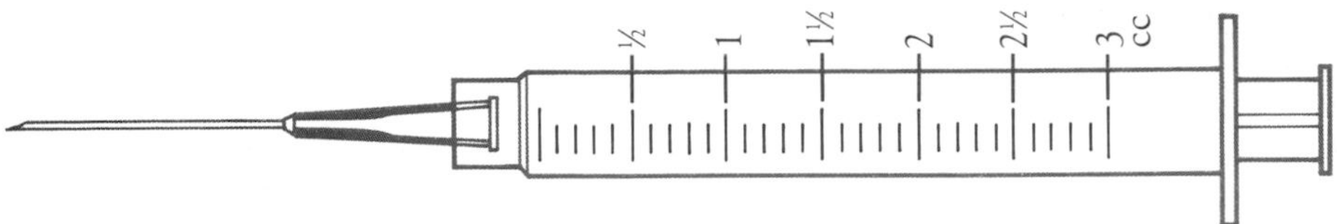

15. Doctor's Order: Chloromycetin 0.5 g I.V. q6h.
    a) What is the volume of diluent used for reconstitution? ________
    b) What is the dose strength of the reconstituted Chloromycetin? ________

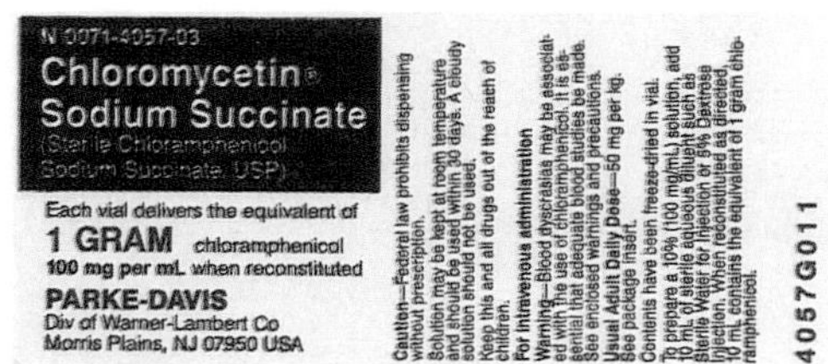

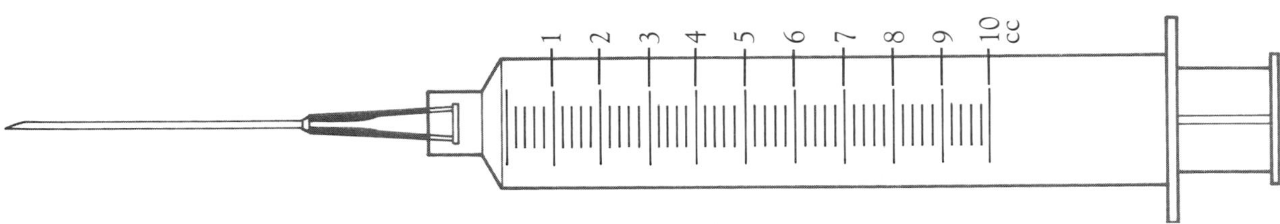

16. Doctor's Order: Penicillin G 400,000 U I.M. q4h.
    Available: Penicillin G 5,000,000 U. Directions state: Add 8 mL diluent to provide 500,000 U/mL.

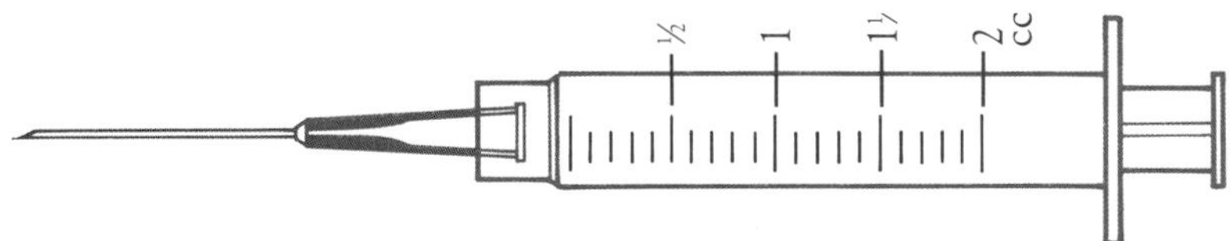

17. Doctor's Order: Penicillin G Potassium 600,000 U I.M. o.d.
    a) What would be the best strength to reconstitute? ________
    b) How many mL of diluent would be used? ________

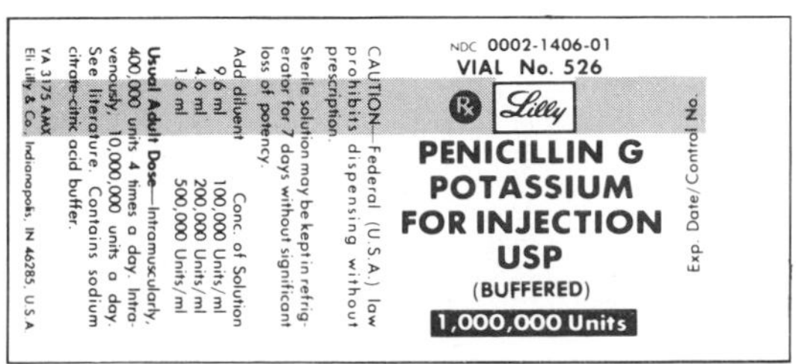

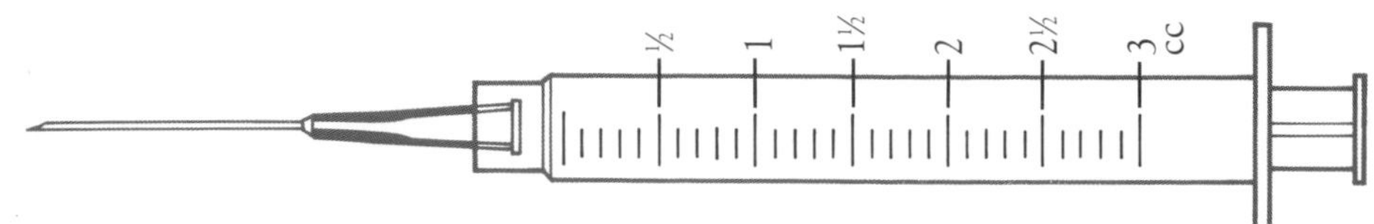

18. Doctor's Order: Ceftazidine 250 mg I.M. q12h.
    Available: Ceftazidime 600 mg. Directions for I.M. use state add 1.5 mL of an approved diluent to provide 300 mg/mL.

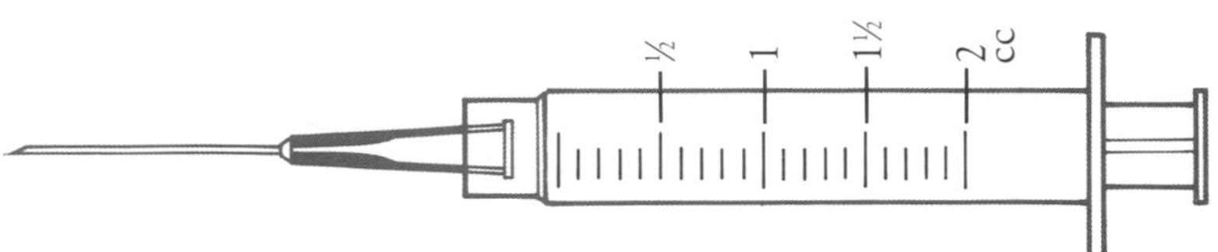

19. Doctor's Order: Ticar 0.5 g I.M. q6h.
    a) How many mL of diluent would be used to reconstitute? __________
    b) What is the dose strength of the reconstituted Ticar? __________

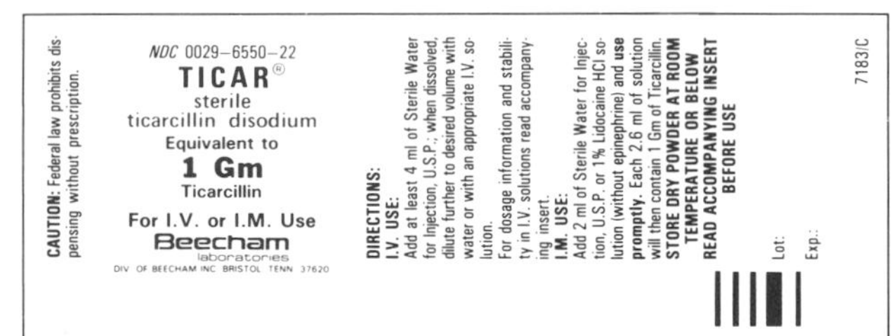

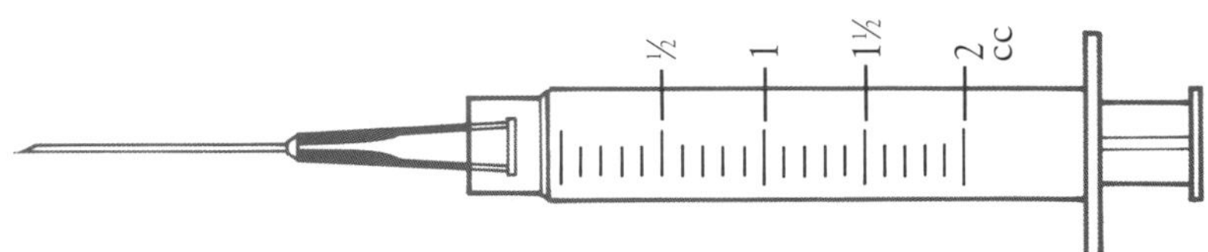

20. Doctor's Order: Staphcillin 1 g I.M. q6h.
    a) How many mL of diluent would be used to reconstitute? __________
    b) What is the dosage strength of the reconstituted Staphcillin? __________

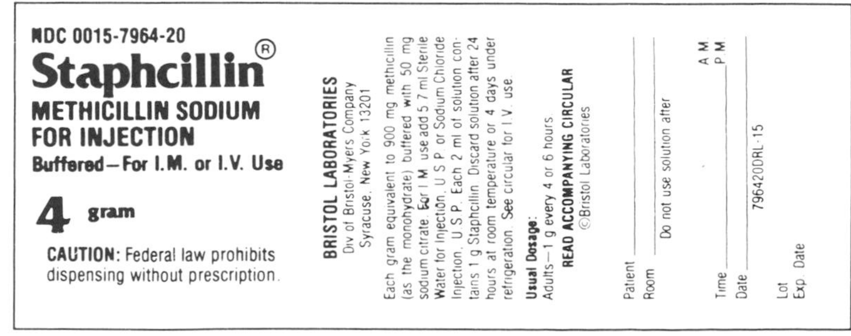

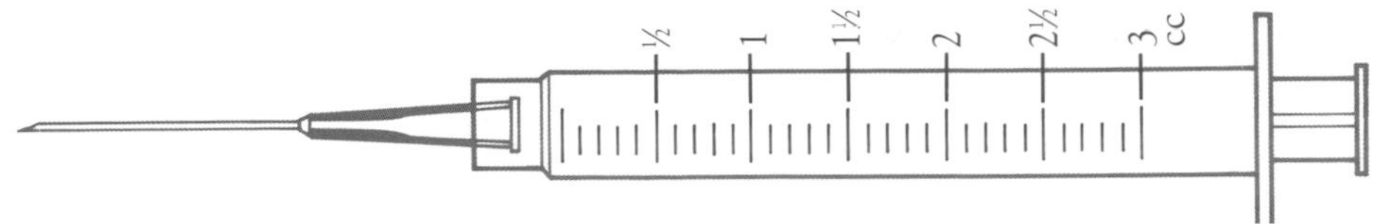

21. Doctor's Order: Tazicef 0.4 g I.V. q8h.
    Directions for I.V. state: Add 10 mL sterile water. Each mL of solution contains 95 mg.

Tazicef Injection
1 gram

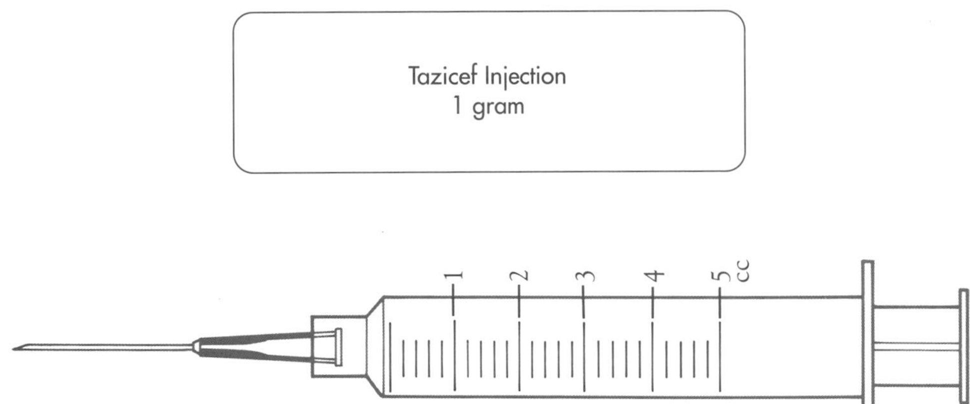

22. Doctor's Order: Vancomycin 0.5 g I.V. q12h.
    Directions for I.V. below.

PREPARATION AND STABILITY
At the time of use, reconstitute by adding either 10 mL of Sterile Water for Injection to the 500-mg vial or 20 mL of Sterile Water for Injection to the 1-g vial of dry, sterile vancomycin powder. Vials reconstituted in this manner will give a solution of 50 mg/mL. FURTHER DILUTION IS REQUIRED.
After reconstitution, the vials may be stored in a refrigerator for 14 days without significant loss of potency. Reconstituted solutions containing 500 mg of vancomycin must be diluted with at least 100 mL of diluent. Reconstituted solutions containing 1 g of vancomycin must be diluted with at least 200 mL of diluent. The desired dose, diluted in this manner, should be administered by intermittent intravenous infusion over a period of at least 60 minutes.

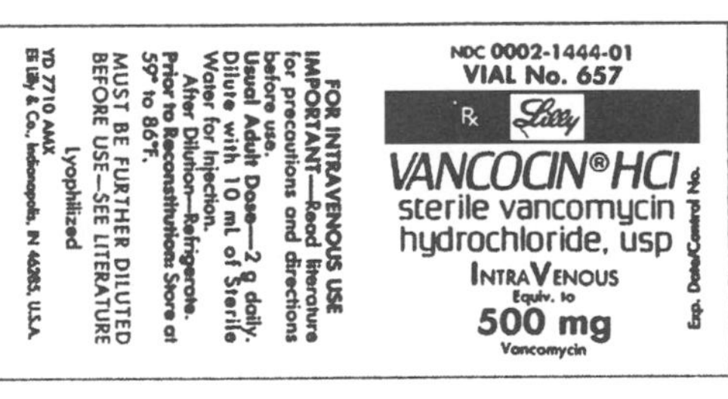

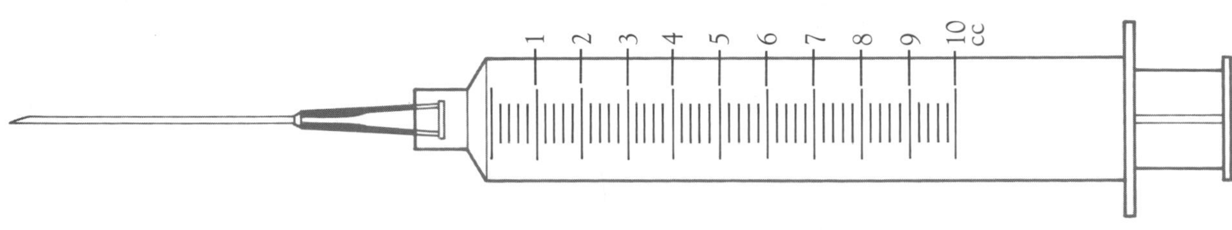

23. Doctor's Order: Levothyroxine sodium 0.05 mg I.V. o.d.
    Available: Levothroxine sodium vial with directions that state: Dilute with 5 mL of sodium chloride to produce 200 mcg.

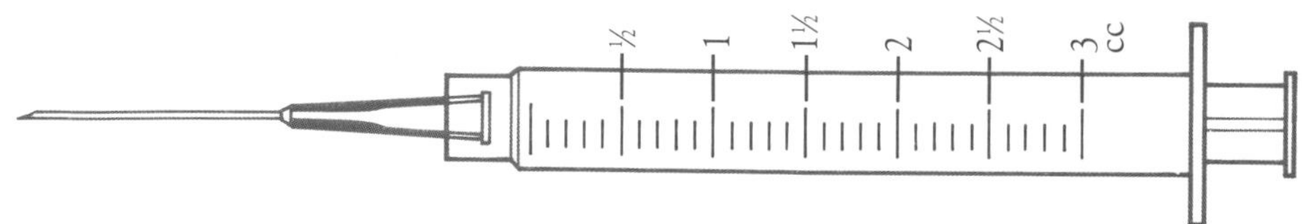

24. Doctor's Order: Zovirax 0.25 g I.V. q8h × 5 days.
    Directions state: Add 10 mL of sterile water to produce 50 mg/mL.

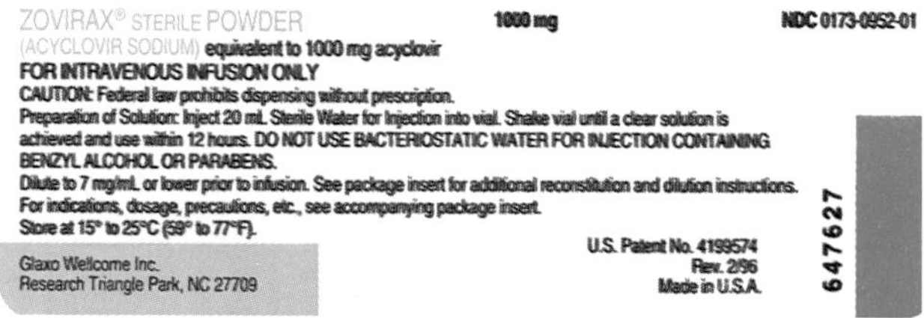

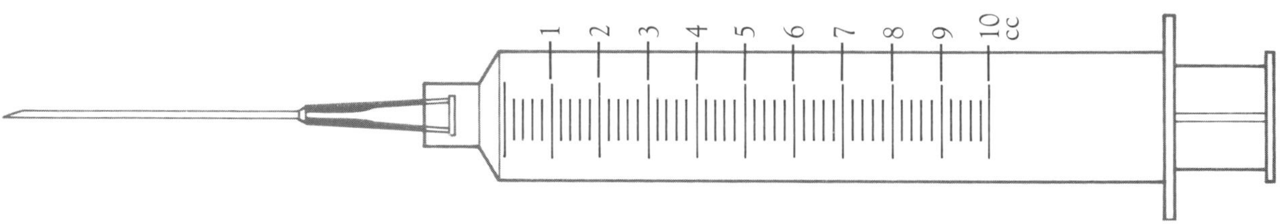

25. Doctor's Order: Suprax 400 mg p.o. q.d.
    a) How many mL of water is needed to reconstitute the powder? ________
    b) How many mL will you administer using an oral syringe? ________

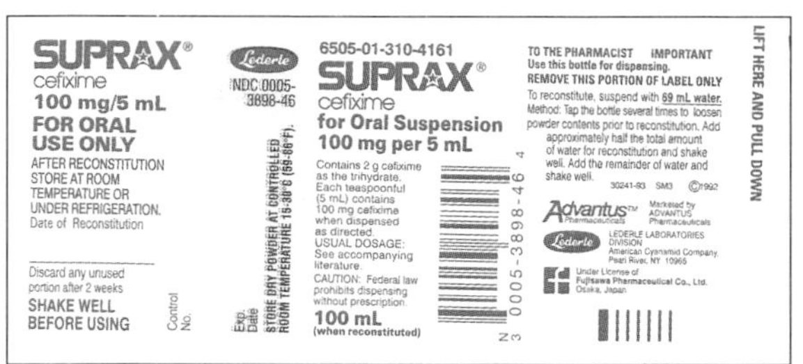

Chapter 18

Insulin

Objectives

After reviewing this chapter the student will be able to do the following:

1. **Identify important information on insulin labels**
2. **Read calibrations on U-100 insulin syringes**
3. **Measure insulin in single doses**
4. **Measure combined insulin doses**
5. **Convert insulin units to milliliters**

Insulin is used in the treatment of diabetes mellitus. Insulin is a hormone secreted by the islets of Langerhans in the pancreas. It is a necessary hormone for glucose use by the body. Individuals who do not produce adequate insulin experience an increase in their blood sugar (glucose) level. These individuals may require the administration of insulin. Accuracy in insulin administration is extremely important since inaccurate doses can lead to serious or life-threatening effects. Insulin doses are measured in units (U) and administered with syringes that correspond to insulin U-100; U-100 insulin means 100 U/mL. The most common type of insulin is supplied in 10-mL vials and labeled U-100. Insulin is also available as U-500 (500 U/mL). U-500 is a more concentrated strength and is used for diabetic clients who have blood sugars that fluctuate to extremely high levels.

Types of Insulin

Different types of insulin are available today. Choice of dose and insulin preparation are dependent on the needs of the client. Insulin is obtained from human and animal sources. The origin of insulin is indicated on the label. Human insulin is identified as semisynthetic, while the animal sources are identified as pork or beef on the label. Due to the variations, the doctor should specify the origin of insulin when writing insulin orders. **Be sure to read the label carefully to administer insulin of the correct origin.** The other information that can be found on the label is the type of insulin. This is indicated by a letter that follows the trade name (Figures 18-1 and 18-2).

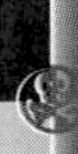

Think Critically to Avoid Errors in Administration

Careful reading of insulin labels is essential for correct identification and avoiding medication errors. If mixing of insulins is necessary, only the same species can be mixed. Example: Pork and pork.

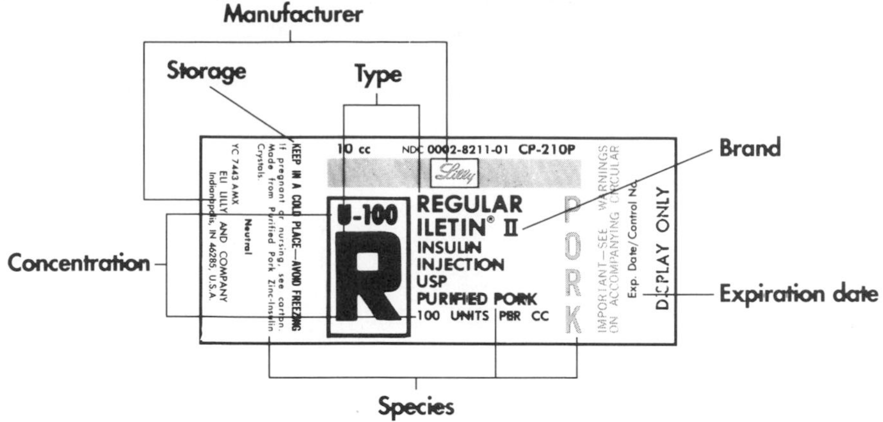

Figure 18-1. Regular insulin. (From Dison N: *Simplified drugs and solutions for nurses,* ed 11, St Louis, 1996, Mosby.)

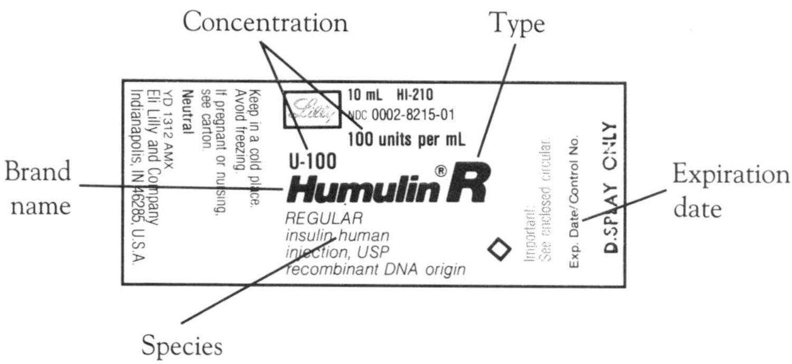

Figure 18-2. Humulin. (From Dison N: *Simplified drugs and solutions for nurses,* ed 11, St Louis, 1992, Mosby.)

The letter that follows the trade name on insulin labels, for example, Humulin R, tells you the type and action time. Nurses must be familiar with onset of action, peak, and duration, which vary depending on the type of insulin. Insulins are classified as rapid-acting (regular), intermediate-acting (NPH), and long-acting (PZI). The expiration date is also indicated on the label and is important to check, as well as the concentration, 100 U/mL. On insulins manufactured under the trade name of Humulin, an international symbol is also indicated on the label, so insulins can be identified worldwide.

Example: (◇) = Regular, (□) = NPH. See insulin labels below.

Notice that both labels shown are Humulin (trade name), but they are followed by the letters N and R. N = NPH (intermediate-acting), R = regular (rapid-acting). Note the international symbols on the label as well.

Labels Showing International Symbols on Humulin Insulin

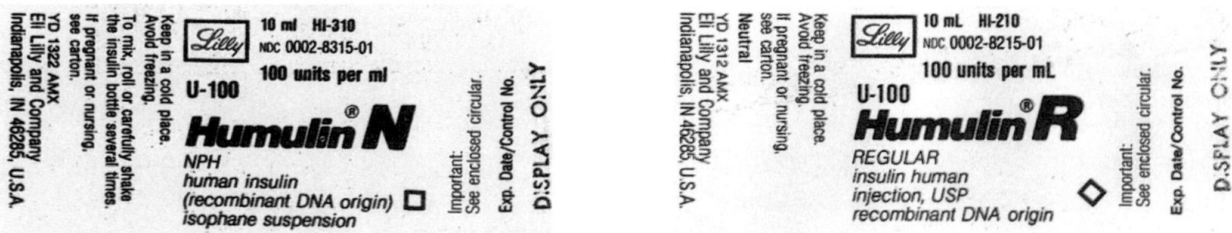

Practice Problems (p. 373)

Using the labels below, identify the type of insulin and its origin. Note the left side of the label indicates whether the insulin is made from beef or pork.

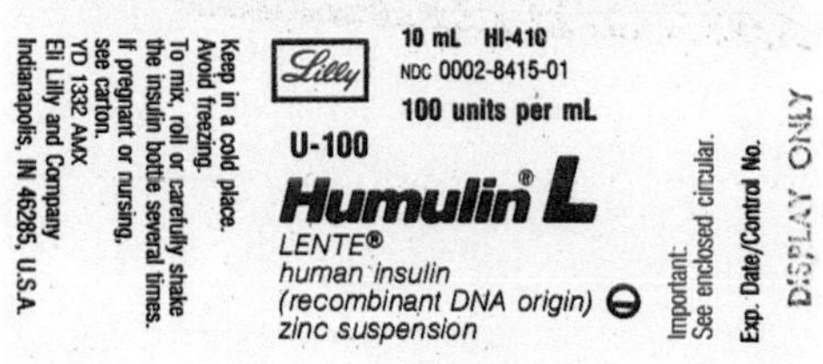

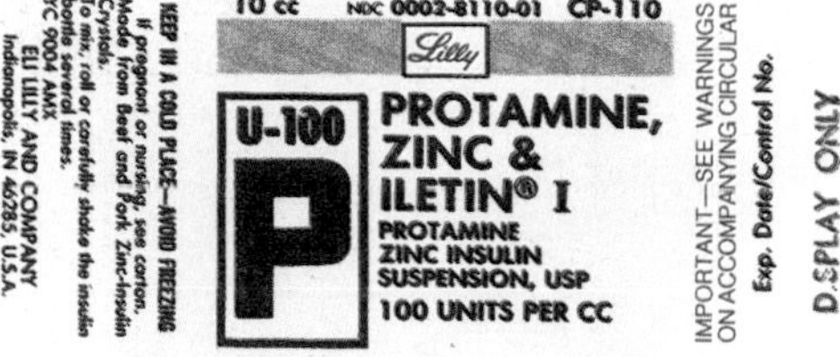

1. ______________________ 2. ______________________

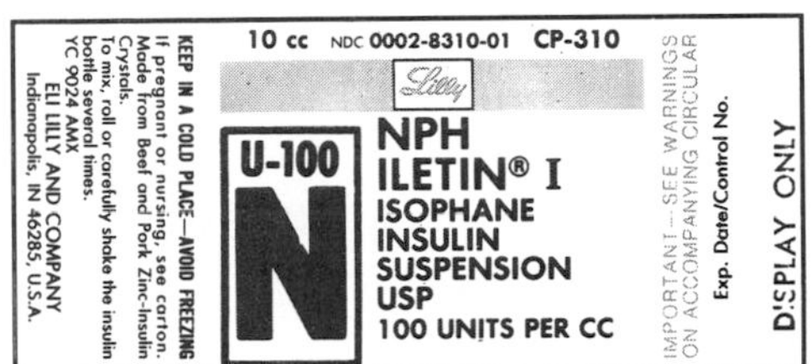

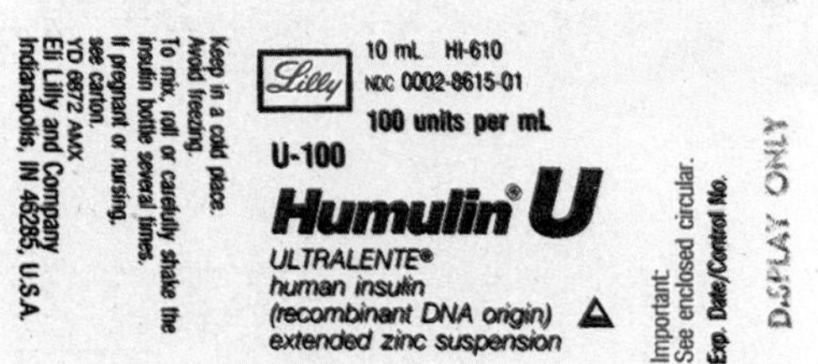

3. ______________________ 4. ______________________

Types of U-100 Insulins

Nurses must be familiar with the three types U-100 insulins.

Fast-Acting (Rapid-Acting)

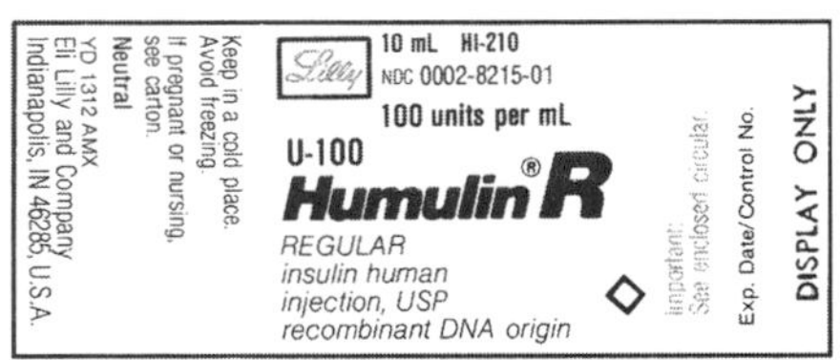

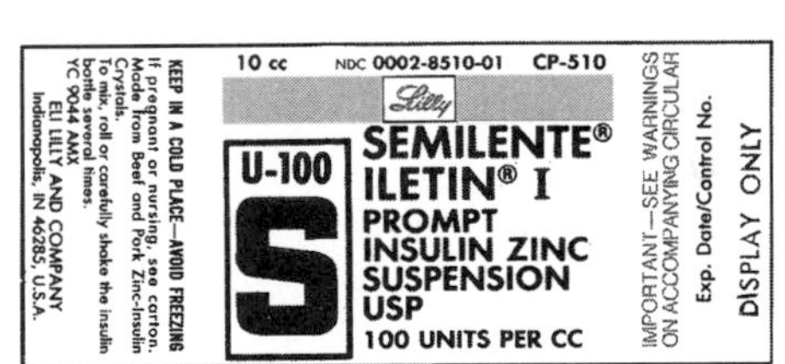

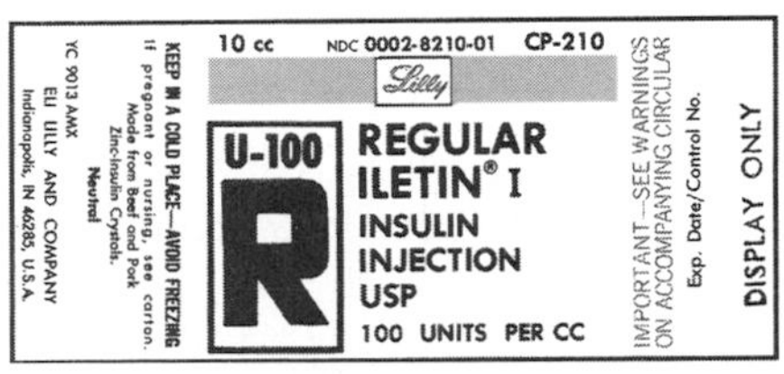

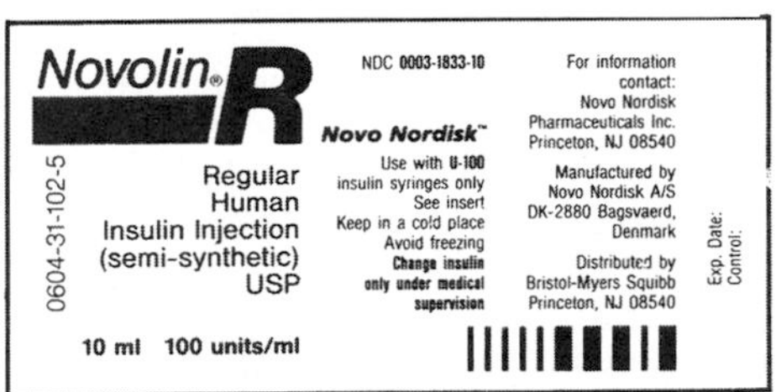

Intermediate-Acting

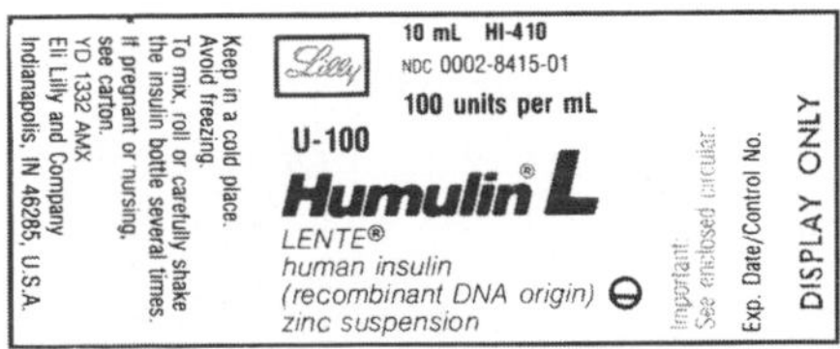

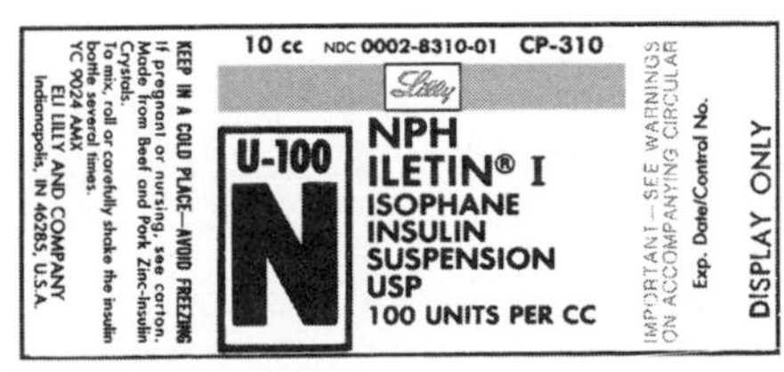

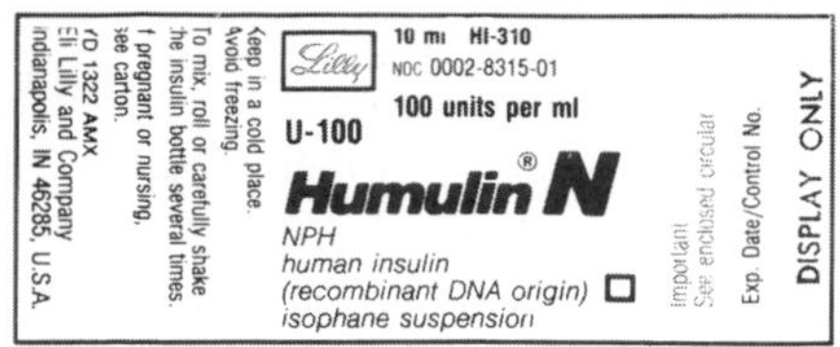

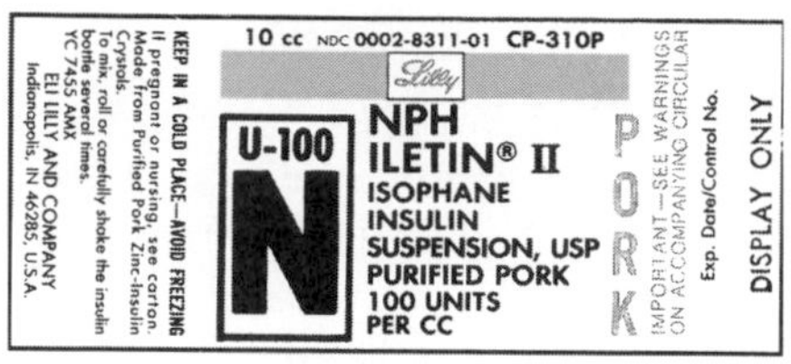

Long-Acting

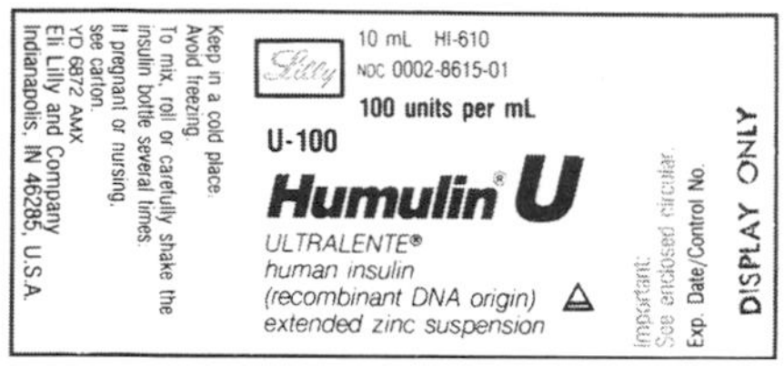

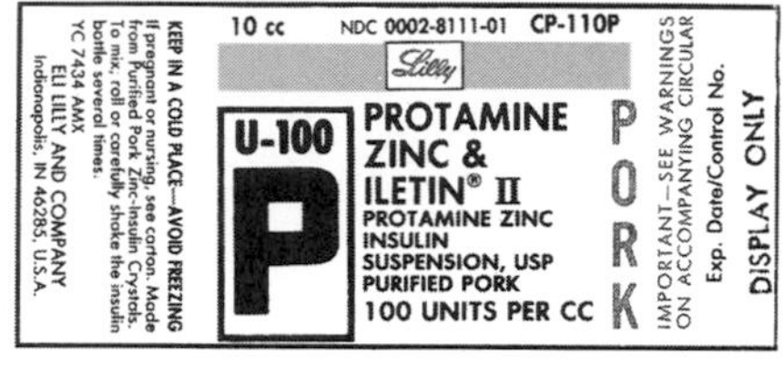

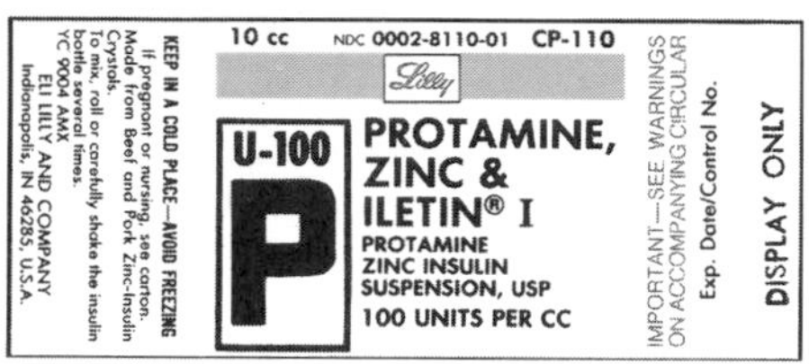

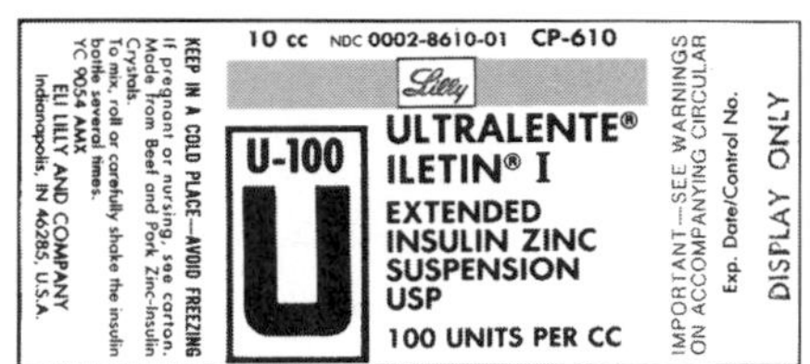

Appearance of Insulin

Regular insulin is clear and is the only insulin that may be given I.V. Other insulin is cloudy and must be rotated between the hands to mix.

Fixed Combination Insulins

Fixed-combination insulins are now available: 70-30 U-100 and 50-50 U-100. The purpose of the fixed-combination insulins is to simulate the varying levels of insulin within the bodies of nondiabetic persons. The fixed-combination insulins are from a human or pork source and are available in the following combinations:

Human Source—50 U of isophane insulin (intermediate-acting) with 50 U of regular (short-acting); 70 U of isophane insulin with 30 U of regular insulin

Pork Source—70 U of pork isophane insulin and 30 U of regular pork insulin

To understand the fixed-combination insulin orders, it is important for the nurse to understand that, for example, 70/30 concentration means there is 70% NPH insulin (isophane) and 30% regular insulin in each unit. Therefore, if the doctor ordered 30 units of Humulin 70/30 insulin, the client would receive 70% or 0.7 × 30 U = 21 U of NPH, and 9 U of regular insulin (30% or 0.3 × 30 U = 9 U), and so on. (See labels of combination insulins below.)

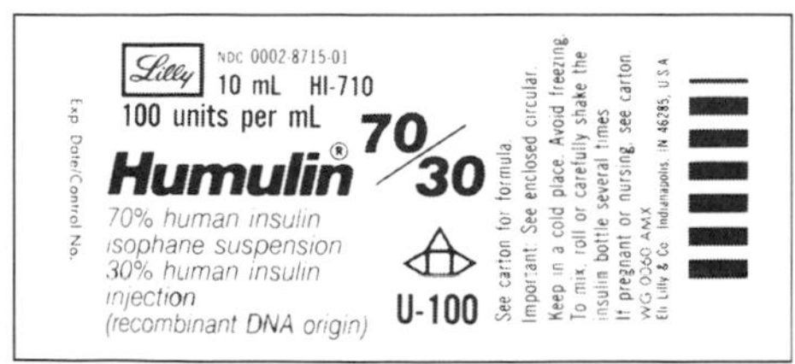

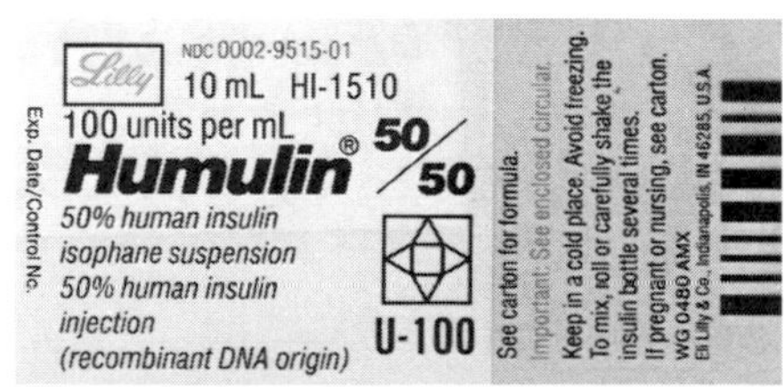

U-100 Syringe

The U-100 syringe was discussed in Chapter 16. As a review, insulin is administered s.c., usually with a syringe marked U-100. There are different types of U-100 syringes:

1. Lo-Dose syringe—It has a capacity of 50 U (0.5 cc). Each calibration on the syringe measures 1 U. There is also a 30-U syringe, which is used to accurately measure very small amounts of insulin. It is marked in units up to 30. Each calibration is 1 U.
2. 1-cc (100 U) capacity syringe—There are two types of 1-cc syringe in current use.
   a) Single-scale syringe is calibrated in 2 U-increments. Any dose measured on this syringe that is an odd number of units is measured between the even calibrations. This would not be the desired syringe for clients with vision problems.
   b) Double-scale syringe has odd number of units on the left and even units on the right. To avoid confusion, the scale on the left should be used for odd units (for example, 13 U) and the scale on the right for even numbers of units (for example, 26 U). When measuring even numbers of units, each calibration then is measured as 2 U.

To review what the syringes look like, see Figure 18.3 for the four types of insulin syringes discussed.

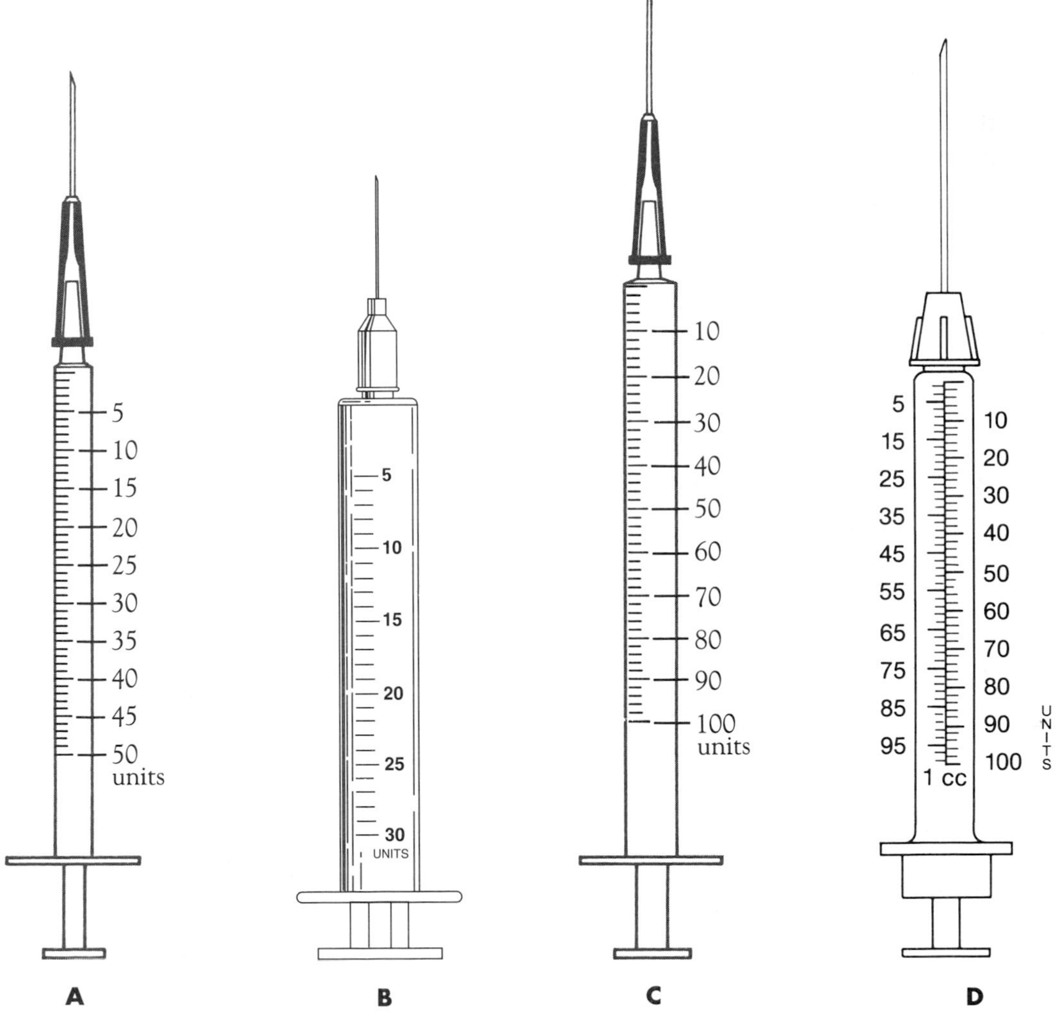

Figure 18-3. **A,** Lo-Dose insulin syringe (50 U). **B,** Lo-Dose insulin syringe (30 U). **C,** Single-scale syringe (100 U). **D,** Double-scale insulin syringe. (**A** and **C** from Dison N: *Simplified drugs and solutions for nurses*, ed 11, St. Louis, 1996, Mosby, and **B** and **D** from Brown M, Mulholland J: *Drug calculations: process and problems for clinical practice,* ed 5, St Louis, 1996, Mosby.)

Lo-Dose Syringe

Let's look at some insulin doses measured in the syringes to help you visualize the amounts in a syringe.

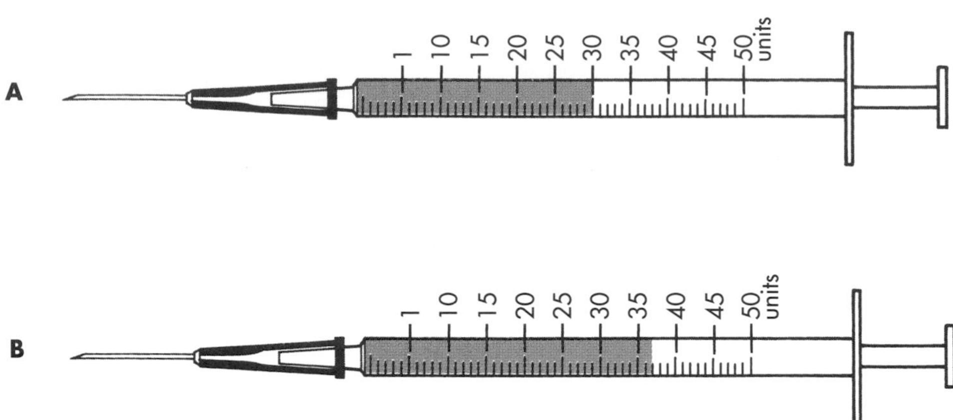

Syringe *A* shows 30 U and syringe *B* shows 37 U on a Lo-Dose syringe.

Practice Problems (p. 373)

Using the syringes below, indicate the doses shown by the arrows.

5. ______________

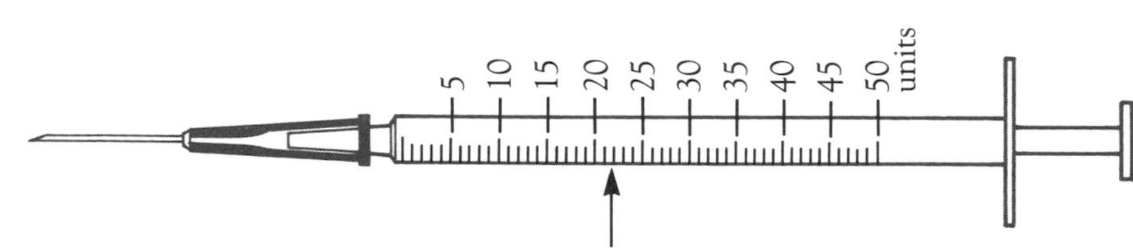

6. ______________

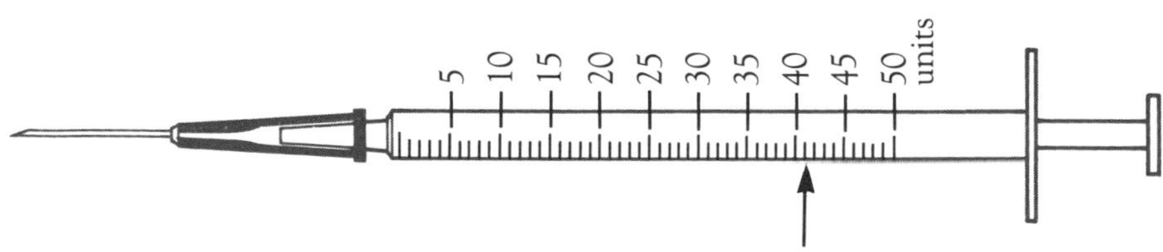

Using the syringes below, measure the following doses. Use an arrow and shading to indicate the doses.

7. 17 U

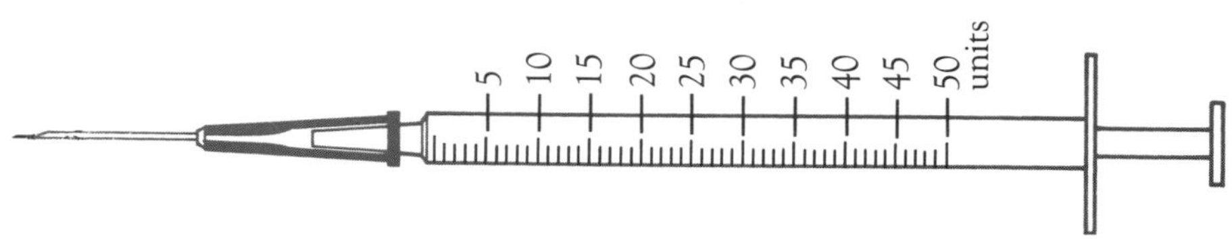

8. 47 U

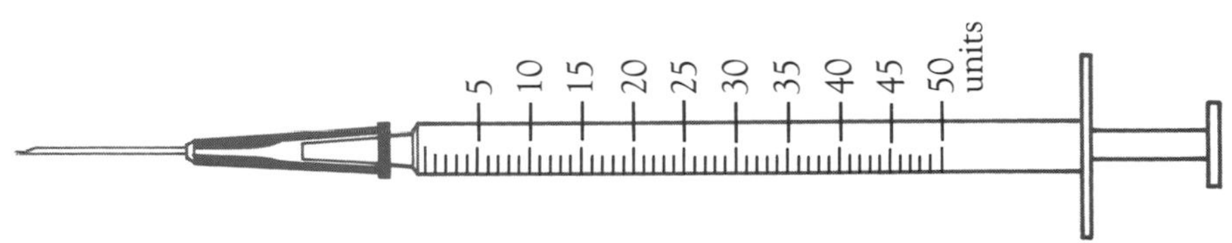

Single-Scale 1-cc Syringe

Now let's look at what doses would look like on a single-scale 1-cc syringe.

The syringes below show 25 U in syringe *A* and 55 U in syringe *B*. Notice the doses are drawn up in between the even calibrations.

A

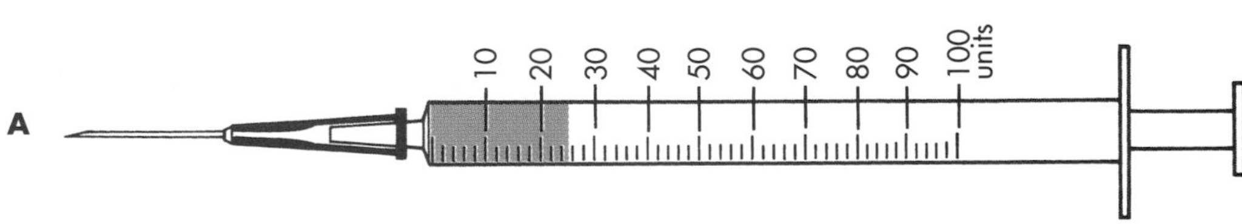

B

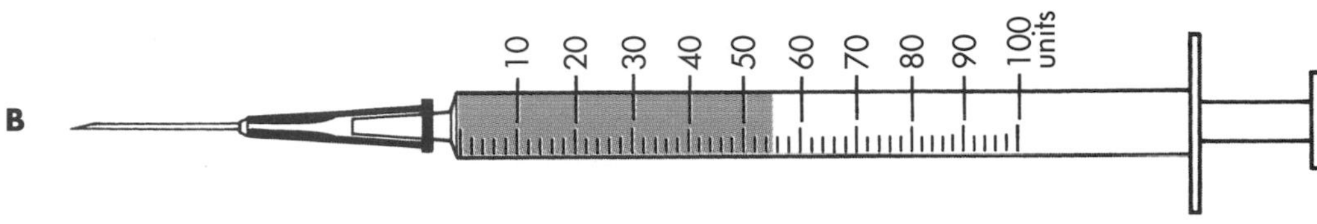

Double Scale 1-cc Syringe

Now let's look at the dose indicated on a double-scale 1-cc syringe. Syringe *C* shows 37 U; notice the scale on the left is used. Syringe *D* shows 54 U; notice the scale on the right is used.

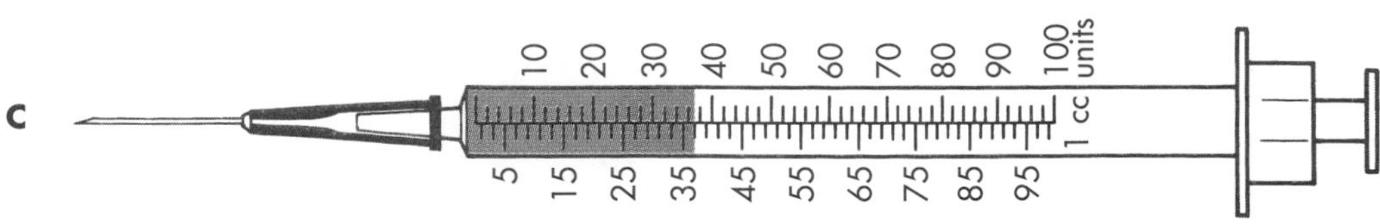

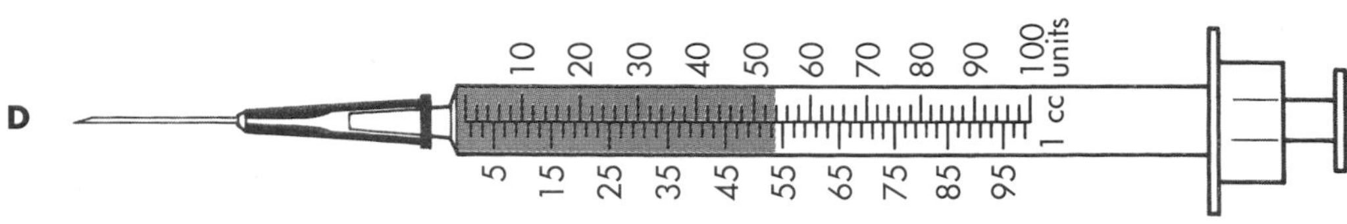

Practice Problems (p. 373)

Read the following doses indicated by the arrows and shaded on the U-100 (1-cc) syringes.

9. ______________

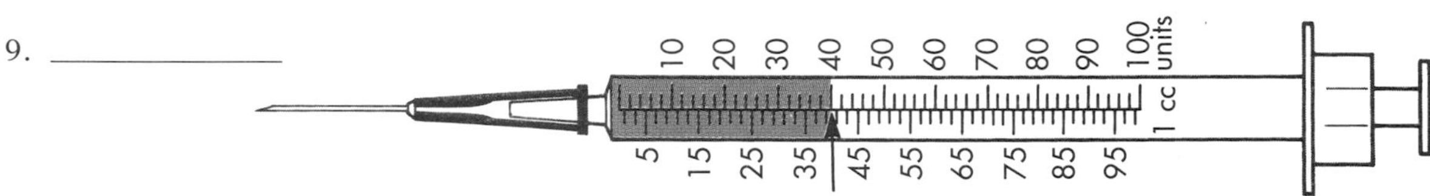

10. ______________

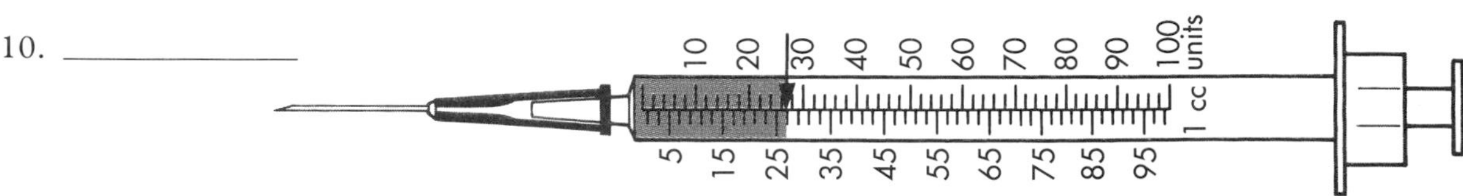

11. ______________

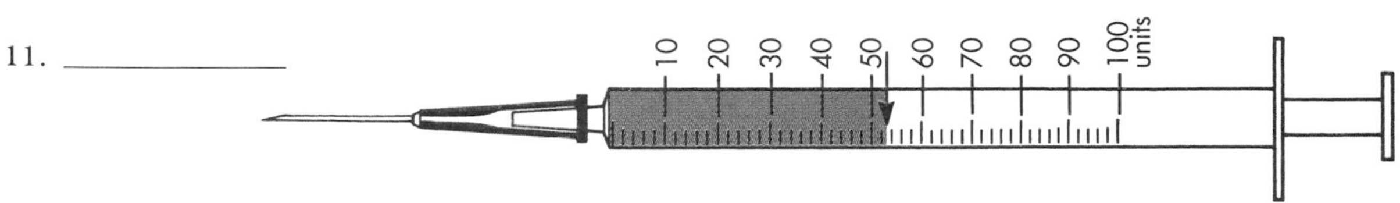

12. ______________

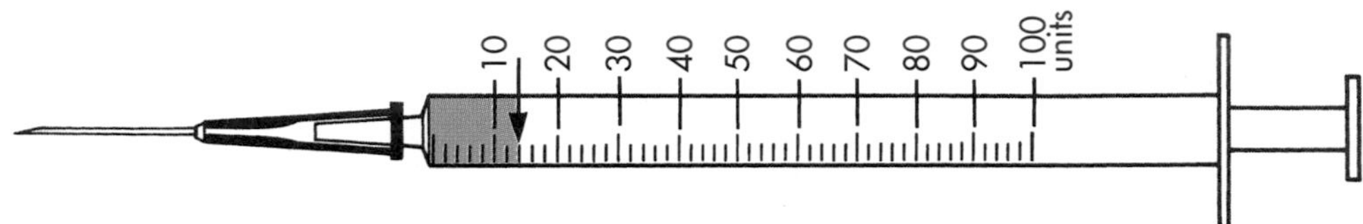

Draw an arrow on each U-100 syringe below to indicate the specified doses and shade in the dose.

13. 88 U

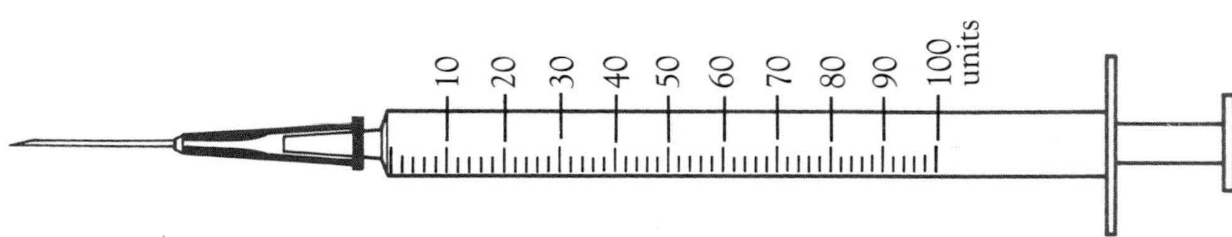

14. 44 U

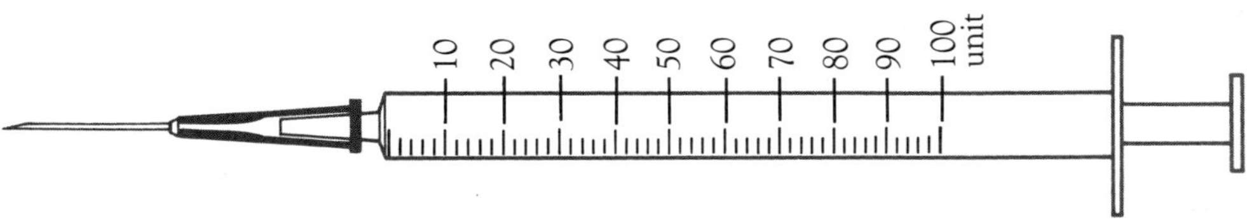

15. 30 U

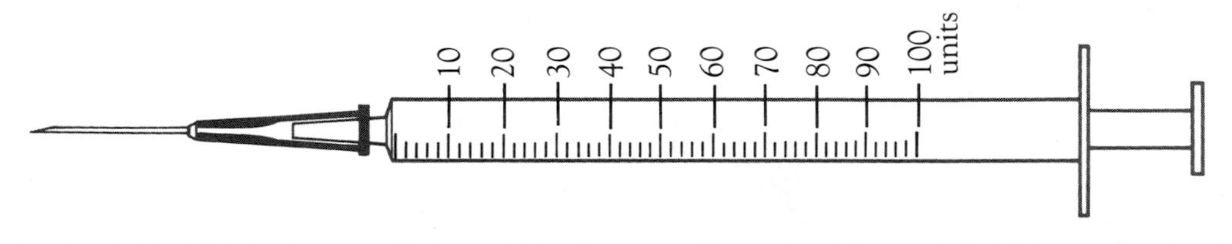

Insulin Orders

Like any medication order that is written, insulin orders must be written clearly and contain certain information to prevent errors in administration. An error in administration can cause harmful effects to a client. Insulin orders should contain the following information:

a) The name of the insulin, including the origin. Example: Humulin Regular; Humulin NPH, pork, beef.
b) The number of units to be administered. Example 20 U, Humulin Regular.
c) The route (s.c.). Insulin is usually administered s.c.; however, regular insulin can be administered I.V. as well.
d) The time it should be given. Example: 1/2 hour before meals.
e) The strength of the insulin to be administered. Example: U-100.

Example of Insulin Order: Regular Humulin insulin U-100 20 U s.c. before breakfast.

Coverage Orders

Sometimes in addition to standing insulin orders clients may have additional insulin ordered to "cover" their increased blood sugar levels. (This is sometimes referred to as sliding scale). Regular insulin is used because of its immediate action and short duration. A coverage order specifies the dose of insulin according to the blood sugar level and the frequency. The amount of insulin and the blood sugar level should be specific. The following is a sample coverage order (sliding scale):

Humulin Regular U-100 according to finger stick q8h.

0–180 no coverage
181–240 2 U s.c.
241–300 4 U s.c.
301–400 6 U s.c.
>400 8 U s.c. stat and notify doctor. Repeat finger stick in 2 hr.

Note: The above sliding scale is an example used in one patient. It is not a standard scale. Sliding scales are individualized for clients.

Preparing a Single Dose of Insulin in an Insulin Syringe

The measurement of insulin in an insulin syringe requires no calculation or conversion.

Example 1: Doctor's Order: Humulin Regular 40 U s.c. in a.m. 1/2 hr a.c.
Available: Humulin Regular labeled 100 U.

To measure 40 U, withdraw U-100 insulin to the 40 mark on the U-100 syringe. A Lo-Dose syringe can also be used to draw up this dose, as shown below.

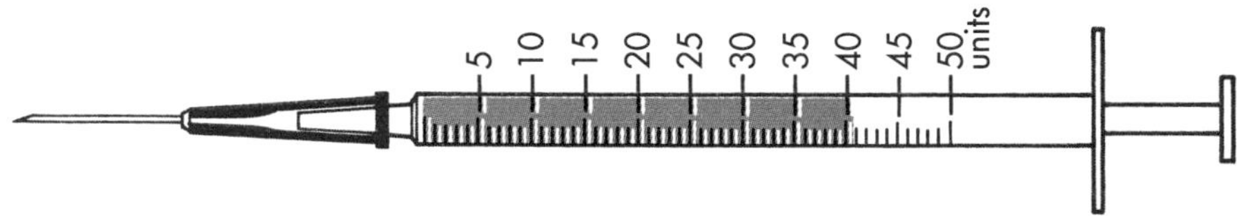

Example 2: Doctor's Order: Humulin NPH 70 U s.c. o.d.
Available: Humulin NPH labeled 100 U.

There is no calculation or conversion required here. Draw up the required amount using a U-100 (1-cc) syringe.

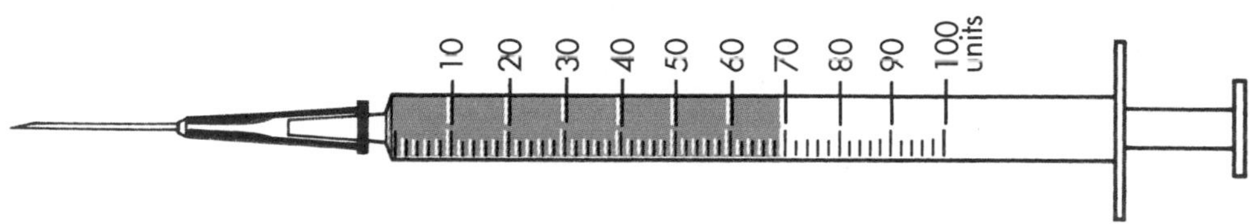

Example 3: Doctor's Order: Humulin Regular 5 U s.c. stat.
Available: Humulin Regular labeled 100 U.

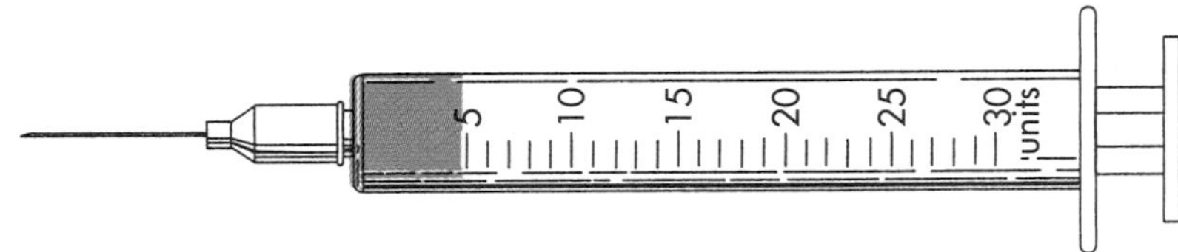

Measuring Two Types of Insulin in the Same Syringe

Sometimes individuals may require two different types of insulin for control of their blood sugar levels, for example, NPH and regular. To decrease the number of injections it is common to mix two insulins in a single syringe. To mix insulin in one syringe remember:

Regular Insulin Is Always Drawn Up in the Insulin Syringe First!

Drawing regular insulin up first prevents contamination of the regular insulin with other insulin.

To prepare insulin in one syringe (mixing insulin), complete the following steps (Figure 18-4):

1. Cleanse tops of both vials with alcohol wipe.
2. Inject air equal to the amount being withdrawn into the vial of cloudy insulin first. When injecting the air, the tip of the needle should not touch the solution.
3. Remove the needle from the vial of cloudy insulin.
4. Using the same syringe, inject an amount of air into the regular insulin (clear) equal to the amount to be withdrawn, invert or turn the bottle up in the air, and draw up the desired amount.
5. Remove the syringe from the regular insulin and check for air bubbles. If air bubbles are present, gently tap the syringe to remove them.
6. Next go back to the cloudy insulin and withdraw the desired dose.
7. The total number of units in the syringe will be the addition of the two insulin orders.

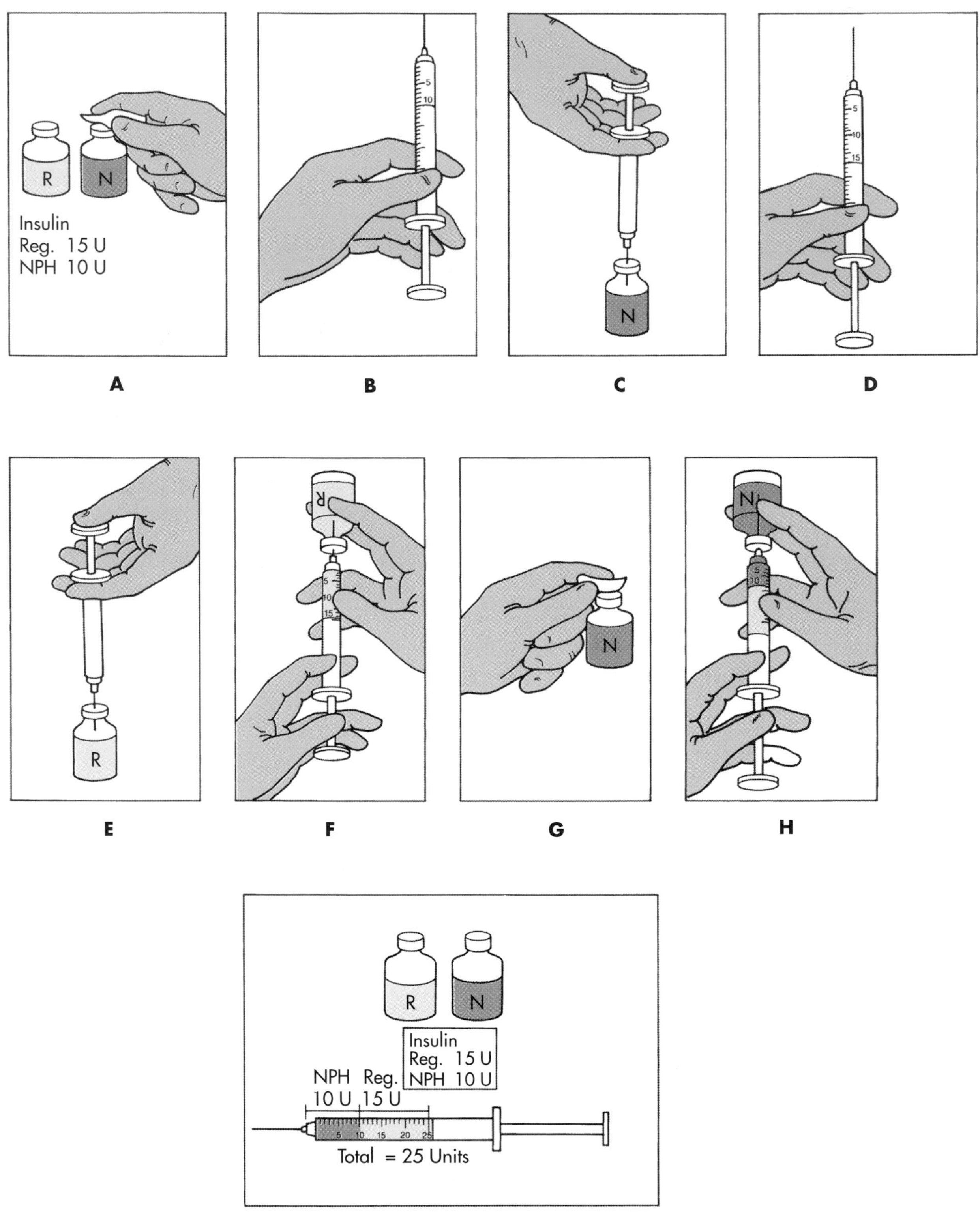

Figure 18-4. Preparing two insulins in one syringe. (From Clayton B, Stock Y: *Basic pharmacology for nurses,* ed 10, St Louis, 1993, Mosby.)

Example: The order is to administer 18 U of regular and 22 U of NPH.

The total amount of insulin is 40 U (18 U + 22 U = 40 U).

To administer this dose a Lo-Dose syringe can be used, as well as the U-100 (1-cc) syringe. However, since the dose is 40 U, the Lo-Dose would be more desirable. (See syringes below illustrating this dosage.)

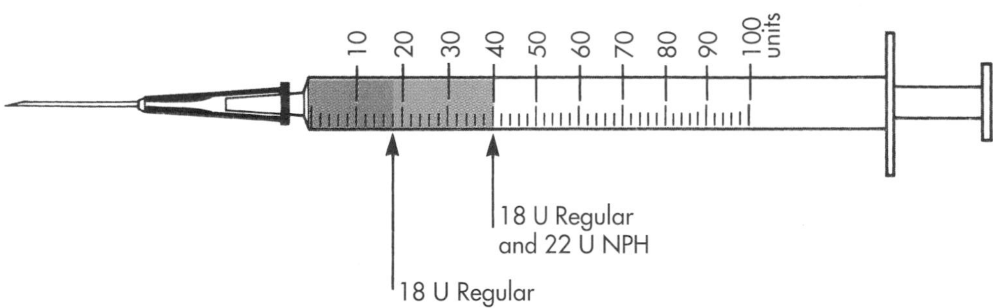

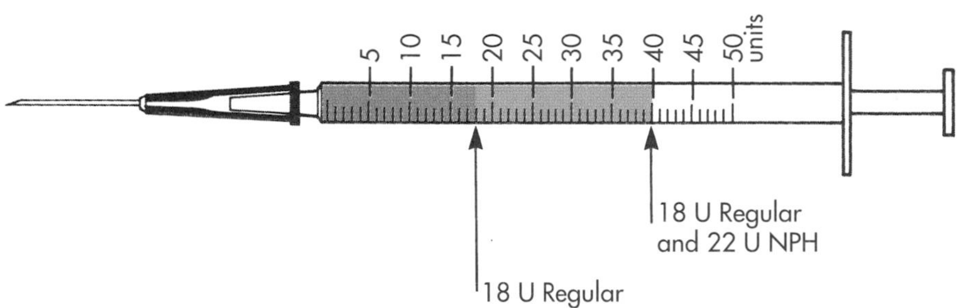

When mixing insulins, it is important to follow the steps outlined to prevent the contamination of regular insulin with other insulins. To help you remember the steps recall: The last one injected is drawn up first, or run fast first (regular), then slow down (NPH).

Measuring Insulin When an Insulin Syringe Is Not Available

Doses of insulin must be exact and therefore should always be measured and administered with an insulin syringe. Only in an emergency or when an insulin syringe is not available, should any other type of syringe be used. A tuberculin syringe or 1-mL syringe can be used to measure insulin because 100 U of insulin = 1 mL.

Example: Doctor's Order: Humulin NPH 40 U s.c. o.d.

Available: Humulin NPH 100 U. No insulin syringes are available. You have a tuberculin syringe.

1. Note: No conversion is necessary in terms of units.
2. Think critically: What answer would be logical based upon the syringe you have?
3. Set up a proportion or formula and solve.

Solution Using the Ratio-Proportion Method

$$100\text{ U} : 1\text{ mL} = 40\text{ U} : x\text{ mL}$$

$$\frac{100}{100}x = \frac{40}{100}$$

$$x = \frac{40}{100} = 0.4\text{ mL}$$

Solution Using the Formula Method

$$\frac{40\text{ U}}{100\text{ U}} \times 1\text{ mL} = x\text{ mL} \quad \textbf{OR} \quad \frac{40\text{ U}}{100\text{ U}} = \frac{x\text{ mL}}{1\text{ mL}}$$

$$x = \frac{40}{100} = 0.4\text{ mL} \qquad x = \frac{40}{100} = 0.4\text{ mL}$$

Tuberculin syringe illustrating this amount:

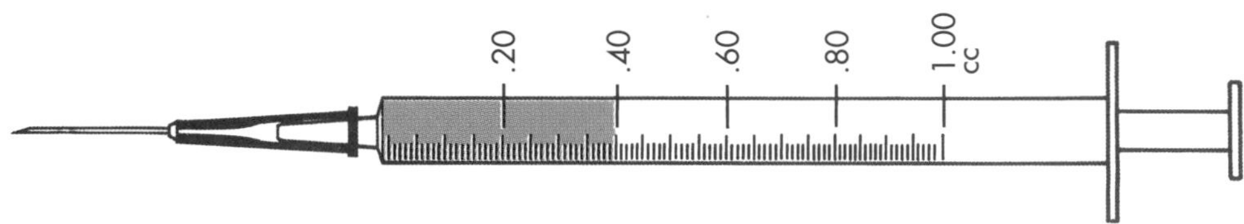

Note: A U-40 strength of insulin is still available, although it is not often used. To administer this insulin you need a syringe calibrated U-40 to measure the dose.

Points to Remember

- U-100 means 100 U/mL.
- To ensure accuracy, insulin should be given only with an insulin syringe. When no insulin syringe is available, a tuberculin syringe may be used in an emergency.
- Insulin doses must be exact.
- Lo-Dose syringes are desirable for small doses up to 50 U. The Lo-Dose 30-U may be used for doses up to 30 U.
- A U-100 (1-cc capacity) syringe is desirable when the dose exceeds 50 U.
- When mixing insulin, regular insulin is always drawn up first.
- The total volume when mixing insulins is the addition of the two insulin amounts.
- Read insulin labels to ensure that you have the correct type of insulin.

Chapter Review (pp. 374-378)

Using the syringes below, indicate the dose you would prepare. Indicate the dose on the syringe with an arrow and shade in.

1. Doctor's Order: Regular Humulin insulin 35 U s.c. o.d.
   Available: Regular Humulin U-100.

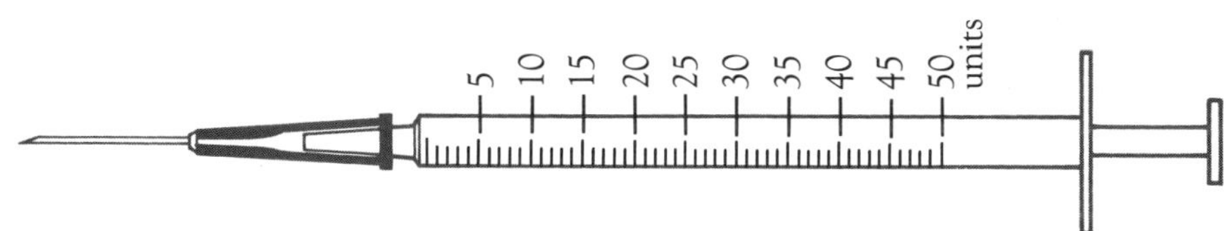

2. Doctor's Order: Humulin NPH 56 U s.c. o.d.
   Available: Humulin NPH U-100.

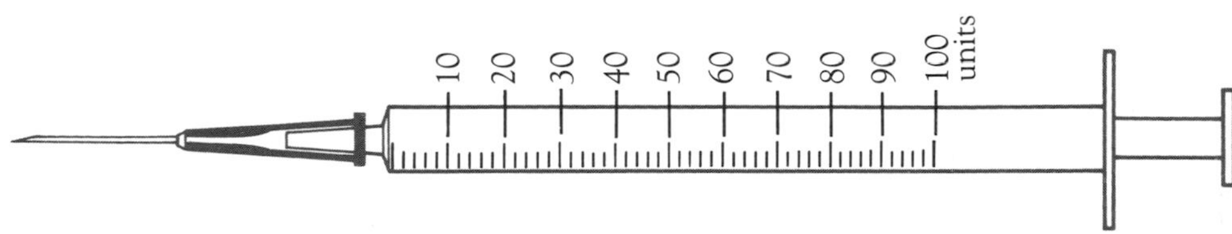

3. Doctor's Order: Humulin Regular 18 U s.c. and NPH 40 U s.c. o.d.
   Available: Humulin Regular U-100, Humulin NPH U-100.

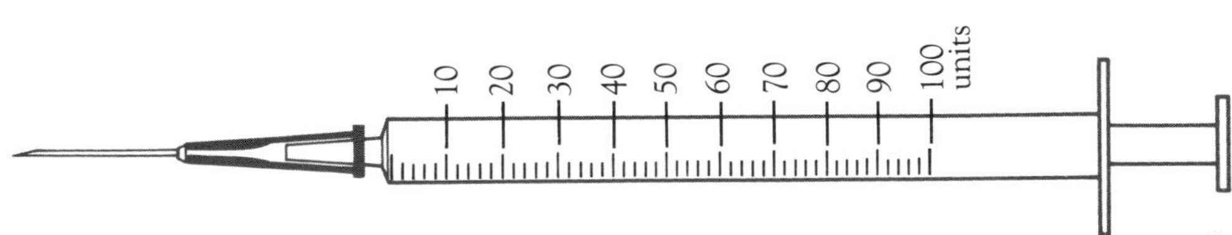

4. Doctor's Order: Regular pork insulin 9 U s.c. o.d.
   Available: Regular pork insulin labeled U-100.

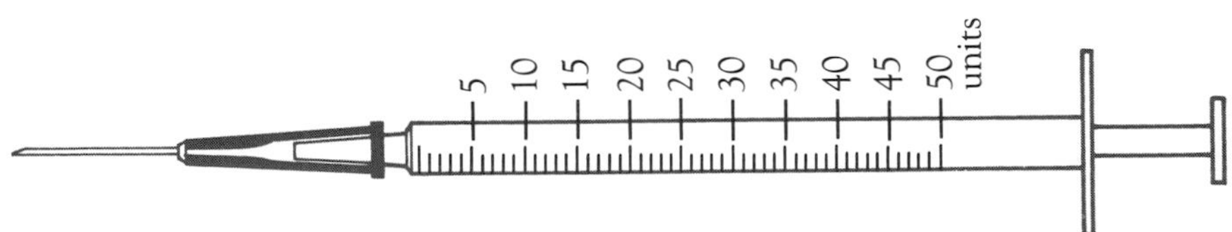

Indicate the number of units measured in the following syringes.

5. Units Measured ____________

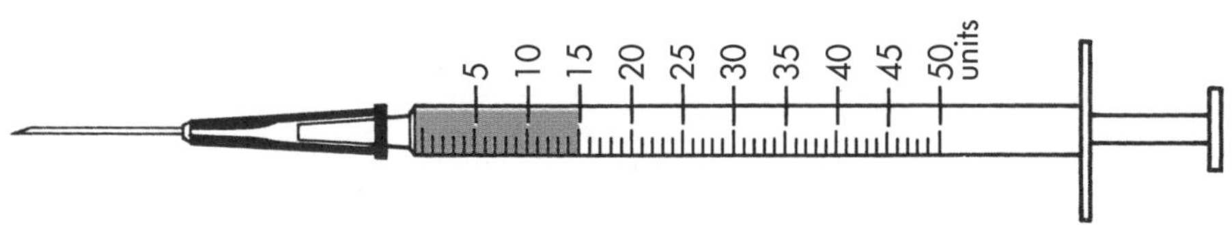

6. Units Measured _______________

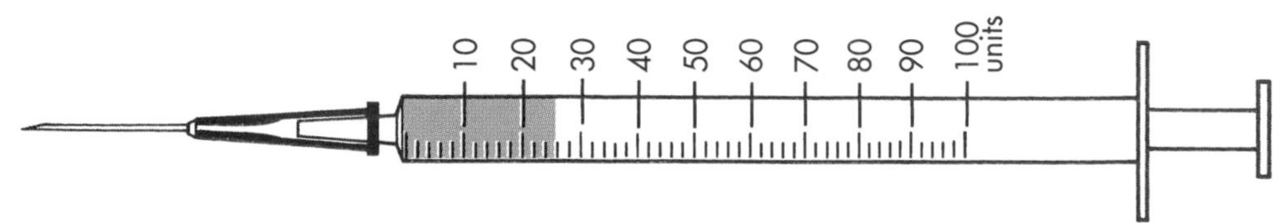

7. Units Measured _______________

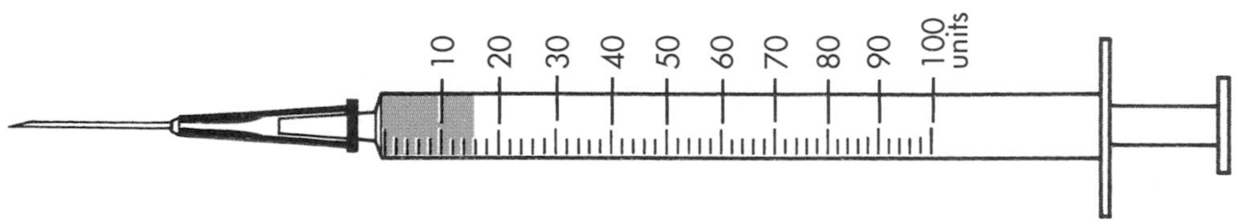

8. Units Measured _______________

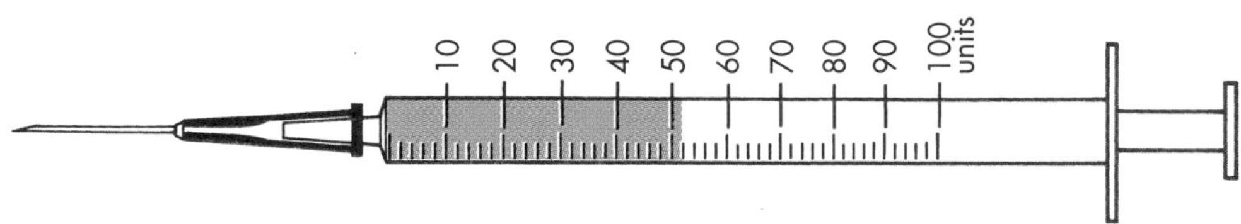

9. Units Measured _______________

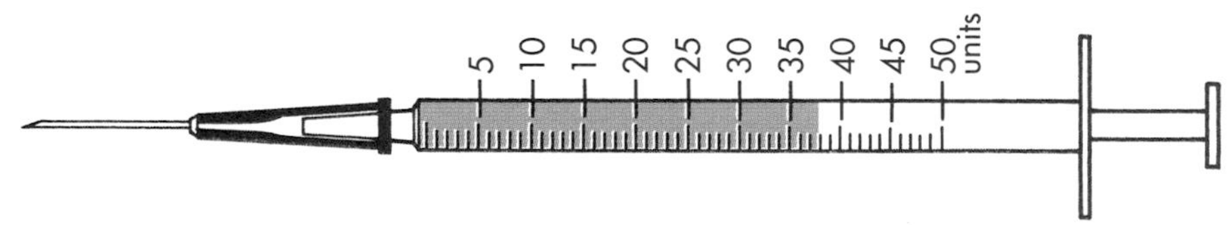

10. Units Measured _______________

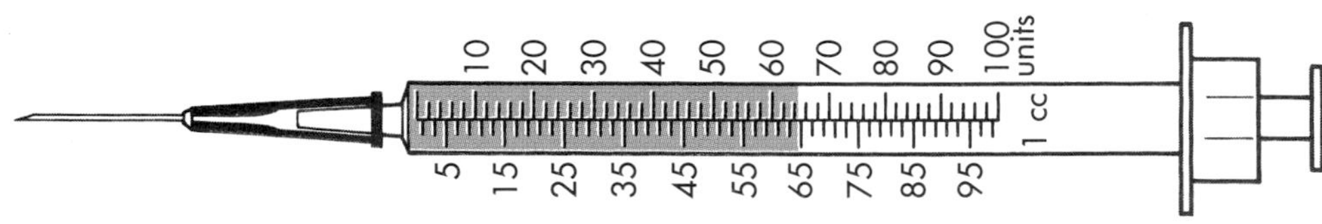

11. Units Measured _______________

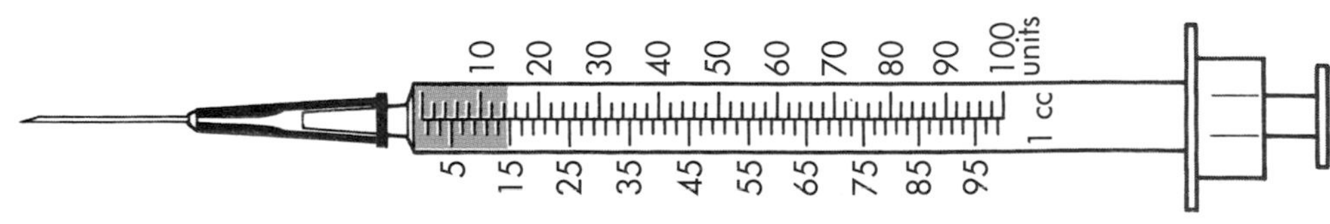

Calculate the dose of insulin where necessary and shade in the dose on the syringe provided. Insulin labeled 100 U/mL is available for all problems regardless of the type of insulin.

12. Doctor's Order: Humulin Regular 10 U s.c. a.c. 7:30 AM.

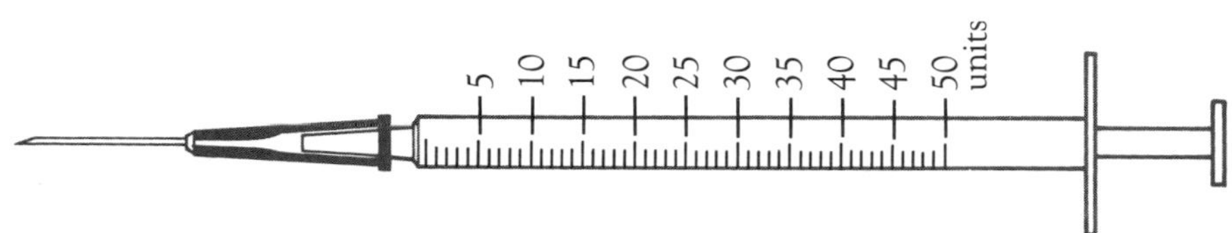

13. Doctor's Order: Humulin Regular 16 U s.c. and 24 U s.c. Humulin NPH a.c. 7:30 AM.

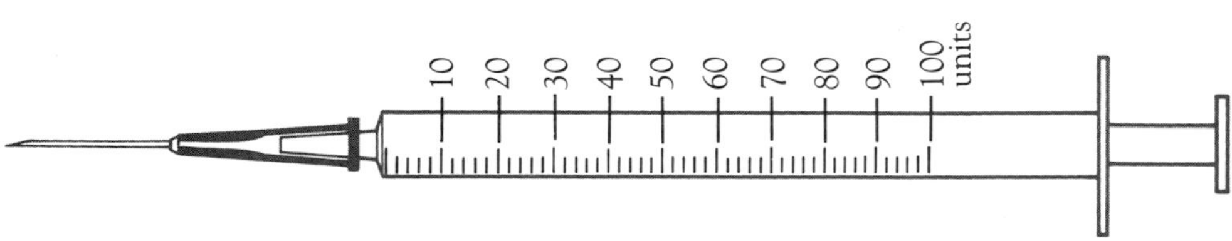

14. Doctor's Order: Lente Insulin 75 U s.c. a.c. 7:30 AM.

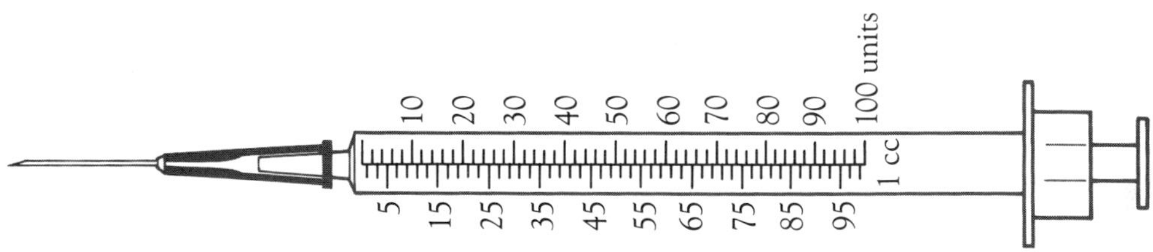

15. Doctor's Order: Regular Iletin II 10 U s.c. and NPH Iletin II 15 U s.c. a.c. 7:30 AM.

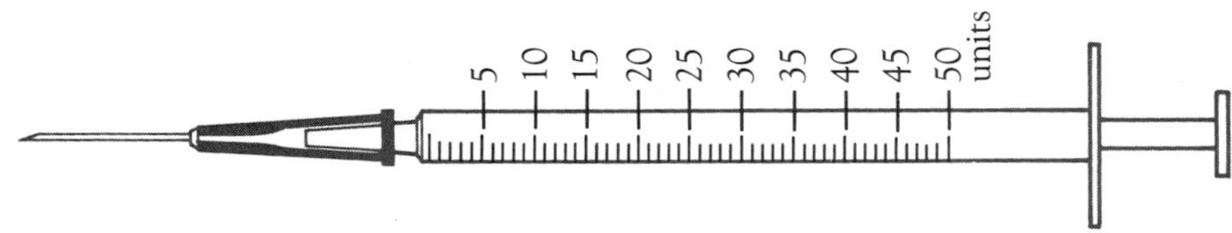

16. Doctor's Order: Humulin Regular 5 U s.c. and Humulin NPH 25 U s.c. a.c. 7:30 AM.

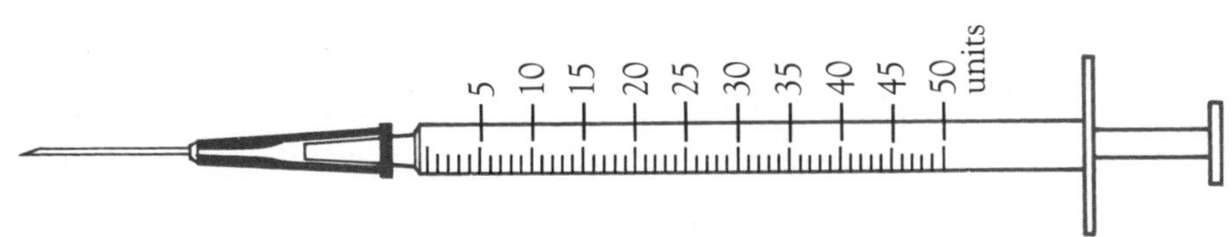

17. Doctor's Order: Humulin Lente 40 U s.c. and Humulin Regular 10 U s.c. at 7:30 AM.

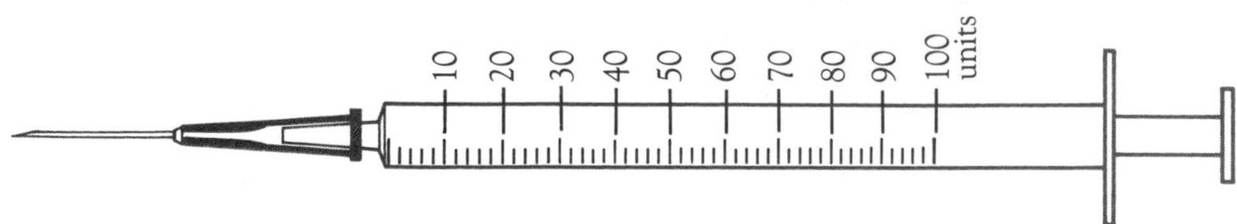

18. Doctor's Order: Humulin NPH 48 U s.c. and Humulin Regular 30 U s.c. a.c. 7:30 AM.

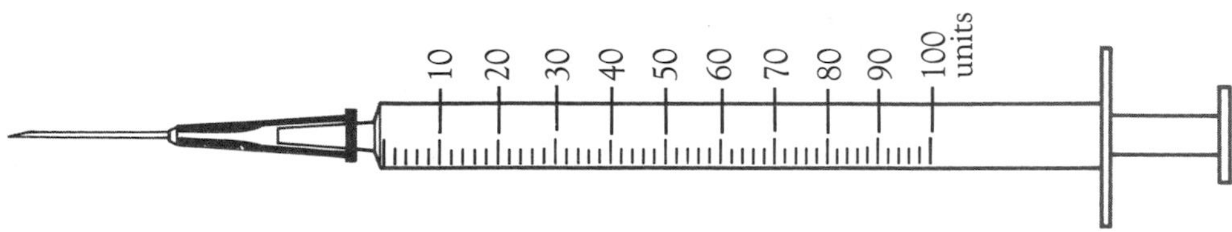

19. Doctor's Order: Humulin Regular 16 U s.c. and Humulin Lente 12 U s.c. 7:30 AM.

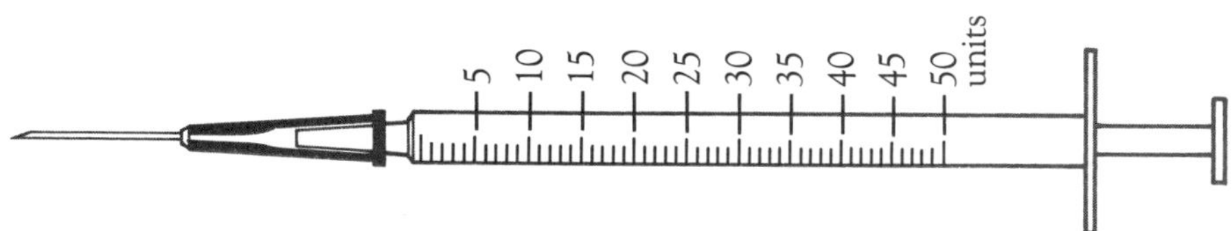

20. Doctor's Order: Humulin Regular 17 U s.c. 5 PM.

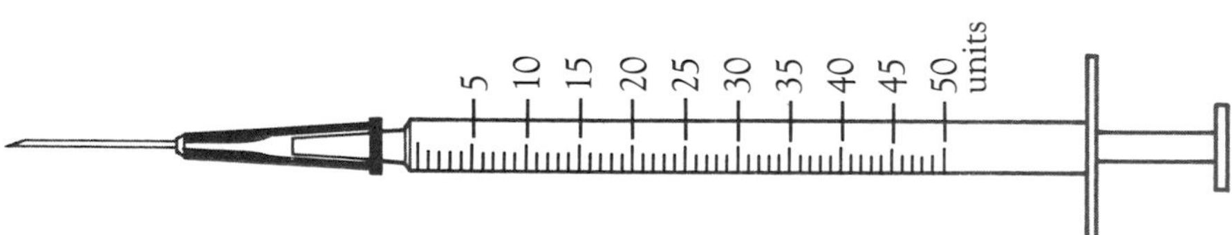

21. Doctor's Order: Iletin II NPH 15 U s.c. 10 PM.

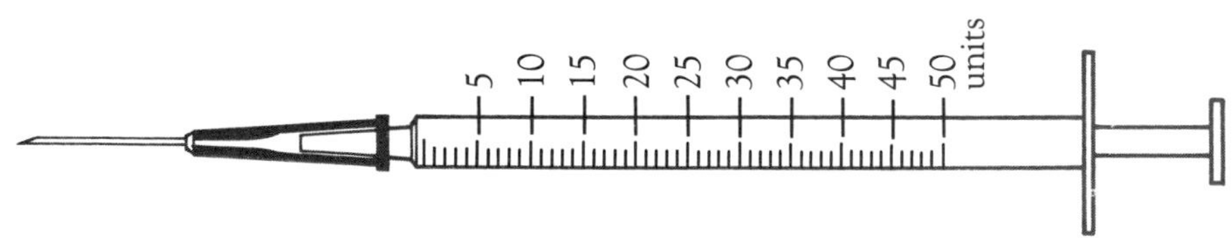

22. Doctor's Order: Humulin Regular 26 U s.c. and Humulin NPH 48 U s.c. q.d.

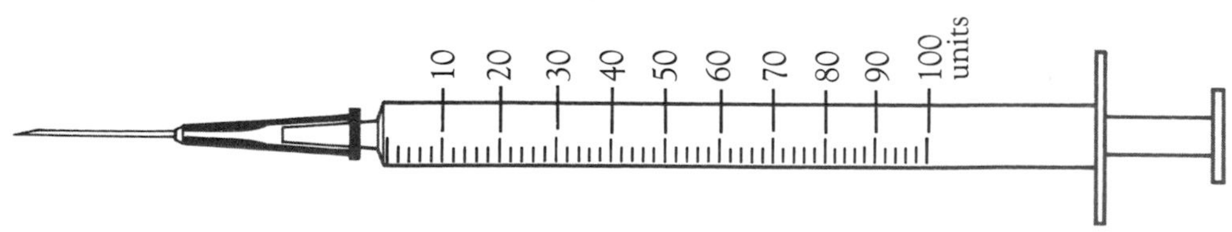

23. Doctor's Order: Iletin Regular II 27 U s.c. at 5 PM.

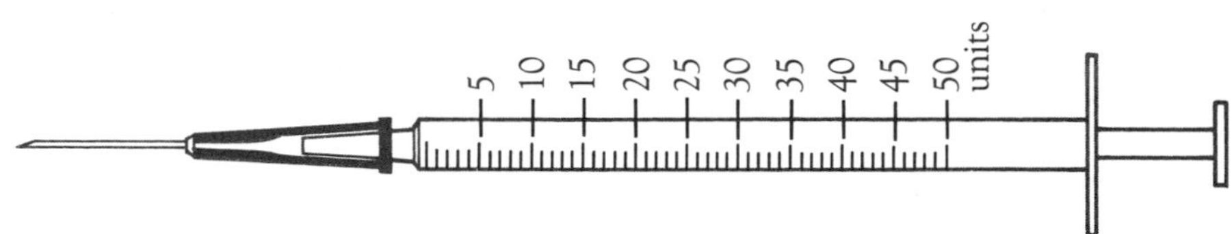

24. Doctor's Order: Regular Iletin I 21 U s.c. and Iletin II NPH 35 U s.c. o.d.

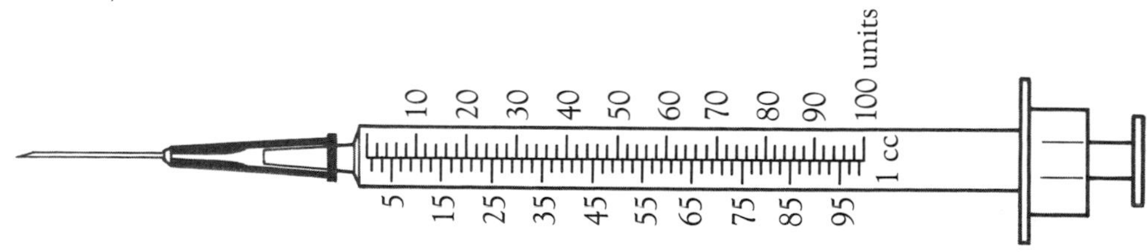

25. Doctor's Order: Novolin Regular 5 U s.c. and Novolin Lente 35 U s.c. 7:30 AM.

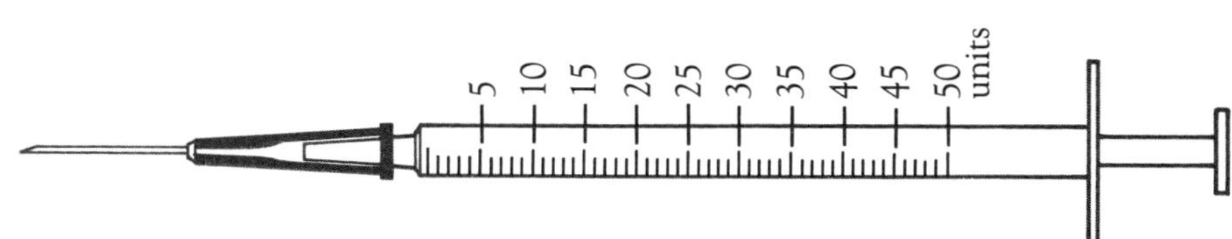

26. Doctor's Order: Humulin NPH 36 U s.c. 10 PM.

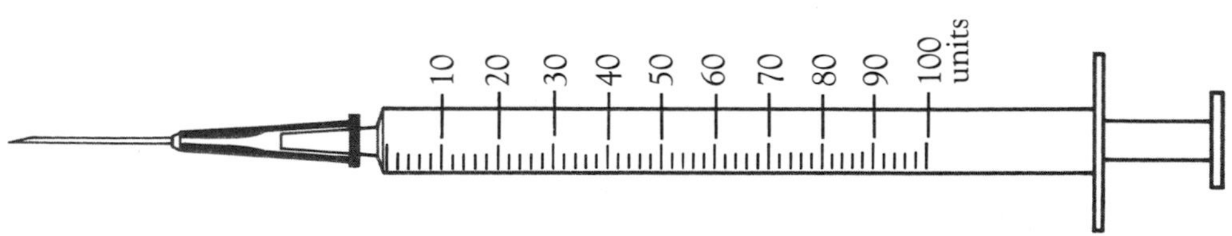

27. Doctor's Order: Regular insulin 8 U s.c. and protamine zinc 20 U s.c. q.d.

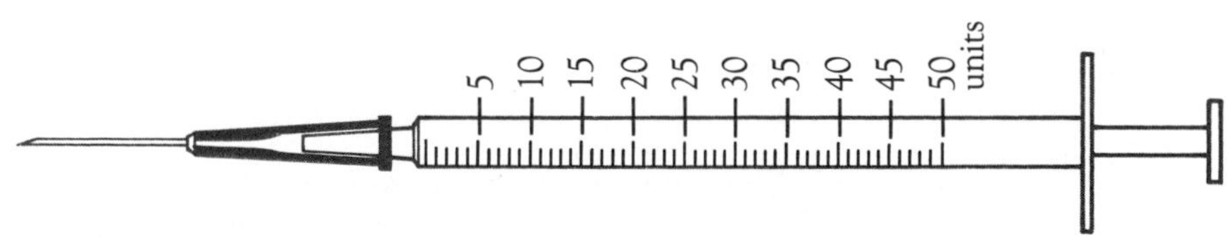

28. A client is on a sliding scale for insulin doses. The doctor ordered Humulin Regular insulin q6h as follows:

Finger stick	0–180	no coverage
	181–240	2 U s.c.
	241–300	4 U s.c.
	301–400	6 U s.c.
	>400	8 U s.c. and repeat finger stick in 2 hr.

At 11:30 AM the client's finger stick is 364. Shade in the syringe to indicate the dose that should be given.

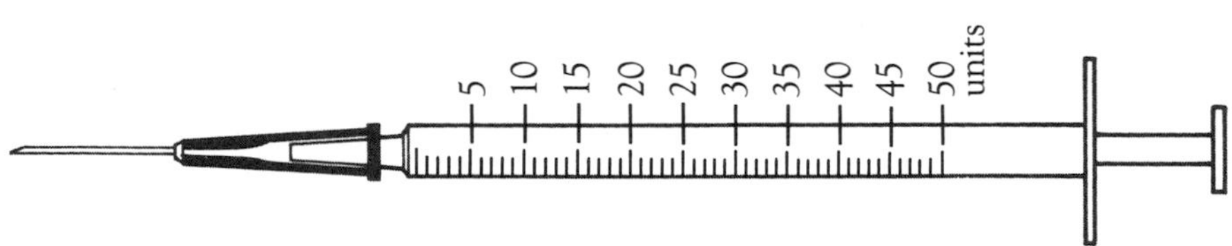

29. Doctor's Order: Humulin NPH 66 U s.c. 10 PM.

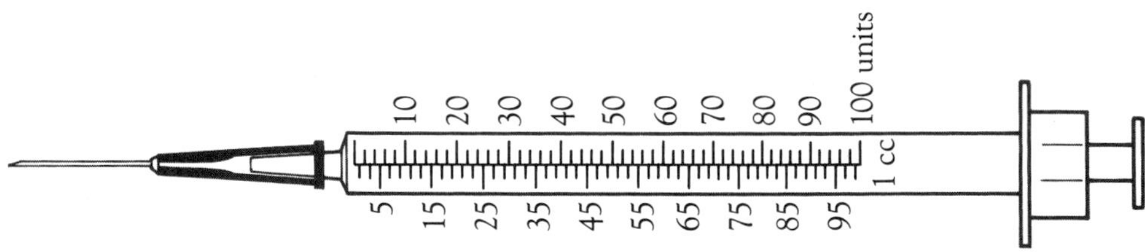

30. Doctor's Order: Ultralente Iletin I 32 U s.c. q AM.

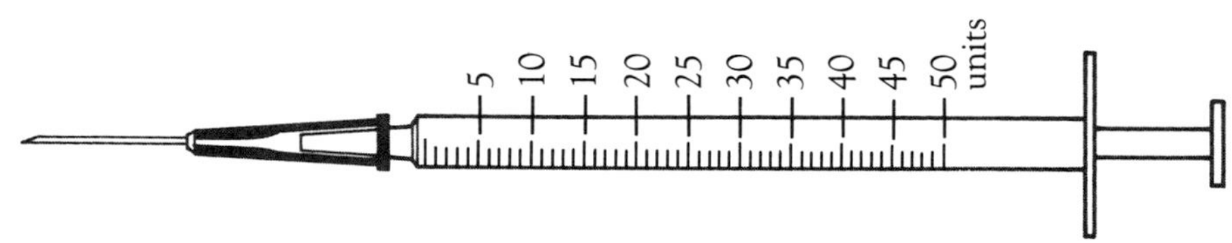

Calculate the amount of insulin to administer in a tuberculin syringe using U-100 insulin (100 U/mL). Shade in the dose on the tuberculin syringe.

31. Doctor's Order: Humulin NPH 38 U s.c. 10 PM.

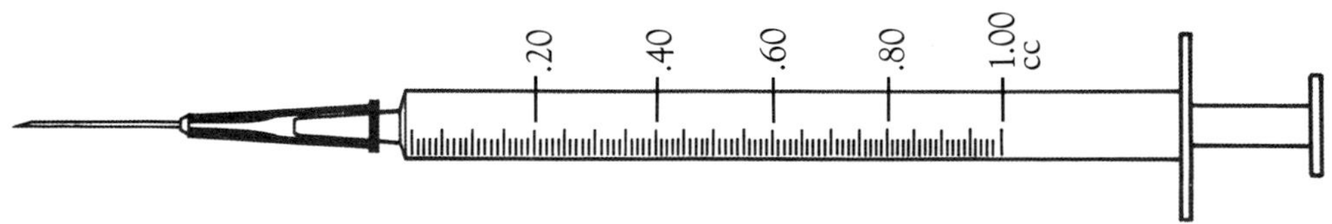

32. Doctor's Order: Humulin Regular 12 U s.c. at 5 PM.

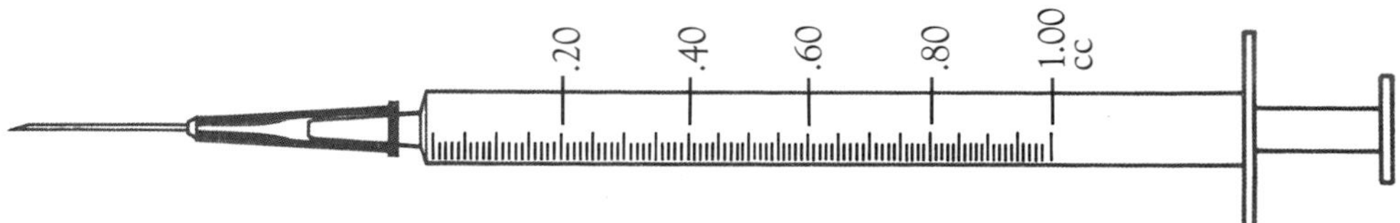

33. Doctor's Order: Lente Iletin I 60 U s.c. q.d.

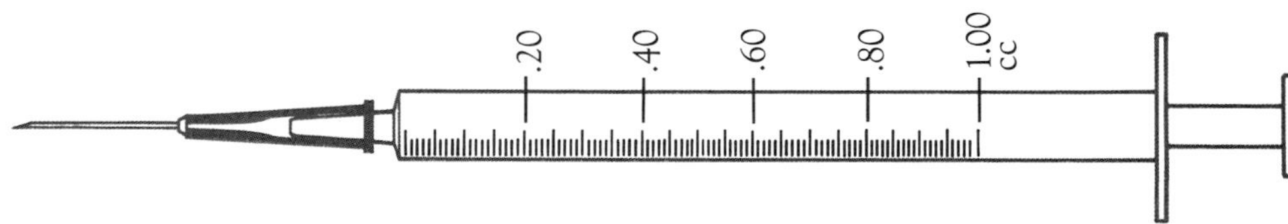

34. Doctor's Order: Humulin NPH 64 U s.c. at 7:30 AM.

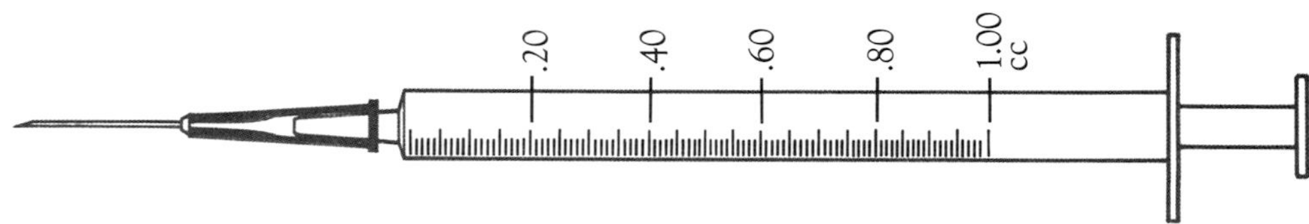

Shade in the dose on the insulin syringe.

35. Doctor's Order: Lente Iletin II 35 U s.c. q.d.

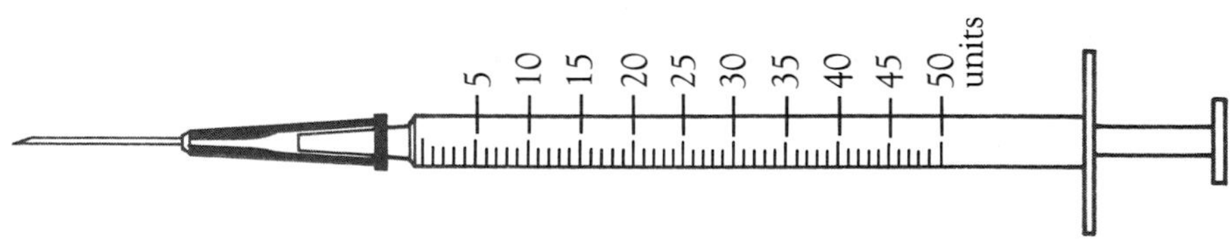

36. Doctor's Order: Humulin Regular 9 U s.c. 5 PM.

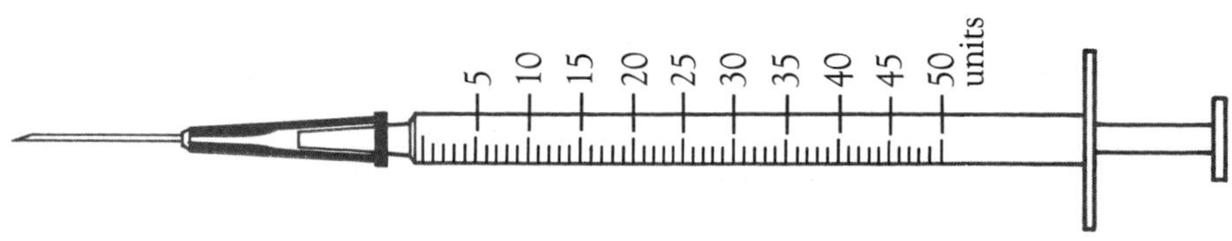

37. Doctor's Order: Humulin NPH 24 U s.c. 10 PM.

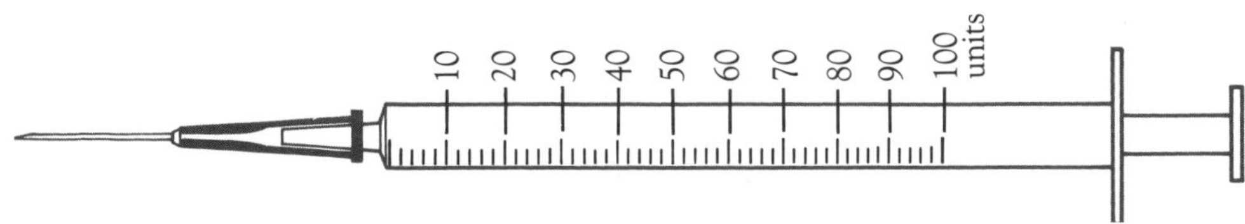

38. Doctor's Order: Humulin Regular 8 U s.c. in AM, and Humulin NPH 18 U in AM.

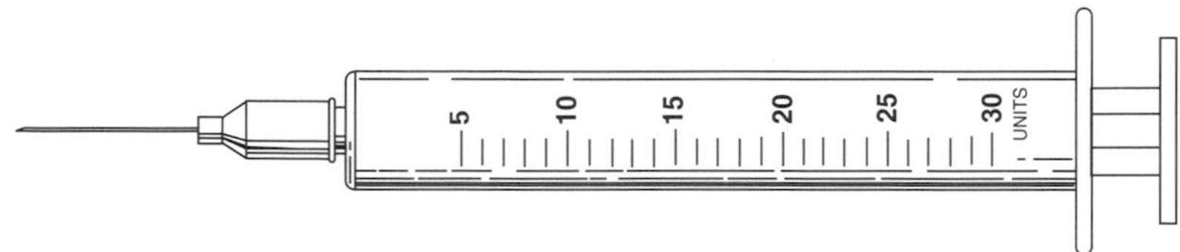

39. Doctor's Order: Humulin NPH 11 U s.c. h.s.

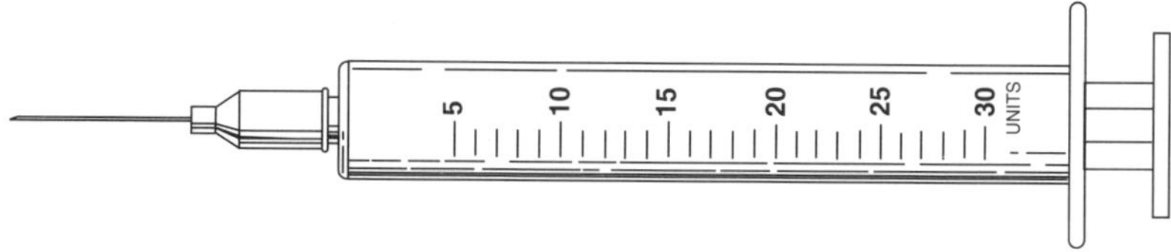

40. Doctor's Order: Humulin 70/30 20 U s.c. 1/2 hr a.c. breakfast.

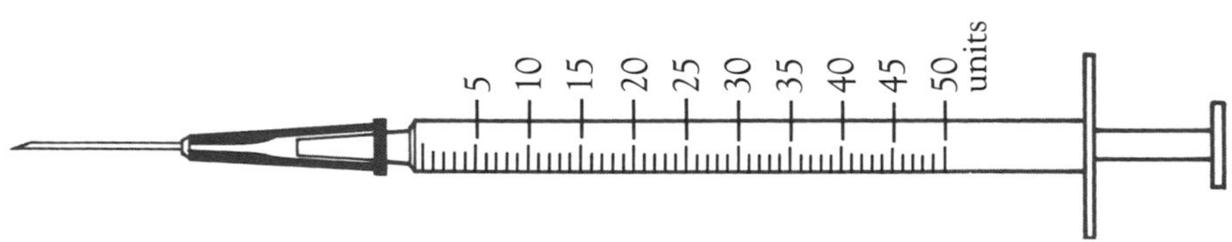

Chapter 19

Pediatric Dose Calculation

Objectives

After reviewing this chapter the student will be able to do the following:

1. **Convert body weight from lb to kg**
2. **Convert body weight from kg to lb**
3. **Calculate doses based on mg per kg**
4. **Determine whether a dose is safe**
5. **Determine body surface area (BSA) using the West nomogram**
6. **Calculate BSA using formulas according to units of measure**
7. **Determine doses using the BSA**

Body weight is an important factor that is used to calculate medication doses for both children and adults. The safe administration of medications to infants and children requires knowledge of the methods used in calculating doses. Because children are smaller than adults, calculating doses for children requires exact and careful mathematics. Exact, accurate doses are especially important since even small discrepancies can be dangerous because of the size, weight, BSA, and physiological capabilities of pediatric clients. (Example: A lessened ability to metabolize drugs because of immaturity of systems, variations in capabilities of metabolism and excretion.) Although the doctor has the responsibility for ordering the medication, **the nurse has the primary responsibility of verifying the dose to be sure it is correct and safe for administration.**

The two methods currently being used to calculate pediatric doses are as follows:

1. According to the weight of the child (mg per kg)
2. According to the child's BSA

Note: These methods can also used to calculate adult medication doses. Of the two methods, the BSA method has been determined to be the most accurate for calculating doses.

Principles Relating to Basic Calculations

Before beginning calculation of medications for the child or infant, there are some guidelines that are helpful to know.

1. Calculation of pediatric doses, as with adult doses, involves the use of ratio-proportion or

the formulas $\frac{D}{H} \times Q = X$ or $\frac{DW}{SW} = \frac{DV}{SV}$ to determine the amount of medication to administer.

2. Pediatric doses are much smaller than those for an adult. Micrograms are used a great deal and occasionally minims are used. The tuberculin syringe (1-cc capacity) is used for the administration of very small doses.
3. I.M. doses are usually not more than 1 cc; however, this can vary with the size of the child.
4. Doses that are less than 1 cc may be measured in minims, tenths of a cc, or with a tuberculin syringe in hundredths of a mL. However, as with adults, the preference is to express an answer using metric measures such as mL or cc instead of minims.
5. Medications in pediatrics generally are not rounded off to the nearest tenth but may be administered with a tuberculin syringe to ensure accuracy. Again, answers may be changed to minims, but the preference is for metric measures since they are more accurate.
6. All answers must be labeled.

Calculation of Doses Based on Body Weight

Let's begin our discussion with calculation of doses according to mg/kg of body weight. Before calculating doses according to mg/kg of body weight, it is essential that you be able to convert a child's weight. Most drug references state doses in terms of kg. Therefore the most common conversion you will encounter will involve the conversion of lb to kg. To do this remember the conversion 1 kg = 2.2 lb.

Converting Lb to Kg

Let's do some sample problems with the conversion of weights.

Example 1: Convert 30 lb to kg.

2.2 lb = 1 kg

2.2 lb : 1 kg = 30 lb : x kg

$$\frac{2.2}{2.2}x = \frac{30}{2.2}$$

30 ÷ 2.2 = 13.63 (rounded to the nearest tenth = 13.6 kg)

Example 2: Convert an infant's weight of 14 lb and 6 oz to kg.

1. Convert oz to lbs.

   16 oz : 1 lb = 6 oz : x lb

   $$\frac{16x}{16} = \frac{6}{16}$$

   6 ÷ 16 = 0.37 lb (0.4 lb to nearest tenth)

   Infant's weight = 14.4 lb

2. Convert total lb to kg.

   2.2 lb : 1 kg = 14.4 lb : x kg

   $$\frac{2.2\,x}{2.2} = \frac{14.4}{2.2}$$

   14.4 ÷ 2.2 = 6.54 (6.5 kg to nearest tenth)

   Infant's weight = 6.5 kg

Remember the Following When Converting Weights

1. 2.2 lb = 1 kg.
2. To convert from lb to kg divide the number of lb by 2.2. Carry the division out to the hundredths place and round off the answer to the nearest tenth. Calculations based on body weight can be rounded off to the nearest tenth.
3. To convert from kg to lb multiply the number of kg by 2.2. and express the answer to the nearest tenth.
4. If the child's weight is in oz and lb, convert the oz to the nearest tenth of a lb, and then add it to the total lb. Convert the total lb to kg to the nearest tenth.

Note: Students should know that although lb is an apothecaries' measure, a decimal may be seen when expressing weight, for example, 65.8 lb.

Practice Problems (p. 378)

Convert the following weights in lb to kg. Round to the nearest tenth where indicated.

1. 20 lb = ______________ kg
2. 64 lb = ______________ kg
3. 22 lb = ______________ kg
4. 52 lb = ______________ kg
5. 71 lb = ______________ kg
6. 12 lb 2 oz = ______________ kg
7. 8 lb 4 oz = ______________ kg
8. 5 lb 6 oz = ______________ kg

Converting Kg to Lb

Example 1: Convert 24 kg to lb.

2.2 lb = 1 kg

2.2 lb : 1 kg = x lb : 24 kg

$x = 24 \times 2.2$

$x = 52.8$ lb

Practice Problems (p. 378)

Convert the following weights in kg to lb. State answer to nearest tenth.

9. 20 kg = ______________ lb
10. 46 kg = ______________ lb
11. 22 kg = ______________ lb
12. 15 kg = ______________ lb
13. 34 kg = ______________ lb
14. 23 kg = ______________ lb
15. 73 kg = ______________ lb
16. 98 kg = ______________ lb

Calculation of medication doses is generally based on mg/kg/day or sometimes mg/lb/day. References often state the safe amount of the drug in mg/kg/day (24-hour period). Once you have determined the child's weight in kg, you are ready to calculate the medication dose. Calculation of the dose involves three steps:

1. Calculation of the daily dose.
2. Division of the daily dose by the number of doses to be administered.
3. Use of either ratio-proportion or the formula method to calculate the number of tablets or capsules or the volume to give to administer the ordered dose.

Example 1: Refer to label.

Pediatric Dose—Initially, 5 mg/kg daily in two or three equally divided doses, with subsequent dosage individualized to a maximum of 300 mg daily.
See package insert for complete prescribing information.
Keep this and all drugs out of the reach of children.
0365G041

N 0071-0365-24
KAPSEALS®
Dilantin®
(Extended Phenytoin Sodium Capsules, USP)
30 mg
Caution—Federal law prohibits dispensing without prescription.
100 CAPSULES
PARKE-DAVIS
Div of Warner-Lambert Co
Morris Plains, NJ 07950 USA

Dispense in tight, light-resistant container as defined in the USP.
Store below 30°C (86°F). Protect from light and moisture.
NOTE TO PHARMACIST—Do not dispense capsules which are discolored.
Exp date and lot

A child weighs 18 kg and requires Dilantin. The recommended dose is 5 mg/kg/daily in two or three equally divided doses. Now that we have the dosage information and the child's weight, we can calculate the dose for this child. Note: The child's weight is in kg (18 kg), and the average dose range is 5 mg/kg. No conversion of weight is required.

Step 1: Start by calculating the safe total daily dose for this child.

$$5 \text{ mg} \times 18 \text{ kg} = 90 \text{ mg/day}$$

The safe dose for this child (total) is 90 mg/day.

The calculation of the safe daily dose could also be done by setting up a ratio-proportion using the format of fractions or colons. Using this example, the setup as a ratio-proportion might be:

$$\frac{5 \text{ mg}}{x \text{ mg}} = \frac{1 \text{ kg}}{18 \text{ kg}} \qquad x = 90 \text{ mg/day}$$

OR

$$5\text{mg} : 1 \text{ kg} = x \text{ mg} : 18 \text{ kg}$$

$$x = 90 \text{ mg/day}$$

Step 2: Now determine the amount of each dose.

The dose is to be given in three equally divided doses. Therefore:

$$\frac{90 \text{ mg}}{3} = 30 \text{ mg per dose}$$

After calculating the safe dose for a child, you can assess whether what the doctor ordered is a safe dose.

The doctor ordered 30 mg q8h. Is this a safe dose?

$$\text{q8h} = 24 \div 8 = 3 \text{ doses}$$

$30 \times 3 = 90$ mg. Compare the ordered daily dose with the safe daily dose you calculated in Step 1. A daily dose of 90 mg is safe.

Step 3: Use the ratio-proportion or formula method to determine the number of capsules to give.

Dilantin is supplied in 30-mg capsules (refer to label). The ordered dose is 30 mg per dose.

$$30 \text{ mg} : 1 \text{ capsule} = 30 \text{ mg} : x \text{ caps}$$

$$\frac{30x}{30} = \frac{30}{30} \quad x = 1 \text{ caps}$$

OR

$$\frac{30 \text{ mg}}{30 \text{ mg}} \times 1 \text{ caps} = x \text{ caps;}$$

$$x = 1 \text{ caps}$$

$$\frac{30 \text{ mg}}{30 \text{ mg}} = \frac{x \text{ caps}}{1 \text{ caps}}$$

$$x = 1 \text{ caps}$$

You would give 1 caps q8h to administer the ordered dose.

Example 2: Doctor orders gentamicin 50 mg IVPB q8h for a child weighing 40 lb. The recommended dose for a child is 6–7.5 mg/kg/24 hr divided q8h.

First, a weight conversion is necessary since you have the child's weight in lb and the reference is in kg. Convert the child's weight in lb to kg to the nearest tenth.

$$\frac{2.2 \text{ lb}}{40 \text{ lb}} = \frac{1 \text{ kg}}{x \text{ kg}}$$

$$\frac{2.2\,x}{2.2} = \frac{40}{2.2}$$

$$x = 18.18 \text{ kg}$$

The weight is 18.2 kg.

Now that you've converted the weight, you can calculate the safe dose. You must calculate and obtain a range. (The recommended dose is 6–7.5 mg/kg/24 hr.)

Therefore calculate the lower and upper range:

$$6 \text{ mg} \times 18.2 \text{ kg} = 109.2 \text{ mg}$$

$$7.5 \text{ mg} \times 18.2 \text{ kg} = 136.5 \text{ mg}$$

The safe range for the child weighing 18.2 kg is 109.2–136.5 mg.

Now divide the total daily dose by the number of times the drug will be given in a day.

$$\text{q8h} = 24 \div 8 = 3$$

$$109.2 \div 3 = 36.4 \text{ mg per dose}$$

$$136.5 \div 3 = 45.5 \text{ mg per dose}$$

The dose range is 36.4–45.5 mg per dose q8h. The ordered dose of 50 mg q8h exceeds the dose of 109.2–136.5 mg total dose for 24 hours.

$$50 \text{ mg q8h} = 50 \times 3 = 150 \text{ mg}$$

Remember that factors such as the child's medical condition might warrant a larger dose. Call the doctor to verify the dose.

Example 3: The recommended dose for dicloxacillin sodium for oral suspension is 12.5 mg/kg/day for children weighing less than 40 kg (88 lb) in equally divided doses q6h. What is the dose for a child weighing 36 lb?

First convert the child's weight in lb to the nearest tenth of a kg.

2.2 lb : 1 kg = 36 lb : x kg (or state ratio as a fraction).

$$\frac{2.2\,x}{2.2} = \frac{36}{2.2}$$

$x = 16.36$ kg. To the nearest tenth the weight is 16.4 kg.

Now that you've converted the weight to kg, you can calculate the safe dose for this child.

$$12.5 \text{ mg} \times 16.4 \text{ kg} = 205 \text{ mg}$$

The safe dose for a child weighing 16.4 kg is 205 mg/day.

If 50 mg is ordered q6h, is this a safe dose?

$$24 \text{ h} \div 6 \text{ h} = 4 \text{ doses per day}$$

$$50 \text{ mg} \times 4 \text{ doses} = 200 \text{ mg per day}$$

The ordered dose is safe.

Next, calculate the amount of medication to give to administer the ordered dose. Dicloxacillin sodium oral suspension is available in a dose strength of 62.5 mg per 5 mL. Use either ratio-proportion or formula method as follows:

$$62.5 \text{ mg} : 5 \text{ mL} = 50 \text{ mg} : x \text{ mL}$$

$$\frac{62.5x}{62.5} = \frac{250 \text{ mg}}{62.5}$$

$$x = 4 \text{ mL}$$

OR

$$\frac{50 \text{ mg}}{62.5 \text{ mg}} \times 5 \text{ mL} = x \text{ mL};$$

$$\frac{250}{62.5} = 4 \text{ mL}$$

$$\frac{50 \text{ mg}}{62.5 \text{ mg}} = \frac{x \text{ mL}}{5 \text{ mL}}$$

$$\frac{250}{62.5} = 4 \text{ mL}$$

You would give 4 mL to administer the ordered dose of 50 mg.

When information concerning a pediatric dose is not present on the drug label, refer to the package insert, the PDR, or other reference text. Now try the following practice problems. Labels or portions of package inserts have been included for some problems.

Remember: It is imperative to calculate safe dosages for a child to avoid medication errors.

Practice Problems: Calculating According to Mg/Kg (pp. 378-380)

Round weights and doses to the nearest tenth where indicated.

17. Refer to the label and answer the following. The child weighs 35 lb.

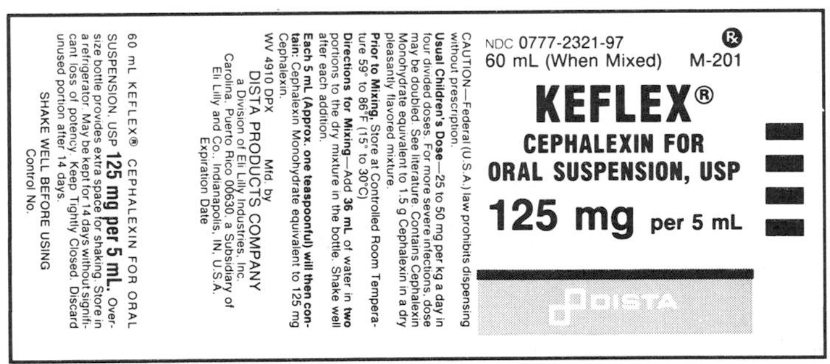

a) What is the recommended dose in mg/kg/day? ____________

b) What is the safe dose range for a child weighing 35 lb? ____________

c) The doctor ordered 150 mg p.o. q6h. Is the dose safe? ____________

d) How many mL will you administer for each dose? ____________

18. Refer to the label. The PDR indicates 15 mg/kg/day q8h of kanamycin. The doctor ordered 200 mg I.V. q8h for a child weighing 35 kg.

a) What is the maximum dose for 24 hours? __________

b) What is the divided dose? __________

c) Is the dose ordered safe? __________

19. The recommended dose of clindamycin oral suspension is 8–25 mg/kg/day in four divided doses. A child weighs 40 kg.

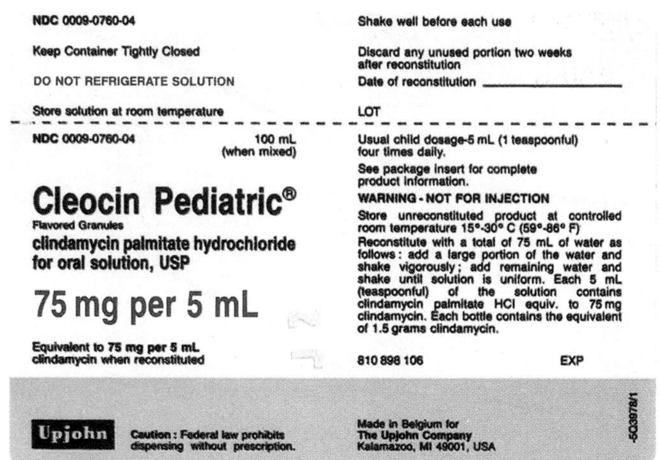

a) What is the maximum dose for 24 hours? __________

b) What is the divided dose? __________

20. The doctor orders phenobarbital 10 mg q12h for a child weighing 9 lb. The recommended maintenance dose is 3–5 mg/kg/day q12h.

a) What is the child's weight in kg to the nearest tenth? __________

b) What is the range of doses that are safe for this child? __________

c) Is the dose ordered safe? ______________

d) Phenobarbital elixer is available in a dose strength of 20 mg per 5 mL.
What will you administer for one dose? ______________

21. The doctor orders morphine sulfate 7.5 mg s.c. q4h p.r.n. for a child weighing 84 lb. The recommended maximum dose for a child is 0.1-0.2 mg/kg/dose.

LOT
EXP
LIGHT SENSITIVE: Keep covered in this box until ready to use.
To open—Cut seal along dotted line

25 DOSETTE® VIALS—Each contains 1 mL
MORPHINE
SULFATE INJECTION, USP
15 mg/mL
FOR SUBCUTANEOUS, INTRAMUSCULAR OR SLOW INTRAVENOUS USE
NOT FOR EPIDURAL OR INTRATHECAL USE
WARNING: May be habit forming
PROTECT FROM LIGHT
DO NOT USE IF PRECIPITATED
CAUTION: Federal law prohibits dispensing without prescription.

NDC 0641-0190-25
Each mL contains morphine sulfate 15 mg, monobasic sodium phosphate, monohydrate 10 mg, dibasic sodium phosphate, anhydrous 2.8 mg, sodium formaldehyde sulfoxylate 3 mg and phenol 2.5 mg in Water for Injection, pH 2.5-6.5; sulfuric acid added, if needed, for pH adjustment. Sealed under nitrogen.
USUAL DOSE: See package insert.
Store at 15°-30° C (59°-86° F). Avoid freezing.
NOTE: Slight discoloration will not alter efficacy. Discard if markedly discolored.
Product Code: 0190-25 B-50190g

ELKINS-SINN, INC. Cherry Hill, NJ 08003-4099
A subsidiary of A. H. Robins Company

a) Is the dose ordered safe? ______________

b) How many mL would you administer for one dose? ______________

22. The recommended dose of Dilantin is 4–8 mg/kg/day q12h. The doctor ordered 15 mg p.o. q12h for a child weighing 11 lb.

a) Is the dose ordered safe? ______________

b) Dilantin suspension is available in a dose strength of 30 mg/5 mL. What would you administer for one dose? ______________

23. The recommended initial dose of mercaptopurine is 2.5 mg/kg/day p.o. What would the recommended daily dose be for a child weighing 44 lb? ______________

24. For a child the recommended dosage of I.V. vancomycin is 40 mg/kg/2 4 hr divided q6h. The doctor ordered 200 mg I.V. q6h for a child weighing 38 lb.

a) What is the child's weight in kg to the nearest tenth? ______________

b) What is the maximum dose for this child in 24 hours? ______________

c) What is the divided dose? ______________

d) Is the dose ordered safe? ______________

25. Use the label below to answer the questions.

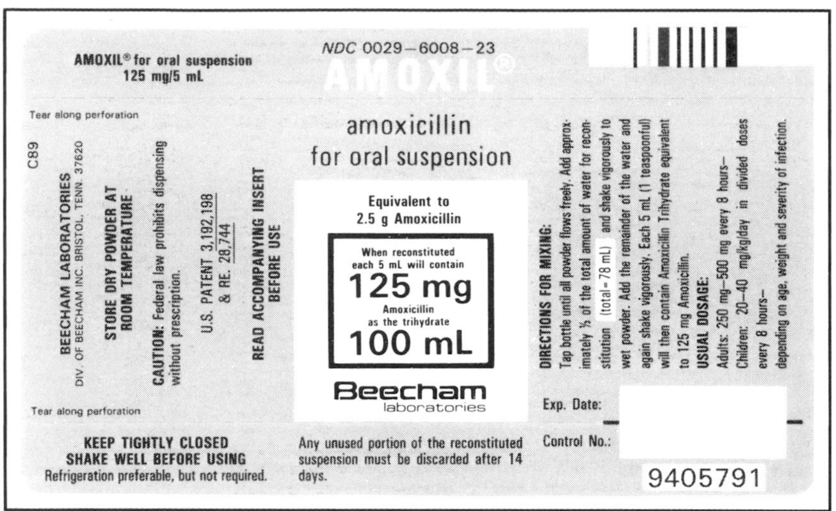

a) What is the recommended dose in mg/kg/day? __________

b) What is the safe dose for a 16-lb child? __________

c) The doctor ordered 125 mg p.o. q8h. Is the dose safe? __________

26. A 44-lb child has an order for Ilosone oral suspension

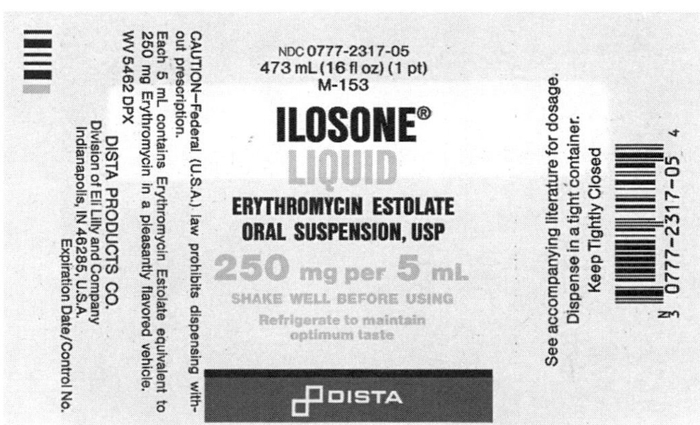

The usual dose for children under 50 lb is 30–50 mg/kg/day in divided doses and for children over 50 lb is 250 mg q6h. The doctor has ordered 250 mg p.o. q6h for this child. Is this dosage safe? __________

27. Refer to the Fungizone insert to calculate the dose for an adult weighing 66.3 kg with good cardiorenal function. ____________

1 vial NDC 0003-0437-30
NSN 6505-01-084-9453

50 mg
FUNGIZONE®
INTRAVENOUS
Amphotericin B for Injection USP

FOR INTRAVENOUS INFUSION IN HOSPITALS ONLY

Caution: Federal law prohibits dispensing without prescription

Read all sides

APOTHECON®
A BRISTOL-MYERS SQUIBB COMPANY

Partial Insert for Fungizone (Amphotericin B)

DOSAGE AND ADMINISTRATION

CAUTION: Under no circumstances should a total daily dose of 1.5 mg/kg be exceeded. Amphotericin B overdoses can result in cardio-respiratory arrest (see OVERDOSAGE).

FUNGIZONE Intravenous should be administered by *slow* intravenous infusion. Intravenous infusion should be given over a period of approximately 2 to 6 hours (depending on the dose) observing the usual precautions for intravenous therapy (see PRECAUTIONS, General). The recommended concentration for intravenous infusion is 0.1 mg/mL (1 mg/10 mL).

Since patient tolerance varies greatly, the dosage of amphotericin B must be individualized and adjusted according to the patient's clinical status (e.g., site and severity of infection, etiologic agent, cardio-renal function, etc.).

A single intravenous **test dose** (1 mg in 20 mL of 5% dextrose solution) administered over 20-30 minutes may be preferred. The patient's temperature, pulse, respiration, and blood pressure should be recorded every 30 minutes for 2 to 4 hours.

In patients with **good cardio-renal function** and a **well tolerated test dose**, therapy is usually initiated with a daily dose of 0.25 mg/kg of body weight. However, in those patients having **severe and rapidly progressive fungal infection**, therapy may be initiated with a daily dose of 0.3 mg/kg of body weight. In patients with **impaired cardio-renal function** or a **severe reaction to the test dose**, therapy should be initiated with smaller daily doses (i.e., 5 to 10 mg).

28. A 200-lb adult is to be treated with Ticar for a complicated urinary tract infection. The recommended dosage is 150 to 200 mg/kg/day I.V. in divided doses every 4 or 6 hours. What is the daily dose range in g for this client? ____________

29. A child weighs 12 lb, 6 oz. The recommended dose for a child of V-Cillin oral solution is 15 to 50 mg/kg/day in four divided doses. What is the safe dose range for this child? ____________

Points to Remember

- To convert lb to kg divide by 2.2; express answer to nearest tenth.
- To convert kg to lb multiply by 2.2; express answer to nearest tenth.
- To calculate doses the child's weight must be converted to the reference.
- To calculate the dose do the following:
  1. Determine the child's weight in kg if needed.
  2. Multiply the child's weight in kg by the dose stated.
  3. Divide the total daily dose by the number of doses needed to administer.
  4. Calculate the number of tablets or volume to administer for each dose by use of ratio-proportion or the formula method.
- When the recommended dose is given as a range, calculate based on the low and high values for each dose.
- Question any discrepancies in doses ordered and remember factors such as age, weight, and medical conditions can cause discrepancies. Ask the doctor to clarify the order when a discrepancy exists.
- Use appropriate resources to determine the safe range for a child's dose.

Calculation of Pediatric Doses Using Body Surface Area (BSA)

A child's BSA is determined by comparing a child's weight and height with what is considered average or the norm. Many pediatric doses are prescribed based on the child's BSA. The BSA is determined from the height and weight of a child and the use of the West nomogram (Figure 19-1).

This information is then applied to a formula for dose calculation. Remember, all children are not the same size at the same age; therefore the West nomogram can be used to determine the BSA of a child. The West nomogram is not easy to use, although it is a tool still employed in some institutions. The nomogram can be used to calculate the BSA for individuals up to 180 lb.

The BSA is used to calculate doses for infants and children up to 12 years of age. It is also possible to determine the BSA from weight alone, if the child is of normal height and weight.

Reading the West Nomogram Chart

Refer to the chart in Figure 19-1. Note: The height is on the left hand side of the chart, and the weight is on the right hand side. To identify the correct values on the BSA chart, you must be able to read it. This entails reading the numbers and determining what the calibration between them is measuring. For example, look at the column indicated by weight and study how it's marked. Looking at the bottom of the chart, notice there are four calibrations between 0.10 and 0.15; those numbers in between are read as 0.11, 0.12, etc. Notice the calibrations between 15 and 20 are 1-lb increments.

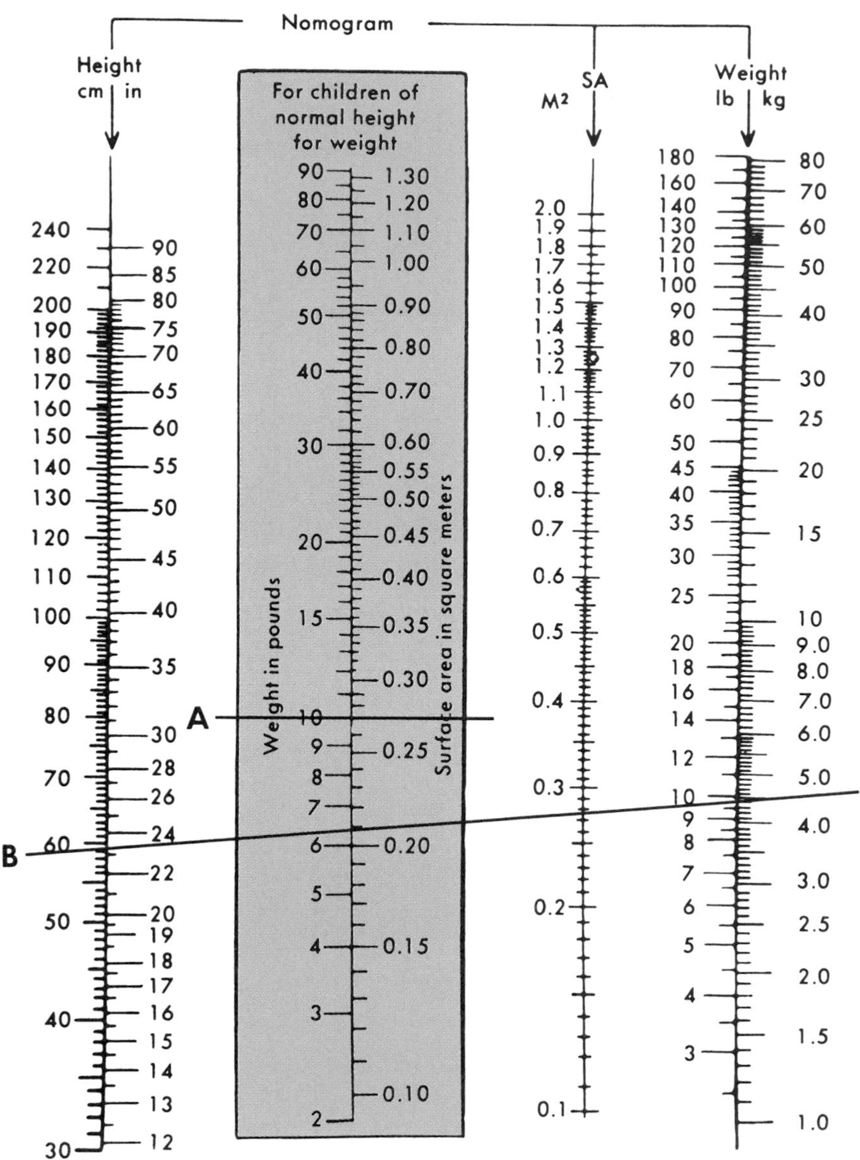

Figure 19-1. West nomogram for estimation of body surface area. (From Dison N: *Simplified drugs and solutions for health care professionals,* ed 11, St. Louis, 1996, Mosby.)

Practice Problems (pp. 380-381)

Refer to the nomogram and determine the BSA from the column marked "Surface area in square meters."

30. For a child weighing 30 lb ____________

31. For a child weighing 10 lb ____________

32. For a child weighing 52 lb ____________

In addition to determining the BSA based on weight, the BSA can also be calculated using both height and weight. If you refer to the chart, notice the columns for height and weight. This chart also includes the weight in lb and kg. Notice the column for height (in cm and inches). To determine the surface area a ruler is placed on the graph from the height to the weight column. The surface area (m^2) is indicated where the line crosses the BSA column, second from right of the nomogram.

Remember: If the ruler is slightly off the height or weight, the BSA will be incorrect.

Practice Problems (p. 381)

Using the nomogram, calculate the following BSAs.

33. A child who is 90 cm long and weighs 50 lb. ____________

34. A child who is 60 cm long and weighs 10 lb. ____________

35. A child who is 100 cm long and weighs 10 kg. ____________

36. A child who is 30 inches long and weighs 20 lb. ____________

37. A child who weighs 60 lb and is 39 inches tall. ____________

38. A baby who weighs 13 lb and is 19 inches long. ____________

39. A child who weighs 30 lb and is 32 inches tall. ____________

40. A child who weighs 13 kg and is 65 cm tall. ____________

Dose Calculation Based on BSA

If you know the child's BSA, the dose is calculated by multiplying the recommended dose by the child's BSA (m^2).

Example 1: The recommended dose is 3 mg per m^2. The child has a BSA of 1.2 m^2.

$$1.2 \times 3 \text{ mg} = 3.6 \text{ mg}$$

Example 2: The recommended dose is 30 mg per m^2. The child has a BSA of 0.75 m^2.

$$0.75 \times 30 = 22.5 \text{ mg.}$$

Formula

$$\frac{\text{BSA of child } (m^2)}{1.7\ (m^2)} \times \text{Adult dose}$$

$$= \text{Estimated child's dose}$$

Calculating Using the Formula

The BSA is expressed in square meters (m^2). The child's BSA is then inserted into the formula below.

If the recommended dose for an adult is cited only, then the formula is used to calculate the child's dose. The formula uses the average adult dose, the average adult BSA (1.7 m^2), and the child's BSA in m^2.

Example 1: The doctor has ordered a medication for which the average adult dose is 125 mg. What will the dose be for a child with a BSA of 1.4 m^2?

$$\frac{1.4}{1.7} \times 125 \text{ mg} = 102.94 \text{ mg} = 102.9 \text{ mg}$$

Example 2: The adult dose for a medication is 100 to 300 mg. What will the dose be for a child with a BSA of 0.5 m²?

$$\frac{0.5}{1.7} \times 100 = 29.4 \text{ mg}$$

$$\frac{0.5}{1.7} \times 300 = 88.2 \text{ mg}$$

The dose range is 29.4–88.2 mg.

Practice Problems: Determining the Dose Using the Formula (pp. 381-382)

Using the West nomogram chart when indicated, calculate the child's dose for the following drugs. Express your answer to the nearest tenth.

41. The child's height is 32 in and weight is 25 lb. The recommended adult dose is 25 mg.

    a) What is the child's BSA? ____________

    b) What is the child's dose? ____________

42. The child's height is 100 cm and weight is 10 kg. The adult dose is 200–400 mg.

    a) What is the child's BSA? ____________

    b) What is the child's dose? ____________

43. The normal adult dose of a drug is 5–15 mg. What will the dose be for a child whose BSA is 1.5 m²? ____________

44. The doctor ordered 5 mg of a drug for a child with a BSA of 0.8 m². The average adult dose is 20 mg. Is this a correct dose? ____________

45. The child's BSA is 0.92 m². The doctor ordered 7 mg of a drug. The average adult dose is 25 mg. Is this correct? ____________

46. The child's BSA is 1.5 m². The doctor ordered an antibiotic for which the average adult dose is 250 mg. What will the child's dose be? ____________

47. The recommended dose is 20 to 30 mg per m². The child has a BSA of 0.74 m². What will the child's dose be? ____________

48. The child has a BSA of 0.67 m². The average adult dose is 20 mg. The doctor ordered 8 mg. Is the dose correct? ____________

49. The child has a BSA of 0.94 m². The recommended adult dose is 10 to 20 mg. What will the child's dose be? ____________

50. The child's weight is 20 lb and height is 30 in. The adult dose is 500 mg.

    a) What is the child's BSA? ____________

    b) What is the child's dose? ____________

51. The recommended adult dose for an antibiotic is 500 mg 4 times a day. The child's BSA is 1.3 m². What will the child's dose be? ____________

52. The child's weight is 30 lb and height is 28 in. The adult dose is 25 mg.

    a) What is the child's BSA? ______________

    b) What is the child's dose? ______________

53. The child's BSA is 0.52 m^2. The average adult dose for a medication is 15 mg. What will the child's dose be? ______________

54. The recommended adult dose for a drug is 150 mg. The child's BSA is 1.10 m^2. What will the child's dose be? ______________

Points to Remember

- BSA is determined from a nomogram using the child's height and weight.
- When you know the child's BSA, the dose is determined by multiplying the BSA by the recommended dose.
- To determine whether a child's dose is safe, a comparison must be made between what is ordered and the calculation of the dose based on BSA.
- The formula for calculating a child's dose is as follows:

$$\frac{\text{BSA of child (m}^2\text{)}}{1.7 \text{ m}^2} \times \text{Adult dose} = \text{Estimated child's dose}$$

Calculating BSA with the Use of a Formula

BSA is used a great deal in calculating doses for children and adults. Calculating BSA is used frequently to determine doses for medications such as chemotherapeutic agents that are used in the treatment of cancer. As already shown, BSA can be calculated using the tool called the West nomogram; however, it is a tool that requires learning to use and can result in an error if the ruler is just slightly off line.

To calculate BSA the client's height and weight are used (adults and children). Instead of using the West nomogram one can calculate the BSA with two tools:

1. Calculator
2. Formula

Calculators are increasingly being used for calculation of critical care doses and in pediatric units where extensive mathematics may be required. It has been determined that the safest way to calculate a BSA is to use a formula and a calculator that can perform square roots ($\sqrt{\ }$). The formula used is based on the units in which the measurements are obtained. (Example: kg, cm, lb, and in.)

Formula for Calculating BSA from kg and cm

Steps

1. Multiply the weight in kg by height in cm.
2. Divide the product obtained in Step 1 by 3,600.
3. Enter the square root sign into the calculator.
4. Round the final m^2 BSA to the nearest hundredth.

Example 1: Calculate the BSA for a child who weighs 23 kg and whose height is 128 cm. Express BSA to the nearest hundredth

$$\sqrt{\frac{23 \text{ (kg)} \times 128 \text{ (cm)}}{3600}} = 0.817$$

$$\sqrt{0.817} = 0.903 = 0.90 \text{ m}^2$$

Formula

$$\text{BSA} = \sqrt{\frac{\text{Weight (kg)} \times \text{Height (cm)}}{3600}}$$

The BSA was calculated as follows: 23 × 128 ÷ 3,600 = 0.817, then the square root ($\sqrt{\ }$) was entered. The final m^2 BSA was rounded to the nearest hundredth.

Example 2: Calculate the BSA for an adult who weighs 100 kg and whose height is 180 cm. Express BSA to the nearest hundredth.

$$\sqrt{\frac{100\text{ (kg)} \times 180\text{ (cm)}}{3600}} = 5$$

$$\sqrt{5} = 2.236 = 2.24\text{ m}^2$$

Formula for Calculating BSA from lb and in

The formula is the same with the exception of the number used in the denominator, which is 3,131.

Example 1: Calculate the BSA for child who weighs 25 lb and is 32 inches tall. Express the BSA to nearest hundredth.

$$\sqrt{\frac{25\text{ (lb)} \times 32\text{ (in)}}{3131}} = 0.255$$

$$\sqrt{0.255} = 0.504 = 0.50\text{ m}^2$$

Example 2: Calculate the BSA for an adult who weighs 143.7 lb and is 61.2 inches tall. Express the BSA to the nearest hundredth.

$$\sqrt{\frac{143.7\text{ (lb)} \times 61.2\text{ (in)}}{3131}} = 2.808$$

$$\sqrt{2.808} = 1.675 = 1.68\text{ m}^2$$

Formula

$$\text{BSA} = \sqrt{\frac{\text{Weight (lb)} \times \text{Height (in)}}{3131}}$$

Practice Problems (p. 382)

Determine the BSA for the following clients using a formula. Express the BSA to the nearest hundredth.

55. An adult whose weight is 95.5 kg and height is 180 cm. ____________

56. A child whose weight is 10 kg and height is 70 cm. ____________

57. A child who weighs 4.8 lb and measures 21 inches. ____________

58. An adult whose weight is 170 lb and height is 67 in. ____________

Note: As already covered in the chapter, once you know the BSA, the dose calculation involves just multiplication.

Example: The recommended dose is 40 mg/m^2. The child's BSA is 0.55 m^2. Express your answer to the nearest whole number. 0.55 × 40 mg = 22 mg

Remember: Always check a dose against m^2 recommendations using appropriate resources. Example: PDR, drug inserts.

Medications, particularly chemotherapy agents, often provide the recommended dose according to m^2 (BSA).

Example: Cisplatin is an antineoplastic agent. The recommended pediatric/adult I.V. dose for bladder cancer is 50–70 mg/m^2 every 3–4 weeks. For carmustine, which is used in Hodgkin's disease, and for brain tumors, the recommended I.V. dose for an adult is 150–200 mg/m^2.

Pediatric Oral and Parenteral Medications

Several methods have been presented to determine doses for children in this chapter. It is important, however, to bear in mind that while the dose may be determined according to weight, BSA, etc., the dose to administer is calculated using the same methods as for adults (ratio-proportion, formula). It is important to remember the following differences with children's doses.

Remember

1. Doses are smaller for children than for adults.
2. Most oral drugs for infants and small children come in liquid form to facilitate easy swallowing.
3. The oral route is preferred; however, when necessary, medications are administered by parenteral route.
4. Not more than 1 mL is injected I.M.
5. Doses are frequently administered using a tuberculin syringe.

Chapter Review (pp. 382-386)

Read the dose information or label given for the following problems. Express body weight conversion to the nearest tenth where indicated and doses to the nearest tenth.

1. The doctor orders Lasix 10 mg I.V. stat for a child weighing 22 lb. The recommended initial dose is 1 mg/kg. Is the dose ordered safe? __________

2. The doctor orders amoxicillin 150 mg p.o. q8h for an infant weighing 23 lb. The maximum daily dosage for an infant is amoxicillin p.o. 20 to 40 mg/kg/24h divided q8h.

   a) What is the child's weight to the nearest tenth? __________

   b) What is the maximum dose for 24 h? __________

   c) What is the divided dose? __________

   d) Is the dose ordered safe? __________

3. The doctor orders Furadantin oral suspension 25 mg p.o. q6h for a child weighing 17 kg. Refer to the Furadantin label below.

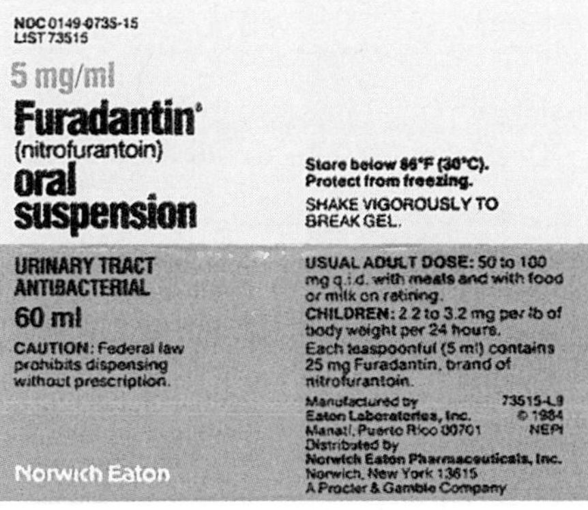

   a) Is this a safe dosage? __________

   b) How many mL must be given per dose to administer the ordered dose? __________

4. The doctor orders 100 mg p.o. q6h of dicloxacillin for a child weighing 35 kg. The recommended dose is 12.5 mg/kg/day for children weighing less than 40 kg in equally divided doses q6h. Is the dosage ordered safe? ____________

5. The doctor orders Vibramycin 75 mg p.o. q12h for a child weighing 30 lb. Refer to the label below and determine if this is a safe dose. ____________

Vibramycin®
SYRUP Calcium
doxycycline calcium
oral suspension
50 mg / 5 ml†
1 PINT (473 ml)
†Each teaspoonful (5 ml) contains doxycycline calcium equivalent to 50 mg of doxycycline.
USUAL DOSAGE:
Adults: 200 mg on the first day (100 mg every 12 hours) followed by a maintenance dose of 100 mg a day.
Children above eight years of age:
Under 100 lbs.—2 mg/lb. of body weight daily divided in two doses on the first day, followed by 1 mg/lb. of body weight on subsequent days in one or two doses.
Over 100 lbs.—See adult dosage.
doxycycline U.S. Pat. No. 3,200,149
READ ACCOMPANYING PROFESSIONAL INFORMATION
RECOMMENDED STORAGE
STORE BELOW 86°F. (30°C.)
Dispense in tight, light resistant containers (USP).
CAUTION: Federal law prohibits dispensing without prescription.
Pfizer LABORATORIES DIVISION
PFIZER INC.,
NEW YORK, N.Y. 10017
MADE IN U.S.A. 2

Pfizer
NDC 0069-0971-93
6188
Vibramycin®
Calcium
SYRUP
doxycycline calcium
oral suspension
50 mg/5ml†
1 PINT
(473 ml)
RASPBERRY/APPLE FLAVORED
For oral use only
SHAKE WELL BEFORE USING
IMPORTANT:
This closure is not child-resistant.

6. The doctor orders oxacillin oral solution 250 mg p.o. q6h for a child weighing 42 lb. The recommended dose is 50 mg/kg/day in equally divided doses q6h. Is the dose ordered safe? ____________

7. The doctor orders Cleocin suspension 150 mg p.o. q8h for a child weighing 36 lb. The recommended dose is 10–25 mg/kg/24h divided q6 to 8h. Is the dosage ordered safe? ____________

8. The doctor orders Keflex suspension 250 mg p.o. q6h for a child weighing 66 lb. The usual child dose is 25–50 mg 1 kg/day in four divided doses. Available: Keflex suspension 125 mg/5 mL.

   a) Is the dosage ordered safe? ____________

   b) How many mL would you give to administer one dose? ____________

9. The doctor orders streptomycin sulfate 400 mg I.M. q12h for a child weighing 35 kg.

   a) The recommended dose is 20-40 mg/kg/day divided q12h I.M. Is the dosage ordered safe? ____________

b) A 1-g vial of streptomycin sulfate is available in powdered form with the following instructions: Dilution with 1.8 mL of sterile water will yield 400 mg per mL. How many mL will you give to administer the ordered dose? ____________

10. A child weighs 46 lb and has a mild infection. The doctor ordered Gantrisin oral suspension 250 mg p.o. q6h. The recommended dose is 120 mg/kg/24h in four equally divided doses. Is the dosage ordered safe? ____________

Using the nomogram on p. 254, determine the BSA and calculate the child's dose by using the formula. Express doses to the nearest tenth.

11. The child's height is 30 inches and weight is 20 lb. The adult dose of an antibiotic is 500 mg.

    a) What is the BSA? ____________

    b) What is the child's dose? ____________

12. The child's height is 32 inches and weight is 27 lb. The adult dose for a medication is 25 mg.

    a) What is the BSA? ____________

    b) What is the child's dose? ____________

13. The child's height is 120 cm and weight is 40 kg. The adult dose for a medication is 250 mg.

    a) What is the BSA? ____________

    b) What is the child's dose? ____________

14. The child's height is 50 inches and weight is 75 lb. The adult dose for a medication is 30 mg.

    a) What is the BSA? ____________

    b) What is the child's dose? ____________

15. The child's height is 50 inches and weight is 70 lb. The adult dose for a medication is 150 mg.

    a) What is the BSA? ____________

    b) What is the child's dose? ____________

Determine the child's dose for the following drugs. Express answers to the nearest tenth.

16. The adult dose of a drug is 50 mg. What will the dose be for a child with a BSA of 0.70 m^2? ____________

17. The adult dose of a drug is 10–20 mg. What will the dose range be for a child whose BSA is 0.66 m^2? ____________

18. The adult dose of a drug is 2,000 U. What will the dose be for a child with a BSA of 0.55 m^2? ____________

19. The adult dose of a drug is 200–250 mg. What will the dose range be for a child with a BSA of 0.55 m^2? ____________

20. The adult dose of a drug is 150 mg. What will the dose be for a child with a BSA of 0.22 m^2? __________

Calculate the child's dose in the following problems. Determine if the doctor's order is correct. If the order is incorrect, give the correct dose. Express answers to the nearest tenth.

21. A child with a BSA of 0.49 m^2 has an order of 25 mg for a drug with an average adult dose of 60 mg. __________

22. A child with a BSA of 0.32 m^2 has an order of 4 mg for a drug with an average adult dose of 10 mg. __________

23. A child with a BSA of 0.68 m^2 has an order of 50 mg for a drug with an average adult dose of 125–150 mg. __________

24. A child with a BSA of 0.55 m^2 has an order of 5 mg for a drug. The adult dose is 25 mg. __________

25. A child with a BSA of 1.2 m^2 has an order for 60 mg of a drug. The adult dose is 75–100 mg. __________

Using the formula method for calculating BSA, determine the BSA in the following clients and express answers to the nearest hundredth.

26. A 15-year-old who weighs 100 lb and is 55 inches tall. __________

27. An adult who weighs 60.9 kg and is 130 cm tall. __________

28. A child who weighs 55 lb and is 45 inches tall. __________

29. A child who weighs 60 lb and is 35 inches tall. __________

30. An adult who weighs 65 kg and 132 cm tall. __________

31. A child who weighs 24 lb and is 28 inches tall. __________

32. An infant who weighs 6 kg and is 55 cm tall. __________

33. A child who weighs 42 lb and is 45 inches tall. __________

34. An infant who weighs 8 kg and is 70 cm tall. __________

35. An adult who weighs 74 kg and is 160 cm tall. __________

Calculate the doses to be given. Use labels where provided.

36. Doctor's Order: AZT 7 mg p.o. q6h × LOS. _______________

    Available: AZT 10 mg/mL.

37. Doctor's Order: Epivir 150 mg p.o. b.i.d. _______________

    Available:

NDC 0173-0471-00

GlaxoWellcome

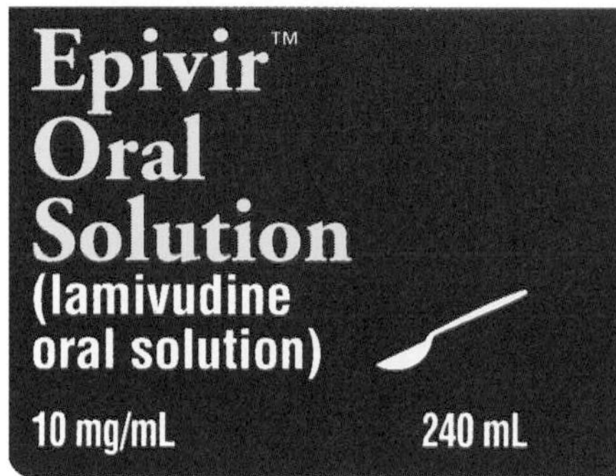

Caution: Federal law prohibits dispensing without prescription.

See package insert for Dosage and Administration.

Store between 2° and 25°C (36° and 77°F) in tightly closed bottles. Contains 6% alcohol.

4 0 5 8 8 9 5

Glaxo Wellcome Inc.
Research Triangle Park,
NC 27709
Manufactured in England
under agreement from
BioChem Pharma Inc.
Laval, Quebec, Canada
Rev. 10/95

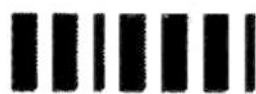

38. Doctor's Order: Digoxin 0.1 mg p.o. o.d. _______________

    Available:

60 mL NDC 0173-0264-27

LANOXIN®
(DIGOXIN)
ELIXIR
PEDIATRIC
Each mL contains
50 μg (0.05 mg)
PLEASANTLY FLAVORED

GlaxoWellcome
Glaxo Wellcome Inc.
Research Triangle Park, NC 27709
Made in U.S.A. Rev. 2/96 542404

Alcohol 10%, Methylparaben 0.1% (added as a preservative)
For indications, dosage, precautions, etc., see accompanying package insert.
Store at 15° to 25°C (59° to 77°F) and protect from light.
CAUTION: Federal law prohibits dispensing without prescription.

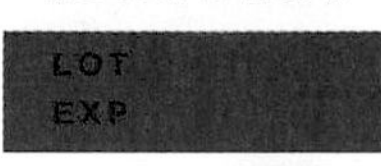

39. Doctor's Order: Retrovir 80 mg p.o. q8h. ______________

    Available: Retrovir 50 mg/5 mL.

240 mL NDC 0173-0113-18

RETROVIR®
(zidovudine)
Syrup

Each 5 mL (1 teaspoonful) contains zidovudine 50 mg and sodium benzoate 0.2% added as a preservative.

CAUTION: Federal law prohibits dispensing without prescription.

U.S. Patent Nos. 4818538 (Product Patent); 4724232, 4833130, and 4837208 (Use Patents)

For indications, dosage, precautions, etc., see accompanying package insert.
Store at 15° to 25°C (59° to 77°F).

Made in U.S.A. Rev. 5/96 587023

GlaxoWellcome
Glaxo Wellcome Inc.
Research Triangle Park, NC 27709

LOT
EXP

40. Doctor's Order: Augmentin 250 mg p.o. q6h. ______________

    Available:

AUGMENTIN®

Tear along perforation

NSN 6505-01-340-0847
Directions for mixing:
Tap bottle until all powder flows freely. Add approximately 2/3 of total water for reconstitution (total = 67 mL); shake vigorously to wet powder. Add remaining water; again shake vigorously.
Dosage: See accompanying prescribing information.

Tear along perforation

Keep tightly closed.
Shake well before using.
Must be refrigerated.
Discard after 10 days.

125mg/5mL
NDC 0029-6085-39

AUGMENTIN®
AMOXICILLIN/
CLAVULANATE POTASSIUM
FOR ORAL SUSPENSION
When reconstituted, each 5 mL contains:
AMOXICILLIN, 125 MG,
as the trihydrate
CLAVULANIC ACID, 31.25 MG,
as clavulanate potassium

75mL *(when reconstituted)*

SB SmithKline Beecham

Use only if inner seal is intact.
Net contents: Equivalent to 1.875 g amoxicillin and 0.469 g clavulanic acid.
Store dry powder at room temperature.
Caution: Federal law prohibits dispensing without prescription.
SmithKline Beecham Pharmaceuticals
Philadelphia, PA 19101

EXP.

LOT

9405804-E

41. Doctor's Order: Tegretol 0.25 g p.o. t.i.d. ______________

    Available:

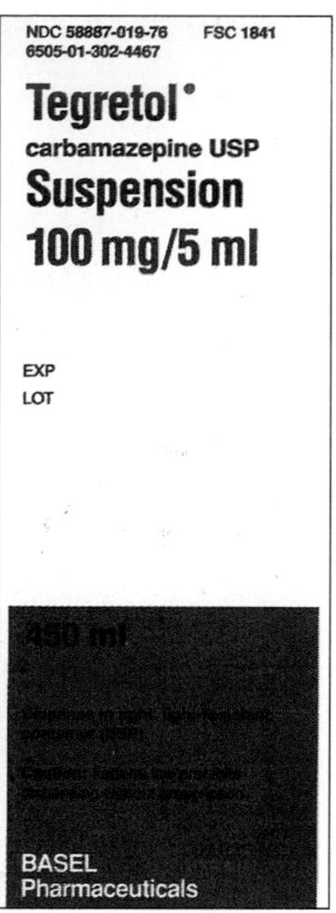

42. Doctor's Order: Amoxicillin 100 mg p.o. t.i.d. ______________

    Available: Amoxicillin 250 mg/5 mL.

Calculate the doses below. Use the labels where provided. Calculate to the nearest hundredths where necessary.

43. Doctor's Order: Gentamycin 7.3 mg I.M. q12h. ______________

    Available: Gentamycin 20 mg/2 mL.

44. Doctor's Order: Atropine 0.1 mg s.c. stat. ______________

    Available: Atropine 400 mcg/mL.

45. Doctor's Order: Ampicillin 160 mg I.M. q12h. ______________

    Available: Ampicillin 250 mg/mL.

46. Doctor's Order: Morphine 3.5 mg s.c. q6h prn for pain. ______________

    Available:

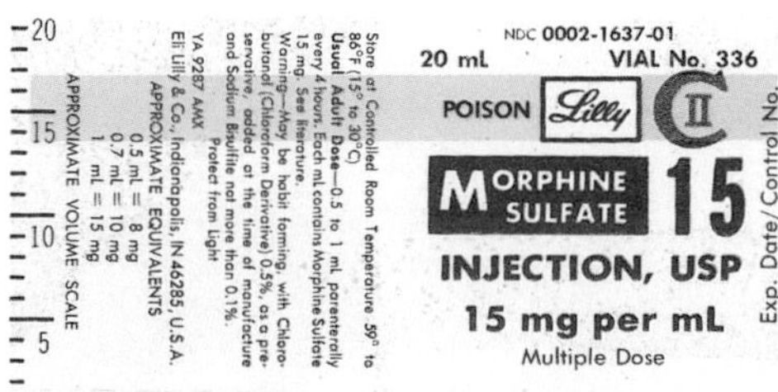

UNIT FIVE

Basic I.V., Heparin, and Critical Care Calculations

The ability to accurately calculate flow rates for I.V. medications is essential to both heparin administration and critical care calculations.

Chapter 20

Basic I.V. Calculations

Objectives

After reviewing this chapter the student will be able to do the following:

1. Differentiate between primary and secondary administration sets
2. Differentiate between various devices used to administer I.V. solutions (Example: Patient-controlled analgesia [PCA] pumps, electronic pumps)
3. Identify the abbreviations used for I.V. fluids
4. Identify the two types of administration tubing
5. Identify from I.V. tubing packages the drop factor in gtt/mL
6. Calculate flow rates using a formula method
7. Calculate infusion times
8. Calculate the flow rate for medications ordered I.V. over a specified time period
9. Calculate flow rates for pediatric I.V. therapy

When clients are receiving I.V. therapy, it is important to make sure they are receiving the correct amount. The doctor is responsible for writing the I.V. order, which must specify the following:

1. The type of I.V. fluid
2. The amount (volume) to be administered
3. The time period the I.V. is to infuse

The nurse often has to perform calculations associated with I.V. therapy. The nursing responsibility includes administration of I.V. fluids at the correct rate and monitoring the client during the therapy. Before turning to calculation aspects of I.V. therapy, let's begin with a general discussion. **I.V. therapy** is the method used to instill fluids or medications directly into the bloodstream. The advantages of administering medications by this route are the immediate availability of the medication to the body and the rapidity of action.

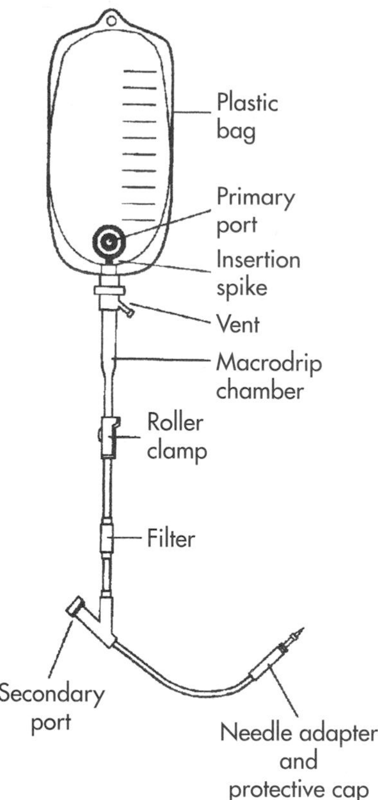

Figure 20-1. Intravenous infusion set. (From Edmunds MW: *Introduction to clinical pharmacology,* ed 2, St Louis, 1995, Mosby.)

The I.V. route is also used to meet nutritional requirements of a client, to replace electrolytes (for example, sodium, potassium), and to administer blood and blood products. Regardless of the purpose of the I.V. therapy, the nurse's primary responsibility is to administer the therapy correctly and at the correct rate.

Methods of Infusion

I.V. fluids are administered by an I.V. infusion set, which includes a sealed bag or bottle containing the fluids. A **drip chamber** is connected to the I.V. bottle or bag. The flow rate is adjusted to drops per minute by use of a **roller clamp.** Some I.V. tubing has a **sliding clamp** attached that can be used to temporarily stop the I.V. infusion. **Injection ports** are located on the I.V. tubing and on most I.V. solution bags. Injection ports allow for injection of medications directly into the bag of solution or line. The injection ports also allow for attachment of secondary I.V. lines containing fluids or medications to the primary line. Figure 20-1 shows a primary line infusion set. I.V. fluids infuse by **gravity flow.** I.V. lines are referred to as peripheral and central lines. A **peripheral line** is one that has an area such as the arm or hand for the infusion site. For a **central line,** a special catheter is used to access a large vein such as the subclavian or jugular. The special catheter is threaded through a large vein into the right atrium.

Secondary lines attach to the primary line at an injection port. The main purpose of secondary lines is to infuse medications on an intermittent basis (for example, antibiotics q6hr). A secondary line is referred to as an I.V. piggyback (IVPB). Notice that the IVPB is hanging higher than the primary line (Figure 20-2).

Another type of secondary medication setup that is used in some institutions is called the **Add Vantage System.** This system requires the use of a special type of I.V. bag that has a port for the insertion of the drug. (The drug is usually in powder form.) It is mixed using the I.V. solution as a diluent. The contents of the vial therefore are mixed into the total solution and then infused.

Volume control devices are used for accurate measurement of small-volume medications and fluids. Most volume control devices have a capacity of 100 to 150 mL. They can be used with secondary or primary lines. They are also used for medication purposes intermittently. They have a port that allows medication to be injected and a certain amount of I.V. fluid added as a diluent. They are referred to by their trade name: Volutrol, Soluset, or Buretrol, depending on the institution. They are used mostly in pediatric and critical care settings (Figure 20-3).

Indwelling infusion ports are used for the purpose of administering I.V. medication intermittently or for access to a vein in an emergency situation. Infusion ports are referred to as medlocks, saline locks, or heplocks. The line is usually kept free from blockage or clotting by irrigation of the line with heparin (anticoagulant) or sterile saline. The solution used and the amount of solution vary from institution to institution (Figure 20-4).

Recently various institutions have purchased a needleless system for administration of medications through the primary line. The needleless system doesn't require attachment of a needle by the nurse. The system allows for administration by I.V. push or bolus or for piggyback use (Figure 20-5).

When medications are administered through indwelling infusion ports (also called access devices), they must be periodically flushed to maintain patency. Due to bolusing of clients with heparin (a potent anticoagulant despite the use of

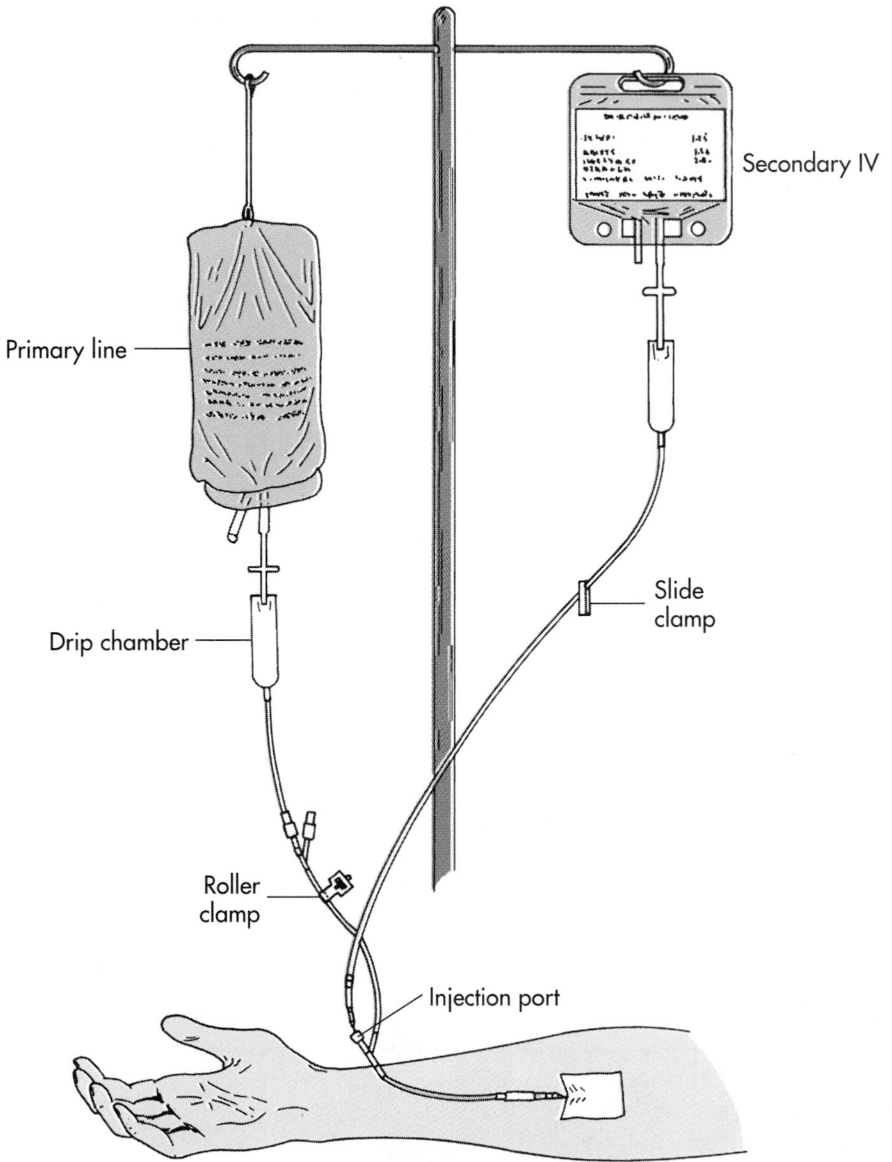

Figure 20-2. **A,** IVPB administration setup. Note that the smaller bag is hung higher than the primary one. (From Dison N: *Simplified drugs and solutions for nurses,* ed 10, St Louis, 1993, Mosby.)

Continued

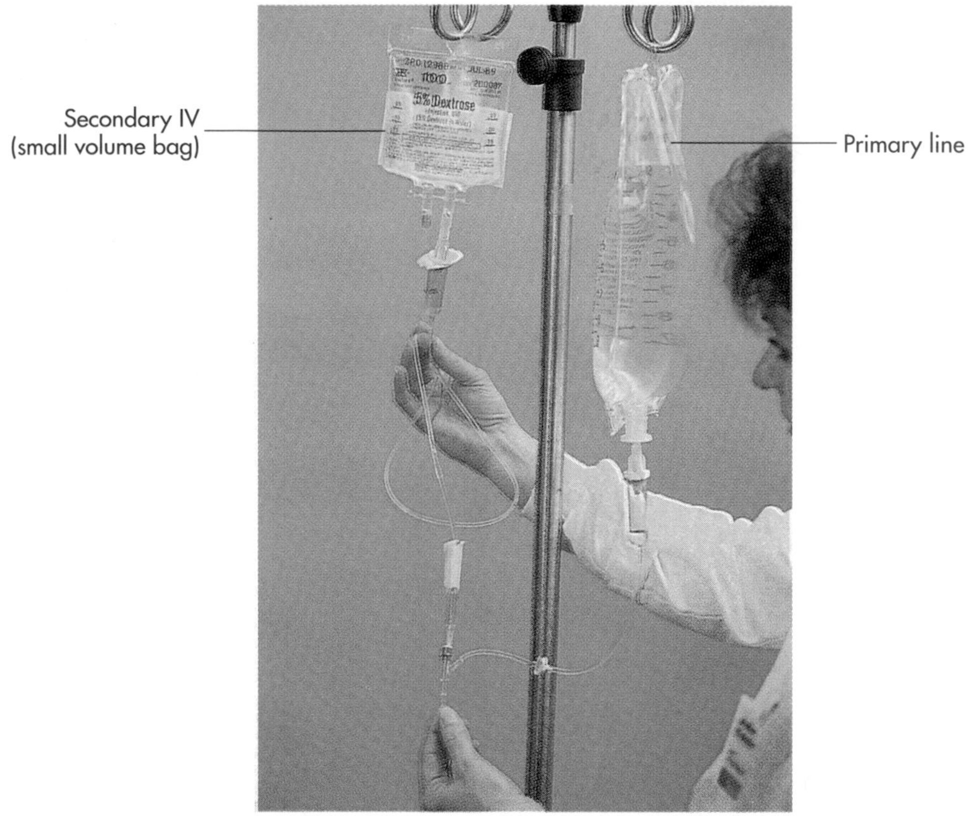

Figure 20-2. **B,** Attach IVPB to main line through injection port away from client. (From Elkin M, Perry A, Potter P: *Nursing interventions and clinical skills,* St Louis, 1996, Mosby.)

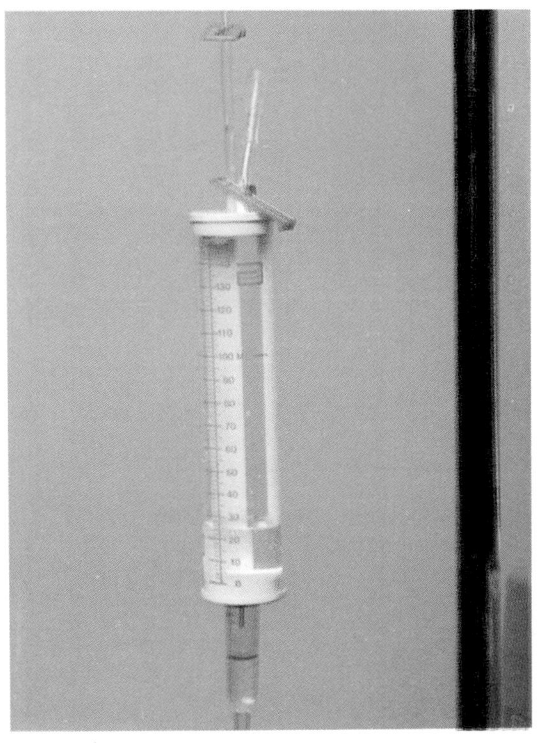

Figure 20-3. Volume control device. (From Elkin M, Perry A, Potter P: *Nursing interventions and clinical skills,* St Louis, 1996, Mosby.)

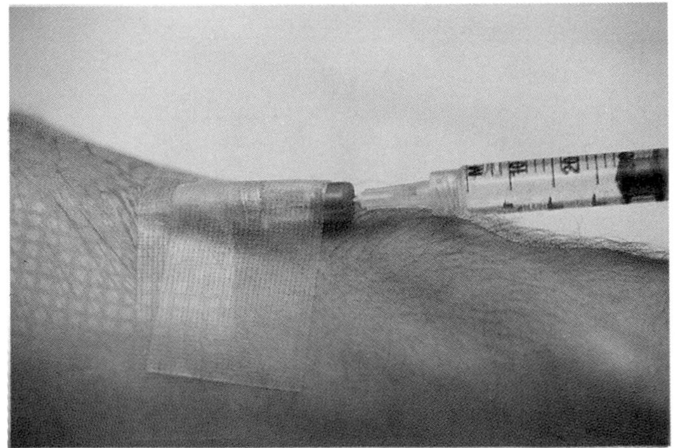

Figure 20-4. An example of an infusion indwelling port. (From Elkin M, Perry A, Potter P: *Nursing interventions and clinical skills,* St Louis, 1996, Mosby.)

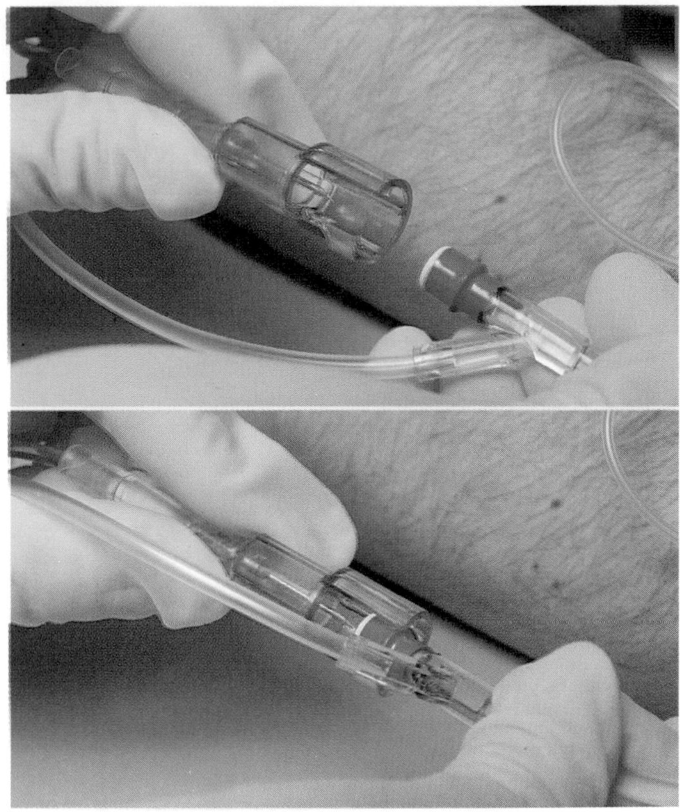

Figure 20-5. Needleless device; piggyback needle-lock device connected to injection port of main I.V. line. (From Potter P, Perry A: *Fundamentals of nursing,* ed 4, St Louis, 1996, Mosby.)

dilute forms of heparin), heparin is now used only on the initial insertion of the catheter. For subsequent flushings of the port, normal saline is used (1 to 2 mL, depending on institution policy). When medications are administered through the infusion port, the port must be flushed before and after medication is given. The letters used in most institutions to remember the technique for medication administration are S, I, S (saline, I.V. medications, saline). With early discharge and an increased number of home care clients discharged with infusion ports in place, it is imperative that clients be taught about the care of the infusion port.

Electronic Infusion Devices

There are several electronic infusion devices on the market today (Figure 20-6).

Electronic rate controllers. The rate of flow of the I.V. solution is maintained by a drop sensor that is connected to the tubing's drip chamber. The sensor monitors the flow rate (see Figure 20-10, *B* for an example of this).

Electronic volumetric pumps. These types of pumps infuse fluids into the vein under pressure and against resistance. The pumps are programmed to deliver a set amount of fluid per hr (Figure 20-6). There is a wide range of electronic pumps.

Syringe pumps. These are electronic devices that deliver medications or fluids by use of a syringe. The drug is measured in a syringe and attached to the special pump, and the medication is infused at the rate set (Figure 20-7).

Patient-controlled analgesia (PCA) devices. This form of pain management allows the client to self-administer I.V. analgesics. This is accomplished by the utilization of a computerized infuser pump that is attached to the I.V. line. The PCA pump is programmed to allow doses of

A

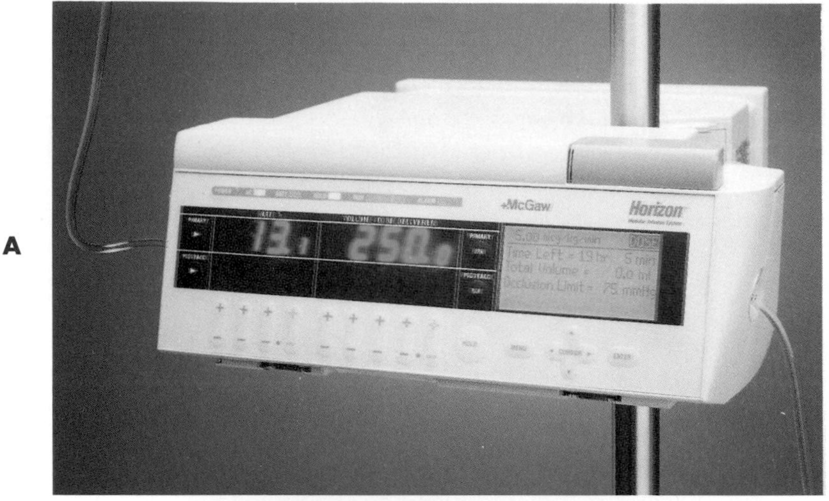

B

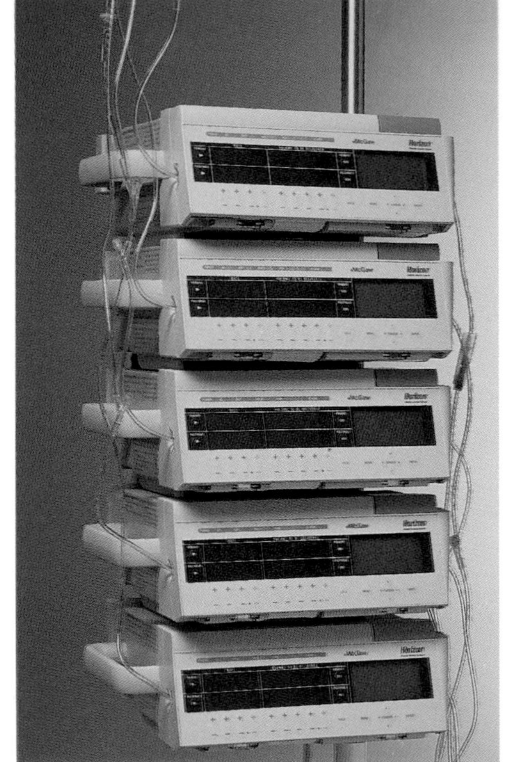

Figure 20-6. **A,** Single-channel unit. **B,** Multichannel unit. (Courtesy McGaw Inc, Irvine, Calif.)

Continued

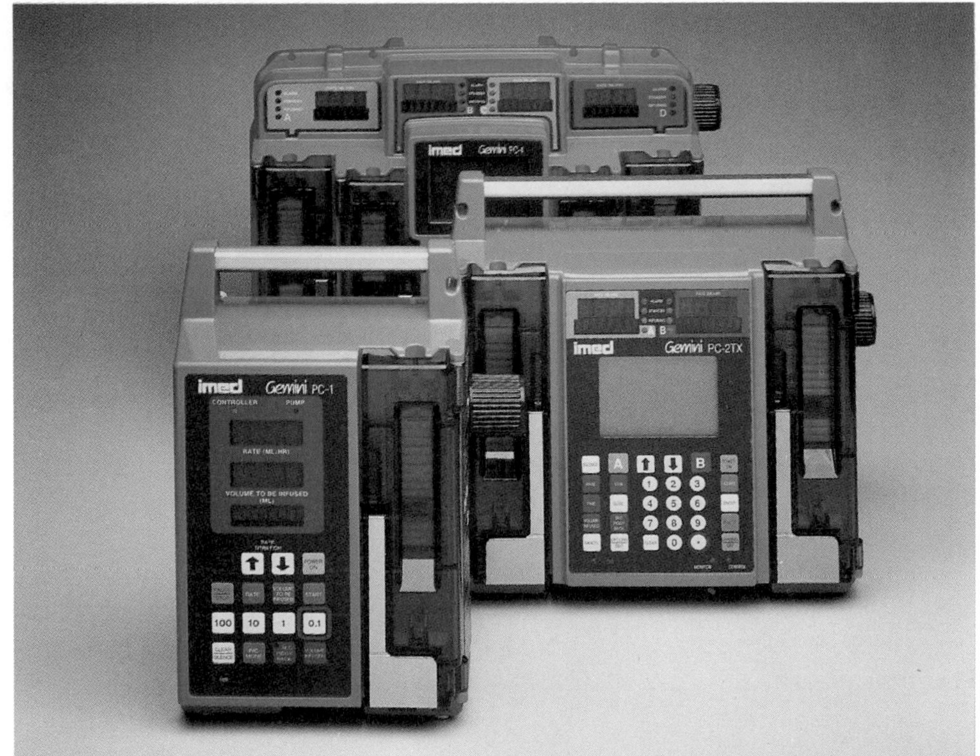

C

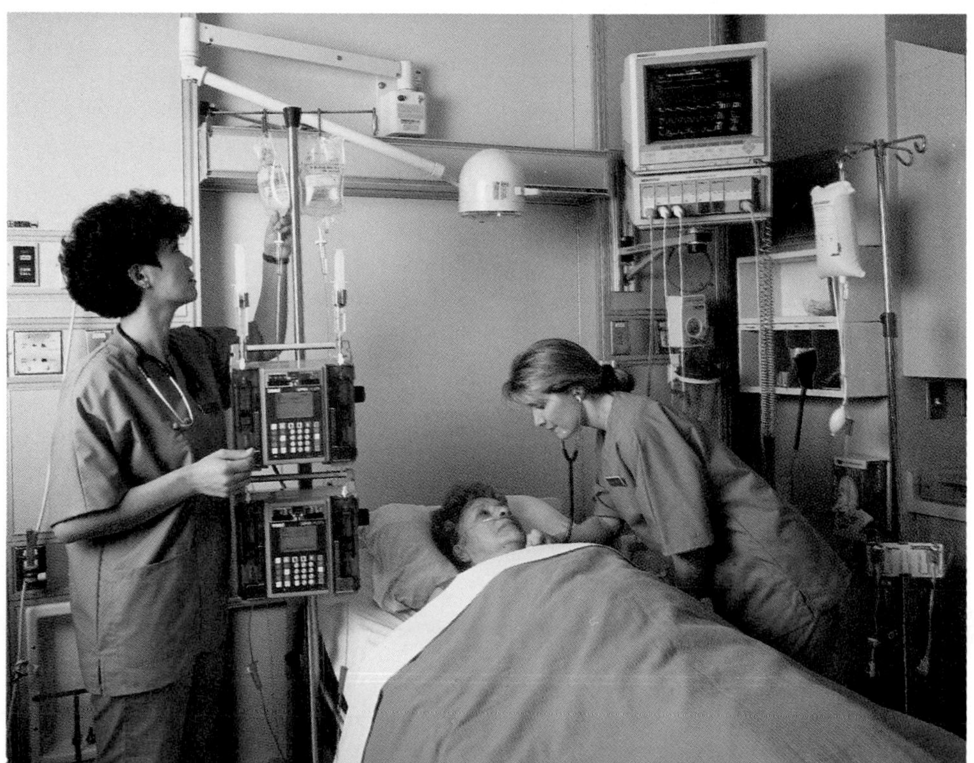

D

Figure 20-6. **C,** One-, two-, and four-channel units. (Courtesy IMED Corporation, San Diego.). **D,** Two-channel models being used on a patient in a critical care setting. (Courtesy IMED Corporation, San Diego.)

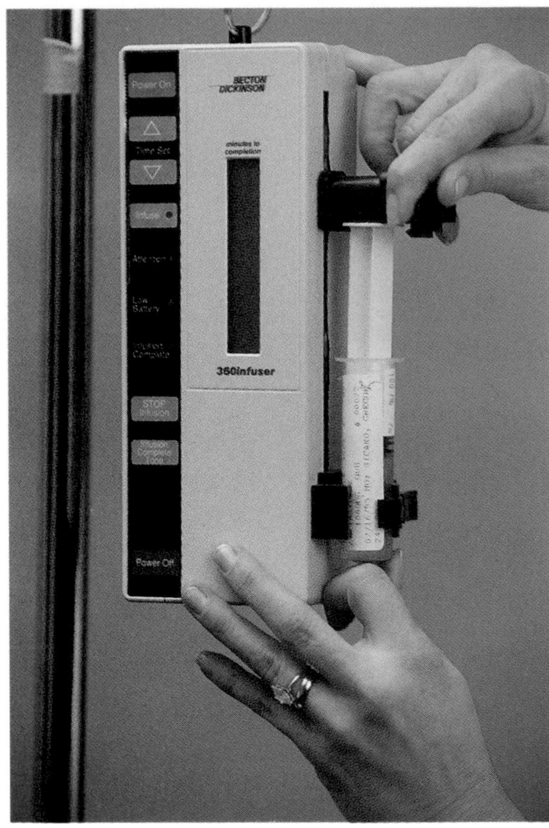

Figure 20-7. Pre-filled syringe being placed into mini-infusion pump. (From Elkin M, Perry A, Potter P: *Nursing interventions and clinical skills,* St Louis, 1996, Mosby.)

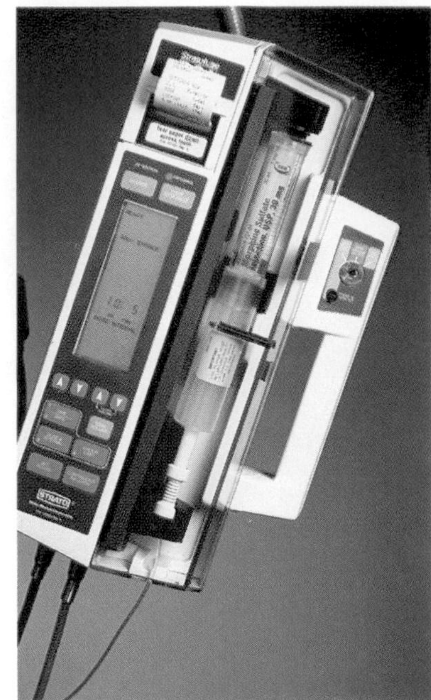

Figure 20-8. PCA pump. (From Potter P, Perry A: *Fundamentals of nursing,* ed 4, St Louis, 1996, Mosby.)

narcotics only within specific limits to prevent overdosage. The dose and frequency of administration are ordered by the doctor and set on the pump. The patient self-medicates by use of a control button. The pump also keeps a record of the number of times the client uses it. The display on the pump lets clients know when they are able to medicate themselves and when it is impossible to give themselves another dose. The pump therefore has what is called a lockout interval. This is an interval during which no medications are delivered. A drug commonly administered by PCA is morphine (30 mg morphine per 30 mL) (Figure 20-8). **Note: Regardless of the electronic device, clients need to be educated about them, the devices must be monitored to ascertain proper functioning, and the client must be monitored.**

I.V. Fluids

There are several types of I.V. fluids. The type of fluid used is individualized according to the client and the reason for its use. I.V. solutions come prepared in plastic bags or glass bottles ranging from 50 mL (bags only) to 1000 mL. When I.V. solutions are written in orders and charts, abbreviations are used. Abbreviations identify the solution, such as D for dextrose, and a number identifies the percentage of solution. Some common abbreviations are listed in Table 20-1.

I.V. fluids are charted on the I & O sheet; in some institutions they are also charted on the MAR. Figure 20-9 is a sample I & O charting record.

Table 20-1 Abbreviations for Common I.V. Solutions

NS	Normal saline 0.9%
$\frac{1}{2}$NS	Normal saline 0.45%
D5RL	Dextrose 5% with Ringer's lactate solution
D5W or 5% D/W	Dextrose 5% in water
RL or RLS	Ringer's lactate solution (electrolytes)
Isolytes	Electrolyte solutions
D5NS	Dextrose 5% in normal saline
D5 and $\frac{1}{2}$NS	Dextrose 5% in $\frac{1}{2}$ normal saline

From Brown M, Mulholland J: *Drug calculations: process and problems for clinical practice,* ed 5, St Louis, 1996, Mosby.

ST. BARNABAS HOSPITAL
BRONX, NEW YORK

DEPARTMENT OF NURSING

Client Addressograph

8 HR INTAKE AND OUTPUT RECORD

DATE: 8/17/96

INTAKE					OUTPUT				
TIME					TIME				
6A-2P	ORAL/TUBE FEEDING TYPE	AMOUNT	I.V. / BLOOD TYPE	AMOUNT	6A-2P	URINE (**CBI)	LIQUID STOOLS	EMESIS	DRAINAGE
7A			LIB* 1000cc 5%D/W	800cc	9A	400cc			
12p			IVPB 100cc	100cc	1p	500cc			
TOTAL				900cc	TOTAL	900cc			

Figure 20-9. Sample of charting I.V. fluids on ITO record. (Courtesy St. Barnabas Hospital, Bronx, New York.)

Calculating Percentage in I.V. Fluids

The amount of each ingredient in an I.V. fluid can be calculated; however, it is not necessary since the label on the I.V. solution indicates the amount of each ingredient. Calculation of the percentage of solutions was presented in the chapter dealing with percentages. As a refresher, remember that the percentage indicates the grams of solute per 100 mL of fluid.

Example: Calculate the amount of dextrose in 1000 mL of 5% dextrose and 0.45% normal saline (D5 and $\frac{1}{2}$NS). This is done by using ratio-proportion.

Percentage = g per 100 mL; therefore 5% = 5 g per 100 mL.

To calculate the percentage of dextrose:

$$5\text{ g} : 100\text{ mL} = x\text{ g} : 1000\text{ mL}$$

$$x = 50\text{ g dextrose}$$

To calculate the percentage of sodium chloride (NaCl) you would use a ratio-proportion as well.

$$0.9\text{ g} : 100\text{ mL} = x\text{ g} : 1000\text{ mL}$$

$$x = 9\text{ g NaCl}$$

I.V. medication protocols are often posted in the medication room of the institution to serve as a reference for nurses concerning specifics about usual medication dosage, dilution for I.V. administration, and compatibility, as well as specific observations that need to be made of a client during medication administration. **Always adhere to the protocol for administering I.V. drugs.**

I.V. Flow Rate Calculation

I.V. fluids are usually ordered on the basis of mL/hr. Example: 3000 mL/24 hr, 1000 mL in 8 hr. Small volumes of fluid are often used when the I.V. contains medications such as antibiotics. Rates for I.V. fluids are usually determined in gtt/mL.

I.V. flow rates are determined by the type of I.V. administration tubing. The drop size is regulated by the size of the tubing. (The larger the tubing, the larger the drops). The first step in calculating I.V. flow rates is to identify the type of tubing and its calibration. The calibration of the tubing is printed on each I.V. administration package.

I.V. Tubing

I.V. tubing has a drip chamber. The nurse determines the flow rate by adjusting the clamp and observing the drip chamber to count the drops per minute (Figure 20-10, *A*). The size of the drop depends on the type of I.V. tubing used. The calibration of I.V. tubing in gtt/mL is known as the *drop factor* and is indicated on the box in which the I.V. tubing is packaged. This calibration is necessary to calculate flow rates (Figure 20-11).

The two common types of tubing used to administer I.V. fluids are as follows:

Macrodrop tubing. This is the standard type of tubing used for general I.V. administration. This type of tubing delivers a certain number of gtt/mL according to the manufacturer. Macrodrop tubing delivers 10, 15, or 20 gtts equal to 1 mL. Macrodrops are large drops; therefore, large amounts of fluid are administered in macrodrops (Figure 20-11, *A*).

Microdrip tubing. Microdrip tubing delivers tiny drops, which can be inferred from *micro.* It is used when small amounts and more exact measurements are needed, for example, in pediatrics, for the elderly, and in critical care settings. Microdrip tubing delivers 60 gtt equal to 1 mL. Since there are 60 minutes in an hour, the number of microdrops per minute is equal to the number of mL/hr. For example, if clients are receiving 100 mL/hr, they are receiving 100 microdrops/min (Figure 20-11, *B*).

Points to Remember

- I.V. orders are written by the doctor.
- Several types of electronic pumps are available on the market. Familiarize yourself with the equipment before use.
- I.V. therapy can be continuous or intermittent.
- Follow the protocol for administration of I.V. medications.

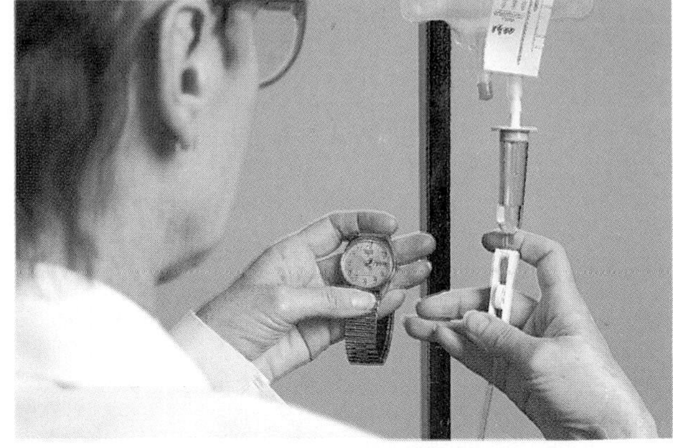

A

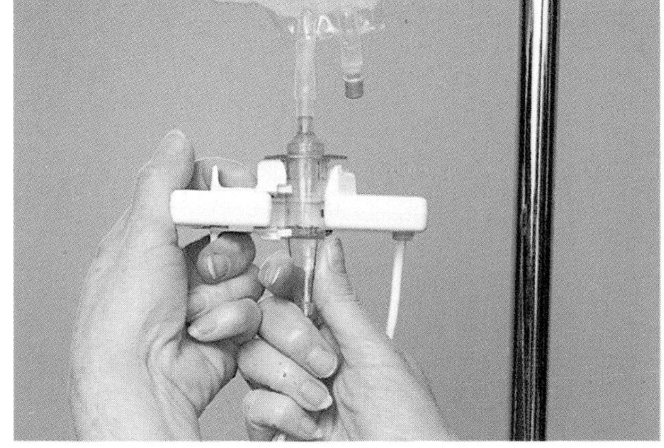

B

Figure 20-10. **A,** Observing the drip chamber to count drops per minute. **B,** Sensor (electronic eye) connected to drip chamber to regulate gtt. (From Potter P, Perry A: *Fundamentals of nursing,* ed 4, St Louis, 1997, Mosby.)

A

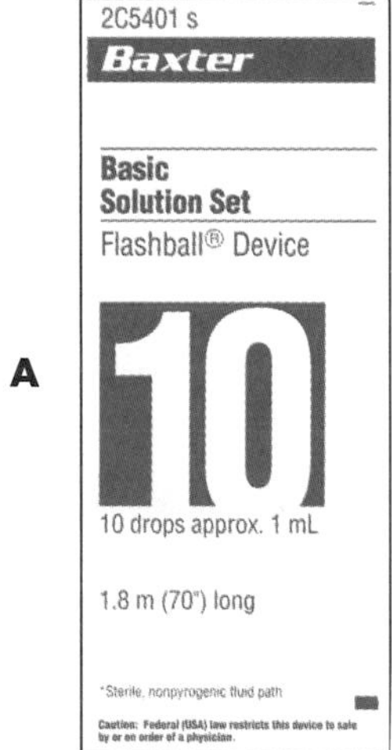

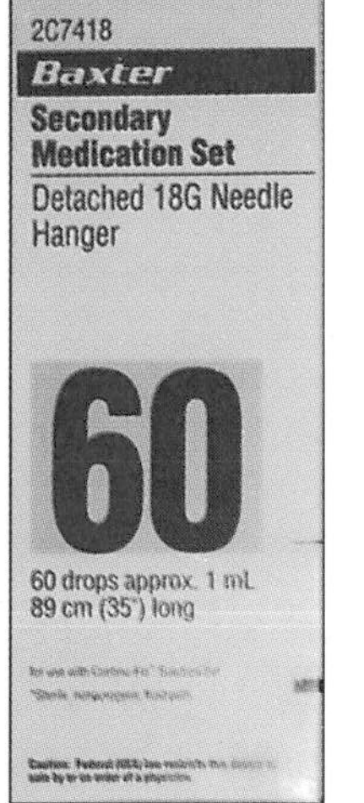

B

Figure 20-11. Types of I.V. administration sets. **A,** Macrodrop set with drop factor of 10. **B,** Microdrip set with drop factor of 60. (From Brown M, Mulholland J: *Drug calculations: process and problems for clinical practice,* ed 5, St Louis, 1996, Mosby.)

Formula Method for Calculating I.V. Flow Rate

To calculate the flow rate or rate at which an I.V. is to infuse, the nurse needs to know the following:

1. The volume or number of mL (cc) to infuse
2. The drop factor
3. The time element (minutes or hours)

This information is placed in the following formula:

Formula

$$\frac{V_1}{T_1} \times \frac{V_2}{T_2} = \text{gtt/min}$$

Note: Numbers have been placed in the formula for the purpose of explanation.

$$\frac{\text{Volume}}{\text{Time}} \times \frac{\text{Volume}}{\text{Time}} = \text{gtt/min}$$

Explanation of Formula

V_1 = Volume (the total number of mL [cc] to infuse)

T_1 = Time in hours (the number of hours the I.V. is to infuse)

V_2 = Drop factor of the tubing used (for example, 10 gtt = 1 mL; 60 gtt = 1 mL)

T_2 = Time in minutes (since there are 60 minutes in an hour, the number is always 60, unless the I.V. is to infuse for a time period less than an hour; then you can place the number of minutes in this position.)

Note: To place the number of minutes in the T_1 position, the number of minutes must be expressed in hours by dividing the number of minutes by 60. It is easier to place the number of minutes directly into the formula in the T_2 position to avoid extra calculation.

Before calculating, let's review some basic principles:

1. Drops per minute are always expressed in whole numbers. You cannot regulate something at a half of a drop. Since drops are expressed in whole numbers, principles of rounding off are applied, for example, 19.5 gtt = 20 gtt.
2. Carry division of the problem one decimal place to round to a whole number of drops.
3. Answers must be labeled. The label is usually drops per minute, unless otherwise specified.

Example: 100 gtt/min or 17 gtt/min

To reinforce the differences in gtt factor, the type of tubing is sometimes included as part of the label.

Example: 100 microgtt/min or 17 macrogtt/min

Let's look at a sample problem and the step-by-step method of using the formula to obtain the answer.

Example 1: The doctor orders an I.V. to infuse at 100 mL/hr. The drop factor is 10 gtt/mL. How many gtt/min should the I.V. infuse?

Solution:

1. Set up the problem, placing the information given in the correct position.

$$\frac{V_1}{T_1} \times \frac{V_2}{T_2} = \frac{100 \text{ mL}}{1 \text{ hr}} \times \frac{10 \text{ gtt/mL}}{60 \text{ min}}$$

2. Reduce where possible to make numbers smaller and easier to manage. Note: Labels are dropped when starting to perform mathematical steps.

$$\frac{100}{1} \times \frac{10}{60} = \frac{100}{1} \times \frac{1}{6} = \frac{100}{6}$$

3. Divide $\frac{100}{6}$ to obtain gtt/min.

   Carry division at least one decimal place and round off to the nearest whole number.

$$\frac{100}{6} = 16.6$$

Answer: 17 gtt/min; 17 macrogtt/min

To deliver 100 mL/hr, with a drop factor of 10 drops/mL, the I.V. rate should be adjusted to 17 drops/min. This answer can also be expressed with the type of tubing as part of the label, for example, 17 macrogtt/min.

Example 2: Administer an I.V. of 50 mL in 20 minutes using a microdrip set (60 gtt/mL).

Solution:

1. $50 \text{ mL} \times \frac{60 \text{ gtt/mL}}{20 \text{ (min)}}$

   Note: Here the 20 minutes is placed in the T_2 position because it represents the time in minutes. The time period is less than an hour. A 1 could also be placed under 50, not to denote 1 hr, but because 50/1 is the same as 50.

   OR

$$\frac{50 \text{ mL}}{1} \times \frac{60 \text{ gtt/mL}}{20 \text{ (min)}}$$

2. $50 \times \frac{3}{1}$ **OR** $\frac{50}{1} \times \frac{3}{1}$

3. Either way of setting the problem up gives 150 as an answer.

Answer: 150 gtt/min

To deliver 50 mL in 20 minutes with a drop factor of 60 drops/mL, the I.V. rate should be adjusted to 150 gtt/min.

This may sound like a lot; however, remember that the tubing used is a microdrip. This answer may be expressed as 150 microdrops/min.

The formula method may also be used to calculate gtt/min for a volume of fluid to be administered in more than 1 hr.

Example 3: 1000 mL dextrose 5% in water (D5W) to infuse in 8 hr. The drop factor is 10 gtt/mL. How many gtt/min should the I.V. be regulated at?

Solution:

$$\frac{1000 \text{ mL}}{8 \text{ hr}} \times \frac{10 \text{ gtt/mL}}{60 \text{ min}}$$

$$\frac{1000}{8} \times \frac{1}{6} = \frac{1000}{48} = 20.8 \text{ or } 21 \text{ drops/min}$$

Another approach to doing this is to first find the mL per hour. Dividing the total volume to be infused by the number of hours equals mL/hr:

$$\frac{V_1}{T_1} = \frac{\text{total volume}}{\text{time}} = \text{mL/hr}$$

$$\frac{1000 \text{ mL}}{8 \text{ hr}} = 125 \text{ mL/hr}$$

After determining the mL/hr, place it into the formula and proceed to calculate gtt/min. This lessens the size of the numbers and makes math calculations easier.

$$\frac{125 \text{ mL/hr}}{1} \times \frac{10 \text{ gtt/mL}}{60 \text{ min}}$$

$$\frac{125}{1} \times \frac{1}{6} = \frac{125}{6} = 20.8$$

Answer: 21 gtt/min; 21 macrogtt/min

As you can see, the formula method can be used for calculating flow rates for less than an hour or for several hours.

Practice Problems (p. 386)

Calculate the flow rate in gtt/min.

1. Administer I.V. at 75 mL/hr. The drop factor is 10 gtt/mL. ______
2. Administer 30 mL/hr. The drop factor is a microdrip. ______
3. Administer 125 mL/hr. The drop factor is 15 gtt/mL. ______
4. Administer 1000 mL in 6 hr. The drop factor is 15 gtt/mL. ______
5. An I.V. medication with a volume of 60 mL is to be administered in 45 minutes using a microdrip set. ______
6. 1000 mL of Ringer's lactate solution (RL) is to infuse in 16 hr. The drop factor is 15 gtt/mL. ______
7. Infuse 150 mL of D5W in 2 hr. The drop factor is 20 gtt/mL. ______
8. Administer 3,000 mL D5 and $\frac{1}{2}$NS in 24 hr. The drop factor is 10 gtt/mL. ______
9. Infuse 2,000 mL D5W in 12 hr. The drop factor is 15 gtt/mL. ______
10. Administer 60 mL of I.V. medication in 30 minutes. The drop factor is a microdrip. ______

Calculating I.V. Flow Rates When Several Solutions Are Ordered

Doctors often write I.V. orders for different amounts or types of fluid to be given in a certain time period. These orders are frequently written for a 24-hr interval and usually are split over three shifts. I.V. solutions may have medications added such as potassium chloride or multivitamins.

Steps to calculating:

1. Add up the total amount of fluid.
2. Proceed as with other I.V. problem calculations.

Note: When medications such as potassium chloride and vitamins are added to I.V. solutions, they are generally not considered in the total volume.

Example 1: The doctor orders the following I.V.s for 24 hours. The drop factor is 15 gtt/mL.

1000 mL D5W with ⓒ 10 mEq potassium chloride (KCl)

500 mL dextrose 5% in normal saline (D5NS) $\bar{c}$ 1 ampule multivitamin (MVI)

500 mL D5W

Solution:

1. Add up total volume.
2. Place information given into formula.
3. Proceed to calculate.

$$\frac{V_1}{T_1} \times \frac{V_2}{T_2} = \frac{2{,}000 \text{ mL}}{24 \text{ hr}} \times \frac{15 \text{ gtt/mL}}{60 \text{ min}}$$

$$\frac{500}{6} \times \frac{1}{4} = \frac{500}{24} = 20.8$$

Answer: 21 gtt/min; 21 macrogtt/min

Remember, this could also have been done by finding the mL/hr first and making the numbers smaller and easier to calculate. Calculating I.V. flow rate when there is more than one I.V. with the hourly rate indicated eliminates the step of adding up the solutions. The hourly rate becomes the total volume.

Example 2: The doctor orders the following I.V.s. The drop factor is 10 gtt/mL to infuse at 150 mL/hr.

1000 mL D5W

1000 mL normal saline (NS)

500 mL D5 and 1/2 NS

The hourly rate is 150 mL/hr. Calculation is done based on this:

$$\frac{150\text{ mL}}{1\text{ hr}} \times \frac{10\text{ gtt/mL}}{60\text{ min}} =$$

$$\frac{150}{1} \times \frac{1}{6} = \frac{150}{6}$$

Answer: 25 gtt/min; 25 macrogtt/min

Practice Problems (pp. 386-387)

Calculate the flow rate in gtt/min.

11. Doctor's order: Dextrose 5% with Ringer's lactate solution (D5RL) $\bar{c}$ 20 U Pitocin × 2 L at 125 mL/hr. The drop factor is 15 gtt/mL. ________

12. Doctor's order: For 16 hr the drop factor is 10 gtt/mL. ________

    a) D5W 500 mL $\bar{c}$ 10 mEq KCl ________

    b) D5W 1000 mL ________

    c) D5W 1000 mL $\bar{c}$ 1 ampule MVI ________

13. Doctor's order: 1000 mL D5NS × 3 L at 100 mL/hr. The drop factor is a microdrip. ________

14. Doctor's order: D5W 1000 mL + 20 mEq KCl × 2 L. For 10 hr the drop factor is 15 gtt/mL. ________

I.V. Medications

As previously discussed in the section on calculating I.V. flow rates, when several solutions are ordered, medications can be added directly to the I.V. solution.

Medications such as antibiotics can also be given by adding a secondary container of solution that contains the medication. The administration of medication by attaching it to a port on the primary line is referred to as piggyback.

The volume of the piggyback container is usually 50 to 100 mL and should infuse over 20, 30, or 60 minutes, depending on the type and amount of medication added. The same formula used to calculate I.V. infusion times is used to calculate the gtt/min.

Sample Problem:

The doctor ordered Keflin 2 g IVPB (piggyback) over 30 minutes. The Keflin is placed in 100 mL of fluid after it is dissolved. The drop factor is 15 gtt/mL. How many gtt/min should the I.V. be regulated at?

To calculate: The 100 mL of fluid the medication is placed in is used as the volume.

$$\frac{100\text{ mL}}{1} \times \frac{15\text{ gtt/mL}}{30\text{ min}}$$

$$\frac{100}{1} \times \frac{1}{2} = \frac{100}{2} = 50$$

The I.V. would be regulated at 50 gtt/min; 50 macrogtt/min

As shown earlier in the chapter, the smaller bag (piggyback) is hung higher than the larger (primary) bag. Since infusion flow is controlled by gravity, the primary bag will resume infusion after the piggyback is empty. The drops per minute will then have to be reset to the correct amount calculated for the primary I.V.

Remember: Electronic pumps can also be used for the administration of I.V. fluids and I.V. medications. The pumps are set to deliver a specific rate of flow per hour. The mechanisms of how the pump works will depend on the manufacturer. Special tubing is usually required for the pump, and calculations are based on that.

Practice Problems (pp. 387-388)

Calculate the gtt/min for the following medications being administered IVPB. Use the labels where provided.

15. Mezlocillin 3 g IVPB in 130 mL NS over 1 hr. The drop factor is 15 gtt/mL. ______________

16. Erythromycin 200 mg in 250 mL D5W to infuse over 1 hr. The I.V. tubing delivers 10 gtt/mL. ______________

17. Ampicillin 1g in 50 mL D5W over 45 minutes. The drop factor is 10 gtt/mL. ______________

18. Clindamycin 900 mg in 75 mL D5W over 30 minutes. The drop factor is 10 gtt/mL. ______________

19. Doctor's Order: Tagamet 300 mg IVPB q8hr. The medication has been added to 50 mL D5W to infuse over 30 minutes. The administration set delivers 10 gtt/mL. ______________

Tagamet HCl Injection
2 mL/300mg

20. Doctor's Order: Vancomycin 500 mg IVPB q24hr. The vancomycin reconstituted provides 50 mg/mL. The medication is placed in 100 mL of D5W to infuse over 60 minutes. The administration set delivers 15 gtt/mL. ______________

    a) How many mL of medication must be added to the solution? ______________

    b) Calculate the gtt/min the I.V. should infuse at. ______________

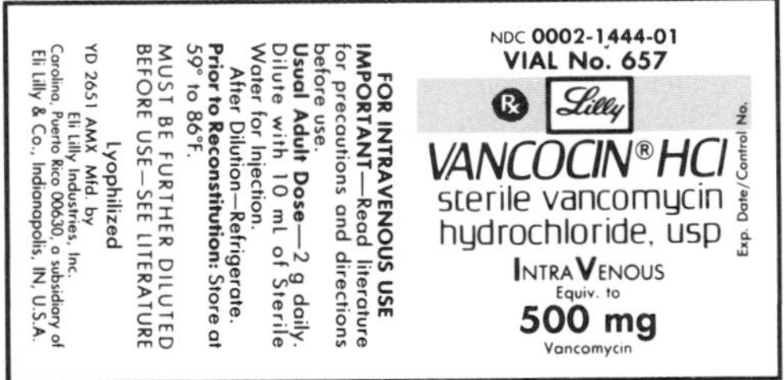

21. Doctor's Order: Fungizone (amphotericin B) 20 mg I.V. Soluset (IVSS) in 300 mL D5W over 6 hr. The reconstituted material contains 50 mg/10 mL. The administration set delivers 60 gtt/mL.

1 vial NDC 0003-0437-30
NSN 6505-01-084-9453
50 mg
FUNGIZONE®
INTRAVENOUS
Amphotericin B
for Injection USP
FOR INTRAVENOUS INFUSION IN HOSPITALS ONLY
Caution: Federal law prohibits dispensing without prescription
Read all sides

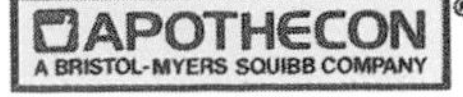

    a) How many mL will you add to the I.V. solution? ______________

    b) How many gtt/min should the I.V. infuse at? ______________

22. Doctor's Order: Septra 300 mg in 300 mL D5W over 1 hr q6h. The administration set delivers 10 gtt/mL.

    Available: Septra in 20-mL vial labeled 320 mg trimethoprim (16 mg/mL) and 1,600 mg sulfamethoxazole (80 mg/mL). (Calculate the dose using trimethoprim.)

    a) How many mL of medication will be added to the I.V.? (Round answer to nearest tenth.) __________

    b) Calculate the gtt/min the I.V. should infuse at. __________

23. Doctor's Order: Retrovir 100 mg I.V. q4h over 1 hr. The medication is placed in 100 mL of D5W. The administration set delivers 10 gtt/mL. __________

20 mL Single-Use Vial NDC 0173-0107-93
RETROVIR® (zidovudine) I.V. INFUSION Sterile
Each mL contains 10 mg zidovudine
FOR INTRAVENOUS INFUSION ONLY. MUST BE DILUTED FOR ADMINISTRATION.
Dilute with 5% Dextrose Injection to a concentration no greater than 4 mg/mL. Contains no preservative. The vehicle contains Water for Injection, qs. Hydrochloric acid and/or sodium hydroxide may have been added to adjust pH.
For indications, dosage, precautions, etc., see accompanying package insert.
Store at 15° to 25°C (59° to 77°F) and protect from light.
CAUTION: Federal law prohibits dispensing without prescription.
Glaxo Wellcome Inc.
Research Triangle Park, NC 27709 Made in U.S.A. Rev. 3/96 U.S. Patent Nos. 4818538 (Product Patent); 4724232, 4833130, and 4837208 (Use Patents)
587152

Determining the Amount of Drug in a Specific Amount of Solution

Sometimes medications are added to I.V. solutions, and the doctor orders a certain amount of the drug to be given in a certain time period.

Example 1: The doctor may order 20 mEq of potassium to be placed in 1000 mL of fluid to be administered at a rate of 2 mEq of potassium per hour. The flow rate (gtt/min) can be determined using the same formula as for other I.V.s, but first the volume to be infused must be calculated by use of ratio-proportion.

Solution:

Step 1: Calculate the number of mL of solution needed to deliver 2 mEq of potassium chloride.

What doctor ordered ↓ (points to 2 mEq)

$$20 \text{ mEq} : 1000 \text{ mL} = 2 \text{ mEq} : x \text{ mL}$$

↑ Total amount of drug in volume of solution (20 mEq : 1000 mL) ↑ Desired volume of solution (x mL)

$$20 : 1000 = 2 : x$$

$$20x = 1000 \times 2$$

$$20x = 2{,}000$$

$$x = \frac{2{,}000}{20}$$

$$x = 100 \text{ mL}$$

Therefore 100 mL of fluid would be needed to administer 2 mEq of potassium chloride per hour.

Step 2: Determine the rate of flow by substituting this information into the formula if 100 mL of solution (containing 2 mEq of potassium chloride) is to be administered over 1 hr using 15 gtt = 1 mL. The rate of flow is determined by the following:

$$\frac{100 \text{ mL}}{1 \text{ hr}} \times \frac{15 \text{ gtt/mL}}{60 \text{ min}}$$

$$\frac{100}{1} \times \frac{1}{4} = \frac{100}{4} =$$

25 gtt/min; 25 macrogtt/min

25 gtt/min would deliver 2 mEq of potassium chloride each hour from this solution.

Example 2: The doctor orders 100 U of regular insulin to be added to 500 mL of 0.45% saline (1/2 NS) to infuse at 10 U per hour. The I.V. flow rate should be how many mL per hour?

Solution:

Step 1: Set up a proportion with the known on one side and the unknown on the other.

$$100 \text{ U} : 500 \text{ mL} = 10 \text{ U} : x$$

$$100x = 500 \times 10$$

$$100x = 5{,}000$$

$$x = \frac{5{,}000}{100}$$

$$x = 50 \text{ mL/hr}$$

For the client to receive 10 U of insulin per hour, 50 mL/hr must be administered.

Step 2: Determine the flow rate in gtt/min using 20 gtt = 1 mL.

$$\frac{50 \text{ mL}}{1 \text{ hr}} \times \frac{20 \text{ gtt/mL}}{60 \text{ min}} = \frac{50}{3} = 16.6 =$$

17 gtt/min; 17 macrogtt/min

17 gtt/min would deliver 10 U of insulin per hour.

Practice Problems (p.388)

Solve the following problems using the steps indicated.

24. 15 mEq of potassium chloride is added to 1000 mL of D5 and $\frac{1}{2}$NS to be administered at a rate of 4 mEq/hr.

    a) How many mL of solution are needed to administer 4 mEq/hr? __________

    b) The administration set delivers 10 gtt/mL; calculate the gtt/min to deliver 4 mEq/hr. __________

25. Doctor's Order: 10 U of regular insulin per hour. 50 U of insulin is placed in 250 mL NS.

    a) How many mL/hr should the I.V. infuse at? __________

    b) Calculate the gtt/min if the administration set delivers 15 gtt/mL. __________

26. Doctor's Order: 15 U of regular insulin per hour. 40 U of insulin is placed in 250 mL of NS.

    a) How many mL/hr should the I.V. infuse at? __________

    b) Calculate the gtt/min if the administration set delivers 60 gtt/mL. __________

Determining Infusion Times and Volumes

You may need to calculate the following:

a) Time in hours—How long it will take a certain amount of fluid to infuse or how long it may last

b) Volume—The total number of mL a client will receive in a certain time period

These unknown elements can be determined by use of the same formula and simple mathematics.

Remember the formula:

$$\frac{\text{Volume } V_1}{\text{Time } T_1} \times \frac{V_2}{T_2} = \text{gtt/min}$$

Steps to Calculating a Problem with an Unknown

1. Take information given in the problem and place it in the formula.
2. Place an x in the formula in the position of the unknown (for example, Volume V_1 position or in T_1 position [time in hours]).
3. Obtain an algebraic equation so that you can solve for x.
4. Solve the equation.
5. Label the answer in hours or mL for volume.

Sample Problem

An I.V. is regulated at 20 microgtt/min. How many hours will it take for 100 mL to infuse?

Note: If it is regulated at 20 microdrops, then the drip factor or apparatus used was a microdrip. You cannot convert macrodrip into a microdrip and vice versa.

Note: In the sample problem, you are being asked the number of hours, or T_1, so therefore when placing the problem into the formula, an x will go in the T_1 position; 60 is in the V_2 position because if regulated at 20 microgtt/min; a microdrip set was used.

Problem Set up in Formula

1. $\frac{V_1}{T_1} \times \frac{V_2}{T_2} = \frac{100 \text{ mL}}{x \text{ hr}} \times \frac{60 \text{ gtt/mL}}{60 \text{ min}} =$

   20 gtt/min; 20 microgtt/min

2. Reduce by cancellation of the fraction 60/60 and get 1.

$$\frac{100}{x} \times \frac{1}{1} = 20$$

3. Obtain an algebraic equation. (You must multiply so you can get rid of the times sign [×].)

a) $\frac{100}{x} \times 1 = 20$

b) $\frac{100}{x} = 20$ (after multiplication)

4. Solve for x by cross multiplying. Now you have the equals sign in between, which is necessary to solve for an unknown.

$$\frac{100}{x} = 20$$

(Note: Placing 20 over 1 doesn't alter value.)

OR

$$\frac{100}{x} = \frac{20}{1}$$

$$20x = 100$$

$$x = 5 \text{ hr}$$

Note: Label is hours since that's what you were asked.

When calculating time intervals and the time or the answer comes out in hours and minutes, express the entire time in hours. For example 1 hour and 30 minutes = 1.5 hr or 1 1/2 hr; 1 1/2 hr is the preferred term.

When calculating volume, proceed with the problem in the same way as calculating time interval except x is placed in a different position (V_1).

Sample Problem

An I.V. is regulated at 17 macrogtt/min. The drop factor is 15 gtt/mL. How much fluid volume in mL will the client receive in 8 hr?

Problem Set up in Formula

1. $\frac{V_1}{T_1} \times \frac{V_2}{T_2} = \frac{x \text{ mL}}{8 \text{ hr}} \times \frac{15 \text{ gtt/mL}}{60 \text{ min}} =$

   17 microgtt/min; 17 gtt/min

2. Reduce by cancellation of the fraction 15/60 and get 1/4.

$$\frac{x}{8} \times \frac{1}{4} = 17$$

3. Multiply to obtain equation and get rid of times sign.

$$\frac{x}{32} = 17$$

4. $x = 32 \times 17$

Answer: 544 mL

Note: Label on this answer is mL.

Some of the problems illustrated in calculating an unknown may be solved without the formula; however, using the formula is recommended.

Practice Problems (p. 388)

Solve the following problems as indicated. Express time in hours.

27. You find that there is 150 mL of fluid left in an I.V. The I.V. is infusing at 60 microgtt/min. How long will the fluid last? ________

28. An I.V. is infusing at 35 gtt/min. The administration equivalency is 15 gtt/mL. How many mL of fluid will the client receive in 5 hr? ________

29. You find that there is 180 mL of fluid left in an I.V. that is infusing at 45 gtt/min. The drop factor is 15 gtt/mL. How many hours will the fluid last? ________

30. An I.V. is infusing at 45 gtt/min. The drop factor is 15 gtt/mL. How many mL will the client receive in 8 hr? __________

31. You find there is 90 mL of fluid left in an I.V. The flow rate is 60 gtt/min. How long will the fluid last? __________

Recalculating an I.V. Flow Rate

Flow rates on I.V.s change when a client stands, sits, or is repositioned in bed. Therefore nurses must frequently check the flow rates. I.V.s generally are labeled with a start and finish time, as well as markings with specific time periods. Sometimes I.V.s infuse ahead of or behind schedule if not monitored closely. When this happens, the I.V. flow rate must be recalculated. To recalculate the flow rate the nurse uses the volume remaining and time remaining.

> **The recalculated flow rate should not vary from the original rate by more than 25%. It is recommended that if the recalculated rate varies more than 25% from the original, the doctor should be notified. The order may have to be revised.**

Example: An I.V. of 1000 mL was to infuse in 8 hr at 31 gtt/min (31 macrogtt/min). The drop factor is 15 gtt/mL. After 4 hr you notice 700 mL of fluid left in the I.V. Recalculate the flow rate for the remaining solution.

Solution:

Time remaining = 4 hr

Volume of solution remaining = 700 mL

$$\frac{700 \text{ ml}}{4 \text{ hr}} \times \frac{15 \text{ gtt/mL}}{60 \text{ min}}$$

$$\frac{700}{4} \times \frac{1}{4} = \frac{700}{16} = 44 \text{ gtt/min; } 44 \text{ macrogtt/min}$$

In this situation the flow rate has to be increased from 31 gtt/min to 44 gtt/min, which is more than 25% of the original. Always assess the client first to determine the client's ability to tolerate an increase in fluid. In addition to assessment of the client's status, the doctor should be notified. This same method can be used if an I.V. is ahead of schedule. An alternate to doing this problem without first calculating mL/hr would be to use the total amount.

Example of I.V. Ahead:

An I.V. of 1000 mL D5W is to infuse from 8 AM to 4 PM (8 hr). The drop factor is 10 gtt/mL. The rate is set at 20 gtt/min (20 macrogtt/min). In 5 hr you notice 700 mL has infused. Recalculate the flow rate for the remaining solution.

Solution:

Time remaining = 3 hr

Volume of solution remaining = 300 mL

$$\frac{300 \text{ mL}}{3 \text{ hr}} \times \frac{10 \text{ gtt/mL}}{60 \text{ min}}$$

$$\frac{300}{3} \times \frac{1}{6} = 16.6$$

In this situation the flow rate has to be decreased from 20 gtt/min (20 macrogtt/min) to 17 gtt/min (17 macrogtt/min), but this is not a change greater than 25% of the original. Although the I.V. is ahead of schedule, it also requires assessment of the client's ability to tolerate the change. The doctor may need to be notified.

Practice Problems (p. 389)

32. An I.V. of 500 mL was ordered to infuse in 8 hr at the rate of 16 gtt/min (16 macrogtt/min). The drip factor is 15 gtt/mL. After 5 hr you find 250 mL of fluid left. Recalculate the flow rate in gtt/min. __________

33. 250 mL of I.V. fluid was to infuse in 3 hr using 15 gtt/mL. With 1 1/2 hr remaining, you find 200 mL left. Recalculate the flow rate in gtt/min. __________

Calculating Total Infusion Times

Despite the fact that the I.V. flow rate is ordered by the doctor, **the nurse needs to be able to determine the number of hours that an I.V. solution takes to infuse.** When the nurse calculates the total time for a certain volume of solution to infuse I.V., this is referred to as **determining total infusion time.** To calculate infusion time it is necessary for the nurse to have knowledge of the following:

a) Amount (volume) to infuse
b) Drip rate (gtt/mL)
c) Set calibration

Knowing the length of time for an infusion helps the nurse in monitoring I.V. therapy, and preparing for the hanging of a new solution as the one infusing is being completed. Determining infusion times helps to avoid such things as a line clotting off due to not knowing when an I.V. was to be completed.

Calculating Infusion Time

This is determined by taking the total number of mL to infuse and dividing it by number of mL/hr solution is infusing at.

Formula

$$\frac{\text{Total number of mL to infuse}}{\text{mL/hr infusing at}} = \text{total infusion time}$$

Example 1: Calculate the infusion time for an I.V. of 1000 mL D5W that is infusing at a rate of 125 mL/hr.

1000 mL (total number of mL to infuse)

125 mL/hr (mL/hr to infuse)

$$\frac{1000}{125} = 1000 \div 25 = 8 \text{ hr}$$

Infusion time = 8 hr

Example 2: 1000 mL of D5 and $\frac{1}{2}$ NS is ordered to infuse at 150 mL/hr. Calculate the infusion time to the nearest hundredth.

$$\frac{1000 \text{ mL}}{150 \text{ mL/hr}} = 6.66$$

Fractions of hours can be changed to minutes: 6 represents the total number of hours; 0.66 represents a fraction of an hour and can be converted to minutes. This is done by multiplying 0.66 by 60 and then rounding off to the nearest whole number.

$$0.66 \times 60 = 39.6 = 40$$

Infusion time = 6 hr and 40 minutes

Once infusion time has been calculated, the nurse can use this information to determine the time an I.V. would be completed. Using Example 2 this would be determined as follows: add the calculated infusion time to the time the infusion was started. If the I.V. in Example 2 was hung at 7:00 AM, add the 6 hr and 40 minutes to that time. The I.V. would be completed at 1:40 PM.

Explanation of Continuous Infusion Administration Record

This form is used to chart continuous I.V. therapy that a client is receiving. I.V. solutions that contain medications and solution without medications are charted on this record. Medications that are administered intermittently by piggyback are charted on other medication sheets according to the order (example: standing medication sheet, p.r.n., or single, stat medication record). Figure 20-12 illustrates charting of I.V. therapy at one institution. The nurse uses arrows and checks on the record. Example: ↑ indicates that I.V. therapy was hung, ↓ indicates that the I.V. was taken down, ✓ indicates the nurse checked the I.V. therapy.

Practice Problems (p. 389)

34. An I.V. of 500 mL NS is to infuse at 60 mL/hr.

    a) Determine the infusion time. __________

    b) The I.V. was started at 10:00 PM. When would the I.V. totally infuse? __________

35. An I.V. of 250 mL D5W is to infuse at 80 mL/hr.

    a) Determine the infusion time. __________

    b) The I.V. was started at 2:00 AM. When would the I.V. totally infuse? __________

WEILER HOSPITAL
BRONX, NEW YORK 10461

CONTINUOUS INFUSION ADMINISTRATION RECORD

ALLERGY: Codeine ☐ NONE

MEDICATION: D5 R/L c̄ 20U Pitocin x2L

DOSE / ROUTE: IV

FREQUENCY / DURATION:

SPECIAL INSTRUCTIONS: 125cc/hr

PRACTITIONER'S SIGNATURE: S. Smith MD DATE/TIME: 5/10/96 4:00 A.M.

M.D. COUNTER SIGNATURE: DATE/TIME: A.M. P.M.

② NOTED BY: Deborah Morris RN DATE/TIME: 5/10/96 4:15 A.M.

DATE 5/10/96	DATE	DATE
TIME/INIT.	TIME/INIT.	TIME/INIT.
4:30 A ↑ #1 DM		
7:00 A ✓ DM		
12:30 P ↓ DM		

Figure 20-12. Continuous infusion administration record. (Courtesy Weiler Hospital, Bronx, New York.)

36. 1000 mL of D5W is to infuse at 40 mL/hr.

   a) Determine the infusion time. ____________

   b) The I.V. was started at 2:10 PM on August 26. When would the I.V. totally infuse? ____________

Calculating Infusion Time When mL/hr Is Not Indicated

There are situations where the doctor may order the I.V. solution and not indicate mL/hr. The only information may be the total number of mL to infuse, the flow rate (gtt/min) of the I.V., and the number of gtt/mL that the tubing delivers. In this situation, before calculating the infusion time, the following must be done:

1. Convert gtt/min to mL/min.
2. Convert mL/min to mL/hr to determine the mL/hr.

After completing these steps, you are ready to calculate the infusion time for the I.V. using the same formula: $\frac{\text{Total number of mL to infuse}}{\text{mL/hr infusing at}}$

Example 1: A client is receiving 1000 mL of RL. The I.V. is infusing at 21 macrogtt/min (20 gtt/min). The administration set delivers 10 gtt/mL. Calculate the infusion time.

Step 1: Use a ratio-proportion stated in any format as discussed in previous chapters to change gtt/min to mL/min.

$$10 \text{ gtt} : 1 \text{ mL} = 21 \text{ gtt} : x \text{ mL}$$

$$10x = 21$$

$$x = 21 \div 10 = 2.1 \text{ mL/min}$$

Step 2: Convert mL/min to mL/hr

$$2.1 \text{ mL/min} \times (60 \text{ min}) = 126 \text{ mL/hr}$$

Step 3: Determine infusion time as already shown.

a) $\frac{1000 \text{ mL}}{126 \text{ mL/hr}} = 7.93 \text{ hr}$

b) $0.93 \times 60 = 55.8 = 56$ minutes

Infusion time = 7 hr and 56 minutes

Note: To determine the time the infusion would be completed you would add the infusion time to the time the I.V. was started.

Practice Problems (p. 389)

37. Determine the infusion time for a client receiving 1000 mL D5W at 25 microgtt/min. The administration set is a microdrip. ____________

38. A client is receiving 250 mL of NS at 17 macrogtt/min. The administration set delivers 15 gtt/mL. Determine the infusion time. ____________

39. A client is receiving 1000 mL D5W. The I.V. is infusing at 30 macrogtt/min. The administration set delivers 20 gtt/mL. Determine the infusion time. ____________

Labeling Solution Bags

The markings on I.V. solution bags are not as precise as, for example, those on a syringe. Most I.V. bags are marked in increments of 50 to 100 mL. After calculating the amount of solution to infuse in 1 hr, the nurse may mark the bag to indicate where the level of fluid should be at each hour. Marking the I.V. bag allows the nurse to check that the fluid is infusing on time. Many institutions have commercially prepared labels for this purpose. In institutions where the commercially prepared labels are not available, regular white surgical tape may be attached to the side of the bag to serve the same purpose (Figure 20-13 shows an I.V. with tape for visualizing the amount infused each hour). The tape should indicate the start and finish time.

I.V. Therapy and Children

Administration of I.V. fluids to children is very specific due to their physiological development and the delicate nature of their veins. Microdrip sets are used for infants and small children; elec-

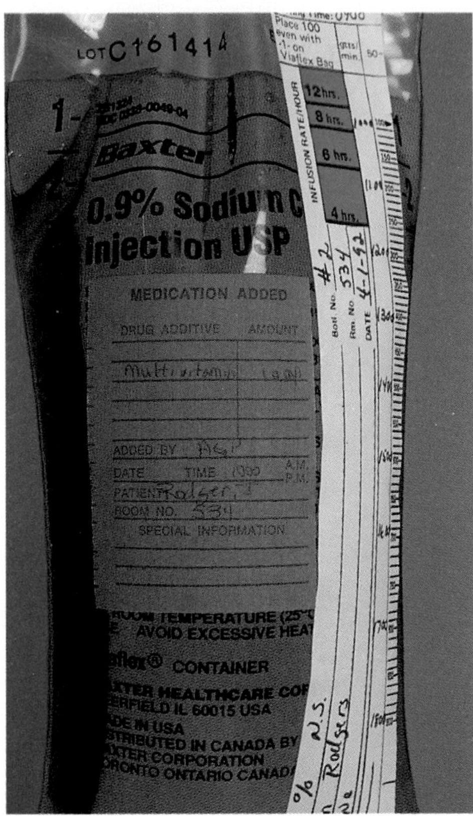

Figure 20-13. I.V. bag with medicine tape. (From Elkin M, Perry A, Potter P: *Nursing interventions and clinical skills,* St Louis, 1996, Mosby.)

tronic devices to control the rate of delivery are also used. For intermittent medication administration several methods of delivery are used, including the following:

Small-volume I.V. bags—These may be used if the child has a primary I.V. line in place. A secondary tubing set is attached to a small-volume I.V. bag and the piggyback method is used.

Calibrated burettes—These are often referred to by their trade names: Buretrol, Volutrol, or Soluset. (Figure 20-14 shows a typical system that consists of a calibrated chamber that can hold a capacity of 100 to 150 mL of fluid.) The burette is calibrated in small increments that allow accuracy and exact measurements of small volume.

Regardless of the method used for medication administration in children, **a solution to flush the I.V. tubing is administered after medication.** The purpose of the flush is to make sure the medication has cleared the tubing, and the total dose is administered. The amount of flush is **15 mL** for peripheral lines and **20 mL** for central lines. The policy for including medication volume as part of the volume specified for dilution varies from institution to institution. **The nurse has the responsibility for checking the protocol at the institution to ensure correct procedure is followed.**

Calculating I.V. Medications by Burette

For the purpose of calculation, use the I.V. formula presented at the beginning of the chapter.

$$\frac{V_1}{T_1} \times \frac{V_2}{T_2} = \text{gtt/min}$$

Note: In doing the calculations, the total volume will include adding the medication to the diluent and the flush to calculate the gtt/min.

Example 1: The doctor orders an antibiotic dose of 100 mg diluted in 20 mL of D5W to infuse over 30 minutes. A 15 mL flush follows. The administration set is a microdrip.

Step 1: Read the drug label and determine what volume the 100 mg is contained in. This is 2 mL.

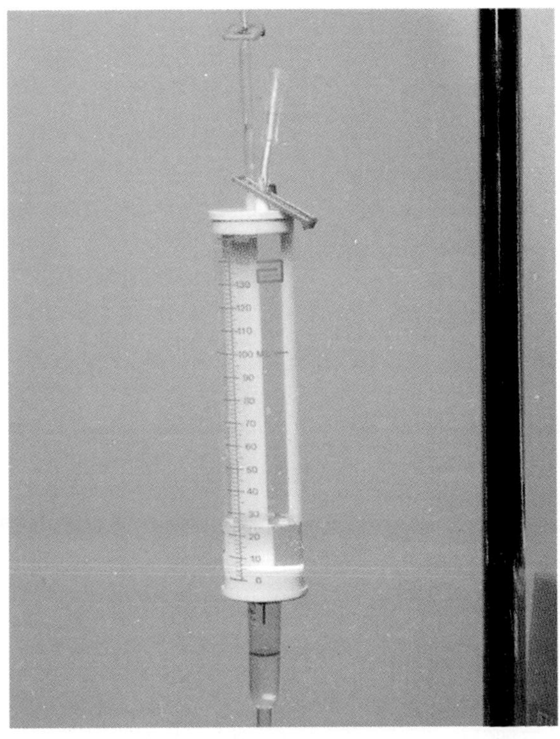

Figure 20-14. Volume control device. (From Elkin M, Perry A, Potter P: *Nursing interventions and clinical skills,* St Louis, 1996, Mosby.)

Step 2: Allow 18 mL D5W to run into the burette and then add the 2 mL containing the 100 mg of medication. Roll the burette between your hands to allow medication to mix thoroughly.

Step 3: Determine the flow rate necessary to deliver the medication plus the flush in 30 minutes.

$$\frac{20 \text{ mL (diluted drug)} + 15 \text{ mL flush}}{1} \times \frac{60 \text{ gtt/mL}}{30 \text{ min}} =$$

$$\frac{35 \text{ mL}}{1} \times \frac{60 \text{ gtt/mL}}{30 \text{ min}} = 35 \times 2 =$$

70 microgtt/min; 70gtt/min

Step 4: Adjust the I.V. flow rate to deliver 70 microgtt/min (70 gtt/min).

Step 5: Label the burette with the drug name, dosage, and medication infusing label.

Step 6: When the medication is completed, add the 15 mL flush, and continue to infuse at 70 microgtt/min. Replace the label with a "flush infusing" label.

Step 7: When the flush is completed, restart the primary line, and remove the flush infusing label. Document the medication on the MAR and the volume of fluid on the I & O according to agency policy.

Note: To express the volume of gtt/min in mL/hr, remember that a microdrip administration set delivers 60 gtt/mL; therefore gtt/min = mL/hr. In this case if the gtt/min = 70, then the mL/hr = 70. For volume controllers mL/hr is set.

Practice Problems (p. 389)

40. An I.V. medication dose of 500 mg is ordered to be diluted to 30 mL and infused over 50 minutes. A 15 mL flush is to follow. The dose of medication is contained in 3 mL. The administration set is a microdrip. Determine the following:

    a) Dilution volume ____________

    b) gtt/min ____________

    c) mL/hr ____________

41. The volume of a 20-mg dose of medication is 2 mL. Dilute to 15 mL and administer over 45 minutes with a 15 mL flush to follow. The adminsitration set is a microdrip. Determine the following:

    a) Dilution volume ____________

    b) gtt/min ____________

    c) mL/hr ____________

Note: Reduction of numbers can make numbers smaller and easier to deal with.

As seen in the chapter on pediatric doses, medications can be calculated based on mg/kg or BSA—I.V. doses for children are calculated on that basis as well. The I.V. medication can be assessed to determine if it is within normal range as well. The safe daily dose is calculated and then compared to the order.

Points to Remember

- Calculation of gtt/min can be done using $\frac{V_1}{T_1} \times \frac{V_2}{T_2}$ = gtt/min.
- To calculate the I.V. flow rate, the nurse must have the volume of solution, the time factor, and the drop factor of the tubing.
- Microdrips always deliver 60 gtt/mL.
- Macrodrops differ according to manufacturer. They can deliver 10, 15, or 20 gtt/mL.
- I.V. flow rates must be monitored by the nurse. When I.V. solutions are behind or ahead of schedule, the flow rate must be recalculated.
- Never increase an I.V. flow rate without recalculating or assessing a client to determine if the client can tolerate a rate increase.
- Read I.V. labels carefully to determine whether the correct solution is being administered.
- Infusion time is calculated by dividing the total volume to infuse by the mL/hr the solution is infusing at.
- Commercial labeling for I.V. bags is used to provide for assessing the volume a client is receiving per hour.
- Pediatric I.V. medications are diluted for administration. It is important to know the hospital policy on whether to include the medication volume as part of the total dilution volume.
- A flush is used following medication administration of I.V. medication in children. A 15-mL flush is used for peripheral lines and a 20-mL flush for central lines.

Chapter Review (pp. 389-393)

Calculate the I.V. flow rate in gtt/min for the following I.V. administrations, unless another unit of measure is stated.

1. 1000 mL D5RL to infuse in 8 hr. The administration set is 20 gtt/mL. __________
2. 2,500 mL D5NS to infuse in 24 hr. The administration set is 10 gtt/mL. __________
3. 500 mL D5W to infuse in 4 hr. The administration set is 15 gtt/mL. __________
4. 300 mL NS to infuse in 6 hr. The administration set is 60 gtt/mL. __________
5. 1000 mL D5W for 24 hr KVO (keep vein open). The administration set is 60 gtt/mL. __________
6. 1000 mL D5 and $\frac{1}{2}$ NS with 20 mEq KCl over 12 hr. The administration set is 10 gtt/mL. __________
7. 1000 mL RL to infuse in 10 hr. The administration set is 20 gtt/mL. __________
8. 1,500 mL NS to infuse in 12 hr. The administration set is 10 gtt/mL. __________
9. A unit of whole blood (500 mL) to infuse in 4 hr. The administration set is 10 gtt/mL. __________

10. A unit of packed cells (250 mL) to infuse in 3 hr. The administration set is 10 gtt/mL. __________

11. 1,500 ml D5W in 8 hr. The administration set is 20 gtt/mL. __________

12. 3,000 mL RL in 24 hr. The administration set is 15 gtt/mL. __________

13. Infuse 2 L RL in 24 hours. The administration set is 15 gtt/mL. __________

14. 1000 mL D5W with 10 mEq KCl to infuse in 7 hr. The administration set is 10 gtt/mL. __________

15. 500 mL D5W in 4 hr. The administration set is 60 gtt/mL. __________

16. 1000 mL D5 and $\frac{1}{2}$ NS in 6 hr. The administration set delivers 20 gtt/mL. __________

17. 250 mL D5W in 8 hr. The administration set delivers 60 gtt/mL. __________

18. 1 L of D5W to infuse at 50 mL/hr. The administration set is 60 gtt/mL. __________

19. 2 L D5RL at 150 mL/hr. The administration set is 15 gtt/mL. __________

20. 500 mL D5W in 6 hr. The administration set is 12 gtt/mL. __________

21. 1,500 mL NS in 12 hr. The administration set is 10 gtt/mL. __________

22. 1,500 mL D5W in 24 hr. The administration set is 12 gtt/mL. __________

23. 2,000 mL D5W in 16 hr. The administration set is 20 gtt/mL. __________

24. 500 mL D5W in 8 hr. The administration set is 15 gtt/mL. __________

25. 250 ml D5W in 10 hr. The administration set is 60 gtt/mL. __________

26. Infuse 300 mL of D5W at 75 mL/hr. The administration set is 60 gtt/mL. __________

27. Infuse 125 mL/hr of D5RL. The administration set is 20 gtt/mL. __________

28. Infuse 40 mL/hr of D5W. The administration set is 60 gtt/mL. __________

29. Infuse an I.V. medication with a volume of 50 mL in 45 minutes. The administration set is a microdrip. __________

30. Infuse 90 mL/hr of NS. The administration set delivers 15 gtt/mL. __________

31. Infuse 150 mL/hr of D5RL. The administration set delivers 10 gtt/mL. __________

32. Infuse 3,000 mL of D5W in 24 hr. The administration set delivers 15 gtt/mL. __________

33. Infuse an I.V. medication with a volume of 50 mL in 40 minutes. The administration set delivers 10 gtt/mL. __________

34. Infuse 100 mL of an I.V. with medication in 30 minutes. The administration set delivers 20 gtt/mL. __________

35. Infuse 250 mL $\frac{1}{2}$ NS in 5 hr. The administration set delivers 20 gtt/mL. ______

36. Infuse 1000 mL of D5W at 80 mL/hr. The administration set delivers 20 gtt/mL. ______

37. Infuse 150 mL of D5RL in 30 minutes. The administration set delivers 12 gtt/mL. ______

38. Infuse Kefzol 0.5 g in 50 mL D5W in 30 minutes. The administration set is a microdrip. ______

39. Infuse Plasmanate 500 mL over 3 hr. The administration set delivers 10 gtt/mL. ______

40. Infuse albumin 250 mL over 2 hr. The administration set delivers 15 gtt/mL. ______

41. The doctor orders the following I.V.s for 24 hr. The administration set delivers 10 gtt/mL.

    a) 1000 mL D5W with 1 ampule MVI (multivitamin)
    500 mL D5W ______

    b) 250 mL D5W ______

42. Infuse vancomycin 1 g IVPB in 150 mL D5W in 1.5 hr. The administration set is a microdrip. ______

43. If 2 L D5W is to infuse in 16 hr, how many mL are to be administered per hour? ______

44. If 500 mL of RL is to infuse in 4 hr, how many mL are to be administered per hour? ______

45. If 200 mL of NS is to infuse in 2 hr, how many mL are to be administered per hour? ______

46. If 500 mL of D5W is to infuse in 8 hr, how many mL are to be administered per hour? ______

47. Infuse 500 mL Intralipids I.V. in 6 hr. The administration set delivers 10 gtt/mL. ______

48. Infuse a hyperalimentation solution of 1,100 mL in 12 hr. The administration set delivers 20 gtt/mL. ______

49. Infuse 3,000 mL D5W in 20 hr. The administration set delivers 20 gtt/mL. ______

50. An I.V. of 500 mL D5W with 200 mg of minocycline is to infuse in 6 hr. The administration set delivers 10 gtt/mL. ______

51. An I.V. of D5W 500 mL was ordered to infuse over 10 hr at a rate of 13 gtt/min. The administration set delivers 15 gtt/mL. After 3 hr you notice that 300 mL of I.V. solution is left. Recalculate the gtt/min for the remaining solution. ______

52. An I.V. of D5W 1000 mL was ordered to infuse over 8 hr at a rate of 42 gtt/min. The administration set delivers 20 gtt/mL. After 4 hr you notice only 400 mL has infused. Recalculate the gtt/min for the remaining solution. ____________

53. An I.V. of 1000 mL D5 and $\frac{1}{2}$ NS has been ordered to infuse at 125 mL/hr. The administration set delivers 15 gtt/mL. The I.V. was hung at 7 AM. At 11 AM you check the I.V., and there is 400 mL left. Recalculate the gtt/min for the remaining solution. ____________

54. An I.V. of 500 mL of NS is to infuse in 6 hr at a rate of 14 gtt/min. The administration set delivers 10 gtt/mL. The I.V. was started at 7 AM. You check the I.V. at 8 AM, and 250 mL has infused. Recalculate the gtt/min for the remaining solution. ____________

55. An I.V. of 1000 mL D5W is to infuse in 10 hr. The administration set delivers 15 gtt/mL. The I.V. was started at 4 AM. At 10 AM 600 mL remains in the bag. Is the I.V. on time? If not, recalculate the gtt/min for the remaining solution. ____________

56. 900 mL of RL is infusing at a rate of 80 gtt/min. The administration set delivers 15 gtt/mL. How long will it take for the I.V. to infuse? (Express time in hours and minutes.) ____________

57. A client is receiving 1000 mL of D5W at 100 mL/hr. How many hours will it take for the I.V. to infuse? ____________

58. 1000 mL of D5W is infusing at 20 gtt/min. The administration set delivers 10 gtt/mL. How long will it take for the I.V. to infuse? (Express time in hours and minutes.) ____________

59. 450 mL of NS is infusing at 25 gtt/min. The administration set delivers 20 gtt/mL. How long will it take for the I.V. to infuse? ____________

60. 100 mL of D5W is infusing at 10 gtt/min. The administration set delivers 15 gtt/mL. How many hours will it take for the I.V. to infuse? ____________

61. An I.V. is regulated at 25 gtt/min. The administration set delivers 15 gtt/mL. How many mL of fluid will the client receive in 8 hr? ____________

62. An I.V. is regulated at 40 gtt/min. The administration set delivers 60 gtt/mL. How many mL of fluid will the client receive in 10 hr? ____________

63. An I.V. is regulated at 30 gtt/min. The administration set delivers 15 gtt/mL. How many mL of fluid will the client receive in 5 hr? ____________

64. 10 mEq of potassium chloride is placed in 500 mL of D5W to be administered at the rate of 2 mEq/hr.

    a) How many mL of solution is needed to administer 2 mEq? ____________

    b) Calculate the gtt/min to deliver 2 mEq/hr. The administration set delivers 20 gtt/mL. ____________

65. 30 mEq of potassium chloride is added to 1000 mL of D5W to be administered at the rate of 4 mEq/hr.

    a) How many mL of solution is needed to administer 4 mEq? __________

    b) Calculate the gtt/min to deliver 4 mEq/hr. The administration set delivers 15 gtt/mL. __________

66. Doctor's order: Regular insulin 7 U/hr. The I.V. solution contains 50 U of regular insulin in 250 mL of NS. How many mL/hr should the I.V. infuse at? __________

67. Doctor's order: Regular insulin 18 U/hr. The I.V. solution contains 100 U of regular insulin in 250 mL of NS. How many mL/hr should the I.V. infuse at? __________

68. Doctor's order: 11 U/hr of regular insulin. The I.V. solution contains 100 U of regular insulin in 100 mL of NS. How many mL/hr should the I.V. infuse at? __________

69. Infuse 150 mL gentamicin IVPB over 1 hr. The administration set delivers 10 gtt/mL. How many gtt/min should the I.V. infuse at? __________

70. Infuse ampicillin 1 g that has been diluted in 40 mL D5W in 40 minutes using a microdrip set. How many gtt/min should the I.V. infuse at? __________

71. Administer I.V. medication with a volume of 35 mL in 30 minutes using a microdrip set. How many gtt/min should the I.V. infuse at? __________

72. Administer I.V. medication with a volume of 80mL in 40 minutes using an administration set that delivers 15 gtt/mL. How many gtt/min would you infuse? __________

73. Administer 50 mL of an antibiotic in 25 minutes. The administration set delivers 10 gtt/mL. How many gtt/min would you regulate the I.V. at? __________

74. An I.V. is to infuse at 65 mL/hr. The administration set delivers 15 gtt/mL. How many gtt/min should infuse? __________

75. 50 mL of D5W with 1 g ampicillin. The I.V. is infusing at 50 microgtt/min. The administration set is a microdrip. Determine the infusion time. (Express time in hours and minutes.) __________

76. 500 mL RL is to infuse at a rate of 80 mL/hr. If the I.V. was started at 7 PM, what time will the I.V. be completed? __________

77. A volume of 150 mL of NS is to infuse at 25 mL/hr.

    a) Calculate the infusion time. __________

    b) The I.V. was started at 3:10 AM. What time will the I.V. be completed? __________

78. The doctor orders 2.5 L of D5W to infuse at 150 mL/hr. Determine the infusion time. __________

79. A child is to receive 10 U of a medication. The dose of 10 U is contained in 1 mL. Dilute to 30 mL and infuse in 20 minutes. A 20 mL flush is to follow.

    a) gtt/min3 ____________

    b) mL/hr ____________

80. A child is to receive 80 mg of a medication. The dose of 80 mg is contained in 2 mL. Dilute to 80 mL and infuse in 60 minutes. A 15 mL flush is to follow.

    a) gtt/min ____________

    b) mL/hr ____________

81. A dose of 250 mg in 5 mL has been ordered diluted to 40 mL and infused in 45 minutes. A 15 mL flush follows.

    a) gtt/min ____________

    b) mL/hr ____________

Chapter 21

Heparin Calculations

Objectives

After reviewing this chapter the student will be able to do the following:

1. **State the importance of calculating heparin doses**
2. **Calculate heparin doses being administered I.V.**
3. **Calculate s.c. doses of heparin**

Heparin is a potent anticoagulant that prevents clot formation and blood coagulation. The therapeutic range for heparin is determined individually by monitoring the client's partial thromboplastin time (PTT). **However, the normal adult heparin dosage is 20,000 to 40,000 U every 24 hours.**

Heparin is always measured in units and can be administered I.V. or s.c. When given I.V., heparin is ordered in units per hour. Heparin comes in different strengths; therefore it is important to read labels carefully when administering it (Figure 21-1).

Calculation of s.c. Doses

Heparin is administered s.c. using a tuberculin syringe to ensure an accurate dose. The same methods of calculating that were presented earlier are used to calculate s.c. heparin, except that the dose is never rounded off.

Example 1: Doctor's Order: Heparin 7,500 U s.c.

Available: Heparin labeled 10,000 U/mL.

What will you administer to the client?

Setup:

1. No conversion is necessary. There is no conversion for units.
2. Think—what would be a logical dose?
3. Set up in ratio-proportion or formula and solve.

A

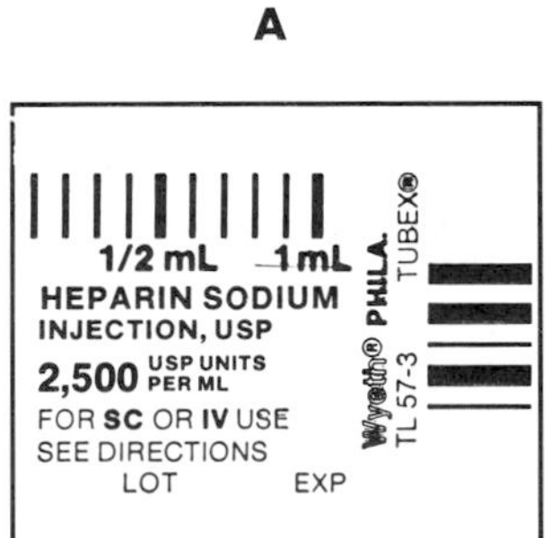

B

N 0469-1262-15 926201
HEPARIN SODIUM
INJECTION, USP
5,000 USP Units/mL
(Derived from Porcine Intestinal Mucosa)
For IV or SC Use
1 mL Multiple Dose Vial
Usual Dosage: See insert.
Lyphomed
Fujisawa USA, Inc.
Deerfield, IL 60015
40213D

Figure 21-1. Heparin labels. **A,** Heparin sodium 2,500 U/mL (From Smith AJ: *Dosages and solutions calculations,* St Louis, 1989, Mosby). **B,** Heparin sodium 5,000 U/mL. (From Brown M, Mulholland J: *Drug calculations,* ed 5, St Louis, 1996, Mosby.)

Solution Using Ratio-Proportion:

$$10{,}000\text{ U} : 1\text{ mL} = 7{,}500\text{ U} : x\text{ mL}$$

$$10{,}000x = 7{,}500$$

$$x = \frac{7{,}500}{10{,}000}$$

$$x = 0.75\text{ mL}$$

Solution Using Formula:

$$\frac{7{,}500\text{ U}}{10{,}000\text{ U}} \times 1\text{ mL} = x\text{ mL}; \frac{7{,}500\text{ U}}{10{,}000\text{ U}} = \frac{x\text{ mL}}{1\text{ mL}}$$

$$x = 0.75\text{ mL}$$

The dose of 0.75 mL is reasonable since the ordered dose is less than what is available. Therefore less than 1 mL will be needed to administer the dose. This dose can be measured accurately only using a tuberculin syringe. This dose would not be rounded to the nearest tenth of a mL. A tuberculin syringe is shown below illustrating the dose to be administered (Figure 21-2).

Calculation of I.V. Heparin Solutions

Using Ratio-Proportion

Calculating mL/hr of heparin can be done by using ratio-proportion.

Example: An I.V. solution of heparin is ordered for a client. D5W 1000 mL containing 20,000 U of heparin is to infuse at 30 mL/hr. Calculate the dose of heparin the client is to receive per hour.

Set up a proportion:

$$20{,}000\text{ U} : 1000\text{ mL} = x\text{ U} : 30\text{ mL}$$

$$1000x = 20{,}000 \times 30$$

$$\frac{1000x}{1000} = \frac{600{,}000}{1000} = 600\text{ U/hr}$$

Using the Set Calibration and Flow Rate

Hourly doses can be calculated when the set calibration and flow rate are given.

Example: A client is receiving 12,500 U of heparin in 250 mL of D5W. The set calibration is 15 gtt/mL, and the flow rate is 30 gtt/min. Calculate the hourly dose the client is receiving. This is solved using a series of steps.

First—Convert the gtt/min to mL/min.

$$15\text{ gtt} : 1\text{ mL} = 30\text{ gtt} : x\text{ mL}$$

$$\frac{15x}{15} = \frac{30}{15}$$

$$x = 2\text{ mL/min}$$

Then—Convert mL/min to mL/hr.

$$2\text{ mL/min} \times 60\text{ min} = 120\text{ mL/hr}$$

After doing these steps, the proportion can be set up to calculate the units per hour that were illustrated.

$$12{,}500\text{ U} : 250\text{ mL} = x\text{ U} : 120\text{ mL}$$

$$250x = 1{,}500{,}000$$

$$x = 6{,}000\text{ U/hr}$$

The client is receiving 6,000 U of heparin per hour.

Since I.V. heparin is ordered in units per hour, after calculating the mL/hr another calculation must be done to determine the flow rate.

Example 1: Infuse 8,000 U/hr of heparin from a solution containing 20,000 U in 250 mL D5W. The administration set delivers 10 gtt/mL.

First calculate mL/hr to be administered:

$$20{,}000\text{ U} : 250\text{ mL} = 8{,}000\text{ U} : x\text{ mL}$$

$$20{,}000x = 8{,}000 \times 250$$

$$\frac{20{,}000}{20{,}000}x = \frac{2{,}000{,}000}{20{,}000} = 100\text{ mL/hr}$$

Then calculate the flow rate in gtt/min:

$$\frac{100\text{ mL}}{1\text{ hr}} \times \frac{10\text{ gtt/mL}}{60\text{ min}} = 16.6$$

Answer: 17 gtt/min; 17 macrogtt/min

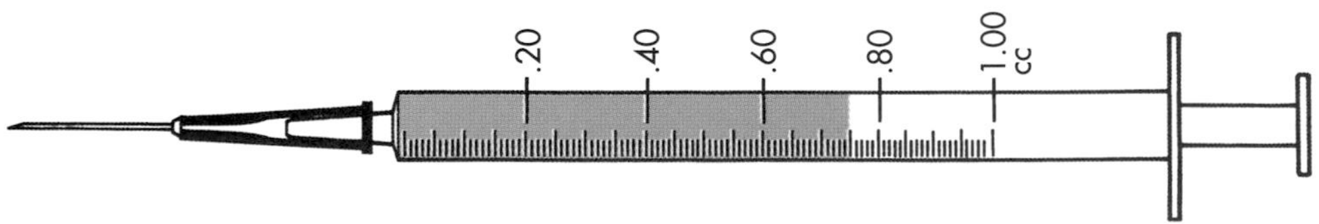

Figure 21-2. Tuberculin syringe illustrating 0.75 mL drawn up. (Syringe from Dison N: *Simplified drugs and solutions for nurses,* ed 10, St Louis, 1992, Mosby.)

Points to Remember

- Doses of heparin must be accurately calculated.
- Heparin doses are administered s.c. and I.V.
- When being administered I.V., calculations involving heparin may involve a series of steps.
- The method of calculating I.V. heparin doses can also be used to calculate I.V. doses of other medications.

Chapter Review (pp. 393-399)

For questions 1 through 12 calculate the dose of heparin you will administer, and shade in the dose on the syringe provided. For questions 13 through 40 calculate the units as indicated by the problem. Use labels where provided to calculate doses.

1. Doctor's Order: Heparin 3,500 U s.c. o.d.
   Available:

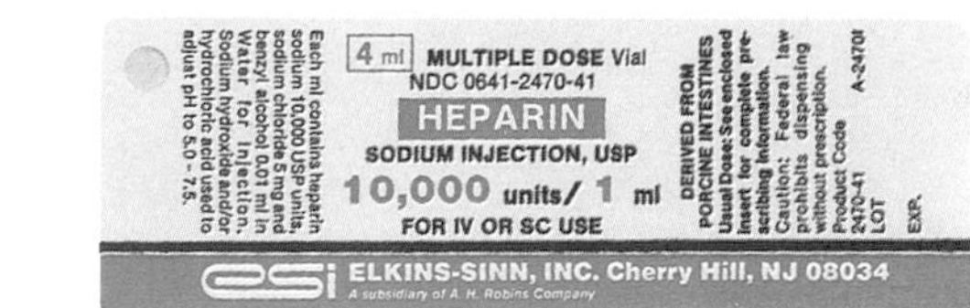

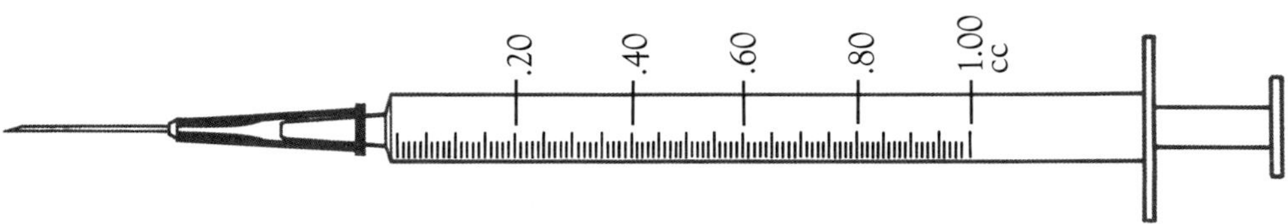

2. Doctor's Order: Heparin 16,000 U s.c. stat.
   Available: Heparin labeled 20,000 U/mL.

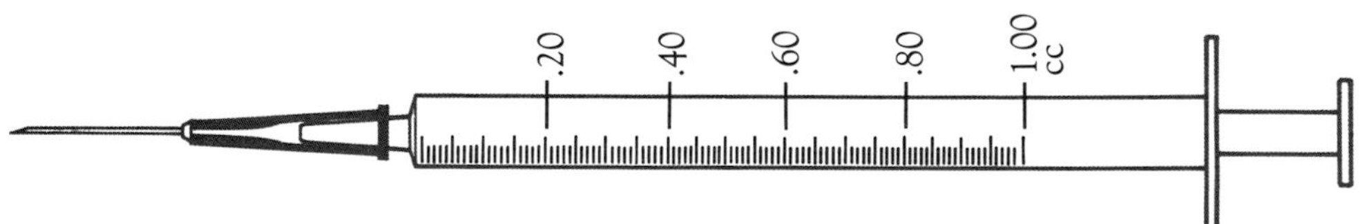

3. Doctor's Order: Heparin 2,000 U s.c. o.d.
   Available: Heparin labeled 2,500 U/mL.

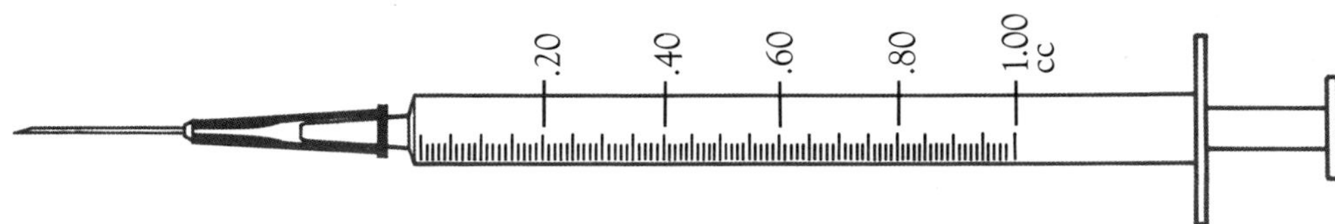

4. Doctor's Order: Heparin 2,000 U s.c. o.d.
   Available: Heparin labeled 5,000 U/mL.

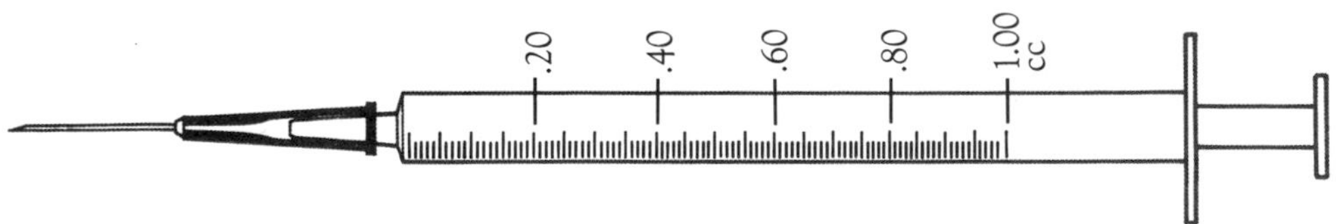

5. Prepare a dose of 500 U of heparin s.c. q4h.
   Available:

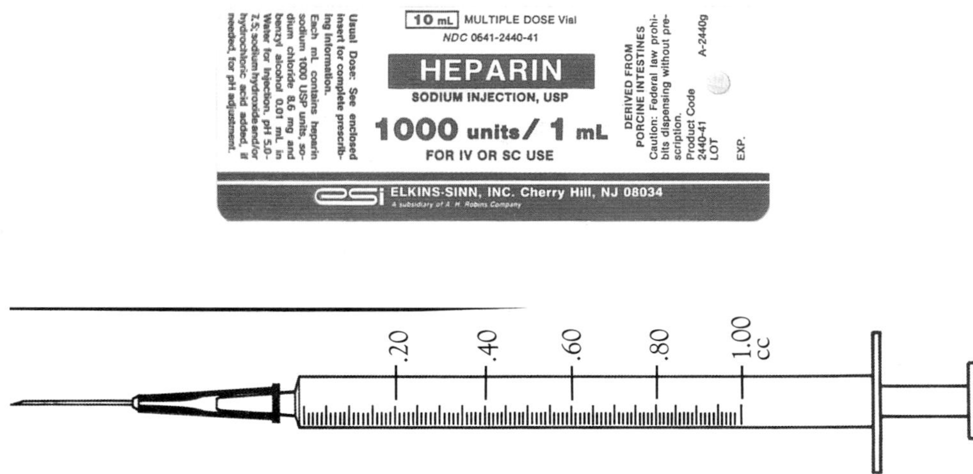

6. Doctor's Order: Heparin flush 10 U q shift to flush a heparin lock.
   Available:

7. Doctor's Order: Heparin 50,000 U in D5W 500 mL.

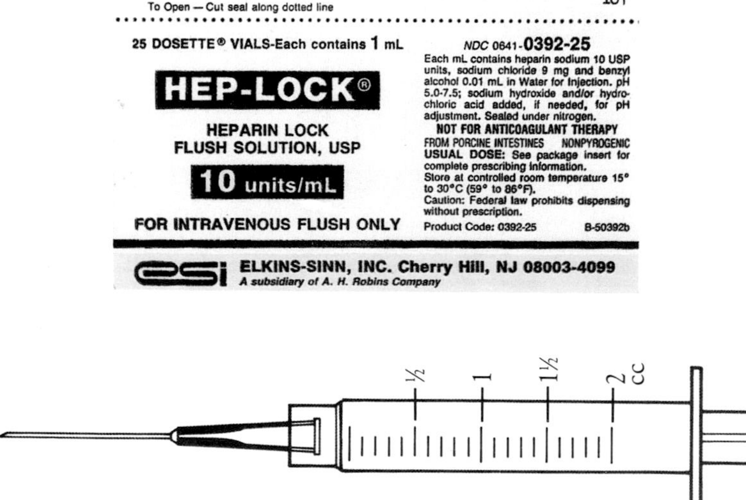

Available: 10,000 U/mL.

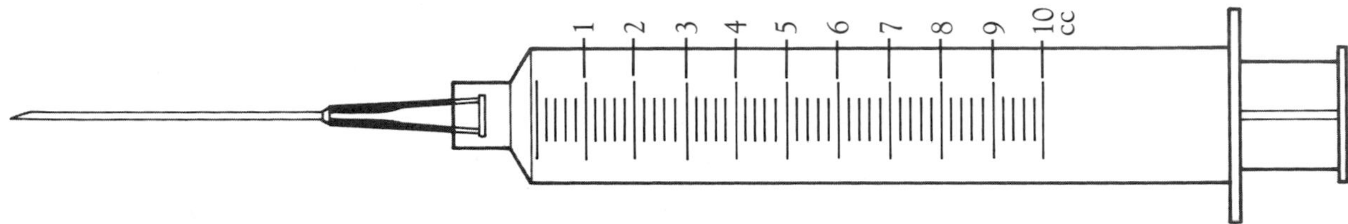

8. Doctor's Order: Heparin 15,000 U s.c. o.d.
   Available: Heparin labeled 20,000 U/mL.

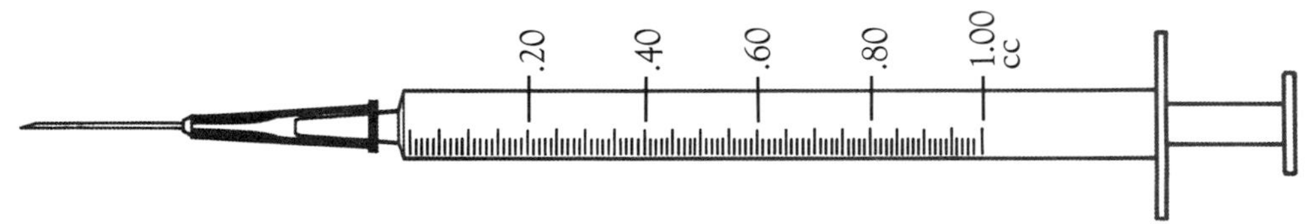

9. Doctor's Order: 3,000 U of heparin to a liter of I.V. solution.
   Available: 2,500 U/mL.

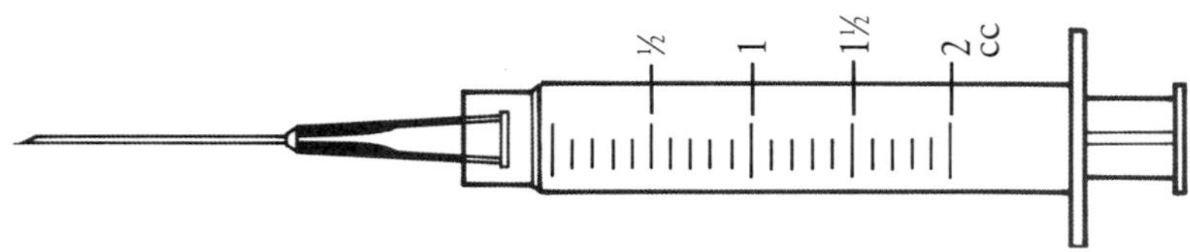

10. Doctor's Order: Heparin 17,000 U s.c. o.d.
    Available: Heparin labeled 20,000 U/mL.

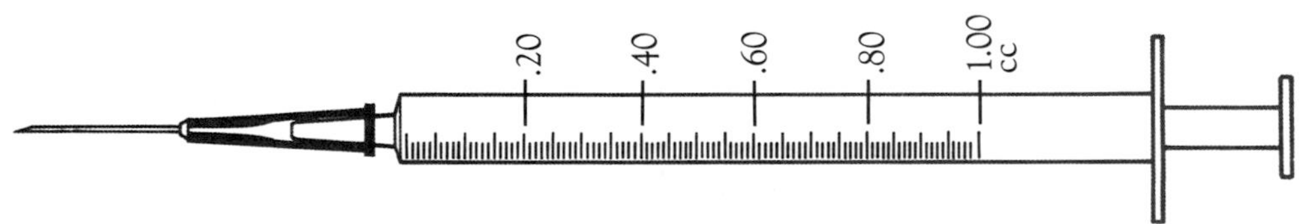

11. Doctor's Order: Heparin bolus of 8,500 U I.V. stat.
    Available: 10,000 U/mL.

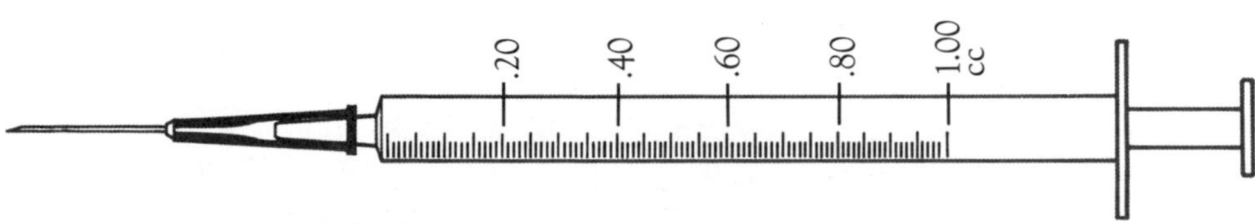

12. Doctor's Order: Heparin 2,500 U s.c. q6h.
    Available: Heparin labeled 10,000 U/mL.

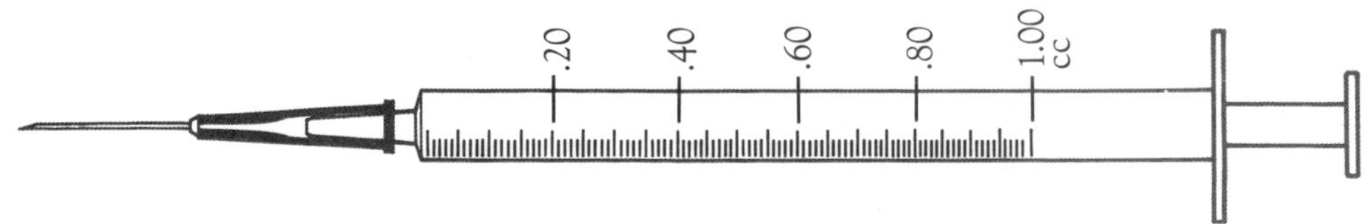

13. Doctor's Order: Heparin 2,000 U/hr I.V. You have 25,000 U per 1000 mL of NS.

    a) How many mL per hour will deliver 2,000 U/hr? ____________

14. Doctor's Order: Heparin 1,500 U/hr I.V.
    Available: 25,000 U per 500 mL of D5W.

    a) How many mL/hr will deliver 1,500 U/hr? ____________

15. Doctor's Order: Heparin 1,800 U/hr I.V.
    Available: 25,000 U per 250 mL of D5W.

    a) How many mL/hr will deliver 1,800 U/hr? ____________

16. Doctor's Order: Add 40,000 U heparin to 1 L NS and infuse at 25 mL/hr.

    a) Calculate the hourly heparin dose. ____________

17. Doctor's Order: Add Heparin 25,000 U to 250 mL D5W and infuse at 11 mL/hr.

    a) Calculate the hourly heparin dose. ____________

18. Doctor's Order: Add 40,000 U heparin to 500 mL D5W and infuse at 30 mL/hr.

    a) Calculate the hourly heparin dose. ____________

19. Doctor's Order: Add 20,000 U to 500 mL D5W to infuse at 12 mL/hr.

    a) Calculate the hourly heparin dose. ____________

20. Doctor's Order: Add heparin 25,000 U to 500 mL D5W to infuse at 15 mL/hr.

    a) Calculate the hourly heparin dose. ____________

21. Doctor's Order: Infuse 1 L of NS with 40,000 U heparin over 24 hr. The administration set delivers 15 gtt/mL.

    a) Calculate the hourly dose of heparin. ____________

    b) Calculate the gtt/min. ____________

22. Doctor's Order: Infuse 1 L of D5W with 15,000 U heparin over 10 hr. Calculate the following:

    a) mL/hr ____________

    b) U/hr ____________

23. Doctor's Order: Infuse 20 mL/hr of 1 L D5W with 35,000 U of heparin.
Calculate the following using a microdrop administration set:

   a) hourly dose ____________

   b) gtt/min ____________

24. Doctor's Order: Infuse 500 mL of NS with 10,000 U heparin at 20 gtt/min. The administration set delivers 10 gtt/mL. Calculate the following:

   a) mL/hr ____________

   b) hourly unit dose ____________

25. Doctor's Order: Infuse 500 mL of D5W with 25,000 U heparin at 25 mL/hr.

   a) Calculate the hourly unit dose of heparin. ____________

26. Doctor's Order: Infuse 500 mL of D5W with 20,000 U heparin at 40 mL/hr.

   a) Calculate the hourly unit dose. ____________

27. Doctor's Order: Infuse 1,400 U/hr of heparin I.V. Heparin 40,000 U is 1000 mL of D5W. The administration set delivers 15 gtt/mL. Calculate the following:

   a) mL/hr ____________

   b) gtt/min ____________

28. Doctor's Order: Infuse 1000 U/hr of heparin I.V. Heparin 40,000 U is in 1 L of NS. The administration set delivers 15 gtt/mL. Calculate the following:

   a) mL/hr ____________

   b) gtt/min ____________

29. Doctor's Order: Administer 1000 U heparin I.V. every hour. Solution available is 25,000 U of heparin in 500 mL D5W. The administration set is a microdrip.

   a) Calculate the gtt/min. ____________

30. Doctor's Order: Administer 2,000 U heparin I.V. every hour. The solution available is 25,000 U of heparin in 1 L NS. The administration set delivers 15 gtt/mL.

   a) Calculate the gtt/min. ____________

31. A client is receiving an I.V. of 1000 mL of D5W with 50,000 U heparin infusing at 15 gtt/min. The administration set delivers 15 gtt/mL.

   a) Calculate the hourly dose of heparin the client is receiving. ____________

32. A client is receiving an I.V. of 250 mL NS with 25,000 U heparin at 20 gtt/min. The administration set delivers 10 gtt/mL.

   a) Calculate the hourly dose of heparin. ____________

33. A client is receiving 500 mL of D5W with 20,000 U of heparin at 20 gtt/min. The administration set is a microdrip.

    a) Calculate the hourly dose of heparin. ____________

34. A client is receiving an I.V. of 25,000 U heparin in 1 L of D5W infusing at 14 gtt/min. The administration set delivers 15 gtt/mL.

    a) Calculate the hourly dose of heparin. ____________

35. A client is receiving an I.V. of 1000 mL D5W with 20,000 U heparin infusing at 24 gtt/min. The administration set delivers 10 gtt/mL.

    a) Calculate the hourly dose of heparin. ____________

Directions: Calculate the following hourly doses of heparin.

36. Doctor's Order: 30,000 U of heparin in 500 mL of D5W to infuse at 25 mL/hr. ____________

37. Doctor's Order: 20,000 U of heparin in 1 L of D5W to infuse at 40 mL/hr. ____________

38. Doctor's Order: 40,000 U of heparin in 500 mL NS to infuse at 25 mL/hr. ____________

39. Doctor's Order: 35,000 U of heparin in 1 L of D5W to infuse at 20 mL/hr. ____________

40. Doctor's Order: 25,000 U of heparin in 1 L of D5W to infuse at 30 mL/hr. ____________

41. Doctor's Order: 40,000 U of heparin in 1 L of D5W to infuse at 30 mL/hr. ____________

42. Doctor's Order: 20,000 U of heparin in 1 L of D5W to infuse at 80 mL/hr. ____________

43. Doctor's Order: 50,000 U of heparin in 1 L of D5W to infuse at 70 mL/hr. ____________

44. Doctor's Order: 20,000 U of heparin in 500 mL NS to infuse at 30 mL/hr. ____________

45. Doctor's Order: 30,000 U of heparin in 1 L of D5W at 25 mL/hr. ____________

Chapter 22

Critical Care Calculations

Objectives

After reviewing this chapter the student will be able to do the following:

1. Calculate doses in mcg/min, mcg/hr, and mg/min
2. Calculate doses in mg/kg/hr, mg/kg/min, and mcg/kg/min

The content in this chapter may not be required as part of the nursing curriculum. It is included as a reference for nurses working in specialty areas.

This chapter will provide basic information on medicated I.V. drips and titration. Critically ill clients receive medications that are potent and require close monitoring. Because of the potency of the medications and their tendency to induce changes in blood pressure and heart rate, accurate calculation of doses is essential. Medications in the critical care area can be ordered by mL/hr, gtt/min, mcg/kg/min, or mg/hr. Infusion pumps and volume control devices are usually used to administer these medications. The process of administering calculated doses of potent drugs is referred to as *titration.* Examples of medicated I.V. drips that require titration are Aramine, nitroprusside, Levophed, and epinephrine.

Titrated medications are added to a specific volume of fluid and then adjusted to infuse at the rate at which the desired effect is obtained. **The drugs that are titrated are potent antiarrhythmic, vasopressor, and vasodilator medications; they must be monitored very carefully by the nurse.** Due to the potency of medications used, minute changes in the infusion can cause an effect on the client. Infusion pumps are used for titration; when one is not available, a microdrip set calibrated at 60 gtt/mL must be used.

An example of an order that involves titration of medication would be "Titrate sodium nitroprusside (Nipride) to maintain the client's blood pressure below 140 mm Hg." The nurses may start, for example, at 3 mcg/kg/min and gradually increase the rate until the systolic blood pressure is maintained below 140 mm Hg. Each time there is a change in rate, the dose of medication the client receives is changed; therefore it is essential that the dose be recalculated each time the nurse changes the rate.

Calculating Critical Care Doses per Hour or per Minute

Example 1: Infuse dopamine 400 mg in 500 mL D5W at 30 mL/hr. Calculate the dose in mcg/min and mcg/hr.

Solution:

1. Use ratio-proportion to determine the dose per hour first.

$$400 \text{ mg} : 500 \text{ mL} = x \text{ mg} : 30 \text{ mL}$$

known unknown

$$500x = 400 \times 30$$
$$500x = 12{,}000$$
$$x = \frac{12{,}000}{500}$$
$$x = 24 \text{ mg/hr}$$

2. The next step is to convert 24 mg to mcg since the question asked for mcg/min and mcg/hr. Change mg to mcg by using the equivalent 1000 mcg = 1 mg. To change mg to mcg multiply by 1000 or move the decimal point three places to the right, since it's a metric measure.

$$24 \text{ mg} = 24{,}000 \text{ mcg/hr}$$

3. Now that you have the mcg per hour, the next step is to change mcg/hr to mcg/min. This is done by dividing the number of mcg/hr by 60 (60 minutes = 1 hour).

$$24{,}000 \text{ mcg/hr} \div 60 = 400 \text{ mcg/min}$$

Remember, accurate math is essential since these medications are extremely potent.

Drugs Ordered in Milligrams per Minute

Drugs such as lidocaine and Pronestyl are ordered in mg/min.

Example 2: A client is receiving Pronestyl at 60 mL/hr. The solution available is Pronestyl 2 g in 500 mL D5W. Calculate the mg/hr and the mg/min the client will receive.

1. A conversion is necessary; g has to be converted to mg. This is what you are being asked for (mg/min, mg/hr).

   Equivalent: 1 g = 1000 mg

   Therefore 2 g = 2,000 mg (1000 × 2)

2. Now determine the mg/hr by setting up a proportion.

$$2{,}000 \text{ mg} : 500 \text{ mL} = x \text{ mg} : 60 \text{ mL}$$
$$500x = 2000 \times 60$$
$$500x = 120{,}000$$
$$x = 240 \text{ mg/hr}$$

3. Convert mg/hr to mg/min.

$$240 \text{ mg/hr} \div 60 = 4 \text{ mg/min}$$

Calculating Doses Based on mcg/kg/min

Drugs are also ordered for clients based on dose per kg per minute. These drugs include Nipride, dopamine, and dobutamine, for example.

Example 3: Doctor's Order: Dopamine 2 mcg/kg/min. The solution available is 400 mg in 250 mL D5W. The client weighs 150 lb.

1. Convert the client's weight in lb to kg.

$$2.2 \text{ lb} = 1 \text{ kg}$$

   To convert the client's weight divide 150 lb by 2.2.

$$150 \text{ lb} \div 2.2 = 68.18 \text{ kg} = 68 \text{ kg}$$

2. Now that you have the client's weight in kg, determine the dose per minute.

$$68 \text{ kg} \times 2 \text{ mcg} = 136 \text{ mcg/min}$$

Titration of Infusions

As already mentioned, critical care medications are ordered within parameters to obtain a desirable response in a client. When a solution is titrated, **the lowest dose of the medication is set first** and increased or decreased as necessary. **The higher dose should not be exceeded without a new order.**

Example: Nipride has been ordered to titrate at 3–6 mcg/kg/min to maintain a client's systolic blood pressure below 140 mm Hg. The solution contains 50 mg Nipride in 250 mL D5W. The client weighs 56 kg. Determine the flow rate setting for a volumetric pump.

1. Convert to **like units.**

   Equivalent: 1000 mcg = 1 mg

   Therefore 50 mg = 50,000 mcg

2. Calculate the concentration of solution in mcg/mL.

   50,000 mcg : 250 mL = x mcg : 1 mL

   $$\frac{250x}{250} = \frac{50,000}{250}$$

   $$x = 200 \text{ mcg/mL}$$

   The concentration of solution is 200 mcg/mL.

3. Calculate the dose range using the upper and lower doses.

   (Lower dose) 3 mcg × 56 kg = 168 mcg/min

   (Upper dose) 6 mcg × 56 kg = 336 mcg/min

4. Convert dose range to mL/min.

   (Lower dose) 200 mcg : 1 mL = 168 mcg : x mL

   $$\frac{200x}{200} = \frac{168}{200}$$

   $$x = 0.84 \text{ mL/min}$$

   (Upper dose) 200 mcg : 1 mL = 336 mcg : x mL

   $$\frac{200x}{200} = \frac{336}{200}$$

   $$x = 1.68 \text{ mL/min}$$

5. Convert mL/min to mL/hr.

   (Lower dose) 0.84 mL × 60 min = 50.4 = 50 mL/hr (gtt/min)

   (Upper dose) 1.68 mL × 60 min = 100.8 = 101 mL/hr (gtt/min)

   A dose range of 3 to 6 mcg/kg/min is equal to a flow rate of 50 to 101 ml/hr (gtt/min).

The client has stabilized and is now maintained at 60 mL/hr. What dose will be infusing per minute?

200 mcg : 1 mL = x mcg : 60 mL

$$x = 12,000 \text{ mcg/hr}$$

12,000 mcg ÷ 60 min = 200 mcg/min

Points to Remember

- When calculating doses to be administered without any type of electronic infusion pumps, always use microgtt tubing (60 gtt = 1 mL). This is preferred because the drops are smaller, so more accurate titration is possible.
- Calculate doses accurately. Double checking math calculations helps to ensure a proper dose.
- Obtain an accurate weight of your client.
- Before determining mL/hr or gtt/min, calculate the dose first.
- Use a calculator whenever possible.
- Use an infusion pump for titration of I.V. drugs in mL/hr.

Practice Problem (p. 399)

1. A client weighing 50 kg has a Dobutrex solution of 250 mg in 500 mL D5W ordered to titrate between 2.5-5 mcg/kg/min

   a) Determine the flow rate setting for a volumetric pump. ______________

   b) If the client's rate is being maintained at 25 mL/hr after several titrations, what is the dose infusing per minute? ______________

Points to Remember

- Always calculate doses first, and check your answers for accuracy.
- The safest way to administer medications is by an infusion device; however, when not available use microgtt tubing (60 gtt = 1 mL).

Practice Problems (pp. 399-400)

2. Doctor's Order: Epinephrine at 30 mL/hr. Solution available is 2 mg in 250 mL D5W. Calculate the following:

   a) mg/hr ____________

   b) mcg/hr ____________

   c) mcg/min ____________

3. Aminophylline 0.25 g is added to 500 mL D5W to infuse in 8 hrs. Calculate the following:

   a) mg/hr ____________

   b) mg/min ____________

4. Doctor's Order: Pitocin at 15 microgtts/min. The solution contains 10 U Pitocin in 1000 mL D5W.

   a) Calculate the number of units per hour the client is receiving. ____________

5. Doctor's Order: 3 mcg/kg/min of Nipride.
   Available: 50 mg of Nipride in 250 mL D5W. Client's weight is 60 kg.

   a) Calculate the flow rate in mL/hr that will deliver this dose. ____________

6. A nitroglycerine drip is infusing at 3 mL/hr. Available solution is 50 mg in 250 cc D5W. Calculate the following:

   a) mcg/hr ____________

   b) mcg/min ____________

Chapter Review (pp. 400-405)

Calculate the doses as indicated. Use the labels where provided.

1. Client is receiving Isuprel at 30 mL/hr. Solution is available in 2 mg of Isuprel in 250 mL D5W. Calculate the following:

   a) mg/hr ____________

   b) mcg/hr ____________

   c) mcg/min ____________

2. Client is receiving epinephrine at 40 mL/hr. Solution is available in 4 mg of epinephrine in 500 mL D5W. Calculate the following:

   a) mg/hr ____________

   b) mcg/hr ____________

   c) mcg/min ____________

3. Infuse dopamine 800 mg in 500 mL D5W at 30 mL/hr. Calculate the dose in mcg/min and mcg/hr.

   a) Calculate the number of mL you will add to the I.V. for this dose. ____________

EXP.
LOT
NDC 0641-0112-25
25 x 5 mL Single Use Vials
DOPAMINE
HCl INJECTION, USP
200 mg/5 mL
(40 mg/mL)
FOR IV INFUSION ONLY
POTENT DRUG: MUST DILUTE BEFORE USING
Each mL contains dopamine hydrochloride 40 mg (equivalent to 32.3 mg dopamine base) and sodium bisulfite 10 mg in Water for Injection. pH 2.5-5.0. Sealed under nitrogen.
USUAL DOSE: See package insert.
Do not use if solution is discolored.
Store at 15° - 30° C (59° - 86° F).
Caution: Federal law prohibits dispensing without prescription.
B-50112c
ELKINS-SINN, INC. Cherry Hill, NJ 08003-4099
A subsidiary of A. H. Robins Company

4. Infuse Nipride at 30 mL/hr. The solution available is 50 mg sodium nitroprusside in D5W 250 mL. Calculate the following:

   a) mcg/hr ____________

   b) mcg/min ____________

Protect from light.
Exp.
Lot
2 mL Single-dose Fliptop Vial NDC 0074-3024-01
NITROPRESS®
Sodium Nitroprusside Injection
50 mg / 2 mL Vial (25 mg/mL)
FOR I.V. INFUSION ONLY.
Monitor blood pressure before and during administration. 06-7378-2/R2-12/93
ABBOTT LABS, NORTH CHICAGO, IL 60064, USA

5. Doctor's Order: 100 mg Aramine in 250 mL D5W to infuse at 25 mL/hr. Calculate the following:

   a) mcg/hr ____________

   b) mcg/min ____________

Protect from light. Store container in carton until contents have been used.
Avoid storage temperatures below −20°C (−4°F) and above 40°C (104°F).
USUAL ADULT DOSAGE: See accompanying circular.
CAUTION: Federal (USA) law prohibits dispensing without prescription.
10 mL | No. 3222X 7217610
MSD NDC 0006-3222-10
10 mL INJECTION
ARAMINE®
(METARAMINOL BITARTRATE, MSD)
1% Metaraminol Equivalent
10 mg per mL
MERCK SHARP & DOHME
DIVISION OF MERCK & CO., INC.
WEST POINT, PA 19486, USA
MULTIPLE DOSE VIAL
Lot
Exp.

6. Doctor's Order: Lidocaine 2 g in 250 mL D5W to infuse at 60 mL/hr. Calculate the following:

   a) mg/hr ____________

   b) mg/min ____________

7. Doctor's Order: Aminophylline 0.25 g to be added to 250 mL of D5W. The order is to infuse over 6 hrs.

   a) Calculate the mg/hr the client will receive. ____________

Aminophylline Injection, USP 500 mg/20 mL (25 mg/mL)

8. A client is receiving Pronestyl at 30 mL/hr. The solution available is 2 g Pronestyl in 250 mL D5W. Calculate the following:

   a) mg/hr ____________

   b) mg/min ____________

9. Doctor's Order: Pitocin (oxytocin) drip at 45 microgtts/min. The solution contains 20 U Pitocin in 1000 mL D5W. Calculate the following:

   a) U/min ____________

   b) U/hr ____________

Oxytocin Label 10 USP Units/mL 1 mL

10. Doctor's Order: 30 U Pitocin (oxytocin) in 1000 mL D5W. Client is receiving oxytocin 40 mL/hr.

    a) How many U/hr of oxytocin is the client receiving? ____________

Oxytocin Label 10 USP Units/mL 1 mL

11. 30 units of Pitocin are added to 500 mL D5RL for an induction. The client is receiving 45 mL/hr.

    a) How many U/hr of Pitocin is the client receiving? __________

12. A client is receiving bretylium at 30 microgtt/min. The solution available is 2 g bretylium in 500 mL D5W. Calculate the following:

    a) mg/hr __________

    b) mg/min __________

13. A client is receiving bretylium at 45 microgtts/min. The solution available is 2 g bretylium in 500 mL D5W. Calculate the following:

    a) mg/hr __________

    b) mg/min __________

14. A client is receiving nitroglycerine 50 mg in 250 mL D5W. The order is to infuse 500 mcg/min.

    a) How many mL/hr would be needed to deliver this amount? __________

15. Dopamine has been ordered to maintain a client's b/p; 400 mg dopamine has been placed in 500 mL D5W to infuse at 35 mL/hr.

    a) How many mg are being administered per hour? __________

16. Doctor's Order: Isuprel at 30 mL/hr. The solution available is 2 mg Isuprel in 250 mL D5W. Calculate the following:

    a) mg/hr __________

    b) mcg/hr __________

    c) mcg/min __________

17. Doctor's Order: 1 g of aminophylline in 1000 mL D5W to infuse over 10 hrs.

    a) Calculate the mg/hr the client will receive. __________

18. Ritodrine (Yutopar) 150 mg is placed in 500 mL D5W to infuse at 30 mL/hr.

    a) Calculate the mg/hr the client is receiving. __________

19. A lidocaine drip is infusing at 22 mL/hr. The solution available is 2 g lidocaine in 250 mL D5W. Calculate the following:

    a) mg/hr __________

    b) mg/min __________

20. Doctor's Order: Epinephrine 8 mL/hr.
    Available: epinephrine 4 mg in 250 mL D5W.
    Calculate the following:

    a) mcg/hr ______________

    b) mcg/min ______________

21. Doctor's Order: Infuse Afronad at 30 mL/hr.
    Available: 500 mg Afronad in 250 mL NS.
    Calculate the following:

    a) mg/hr ______________

    b) mg/min ______________

22. Doctor's Order: Infuse dobutamine at 30 mL/hr. Dobutamine 500 mg is placed in 500 mL D5W.
    Calculate the following:

    a) mcg/hr ______________

    b) mcg/min ______________

23. Doctor's Order: 2 g/hr of magnesium sulfate.
    Available: 25 g of 50% magnesium sulfate in 300 mL D5W.

    a) How many mL/hr would be needed to administer the required dose? ______________

Magnesium Sulfate Injection Label
50% (1 gr/2 mL)
2 mL Vial

24. Doctor's Order: Infuse 200 mcg/min of dopamine I.V. The solution available is 400 mg dopamine in 500 mL NS. A volumetric pump is being used.

    a) Calculate the mL/hr. ______________

25. Doctor's Order: 3 g/hr of magnesium sulfate.
    Available: 25 g of 50% magnesium sulfate in 300 mL D5W.

    a) How many mL/hr would be needed to administer the required dose? __________

26. A client with chest pain has an order for nitroglycerine 10 mcg/min. Solution available is 50 mg nitroglycerine in 250 mL D5W.

    a) Calculate the I.V. rate in gtt/min using a microdrip administration set. __________

27. Doctor's Order: 2 mcg/kg/min of Nipride.
    Solution available: 50 mg Nipride in 250 mL D5W.
    Client's weight is 120 lb.

    a) Calculate the dose per minute. __________

28. Doctor's Order: Infuse 500 mL of D5W with Dobutrex 250 mg at 3 mcg/kg/min. The client weighs 80 kg.

    a) How many mcg/min should the client receive? __________

29. Doctor's Order: Infuse 500 mL D5W with 800 mg theophylline at 0.7 mg/kg/hr. The client weighs 73.5 kg.

    a) How many mg should this patient receive per hour? __________

30. Doctor's Order: Infuse 1 g of aminophylline in 1000 mL of D5W at 0.7 mg/kg/hr. The patient weighs 110 lb.

    a) Calculate the dose in mg/hr. __________

    b) Calculate the dose in mg/min. __________

    c) Reference states no more than 20 mg/min. Is the order safe? __________

31. Norepinephrine (Levophed) 2–6 mcg/min has been ordered to maintain a client's systolic blood pressure at 100. The solution is titrated at 2 mg in 500 mL D5W.

    a) Determine the flow rate setting for a volumetric pump. __________

32. Ritodrine (Yutopar) 150 mg is diluted in 500 mL of D5W. The order is to infuse at 0.15 mg/min.

    a) Calculate the flow rate to deliver this dose by volumetric pump. __________

33. Esmolol is to titrate between 50 and 75 mcg/kg/min. The client weighs 60 kg. The solution strength is 5,000 mg in 500 mL D5W.

    a) Determine the flow rate for a volumetric pump. __________

    b) The titration rate is at 30 mL/hr. What is the dose infusing per minute? __________

34. Doctor's Order: Infuse 10 mcg/kg/min of dobutamine. The solution has a concentration of 500 mg dobutamine in 250 mL D5W. The client weighs 65 kg.

    a) Calculate the flow rate in mL/hr (gtt/min). ____________

35. Aminophylline 0.25g is added to 250 mL D5W. The order is to infuse over 6 hr.

    a) Calculate the mg/hr the client will receive. ____________

36. A client is receiving lidocaine at a rate of 20 mL/hr. The solution available is 1 g lidocaine in 500 mL D5W. Calculate the following:

    a) mg/hr ____________

    b) mg/min ____________

37. A client is receiving Septra at a rate of 15 gtt/min. Tubing is microgtt. The solution available is 300 mg Septra in 500 mL D5W (based on trimethoprim). Calculate the following:

    a) mg/min ____________

    b) mg/hr ____________

Comprehensive Posttest

Directions: Solve the following calculation problems. Remember to apply the principles learned in the text relating to doses. Use labels where provided. Shade in the dose on the syringe where indicated. (See pp. 405-408.)

1. Doctor's Order: Augmentin 300 mg p.o. q8h. ____________________

   Available:

200mg/5mL
NDC 0029-6087-29
AUGMENTIN®
AMOXICILLIN/CLAVULANATE POTASSIUM
FOR ORAL SUSPENSION
When reconstituted, each 5 mL contains:
AMOXICILLIN, 200 MG, as the trihydrate
CLAVULANIC ACID, 28.5 MG, as clavulanate potassium
Caution: Federal law prohibits dispensing without prescription.
50mL (when reconstituted)
SB SmithKline Beecham

SmithKline Beecham Pharmaceuticals
Philadelphia, PA 19101

Directions for mixing: Tap bottle until all powder flows freely. Add approximately 2/3 of total water for reconstitution (total = 47 mL); shake vigorously to wet powder. Add remaining water; again shake vigorously. Keep tightly closed. Shake well before using. Must be refrigerated. Discard after 10 days. Phenylketonurics: Contains phenylalanine 7 mg per 5 mL. Net contents: Equivalent to 2 g amoxicillin and 0.285 g clavulanic acid. Use only if inner seal is intact. Store dry powder at or below 25°C (77°F).

9405808-A
EXP.
LOT Pc# 14078

Dosage: Administer every 12 hours.
See accompanying prescribing information.

2. Doctor's Order: Procan SR 1 g p.o. q6h for a client with atrial fibrillation. ____________________

   Available:

Procan SR
500 mg/100 tablets

3. Doctor's Order: Lanoxicaps 0.2 mg p.o. q.d. ____________________
   Available:

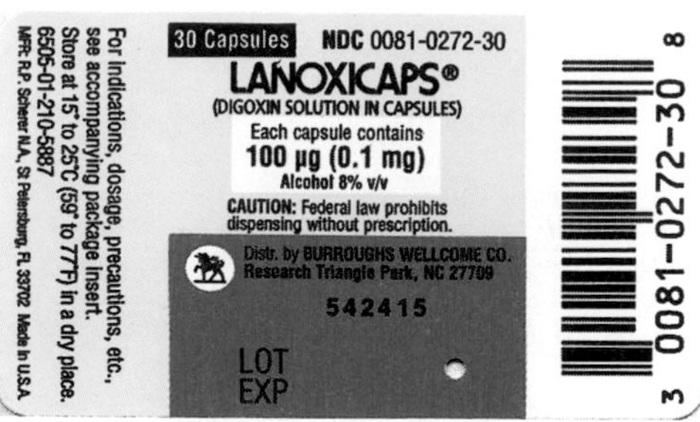

4. Doctor's Order: Septra DS 1 tab p.o. q12h × 14 days. ____________________
   Available:

100 Tablets NDC 0173-0852-55
SEPTRA® TABLETS
(trimethoprim and sulfamethoxazole)
Each scored tablet contains
80 mg trimethoprim and
400 mg sulfamethoxazole.
CAUTION: Federal law prohibits dispensing without prescription.
Glaxo Wellcome Inc.
Research Triangle Park, NC 27709
Rev. 2/96
596154
LOT
EXP
For indications, dosage, precautions, etc., see accompanying package insert.
Store at 15° to 25°C (59° to 77°F) in a dry place.
Dispense in a tight, light-resistant container as defined in the U.S.P.
Made in U.S.A. U.S. Patent No. 4,209,513 (tablet)
N 3 0173-0852-55 7
6505-00-501-6452

A

100 Tablets NDC 0173-0853-55
SEPTRA® DS
Double Strength
(trimethoprim and sulfamethoxazole)
Each scored tablet contains
160 mg trimethoprim and
800 mg sulfamethoxazole.
CAUTION: Federal law prohibits dispensing without prescription.
U.S. Patent No. 4,209,513 (Tablet)
Glaxo Wellcome Inc.
Research Triangle Park, NC 27709
595493
LOT
EXP
Store at 15° to 25°C (59° to 77°F) in a dry place.
Dispense in tight, light-resistant container as defined in the U.S.P.
For indications, dosage, precautions, etc., see accompanying package insert.
6505-01-016-1470
Rev. 5/96
Made in U.S.A.
N 3 0173-0853-55 4

B

   a) Indicate by letter which tablets you would choose to administer to the client based on the order and why. ____________________

5. Doctor's Order: Corvert 1 mg I.V. stat for a client with atrial arrhythmia; repeat in 10 minutes if arrhythmia does not terminate. ____________________
   Available:

Caution: Federal law prohibits dispensing without prescription.
See package insert for complete product information. Store at controlled room temperature (20° to 25° C or 68° to 77° F) [see USP].
Each mL contains:
Ibutilide fumarate, 0.1 mg; sodium chloride, 8.90 mg; sodium acetate trihydrate, 0.189 mg; water for injection. When necessary, pH was adjusted with sodium hydroxide and/or hydrochloric acid.
816 416 000
The Upjohn Company
Kalamazoo, MI 49001, USA

NDC 0009-3794-01 10 mL
Corvert™
Injection
ibutilide fumarate injection
0.1 mg per mL
For IV use only

6. Doctor's Order: Heparin 6,500 U s.c.o.d. (Express your answer in hundredths.) ________________
   Available:

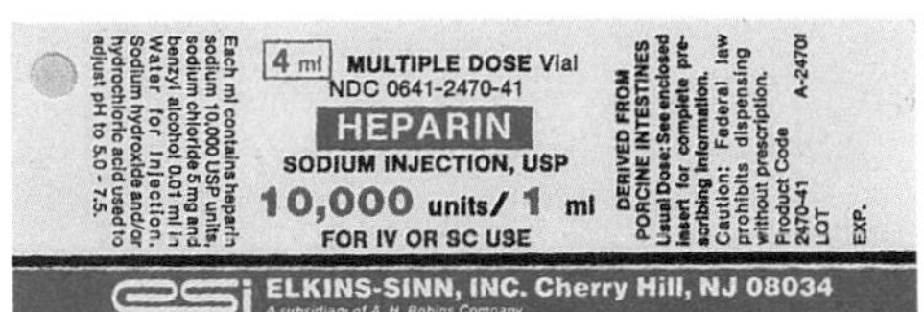

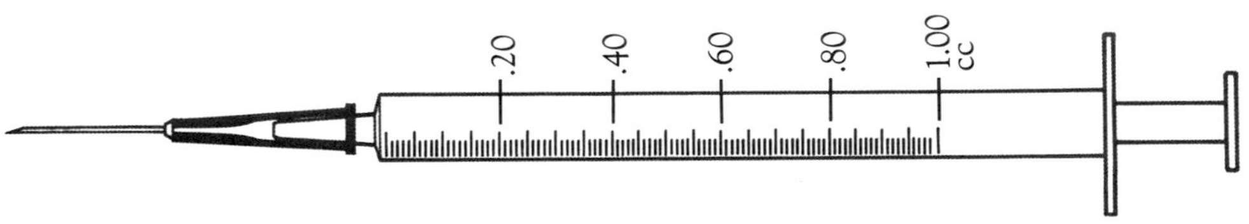

7. Doctor's Order: Cipro 0.75 g I.V. q12h × 7 days. ________________
   Available

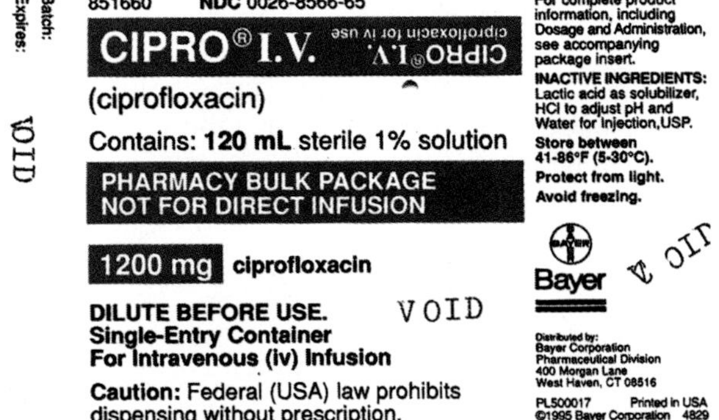

8. Doctor's Order: Amphotericin B 75 mg in 1000 mL D5W to infuse over 6 hr o.d. The reconstituted solution contains 50 mg/10 mL.
   Available:

   1 vial NDC 0003-0437-30
   NSN 6505-01-084-9453
   50 mg
   FUNGIZONE®
   INTRAVENOUS
   Amphotericin B
   for Injection USP
   FOR INTRAVENOUS INFUSION
   IN HOSPITALS ONLY
   Caution: Federal law prohibits dispensing without prescription
   Read all sides
   APOTHECON®
   A BRISTOL-MYERS SQUIBB COMPANY

   a) How many mL will you add to the I.V. solution? __________

   b) The I.V. is to infuse in 6 hr. The administration set delivers 10 gtt/mL. How many gtt/min should the I.V. infuse at? __________

9. The recommended dose of Retrovir for adults with symptomatic HIV infection is 1 mg/kg infused over 1 hour q4hr. Determine dose for a client weighing 110 lb. __________
   Available:

   20 mL Single-Use Vial NDC 0173-0107-93
   RETROVIR® (zidovudine) I.V. INFUSION Sterile
   Each mL contains 10 mg zidovudine
   FOR INTRAVENOUS INFUSION ONLY. MUST BE DILUTED FOR ADMINISTRATION.
   Dilute with 5% Dextrose Injection to a concentration no greater than 4 mg/mL. Contains no preservative. The vehicle contains Water for Injection, qs. Hydrochloric acid and/or sodium hydroxide may have been added to adjust pH.
   For indications, dosage, precautions, etc., see accompanying package insert.
   Store at 15° to 25°C (59° to 77°F) and protect from light.
   CAUTION: Federal law prohibits dispensing without prescription.
   Glaxo Wellcome Inc.
   Research Triangle Park, NC 27709 Made in U.S.A. Rev. 3/96
   U.S. Patent Nos. 4818538 (Product Patent); 4724232, 4833130, and 4837208 (Use Patents)
   587152

10. Doctor's Order: Epivir 0.3 g p.o. q.d. ____________________
    Available:

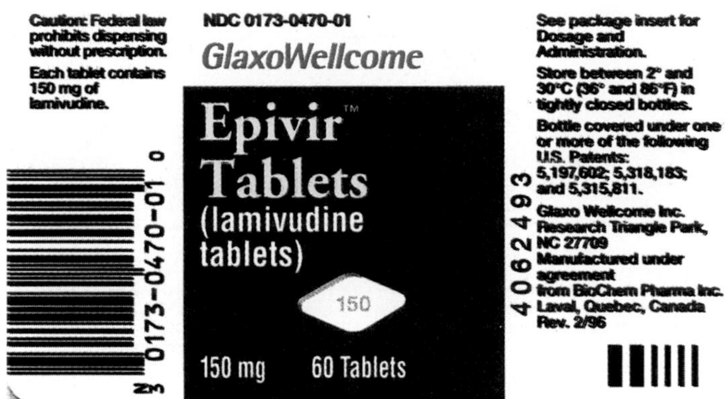

11. Doctor's Order: Tazicef 0.25 g I.V. q12h. ____________________
    Available:

Tazicef Injection Label
Available: 1 gram

Directions for reconstitution state the following for I.V. infusion: 1-g vial, add 10 mL sterile water to provide 95 mg/mL; 2-g vial, add 10 mL sterile water to provide 180 mg/mL.

a) Using the label provided, what concentration will you prepare? ____________________

b) How many mL will you administer? ____________________

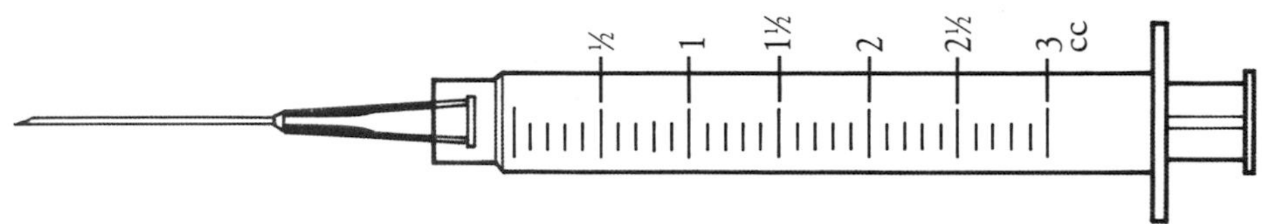

12. Doctor's Order: Thorazine 75 mg p.o. b.i.d.

Thorazine
25 mg/100 Tablets

Thorazine
50 mg/100 Tablets

a) How many of which tablets would be best to administer to the client? ______________

13. Doctor's Order: Transfuse 1 U packed red blood cells (250 mL) over 3 hr. The administration set delivers 20 gtt/mL. How many gtt/min should the I.V. infuse at? ______________

14. Doctor's Order: Lactated Ringer's solution 1000 mL to infuse at 80 mL/hr. The administration set delivers 15 gtt/mL. How many gtt/min should the I.V. infuse at? ______________

15. A client is receiving 500 mg of Flagyl IVPB q8h. The Flagyl has been placed in 100 mL D5W to infuse over 45 minutes. The administration set delivers 10 gtt/mL. How many gtt/min should the I.V. infuse at? ______________

16. Calculate the infusion time for an I.V. of 1000 mL of D5NS infusing at 60 mL/hr. Express time in hours and minutes. ______________

17. The doctor orders Septra Suspension 60 mg p.o. q12h for a child weighing 12 kg. The pediatric drug reference states that Septra Suspension contains trimethoprim (TMP) 40 mg and sulfamethoxazole (SMZ) 200 mg in 5 mL oral suspension, and the safe dose of the medication is based on trimethoprim. The safe dose is 6 to 12 mg/kg/day of TMP given q12h. Is the dose ordered safe? ______________

18. A medicated I.V. of 100 mL is to infuse at a rate of 50 mL/hr.

    a) Determine the infusion time. ________________

    b) The I.V. was started at 10:00 AM. When will it be completed? ________________

19. A client is to receive 10 mcg/min of nitroglycerine I.V. The concentration of solution is 50 mg in 250 mL D5W. What should the flow rate be (in mL/hr) to deliver 10 mcg/min? ________________

20. Doctor's Order: 6 U Humulin Regular and 16 U Humulin NPH s.c. at 7:30 AM.

    What is the total volume you will administer? ________________

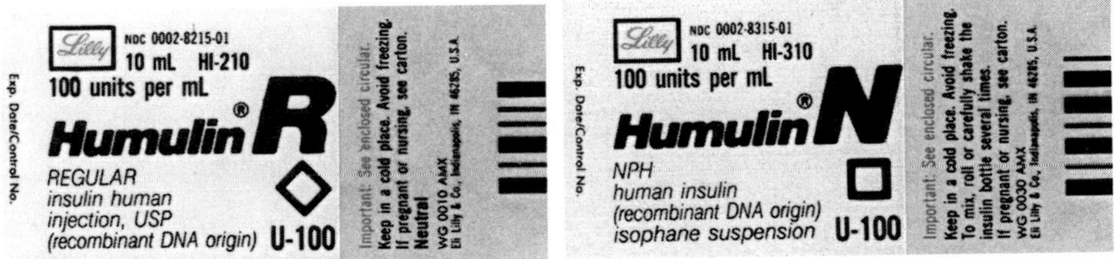

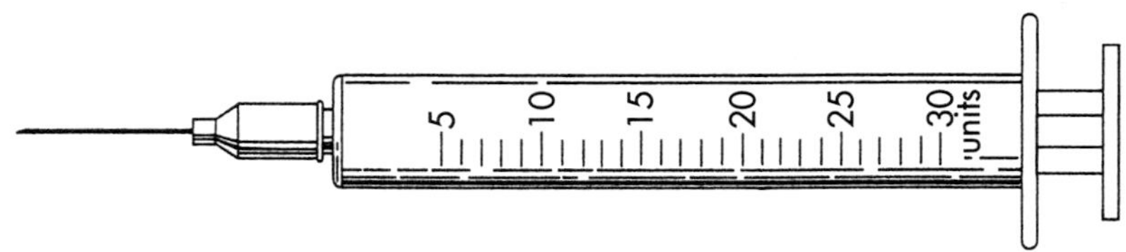

21. A dose of 500 mg in a volume of 3 mL is ordered to dilute 55 mL to infuse over 50 minutes. A 20-mL flush is to follow.

    a) What is the dilution volume? ________________

    b) How many gtt/min should the I.V. infuse at? (Administration set is a microdrip.) ________________

    c) Indicate the mL/hr. ________________

22. Doctor's Order: Augmentin 125 mg p.o. q8h. ________________
    Available:

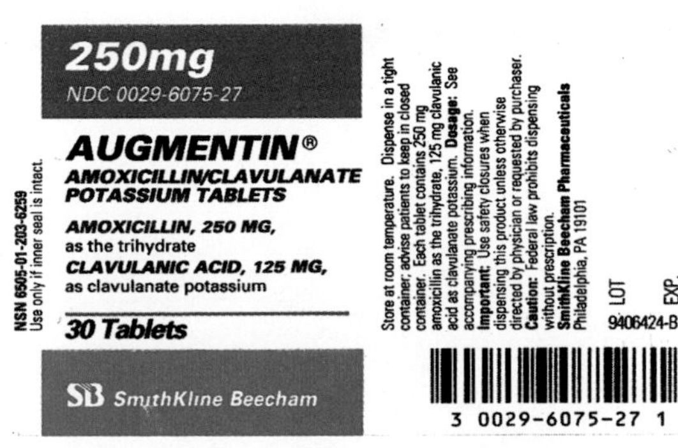

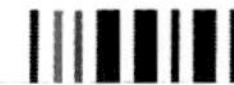

23. Calculate the BSA using the formula for a child who weighs 102 lb and is 51 inches tall. Calculate the BSA to the nearest hundredth. ____________________

24. Zovirax I.V. is to be administered to a child who has herpes simplex encephalitis. The child weighs 13.6 kg and is 60 cm tall. The recommended dose is 500 mg/m². Use the formula to calculate the BSA.

    a) What is the BSA? (nearest hundredth) ____________________

    b) What will the dose be? (nearest whole number) ____________________

    c) The reconstituted material provides 50 mg/mL. Calculate the number of mL to administer. ____________________

ZOVIRAX® STERILE POWDER 1000 mg NDC 0173-0952-01
(ACYCLOVIR SODIUM) equivalent to 1000 mg acyclovir
FOR INTRAVENOUS INFUSION ONLY
CAUTION: Federal law prohibits dispensing without prescription.
Preparation of Solution: Inject 20 mL Sterile Water for Injection into vial. Shake vial until a clear solution is achieved and use within 12 hours. DO NOT USE BACTERIOSTATIC WATER FOR INJECTION CONTAINING BENZYL ALCOHOL OR PARABENS.
Dilute to 7 mg/mL or lower prior to infusion. See package insert for additional reconstitution and dilution instructions.
For indications, dosage, precautions, etc., see accompanying package insert.
Store at 15° to 25°C (59° to 77°F).
Glaxo Wellcome Inc.
Research Triangle Park, NC 27709
U.S. Patent No. 4199574
Rev. 2/96
Made in U.S.A.
647627

25. Doctor's Order: Capoten 50 mg p.o. t.i.d. Hold if systolic blood pressure (SBP) ≤100.

    a) How many tabs will you give? ____________________

    b) The client's blood pressure is 90/60. What should the nurse do? ____________________

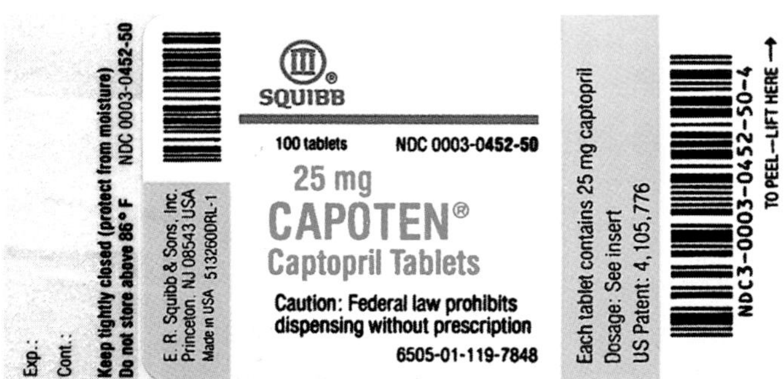

Answer Key

Answers to Pretest for Unit One

1. ix, $\overline{\text{ix}}$, IX
2. xvi, $\overline{\text{xvi}}$, XVI
3. xxiii, $\overline{\text{xxiii}}$, XXIII
4. xss, $\overline{\text{xss}}$
5. xxii, $\overline{\text{xxii}}$, XXII
6. $11\frac{1}{2}$
7. 12
8. 18
9. 24
10. 6
11. $\frac{2}{3}$
12. $\frac{1}{4}$
13. $\frac{1}{75}$
14. $\frac{4}{5}$
15. $\frac{4}{6} = \frac{2}{3}$
16. 2
17. $5\frac{1}{3}$
18. $\frac{23}{45}$
19. $4\frac{13}{42}$
20. $18\frac{2}{3}$
21. 0.9
22. 0.3
23. 0.7
24. 0.9
25. $\frac{7}{8}$
26. $\frac{11}{12}$
27. 87.45
28. 5.008
29. 40.112
30. 47.77
31. 1,875
32. 23.7
33. 36.8
34. 0.674
35. 0.375
36. 0.6
37. $x = 12$
38. $x = 2$
39. $x = 3$
40. $x = 0.5$ or $\frac{1}{2}$
41. 0.4
42. 0.7
43. 1.5
44. 0.74
45. 0.83
46. 1.23

	Percent	Decimal	Ratio	Fraction
47.	6%	0.06	3 : 50	$\frac{3}{50}$
48.	35%	0.35	7 : 20	$\frac{7}{20}$
49.	525%	5.25	21 : 4	$5\frac{1}{4}$
50.	1.5%	0.015	3 : 200	$\frac{3}{200}$

Chapter 1

Answers to Practice Problems

1. xv, $\overline{\text{xv}}$, XV
2. xiii, $\overline{\text{xiii}}$, XIII
3. xxx, $\overline{\text{xxx}}$, XXX
4. xi, $\overline{\text{xi}}$, XI
5. xvii, $\overline{\text{xvii}}$, XVII
6. xiv, $\overline{\text{xiv}}$, XIV
7. xxix, $\overline{\text{xxix}}$, XXIX
8. iv, $\overline{\text{iv}}$, IV
9. xix, $\overline{\text{xix}}$, XIX
10. xxxiv, $\overline{\text{xxxiv}}$, XXXIV

Answers to Chapter Review

1. vi, $\overline{\text{vi}}$, VI
2. xxx, $\overline{\text{xxx}}$, XXX
3. iss, $\overline{\text{iss}}$
4. xxvii, $\overline{\text{xxvii}}$, XXVII
5. xii, $\overline{\text{xii}}$, XII
6. xviii, $\overline{\text{xviii}}$, XVIII
7. xx, $\overline{\text{xx}}$, XX
8. iii, $\overline{\text{iii}}$, III
9. xxi, $\overline{\text{xxi}}$, XXI
10. xxvi, $\overline{\text{xxvi}}$, XXVI
11. $7\frac{1}{2}$
12. 19
13. 15
14. 30
15. $\frac{1}{2}$
16. 3
17. 22
18. 16
19. 5
20. 27

Chapter 2

Answers to Practice Problems

1. LCD = 30; therefore $\frac{6}{30}$ has the lesser value.
2. LCD = 8; therefore $\frac{6}{8}$ has the lesser value.
3. $\frac{1}{150}$ has the lesser value; the denominator (150) is larger.
4. $\frac{6}{18}$ has the lesser value; the numerator (6) is smaller.
5. $\frac{3}{5}$ has the lesser value; the numerator (3) is smaller.
6. $\frac{1}{8}$ has the lesser value; the numerator (1) is smaller.
7. $\frac{1}{40}$ has the lesser value; the denominator (40) is larger.
8. $\frac{1}{300}$ has the lesser value; the denominator (300) is larger.
9. $\frac{4}{24}$ has the lesser value; the numerator (4) is smaller.
10. LCD = 6; therefore $\frac{1}{6}$ has the lesser value.
11. LCD = 72; therefore $\frac{6}{8}$ has the higher value.
12. LCD = 6; therefore $\frac{7}{6}$ has the higher value.
13. LCD = 72; therefore $\frac{6}{12}$ has the higher value.

14. LCD = 120; therefore $\frac{1}{6}$ has the higher value.

15. $\frac{1}{75}$ has the higher value; the denominator (75) is smaller.

16. $\frac{6}{5}$ has the higher value; the numerator (6) is larger.

17. LCD = 24; therefore $\frac{4}{6}$ has the higher value.

18. $\frac{8}{9}$ has the higher value; the numerator (8) is larger.

19. LCD = 150; therefore $\frac{1}{10}$ has the higher value.

20. $\frac{6}{15}$ has the higher value; the denominator (6) is larger.

21. $\frac{10 \div 5}{15 \div 5} = \frac{2}{3}$

22. $\frac{7 \div 7}{49 \div 7} = \frac{1}{7}$

23. $\frac{64 \div 2}{128 \div 2} = \frac{32}{64} = \frac{1}{2}$

24. $\frac{100 \div 2}{150 \div 2} = \frac{50}{75} = \frac{2}{3}$

25. $\frac{20 \div 4}{28 \div 4} = \frac{5}{7}$

26. $\frac{14 \div 2}{98 \div 2} = \frac{7}{49} = \frac{1}{7}$

27. $\frac{10 \div 2}{18 \div 2} = \frac{5}{9}$

28. $\frac{24 \div 12}{36 \div 12} = \frac{2}{3}$

29. $\frac{10 \div 10}{50 \div 10} = \frac{1}{5}$

30. $\frac{9 \div 9}{27 \div 9} = \frac{1}{3}$

31. $\frac{9 \div 9}{9 \div 9} = \frac{1}{1} = 1$

32. $\frac{15 \div 15}{45 \div 15} = \frac{1}{3}$

33. $\frac{124 \div 31}{155 \div 31} = \frac{4}{5}$

34. $\frac{12 \div 6}{18 \div 6} = \frac{2}{3}$

35. $\frac{36 \div 4}{64 \div 4} = \frac{9}{16}$

Answers to Chapter Review

1. $1\frac{2}{8} = 1\frac{1}{4}$

2. $7\frac{2}{4} = 7\frac{1}{2}$

3. $3\frac{4}{6} = 3\frac{2}{3}$

4. $2\frac{3}{4}$

5. $4\frac{3}{14}$

6. $6\frac{7}{10}$

7. $4\frac{1}{2}$

8. $2\frac{1}{5}$

9. $4\frac{4}{15}$

10. $7\frac{9}{13}$

11. $\frac{5}{2}$

12. $\frac{59}{8}$

13. $\frac{43}{5}$

14. $\frac{65}{4}$

15. $\frac{16}{5}$

16. $\frac{13}{5}$

17. $\frac{84}{10}$

18. $\frac{37}{4}$

19. $\frac{51}{4}$

20. $\frac{47}{7}$

21. LCD = 30. $1\frac{13}{30}$

22. LCD = 24. $\frac{13}{24}$

23. LCD = 4. $\frac{88}{4} = 22$

24. LCD = 10. $\frac{7}{10}$

25. LCD = 36. $\frac{234}{36} = 6\frac{18}{36} = 6\frac{1}{2}$

26. LCD = 4. 1

27. LCD = 4. $\frac{3}{4}$

28. $2\frac{2}{4} = 2\frac{1}{2}$

29. LCD = 30. $\frac{19}{30}$

30. $\frac{1}{9}$

31. LCD = 20. $\frac{11}{20}$

32. LCD = 24. $\frac{7}{24}$

33. LCD = 6. $\frac{17}{6} = 2\frac{5}{6}$

34. LCD = 15. $\frac{19}{15} = 1\frac{4}{15}$

35. LCD = 21. $\frac{5}{21}$

36. $\frac{4}{36} = \frac{1}{9}$

37. $9\frac{11}{32}$

38. 14

39. 10

40. 27

41. $\frac{10}{16} = \frac{5}{8}$

42. $\frac{2}{30} = \frac{1}{15}$

43. $\frac{12}{120} = \frac{1}{10}$

44. $\frac{7}{27}$

45. $\frac{50}{75} = \frac{2}{3}$

46. $\frac{42}{75} = \frac{14}{25}$

47. $\frac{2}{3}$

48. 2

49. $\frac{28}{72} = \frac{7}{18}$

50. $\frac{24}{6} = 4$

51. $\frac{8}{6} = \frac{4}{3} = 1\frac{1}{3}$

52. $1\frac{25}{50} = 1\frac{1}{2}$

53. $7\frac{1}{2}$

54. $\frac{15}{300} = \frac{1}{20}$

55. 1

Chapter 3

Answers to Practice Problems

1. eight and thirty-five hundredths
2. eleven and one thousandth
3. four and fifty-seven hundredths
4. five and seven ten thousandths
5. ten and five tenths
6. one hundred sixty-three thousandths
7. 0.4
8. 84.07
9. 0.07
10. 2.23
11. 0.05
12. 0.009
13. 0.5
14. 2.87
15. 0.375
16. 0.175
17. 7.35
18. 0.087
19. 18.4
20. 40.449
21. 3.95
22. 3.87
23. 2.92
24. 43.1
25. 0.035
26. 5.88
27. 0.04725
28. 0.9125
29. 9,650
30. 1.78
31. 100.8072
32. 4
33. 1.16
34. 70.88
35. 30.46
36. 0.59
37. 3.6
38. 1
39. 2
40. 3.55
41. 0.61
42. 0.74
43. 0.0005
44. 0.00004
45. 584
46. 500
47. 0.75
48. 0.555
49. 0.5
50. $\frac{3}{4}$
51. $\frac{1}{2{,}000}$
52. $\frac{1}{25}$

Answers to Chapter Review

1. 0.444
2. 0.8
3. 1.5
4. 0.2
5. 0.725
6. 9.783
7. 28.9
8. 2.743
9. 5.12
10. 2.5
11. 6.33
12. 1.5
13. 1.5
14. 15
15. 31.2
16. 0.9448
17. 1.8

18. 0.1
19. 1.43
20. 0.15
21. 0.125
22. 0.06
23. 6.5
24. $1\frac{1}{100}$
25. $\frac{13}{200}$

Chapter 4

Answers to Chapter Review

1. 2 : 3
2. 1 : 9
3. 3 : 4
4. 1 : 5
5. 1 : 2
6. 1 : 5
7. $\frac{3}{7}$
8. $\frac{2}{3}$
9. $\frac{1}{7}$
10. $1\frac{1}{3}$
11. $\frac{3}{4}$
12. $x = 5$
13. $x = 2$
14. $x = 4$
15. $x = 3.33$ or $3\frac{1}{3}$
16. $x = 4.5$
17. $x = 0.8$ or $\frac{4}{5}$
18. $x = 1.33$ or $1\frac{1}{3}$
19. $x = 0.16$
20. $x = 0.1$
21. 1000 U : 1 mL; 1 mL : 1000 U; $\frac{1000 \text{ U}}{1 \text{ mL}}$; $\frac{1 \text{ mL}}{1000 \text{ U}}$
22. 1 tab : 0.2 mg; 0.2 mg : 1 tab; $\frac{1\text{tab}}{0.2}$ mg; $\frac{0.2 \text{ mg}}{1 \text{ tab}}$
23. 1 cap : 250 mg; 250 mg : 1 cap; $\frac{1 \text{ cap}}{250 \text{ mg}}$; $\frac{250 \text{ mg}}{1 \text{ cap}}$
24. 125 mg : 5 mL; 5 mL : 125 mg; $\frac{125 \text{ mg}}{5 \text{ mL}}$; $\frac{5 \text{ mL}}{125 \text{ mg}}$
25. 40 mg : 1 mL; 1 mL : 40 mg; $\frac{40 \text{ mg}}{1 \text{ mL}}$; $\frac{1 \text{ mL}}{40 \text{ mg}}$

Chapter 5

Answers to Practice Problems

1. 50 grams
2. 100 grams
3. 12.5 grams
4. 50 grams
5. 7.5 grams
6. $\frac{1}{100}$
7. $\frac{1}{50}$
8. $\frac{1}{2}$
9. $\frac{4}{5}$
10. $\frac{3}{100}$
11. 0.1
12. 0.35
13. 0.5
14. 0.142

15. 0.0025
16. 1 : 4
17. 11 : 100
18. 3 : 4
19. 9 : 200
20. 1 : 250
21. 40%
22. 275%
23. 50%
24. 25%
25. 70%
26. 4%
27. 75%
28. 10%
29. 1%
30. 50%

Answers to Chapter Review

	Percent	Ratio	Fraction	Decimal
1.	0.25%	1 : 400	$\frac{1}{400}$	0.0025
2.	71%	71 : 100	$\frac{71}{100}$	0.71
3.	7%	7 : 100	$\frac{7}{100}$	0.07
4.	2%	1 : 50	$\frac{1}{50}$	0.02
5.	6%	3 : 50	$\frac{3}{50}$	0.06
6.	3.3%	1 : 30	$\frac{1}{30}$	0.033
7.	61%	61 : 100	$\frac{61}{100}$	0.61
8.	0.7%	7 : 1000	$\frac{7}{1000}$	0.007
9.	5%	1 : 20	$\frac{1}{20}$	0.05
10.	2.5%	1 : 40	$\frac{1}{40}$	0.025

Answers to Posttest for Unit One

1. v, $\overline{\text{v}}$, V
2. xvii, $\overline{\text{xvii}}$, XVII
3. xxvii, $\overline{\text{xxvii}}$, XXVII
4. xxix, $\overline{\text{xxix}}$, XXIX
5. xxx, $\overline{\text{xxx}}$, XXX
6. $6\frac{1}{2}$
7. 24
8. 19
9. 25
10. 15
11. $1\frac{1}{3}$
12. $\frac{2}{3}$
13. $\frac{3}{7}$
14. $\frac{2}{3}$
15. $1\frac{3}{5}$
16. $1\frac{4}{21}$
17. $1\frac{2}{9}$
18. $25\frac{1}{3}$
19. $1\frac{22}{35}$
20. $1\frac{17}{36}$
21. 1.1
22. 0.1
23. 0.1
24. 0.9
25. $\frac{2}{3}$
26. $\frac{3}{4}$
27. 37.7
28. 17.407
29. 105.7
30. 32.94
31. 84.8
32. 22.5
33. 0.5
34. 0.850
35. 3.002
36. 0.493
37. $x = 4$
38. $x = 2.5$ or $2\frac{1}{2}$
39. $x = 0.1$ or $\frac{1}{10}$
40. $x = 4$
41. 0.6
42. 1

43. 1.4
44. 0.68
45. 0.83
46. 1.22

	Percent	Decimal	Ratio	Fraction
47.	10%	0.1	1 : 10	$\frac{1}{10}$
48.	60%	0.6	3 : 5	$\frac{3}{5}$
49.	$66\frac{2}{3}\%$	0.67	2 : 3	$\frac{2}{3}$
50.	25%	0.25	1 : 4	$\frac{1}{4}$

Chapter 6

Answers to Practice Problems

1. 0.3 g
2. 6,000 mcg
3. 700 mL
4. 0.18 mg
5. 20 mcg
6. 4,500 mL
7. 4,200 mg
8. 900 mg
9. 3.25 L
10. 0.042 kg

Answers to Chapter Review

1. gram (g), liter (L), meter (m)
2. kilogram (kg)
3. 0.001 L
4. a) L (liter), mL (milliliter), cc (cubic centimeter)

   b) g (gram), mg (milligram), mcg (microgram), kg (kilogram)
5. 1 g
6. 1 cc
7. 1 mg
8. 1 L
9. 10 mL
10. mcg or μg
11. mL
12. g
13. cc
14. 1000 times
15. the thousandth part of
16. 0.6 g
17. 50 kg
18. 0.4 mg
19. 0.04 L
20. 4.2 mcg
21. 0.005 g
22. 0.06 g
23. 2.6 mL
24. 100 mL
25. 0.03 mL
26. 0.95 mg
27. 58,500 mL
28. 130 cc
29. 276,000 mg
30. 0.55 L
31. 56,500 mL
32. 0.205 kg
33. 25 g
34. 1000 mL
35. 15 mg

Chapter 7

Answers to Chapter Review

1. gr $8\frac{1}{2}$, gr $\overline{\text{viiiss}}$
2. m 3, m $\overline{\text{iii}}$
3. dr 5, ʒ v
4. oz 8, ℥ $\overline{\text{viii}}$
5. qt
6. pt
7. gr $\frac{1}{125}$
8. fʒ viss, fʒ $\overline{\text{viss}}$, fʒ $6\frac{1}{2}$
9. f℥ ii, f℥ $\overline{\text{ii}}$, f℥ 2

10. oz 5, ℥ v, ℥ 5
11. ♏ i, ♏ i̇, ♏ 1
12. ♏ 60, ♏lx
13. fʒ $\overline{\text{viii}}$, fʒ 8
14. f℥ $\overline{\text{xvi}}$, f℥ 16
15. f℥ $\overline{\text{xxxii}}$, f℥ 32
16. f℥ $\frac{1}{2}$, f℥ ss
17. gtt
18. tablespoon
19. teaspoon
20. 5mL
21. 60 gtt
22. 8 ounces
23. 15 mL
24. 16 ounces
25. 32 ounces

Chapter 8

Answers to Practice Problems

1. 0.6 L
2. 16 mg
3. 4,000 g
4. 0.003 mg
5. 0.0003 g
6. 10 g
7. 1,900 mL
8. 0.0005 kg
9. 70 mcg
10. 0.65 L
11. 40 mg
12. 0.00012 kg
13. 0.18 g
14. 1.7 L
15. 15,000 g
16. 0.5 L
17. 4,000 g
18. 1,400 cc
19. ℥ $\frac{3}{4}$
20. ʒ ii, ʒ 2, ʒ $\overline{\text{ii}}$
21. ʒ iv, ʒ 4, ʒ $\overline{\text{iv}}$
22. $\frac{1}{6}$ tsp
23. 0.06 kg
24. 0.6 g
25. 736 mcg
26. 1.6 L
27. 15 mL
28. 180 mg
29. 0.025 mg
30. 0.0052 kg
31. 27.27 kg
32. gr $\frac{1}{4}$
33. 20 cc (25 cc if conversion is 5 cc)
34. 300 mg
35. 210 cc
36. $\frac{1}{4}$ qt
37. 3 tbs
38. 3 g
39. 90 mg
40. 3 mL
41. 1000 mg (900 mg if gr 1 = 60 mg)
42. 4,000 mL
43. 158.4 lb or 158 $\frac{2}{5}$ lb
44. 0.48 mg
45. 2,400 cc

Answers to Chapter Review

1. 7 mg
2. 0.001 g
3. 6 kg
4. 0.005 L
5. 450 cc
6. ℥ ii or ℥ 2
7. 0.2 mg
8. gr $\frac{1}{60}$
9. ʒ 3, ʒ iii, ʒ $\overline{\text{iii}}$
10. 120 mg
11. 1,500 mL
12. gr ss, gr $\overline{\text{ss}}$, gr $\frac{1}{2}$
13. 1,600 mL
14. 103.4 lb or 103$\frac{2}{5}$ lb
15. ♏ 15 or ♏ 16
16. 34.09 kg
17. 8 mg
18. ♏ 45 (♏ 48 if conversion is ♏ 16)
19. 30 mg
20. 0.4 mg
21. 6.172 kg
22. 40 tsp (50 tsp if conversion is 4 mL)
23. 46.36 kg
24. 0.204 kg
25. 1,500 cc
26. 0.2 mg
27. 48,600 cc
28. 700 cc
29. 165 mL
30. 20 cc (16 cc if conversion is 4 cc)
31. 240 mg (using gr i = 60 mg)
32. 30 mL (32 mL if conversion is 16 mL)
33. 10 mL (8 mL if conversion is 4 mL; 10 mL if conversion is 5 mL)
34. gr $\frac{3}{4}$

35. 3 g
36. 600 mL
37. 150 mg
38. 22.5 mg
39. 600 mg (gr i = 60 mg)
40. 8.8 lb or $8\frac{4}{5}$ lb
41. 3,250 mcg
42. ℥ iiss, ℥ i̅i̅ss, ℥ $2\frac{1}{2}$
43. 0.5 mg
44. 6,653 mg
45. 4,000 mg
46. 0.036 g
47. 800 mg
48. gr 135 or gr cxxxv
49. gr $\frac{1}{120}$
50. 2 L
51. 245 cc
52. 1,310 cc

Chapter 9

Answers to Chapter Review

1. drug, dose, client, route, time, documentation
2. identification band, asking the name, getting a staff member to help identify the client
3. three
4. after
5. parenteral

Chapter 10

Answers to Chapter Review

1. name of the client
2. date and time the order was written
3. name of the medication
4. dose of medication
5. route by which medication is to be administered
6. time and/or frequency of administration
7. signature of the person writing the order
8. twice a day
9. both eyes
10. as desired
11. subcutaneous
12. with
13. before meals
14. four times a day
15. twice a week
16. hour of sleep (bedtime)
17. once a day
18. elixir
19. left eye
20. syrup
21. nothing by mouth
22. sublingual
23. p.c. or pc
24. t.i.d. or tid
25. I.M. or IM
26. q.8.h. or q8h
27. supp
28. I.V. or IV
29. s.o.s. or sos
30. $\bar{s}$
31. stat or STAT
32. OD or O. D.
33. ung or oint
34. ss or $\overline{ss}$
35. mEq
36. q.h.s. or qhs
37. p.r. or pr
38. Give 0.2 milligrams of Methergine orally (by mouth) every 4 hours for six doses.
39. Give 0.125 milligrams of digoxin orally (by mouth) once a day.
40. Give 14 units of regular Humulin insulin by subcutaneous injection every day at 7:30 AM.
41. Give 50 milligrams of Demerol by intramuscular injection and $\frac{1}{150}$ grains of atropine by intramuscular injection on call to the operating room.
42. Give 500 milligrams of ampicillin orally (by mouth) immediately and then 250 milligrams orally (by mouth) four times a day thereafter.
43. Give 40 milligrams of Lasix by intramuscular injection immediately.
44. Give 50 milligrams of Librium orally (by mouth) every 4 hours when necessary for agitation.
45. Give 20 milliequivalents of potassium chloride intravenously times 2 liters. (Place 20 milliequivalents in a 1 liter bag and then another 20 milliequivalents in another 1 liter bag. Total is 2 liters, which is 2,000 milliliters.)
46. Give 10 grains of Tylenol orally (by mouth) every 4 hours whenever necessary for pain.
47. Give 80 milligrams of Mylicon orally (by mouth) after meals and at bedtime.
48. Give 1 milligram of folic acid orally (by mouth) once a day.

49. Give 100 milligrams of Nembutal orally (by mouth) at bedtime when necessary/required.
50. Give 10 grains of aspirin orally (by mouth) every 4 hours when necessary/required for temperature greater than 101° F.
51. Give 100 milligrams of Dilantin orally (by mouth) three times a day.
52. Give 2 milligrams of Minipress orally (by mouth) two times a day. Hold for systolic blood pressure less than 120.
53. Give 10 milligrams of Compazine by intramuscular injection every 4 hours as needed/required for nausea and vomiting.
54. Give 1 gram of ampicillin intravenous piggyback every 6 hours for 4 doses.
55. Give 5,000 units of heparin by subcutaneous injection every 12 hours.
56. Give 200 milligrams of Dilantin suspension every morning and 300 milligrams at bedtime (hour of sleep) through a nasogastric tube.
57. Give 50 milligrams of Benadryl orally (by mouth) immediately.
58. Give 1000 micrograms of vitamin B_{12} by intramuscular injection three times a week.
59. Give 1 ounce of milk of magnesia orally (by mouth) at bedtime (hour of sleep) whenever necessary (as needed).
60. Give 1 double-strength tablet of Septra orally (by mouth) every day.
61. Apply 1 percent Neomycin ophthalmic ointment to the right eye three times a day.
62. Give 1 gram of Carafate by nasogastric tube four times a day.
63. Give 15 milligrams of morphine sulfate by subcutaneous injection immediately and 10 milligrams by subcutaneous injection every 4 hours when necessary (as needed).
64. Give 120 milligrams of ampicillin by intravenous Soluset every 6 hours for 7 days.
65. Give 10 milligrams of prednisone orally (by mouth) every other day.
66. route of administration
67. frequency/time interval of administration
68. dose of medication (drug)
69. name of medication (drug)
70. dose of medication (drug) and route of administration

Chapter 11

Answers to Practice Problems

1. 0730
2. 1030
3. 2010
4. 1745
5. 0016
6. 2:07 AM
7. 5:43 PM
8. 12:04 AM

Answers to Practice Exercise 1 (Reading of Medication Record, Figure 11-6)

Date

4/6/92	**Medication**	**Dosage**	**Route**	**Time**
	Procardia	10 mg	p.o.	5 PM

Date

4/8/92

	Medication	Dosage	Route	Time
1.	Digoxin	0.25 mg	p.o.	9 AM
2.	Lasix	20 mg	p.o.	9 AM, 5 PM
3.	Procardia	10 mg	p.o.	9 AM, 1 PM, 5 PM
4.	Colace	100 mg	p.o.	9 AM, 5 PM
5.	Heparin	5,000 U	s.c.	9 AM

Answer to Practice Exercise 2 (Figure 11-7)

MONTEFIORE MEDICAL CENTER
JACK D. WEILER HOSPITAL OF THE ALBERT EINSTEIN COLLEGE OF MEDICINE DIVISION

STANDING ORDERS MEDICATION RECORD

INIT.	SIGNATURE	INIT.	SIGNATURE	INIT.	SIGNATURE
DG	Deborah C. Gray				

Addressograph with Client Identification

ADDRESSOGRAPH

DRUG SENSITIVITIES ☒ NONE KNOWN

☐ PATIENT DISCHARGED

	MEDICATIONS	DATE 4/9/92 TIME AND INITIALS	DATE TIME AND INITIALS	DATE TIME AND INITIALS	DATE TIME AND INITIALS	DATE TIME AND INITIALS	DATE TIME AND INITIALS	DATE TIME AND INITIALS
1	DRUG: Potassium Chloride; DOSE: 20mEq; FREQUENCY: od; ADMINISTRATION TIMES: 10A; ROUTE: p.o.; DATE ORDERED: 4-9-92	10A						
2	DRUG: Digoxin; DOSE: 0.125mg; FREQUENCY: od; ADMINISTRATION TIMES: 10A; ROUTE: p.o.; DATE ORDERED: 4-9-92	10A						
3	DRUG: Lasix; DOSE: 30 mg; FREQUENCY: b.i.d; ADMINISTRATION TIMES: 10A - 6P; ROUTE: p.o.; DATE ORDERED: 4-9-92	10A 6P						
4	DRUG: Aldomet; DOSE: 500mg; FREQUENCY: bid.; ADMINISTRATION TIMES: 10A - 6P; ROUTE: p.o.; DATE ORDERED: 4-9-92	10A 6P.						
5	DRUG: Restoril; DOSE: 30mg; FREQUENCY: H.S.; ADMINISTRATION TIMES: 10P; ROUTE: p.o.; DATE ORDERED: 4-9-92	10P						
6	DRUG: ; DOSE: ; FREQUENCY: ; ADMINISTRATION TIMES: ; ROUTE: ; DATE ORDERED:							

STANDING ORDERS

Answer to Practice Exercise 2 (Figure 11-8)

MONTEFIORE MEDICAL CENTER
HOSPITAL OF THE ALBERT EINSTEIN COLLEGE OF MEDICINE DIVISION
PRE-OP, STAT AND PRN MEDICATION RECORD

ADDRESSOGRAPH

INIT.	SIGNATURE	INIT.	SIGNATURE	INIT.	SIGNATURE
DG	Deborah C. Gray				

DRUG SENSITIVITIES ☐ NONE KNOWN

☐ PATIENT DISCHARGED

SEND 2ND COPY TO PHARMACY WHEN COMPLETED

PRE-OP AND STAT

MEDICATIONS	DATE 4-9-92	DATE	DATE	DATE	DATE	DATE	DATE
	TIME AND INITIALS	TIME AND INITIALS	TIME AND INITIALS	TIME AND INITIALS	TIME AND INITIALS	TIME AND INITIALS	TIME AND INITIALS

PRN

#	DRUG	DOSE	FREQUENCY	ADMINISTRATIVE TIMES	ROUTE	DATE ORDERED	4-9-92
1	Tylenol	650 mg.	q4h	prn T > 38²	p.o.	4-9-92	
2	Percocet	2 tabs	q3-4h x 2days	prn pain	p.o.	4-9-92	2p DG
3							
4							
5							
6							

Chapter 12

Answers to Chapter Review

1. Generic name: prazosin hydrochloride

   Trade name: Minipress

   Form: capsules

   Dose strength: 1 mg per capsule

2. Generic name: digoxin

   Trade name: Lanoxin

   Total volume: 2 mL

   Form: injectable

   Dose strength: 500 mg (0.5 mg) in 2 mL, 250 mg (0.25 mg)/mL

3. Generic name: dexamethasone, MSD

   Trade name: Decadron

   Form: tablets

   Dose strength: 0.25 mg per tablet

4. Generic name: gentamicin sulfate

   Trade name: Garamycin

   Total volume: 20 mL

   Form: injectable

   Dose strength: 40 mg/mL

   Instructions: should not be physically premixed with other drugs

5. Generic name: digitoxin

   Trade name: Crystodigin

   Form: tablets

   Dose strength: 0.1 mg per tablet

6. Generic name: levothyroxine sodium

   Trade name: Synthroid

   Form: tablets

   Dose strength: 50 mcg per tablet, 0.05 mg per tablet

7. Generic name: penicillin V potassium

   Trade name: V-Cillin K

   Total volume: 100 mL

   Dose strength: 125 mg/5 mL, 200,000 U/5 mL

   Directions for storage: 59° to 86° F (15° to 30° C). Store in refrigerator after mixing.

8. Generic name: potassium chloride

   Trade name: none

   Form: injectable

   Dose strength: 2 mEq/mL

9. Generic name: docusate calcium

   Trade name: Surfak

   Form: capsules

   Dose strength: 50 mg per capsule

10. Generic name: streptomycin sulfate

    Trade name: none

    Form: injectable (I.M. use only)

    Directions for mixing: The dry powder is dissolved by adding 9 mL water, USP or sodium chloride for injection.

    Dose strength after reconstitution: 400 mg/mL.

    Storage instructions: In dry form store below 86° F (30° C). Protect reconstituted solution from light, may store at room temperature for 4 weeks.

11. Generic name: lamivudine

    Trade name: Epivir

    Total volume: 240 mL

    Form: oral solution

    Dose strength: 10 mg/mL

12. Generic name: acyclovir sodium

    Trade name: Zovirax

    Directions for mixing: Inject 20 mL sterile water for injection into vial. Shake vial until a clear solution is achieved and use within 12 hours. Do not use bacteriostatic water for injection containing benzyl alcohol or Parabens.

    Storage: Store at 15° to 25° C (59° to 77° F)

    Form: injectable (I.V. infusion only)

    Dose strength: 1000 mg/20 mL

13. Generic name: ranitidine hydrochloride

    Trade name: Zantac

    NDC number: 0173-0363-00

    Form: injectable

    Dose strength: 25 mg/mL

14. Generic name: ciprofloxacin hydrochloride

    Trade name: Cipro

    Amount: 50 tablets

    Form: tablets

    Dose strength: 750 mg per tablet

15. Generic name: amphotericin B

    Trade name: Fungizone

    Form: injectable (I.V. only)

    Drug manufacturer: Apothecon

16. Generic name: medroxyprogesterone acetate

    Trade name: Depo-Provera

    Form: injectable

    Dose strength: 150 mg/mL

    Use: contraceptive (intramuscular use only)

17. Generic name: medroxyprogesterone acetate

    Trade name: Depo-Provera

    Dose strength: 400 mg/mL

    Directions for use: for intramuscular use only

18. Generic name: diltiazem hydrochloride (HCL)

    Trade name: Cardizem

    Amount: 100 tablets

    Form: tablets

    Dose strength: 120 mg/per tablet

19. Generic name: ibutilide fumarate

    Trade name: Corvert

    Directions for use: for I.V. use only

    Form: Injectable (intravenous infusion only)

    Dose strength: 0.1 mg/mL

20. Generic name: heparin sodium

    Trade name: none

    Directions for use: s.c. or I.V. use

    Dose strength: 1000 U/mL

    Total volume: 30 mL

Chapter 13

Answers to Practice Problems

1. Less than 1 tab
2. More than 1 tab
3. Less than 1 tab
4. More than 1 tab
5. More than 1 tab

Answers to Problems Using Ratio-Proportion

6. $5 \text{ mg} : 1 \text{ tab} = 7.5 \text{ mg} : x \text{ tab}$

$$\frac{5x}{5} = \frac{7.5}{5}$$

$$x = \frac{7.5}{5}$$

OR

$$\frac{5 \text{ mg}}{1 \text{ tab}} = \frac{7.5 \text{ mg}}{x \text{ tab}}$$

$$\frac{5x}{5} = \frac{7.5}{5}$$

$x = 1.5$ tabs or $1\frac{1}{2}$ tabs (5 mg is smaller than 7.5 mg; therefore you will need more than 1 tab to administer the dose.)

7. equivalent: 60 mg = gr 1 (gr $\frac{1}{4}$ = 15 mg)

$$15 \text{ mg} : 1 \text{ tab} = 15 \text{ mg} : x \text{ tab}$$

$$\frac{15x}{15} = \frac{15}{15}$$

$$x = \frac{15}{15}$$

OR

$$\frac{15 \text{ mg}}{1 \text{ tab}} = \frac{15 \text{ mg}}{x \text{ tab}}$$

$$\frac{15x}{15} = \frac{15}{15}$$

$$x = \frac{15}{15}$$

$x = 1$ tab (15 mg is equal to 1 tab)

8. equivalent: 60 mg = gr 1

$$\left(\text{gr } 1\frac{1}{2} = 90 \text{ mg}\right)$$

$$100 \text{ mg} : 1 \text{ caps} = 90 \text{ mg} : x \text{ caps}$$

$$\frac{100x}{100} = \frac{90}{100}$$

$$x = \frac{90}{100}$$

OR

$$\frac{100 \text{ mg}}{1 \text{ caps}} = \frac{90 \text{ mg}}{x \text{ caps}}$$

$$\frac{100x}{100} = \frac{90}{100}$$

$$x = \frac{90}{100}$$

$x = 1$ caps. It would be impossible to administer 0.9 of a capsule. A 10% margin of difference is allowed between what is ordered and what is administered. Using this 10% safety margin, no more than 110 mg and no less than 90 mg may be given. The doctor ordered gr iss (90 mg). The capsules available are 100 mg. Capsules are not dividable. Administering 1 caps is within the 10% margin of difference allowed.

9. 0.5 mg : 1 cc = 0.25 mg : x cc

$$\frac{0.5x}{0.5} = \frac{0.25}{0.5}$$

$$x = \frac{0.25}{0.5}$$

OR

$$\frac{0.5 \text{ mg}}{1 \text{ cc}} = \frac{0.25 \text{ mg}}{x \text{ cc}}$$

$$\frac{0.5x}{0.5} = \frac{0.25}{0.5}$$

$$x = \frac{0.25}{0.5}$$

$x = 0.5$ cc, $\frac{1}{2}$ cc (0.25 mg is less than 0.5 mg; you will need less than 1 cc to administer the dose.)

10. gr $\frac{3}{4}$: 1 cc = gr $\frac{1}{4}$: x cc

$$\frac{\frac{3}{4}x}{\frac{3}{4}} = \frac{\frac{1}{4}}{\frac{3}{4}}$$

$$x = \frac{1}{4} \div \frac{3}{4} = \frac{1}{4} \times \frac{4}{3} = \frac{4}{12} = \frac{1}{3}$$

OR

$$\frac{\text{gr } \frac{3}{4}}{1 \text{ cc}} = \frac{\text{gr } \frac{1}{4}}{x \text{ cc}}$$

$$\frac{\frac{3}{4}x}{\frac{3}{4}} = \frac{\frac{1}{4}}{\frac{3}{4}}$$

$$x = \frac{\frac{1}{4}}{\frac{3}{4}}$$

$$x = \frac{1}{4} \div \frac{3}{4} = \frac{1}{4} \times \frac{4}{3} = \frac{4}{12} = \frac{1}{3}$$

$x = 0.33 = 0.3$ cc (gr $\frac{1}{4}$ is less than gr $\frac{3}{4}$; therefore you will need less than 1 cc to administer the dose.)

11. 40 mEq : 10 cc = 20 mEq : x cc

$$\frac{40x}{40} = \frac{200}{40}$$

$$x = \frac{200}{40}$$

OR

$$\frac{40 \text{ mEq}}{10 \text{ cc}} = \frac{20 \text{ mEq}}{x \text{ cc}}$$

$$\frac{40x}{40} = \frac{200}{40}$$

$x = 5$ cc (20 mEq is less than 40 mEq; you will need less than 10 cc to administer the dose.)

12. 10,000 U : 1 cc = 5,000 U : x cc

$$\frac{10{,}000x}{10{,}000} = \frac{5{,}000}{10{,}000}$$

$$x = \frac{5{,}000}{10{,}000}$$

OR

$$\frac{10{,}000 \text{ U}}{1 \text{ cc}} = \frac{5{,}000 \text{ U}}{x \text{ cc}}$$

$$\frac{10{,}000x}{10{,}000} = \frac{5{,}000}{10{,}000}$$

$$x = \frac{5{,}000}{10{,}000}$$

$x = 0.5$ cc, $\frac{1}{2}$ cc (10,000 U is more than 5,000 U; therefore you will need less than 1 cc to administer the dose.)

13. 80 mg : 2 cc = 50 mg : x cc

$$\frac{80x}{80} = \frac{100}{80}$$

$$x = \frac{100}{80}$$

OR

$$\frac{80 \text{ mg}}{2 \text{ cc}} = \frac{50 \text{ mg}}{x \text{ cc}}$$

$$\frac{80x}{80} = \frac{100}{80}$$

$$x = \frac{100}{80}$$

$x = 1.25 = 1.3$ cc (50 mg is less than 80 mg; therefore you will need less than 2 cc to administer the dose.)

14. equivalent : 1000 mg = 1 g (0.5 g = 500 mg)

250 mg : 1 caps = 500 mg : x caps

$$\frac{250x}{250} = \frac{500}{250}$$

$$x = \frac{500}{250}$$

OR

$$\frac{250 \text{ mg}}{1 \text{ caps}} = \frac{500 \text{ mg}}{x \text{ caps}}$$

$$\frac{250x}{250} = \frac{500}{250}$$

$x = 2$ caps (500 mg is more than 250 mg; therefore you will need more than 1 caps to administer the dose.)

15. 125 mg : 5 cc = 400 mg : x cc

$$\frac{125x}{125} = \frac{2{,}000}{125}$$

$$x = \frac{2{,}000}{125}$$

OR

$$\frac{125 \text{ mg}}{5 \text{ cc}} = \frac{400 \text{ mg}}{x \text{ cc}}$$

$$\frac{125x}{125} = \frac{2{,}000}{125}$$

$$x = \frac{2{,}000}{125}$$

$x = 16$ cc (400 mg is larger than 125 mg; therefore you will need more than 5 cc to administer the dose.)

16. 80 mg : 1 mL = 50 mg : x mL

$$\frac{80x}{80} = \frac{50}{80}$$

$$x = \frac{50}{80}$$

OR

$$\frac{80 \text{ mg}}{1 \text{ mL}} = \frac{50 \text{ mg}}{x \text{ mL}}$$

$$\frac{80x}{80} = \frac{50}{80}$$

$$x = \frac{50}{80}$$

$x = 0.62 = 0.6$ mL (50 mg is less than 80 mg; therefore you will need less than 1 mL to administer the dose.)

17. gr$\overline{ss}$: 1 mL = gr 1 : x mL

gr $\frac{1}{2}$: 1 mL = gr 1 : x mL

$$\frac{\frac{1}{2}x}{\frac{1}{2}} = \frac{1}{\frac{1}{2}}$$

$$x = 1 \div \frac{1}{2} = 1 \times \frac{2}{1}$$

$$\frac{2}{1} = 2$$

OR

$$\frac{\text{gr}\overline{\text{ss}}}{1 \text{ mL}} = \frac{\text{gr } 1}{x \text{ mL}} \left(\frac{\text{gr } \frac{1}{2}}{1 \text{ mL}} = \frac{\text{gr } 1}{x \text{ mL}} \right)$$

$$\frac{\frac{1}{2}x}{\frac{1}{2}} = \frac{1}{\frac{1}{2}}$$

$$x = \frac{1}{\frac{1}{2}}$$

$$x = 1 \div \frac{1}{2} = 1 \times \frac{2}{1}$$

$$\frac{2}{1} = 2$$

$x = 2$ mL (gr$\overline{ss}$ is less than gr 1; therefore you will need more than 1 mL to administer the dose.)

18. gr v : 1 tab = gr xv : x tab

gr 5 : 1 tab = gr 15 : x tab

$$\frac{5x}{5} = \frac{15}{5}$$

$$x = \frac{15}{5}$$

OR

$$\frac{\text{gr } 5}{1 \text{ tab}} = \frac{\text{gr } 15}{x \text{ tab}}$$

$$\frac{5x}{5} = \frac{15}{5}$$

$x = 3$ tabs (gr 15 is more than gr 5; therefore you will need more than 1 tab to administer the dose.)

19. $\text{gr } \frac{1}{150} : 1 \text{ tab} = \text{gr } \frac{1}{300} : x \text{ tab}$

$$\frac{\frac{1}{150}x}{\frac{1}{150}} = \frac{\frac{1}{300}}{\frac{1}{150}}$$

$$x = \frac{1}{300} \div \frac{1}{150} = \frac{1}{300} \times \frac{150}{1}$$

$$x = \frac{150}{300}$$

$$x = 0.5$$

OR

$$\frac{\text{gr } \frac{1}{150}}{1 \text{ tab}} = \frac{\text{gr } \frac{1}{300}}{x \text{ tab}}$$

$$\frac{\frac{1}{150}x}{\frac{1}{150}} = \frac{\frac{1}{300}}{\frac{1}{150}}$$

$$x = \frac{1}{300} \div \frac{1}{150} = \frac{1}{300} \times \frac{150}{1}$$

$$x = \frac{150}{300}$$

$x = 0.5$ tab or $\frac{1}{2}$ tab (gr $\frac{1}{150}$ is larger than gr $\frac{1}{300}$; therefore you will need less than 1 tab to administer the dose.)

20. $\text{gr } \frac{1}{4} : 1 \text{ mL} = \text{gr } \frac{1}{6} : x \text{ mL}$

$$\frac{\frac{1}{4}x}{\frac{1}{4}} = \frac{\frac{1}{6}}{\frac{1}{4}}$$

$$x = \frac{1}{6} \div \frac{1}{4} = \frac{1}{6} \times \frac{4}{1} = \frac{4}{6} = \frac{2}{3}$$

OR

$$\frac{\text{gr } \frac{1}{4}}{1 \text{ mL}} = \frac{\text{gr } \frac{1}{6}}{x \text{ mL}} = \frac{\frac{1}{4}x}{\frac{1}{4}} = \frac{\frac{1}{6}}{\frac{1}{4}}$$

$$x = \frac{1}{6} \div \frac{1}{4} = \frac{1}{6} \times \frac{4}{1} = \frac{4}{6} = \frac{2}{3}$$

$$\begin{array}{r} 0.66 \\ 3\,\overline{)2.00} \\ -\,18 \\ \hline 20 \end{array}$$

$x = 0.66 = 0.7$ mL (gr $\frac{1}{4}$ is larger than gr $\frac{1}{6}$; therefore you will need less than 1 mL to administer the dose.)

21. $0.5 \text{ mg} : 2 \text{ mL} = 0.125 \text{ mg} : x \text{ mL}$

$$\frac{0.5}{0.5}x = \frac{0.25}{0.5}$$

$$x = \frac{0.25}{0.5}$$

OR

$$\frac{0.5 \text{ mg}}{2 \text{ mL}} = \frac{0.125}{x \text{ mL}}$$

$$\frac{0.5x}{0.5} = \frac{0.25}{0.5}$$

$x = 0.5$ mL, $\frac{1}{2}$ mL. (0.125 mg is less than 0.5 mg; therefore you will need less than 2 mL to administer the dose.)

22. $0.25 \text{ mg} : 1 \text{ mL} = 0.75 \text{ mg} : x \text{ mL}$

$$\frac{0.25x}{0.25} = \frac{0.75}{0.25}$$

$$x = \frac{0.75}{0.25}$$

OR

$$\frac{0.25 \text{ mg}}{1 \text{ mL}} = \frac{0.75 \text{ mg}}{x \text{ mL}}$$

$$\frac{0.25x}{0.25} = \frac{0.75}{0.25}$$

$x = 3$ mL (0.75 mg is more than 0.25 mg; therefore you will need more than 1 mL to administer the dose.)

23. $125 \text{ mg} : 5 \text{ mL} = 375 \text{ mg} : x \text{ mL}$

$$\frac{125x}{125} = \frac{375 \times 5}{125}$$

$$x = \frac{1875}{125}$$

OR

$$\frac{125 \text{ mg}}{5 \text{ mL}} = \frac{375 \text{ mg}}{x \text{ mL}}$$

$$\frac{125x}{125} = \frac{375 \times 5}{125}$$

$x = 15$ mL (375 mg is more than 125 mg; therefore you will need more than 5 mL to administer the dose.)

24. 7,500 U : 1 mL = 10,000 U : x mL

$$\frac{7{,}500x}{7{,}500} = \frac{10{,}000}{7{,}500}$$

$$x = \frac{10{,}000}{7{,}500}$$

OR

$$\frac{7{,}500 \text{ U}}{1 \text{ mL}} = \frac{10{,}000 \text{ U}}{x \text{ mL}}$$

$$\frac{7{,}500x}{7{,}500} = \frac{10{,}000}{7{,}500}$$

$x = 1.33 = 1.3$ mL (10,000 U is more than 7,500 U; therefore you will need more than 1 mL to administer the dose.)

25. 0.3 mg : 1 tab = 0.45 mg : x tab

$$\frac{0.3x}{0.3} = \frac{0.45}{0.3}$$

$$x = \frac{0.45}{0.3}$$

OR

$$\frac{0.3 \text{ mg}}{1 \text{ tab}} = \frac{0.45 \text{ mg}}{x \text{ tab}}$$

$$\frac{0.3x}{0.3} = \frac{0.45}{0.3}$$

$x = 1.5$ tab or $1\frac{1}{2}$ tab (0.45 mg is more than 0.3 mg; therefore you will need more than 1 tab to administer the dose.)

Chapter 13

Answers to Chapter Review Part I

1. 1 tab
2. 1 caps
3. 2 caps
4. 2 tabs
5. 2 tabs
6. 0.5 tab or $\frac{1}{2}$ tab
7. 1 tab
8. 1 tab
9. 1 tab
10. 1 tab
11. 2 caps
12. 1 tab
13. 2 caps
14. 2 caps
15. 2 tabs
16. 1 tab
17. 2 caps
18. 2 caps
19. 1 tab
20. 2 tabs
21. 0.5 tab or $\frac{1}{2}$ tab
22. 1 tab
23. 2 tabs
24. 2 caps
25. 1 caps
26. 3 tabs
27. 1 tab

Answers to Chapter Review Part II

28. 4 mL
29. 20 mL
30. 1.3 mL
31. 10 mL
32. 0.7 mL
33. 2.3 mL
34. 1 mL
35. 1 mL
36. 0.66 mL
37. 7.5 mL
38. 1 mL
39. 0.5 mL
40. 0.5 mL
41. 10 mL
42. 0.75 mL
43. 1.1 mL
44. 0.5 mL
45. 0.5 mL
46. 0.8 mL
47. 4 mL
48. 6 mL
49. 6.3 mL
50. 0.8 mL
51. 20 mL
52. 30 mL
53. 40 mL
54. 10 mL
55. 1 mL

Chapter 14

Answers to Chapter Review

1. $$\frac{\text{gr } \frac{1}{150}}{\text{gr } \frac{1}{300}} \times 1 \text{ tab} = x \text{ tab}$$

$$\frac{1}{150} \div \frac{1}{300} = \frac{1}{150} \times \frac{300}{1} = \frac{300}{150} = 2$$

$x = 2$ tabs (gr $\frac{1}{300}$ is smaller than gr $\frac{1}{150}$; therefore you will need more than 1 tab to administer the dose.)

OR

$$\frac{\text{gr } \frac{1}{150}}{\text{gr } \frac{1}{300}} = \frac{x \text{ tab}}{1 \text{ tab}}$$

$$\frac{\frac{1}{300}x}{\frac{1}{300}} = \frac{1}{150} \div \frac{1}{300}$$

$$x = \frac{1}{150} \div \frac{1}{300} = \frac{1}{150} \times \frac{300}{1} = \frac{300}{150} = 2$$

2. equivalent: 1000 mg = 1 g

(0.75 g = 750 mg)

$$\frac{750 \text{ mg}}{250 \text{ mg}} \times 1 \text{ caps} = x \text{ caps}$$

$x = 3$ caps (750 mg is larger than 250 mg; therefore you will need more than 1 caps to administer the dose.)

OR

$$\frac{750 \text{ mg}}{250 \text{ mg}} = \frac{x \text{ caps}}{1 \text{ caps}}$$

$$\frac{250x}{250} = \frac{750}{250}$$

$$x = \frac{750}{250} = 3$$

3. $$\frac{90 \text{ mg}}{60 \text{ mg}} \times 1 \text{ tab} = x \text{ tabs}$$

$x = 1.5$ or $1\frac{1}{2}$ tabs (90 is larger than 60 mg; therefore you will need more than 1 tab to administer the dose.)

OR

$$\frac{90 \text{ mg}}{60 \text{ mg}} = \frac{x \text{ tab}}{1 \text{ tab}}$$

$$\frac{60x}{60} = \frac{90}{60}$$

$$x = \frac{90}{60} = 1.5$$

4. $$\frac{7.5 \text{ mg}}{2.5 \text{ mg}} \times 1 \text{ tab} = x \text{ tabs}$$

$x = 3$ tabs (7.5 mg is larger than 2.5 mg; therefore you will need more than 1 tab to administer the dose.)

OR

$$\frac{7.5 \text{ mg}}{2.5 \text{ mg}} = \frac{x \text{ tab}}{1 \text{ tab}}$$

$$\frac{2.5x}{2.5} = \frac{7.5}{2.5}$$

$$x = \frac{7.5}{2.5}$$

5. equivalent: 1000 mcg = 1 mg

(0.05 mg = 50 mcg)

$$\frac{50 \text{ mcg}}{25 \text{ mcg}} \times 1 \text{ tab} = x \text{ tabs}$$

$x = 2$ tabs (50 mcg is larger than 25 mcg; therefore you will need more than 1 tab to administer the dose.)

OR

$$\frac{50 \text{ mcg}}{25 \text{ mcg}} = \frac{x \text{ tab}}{1 \text{ tab}}$$

$$\frac{25x}{25} = \frac{50}{25}$$

$$x = \frac{50}{25} = 2$$

6. $$\frac{40 \text{ mg}}{80 \text{ mg}} \times 2 \text{ mL} = x \text{ mL}$$

$x = 1$ mL (40 mg is one half of the dose available; you will need less than 2 mL to administer the dose.)

OR

$$\frac{40 \text{ mg}}{80 \text{ mg}} = \frac{x \text{ mL}}{2 \text{ mL}}$$

$$\frac{80x}{80} = \frac{80}{80}$$

$$x = \frac{80}{80} = 1$$

7. $\frac{4{,}500\text{ U}}{5{,}000\text{ U}} \times 1\text{ mL} = x\text{ mL}$

$$\frac{4{,}500}{5{,}000} = x$$

$x = 0.9$ mL (4,500 U is less than 5,000 U; you will need less than 1 mL to administer the dose.)

OR

$$\frac{4{,}500\text{ U}}{5{,}000\text{ U}} = \frac{x\text{ mL}}{1\text{ mL}}$$

$$\frac{5{,}000x}{5{,}000} = \frac{4{,}500}{5{,}000}$$

$$x = \frac{4{,}500}{5{,}000} = 0.9$$

8. equivalent: 60 mg = gr 1

$$\left(\text{gr } \frac{1}{200} = 0.3\text{ mg}\right)$$

$$\frac{0.3\text{ mg}}{0.3\text{ mg}} \times 1\text{ mL} = x\text{ mL}$$

$x = 1$ mL (0.3 mg is equal to 1 mL; therefore you will need 1 mL to administer the dose.)

OR

$$\frac{0.3\text{ mg}}{0.3\text{ mg}} = \frac{x\text{ mL}}{1\text{ mL}}$$

$$\frac{0.3x}{0.3} = \frac{0.3}{0.3}$$

$$x = \frac{0.3}{0.3} = 1$$

9. $\frac{0.75\text{ mg}}{0.25\text{ mg}} \times 1\text{ mL} = x\text{ mL}$

$x = 3$ mL (0.75 mg is larger than 0.25 mg; you will need more than 1 mL to administer the dose.)

OR

$$\frac{0.75\text{ mg}}{0.25\text{ mg}} = \frac{x\text{ mL}}{1\text{ mL}}$$

$$\frac{0.25x}{0.25} = \frac{0.75}{0.25}$$

10. equivalent: 60 mg = gr 1

$$\left(\text{gr } \frac{1}{6} = 10\text{ mg}\right)$$

$$\frac{10\text{ mg}}{15\text{ mg}} \times 1\text{ mL} = x\text{ mL}$$

$x = 0.66 = 0.7$ mL (10 mg is less than 15 mg; you will need less than 1 mL to administer the dose.)

OR

$$\frac{10\text{ mg}}{15\text{ mg}} = \frac{x\text{ mL}}{1\text{ mL}}$$

$$\frac{15x}{15} = \frac{10}{15}$$

$$x = \frac{10}{15} = 0.66$$

11. 1 tab
12. 1 tab
13. 2 caps
14. 1 tab
15. 2 tabs
16. $1\frac{1}{2}$ tabs or 1.5 tabs
17. 1 caps
18. 1 caps
19. 2 caps
20. 2 tabs
21. $1\frac{1}{2}$ tabs or 1.5 tabs
22. 2 caps
23. 1 tab
24. 3 tabs
25. 2 caps
26. 0.7 mL
27. 1 mL
28. 0.4 mL
29. 12 mL
30. 7.5 mL or $7\frac{1}{2}$ mL
31. 11.3 mL
32. 0.6 mL
33. 2 mL
34. 1.8 mL
35. 10 mL
36. 0.8 mL
37. 2 mL

38. 0.6 mL
39. 0.8 mL
40. 0.5 mL or $\frac{1}{2}$ mL
41. 0.3 mL
42. 1 mL
43. 2 mL
44. 3.2 mL
45. 5 mL
46. 1 tab
47. 1 tab
48. 2 caps (pulvules)
49. 5 mL
50. 1 tab
51. 2 tabs
52. 1.3 mL
53. 2 mL
54. 3 mL
55. 2 tabs

Chapter 15

Answers to Practice Problems on Tablets and Capsules

The answers to the practice problems include the rationale for the answer where indicated. Where necessary, the methods for calculation of the dose are shown as well. Note: In problems that required a conversion before calculating the dose, the problem setup shown illustrates the problem after appropriate conversions have been made.

1. 0.025 mg = 25 mcg
   50 mcg : 1 tab = 25 mcg : x tab

   OR

   $$\frac{25\text{ mcg}}{50\text{ mcg}} \times 1\text{ tab} = x\text{ tab}; \frac{25\text{ mcg}}{50\text{ mcg}} = \frac{x\text{ tab}}{1\text{ tab}}$$

   Answer: 0.5 or $\frac{1}{2}$ tab. This is an acceptable answer since the tabs are scored. (For administration purposes state as $\frac{1}{2}$ tab.)

2. 25 mg : 1 tab = 6.25 mg : x tab

   OR

   $$\frac{6.25\text{ mg}}{25\text{ mg}} \times 1\text{ tab} = x\text{ tab}; \frac{6.25\text{ mg}}{25\text{ mg}} = \frac{x\text{ tab}}{1\text{ tab}}$$

   Answer: $\frac{1}{4}$ tab. This is logical since the tablets are scored in quarters; therefore you could accurately administer the dose.

3. Conversion is necessary: 1000 mg = 1 g.

   Therefore 1.2 g = 1,200 mg

   400 mg : 1 tab = 1,200 mg : x tab

   OR

   $$\frac{1{,}200\text{ mg}}{400\text{ mg}} \times 1\text{ tab} = x\text{ tab}; \frac{1{,}200\text{ mg}}{400\text{ mg}} = \frac{x\text{ tab}}{1\text{ tab}}$$

   Answer: 3 tabs. The dose ordered is greater than what is available. You will need more than 1 tab to administer the dose. The maximum number of tabs that can be given is 3.

4. It would be best to administer one of the 5-mg tablets and one of the 2.5-mg tablets (5 mg + 2.5 mg = 7.5 mg).

5. a) 125-mcg tablet is the appropriate strength to use (0.125 mg = 125 mcg).

   b) 1 tab. Even though the tablets are scored, $\frac{1}{2}$ of 500 mcg would still be twice the dose desired.

   125 mcg : 1 tab = 125 mcg : x tab

   OR

   $$\frac{125\text{ mcg}}{125\text{ mcg}} \times 1\text{ tab} = x\text{ tab}; \frac{125\text{ mcg}}{125\text{ mcg}} = \frac{x\text{ tab}}{1\text{ tab}}$$

   Answer: 1 tab

6. a) 500-mg caps would be appropriate to use.

   b) 2 caps (500 mg each). 1000 mg = 1 g; therefore 2 caps of 500 mg each would be the least number of capsules. Using the 250-mg strength capsules would require 4 caps.

   c) 2 caps q6h = 8 caps. Multiplying the number of caps needed by the number of days gives you the number of capsules required.

   8 (number of caps per day) $\times$ 7 (number of days) = 56 (total caps needed)

   500 mg : 1 caps = 1000 mg : x caps

   $$\frac{1000\text{ mg}}{500\text{ mg}} \times 1\text{ caps} = x\text{ caps}; \frac{1000\text{ mg}}{500\text{ mg}} = \frac{x\text{ caps}}{1\text{ caps}}$$

   x = 2 caps $\qquad$ x = 2 caps

7. 5 mg : 1 tab = 10 mg : x tab

$$\frac{10 \text{ mg}}{5 \text{ mg}} \times 1 \text{ tab} = x \text{ tab}; \frac{10 \text{ mg}}{5 \text{ mg}} = \frac{x \text{ tab}}{1 \text{ tab}}$$

Answer: 2 tabs. The dose ordered is greater than what is available. You will need more than 1 tab to administer the dose.

8. a) $1\frac{1}{2}$ tabs; the tablets are scored. (State as $1\frac{1}{2}$ tabs for administration purposes.)

10 mg : 1 tab = 15 mg : x tab

$$\frac{15 \text{ mg}}{10 \text{ mg}} \times 1 \text{ tab} = x \text{ tab}; \frac{15 \text{ mg}}{10 \text{ mg}} = \frac{x \text{ tab}}{1 \text{ tab}}$$

$$x = 1\frac{1}{2} \text{ tab} \qquad x = 1\frac{1}{2} \text{ tab}$$

b) 15 mg × 3 (t.i.d.) = 45 mg/day. The total number of mg received for 3 days = 135 mg.

45 mg × 3 = 135 mg

9. 0.075 mg = 75 mcg

50 mcg : 1 tab = 75 mcg : x tab

OR

$$\frac{75 \text{ mg}}{50 \text{ mg}} \times 1 \text{ tab} = x \text{ tab}; \frac{75 \text{ mg}}{50 \text{ mg}} = \frac{x \text{ tab}}{1 \text{ tab}}$$

Answer: 1.5 or $1\frac{1}{2}$ tabs, since the tabs are scored. (State as $1\frac{1}{2}$ tabs for administration purposes.)

10. 1.3 g = 1,300 mg

650 mg : 1 tab = 1,300 mg : x tab

OR

$$\frac{1{,}300 \text{ mg}}{650 \text{ mg}} \times 1 \text{ tab} = x \text{ tab}; \frac{1{,}300 \text{ mg}}{650 \text{ mg}} = \frac{x \text{ tab}}{1 \text{ tab}}$$

Answer: 2 tabs. The dose ordered is more than what is available; therefore more than 1 tab will be needed to administer the dose.

11. No conversion is necessary.

30 mg : 1 caps = 90 mg : x caps

$$\frac{30x}{30} = \frac{90}{30}$$

OR

$$\frac{90 \text{ mg}}{30 \text{ mg}} \times 1 \text{ caps} = x \text{ caps}; \frac{90 \text{ mg}}{30 \text{ mg}} = \frac{x \text{ caps}}{1 \text{ caps}}$$

Answer: 3 caps. The dose ordered is greater than what is available. You will need more than 1 caps to administer the dose.

12. No conversion is necessary.

100 mg : 1 tab = 200 mg : x tab

$$\frac{100x}{100} = \frac{200}{100}$$

OR

$$\frac{200 \text{ mg}}{100 \text{ mg}} \times 1 \text{ tab} = x \text{ tab}; \frac{200 \text{ mg}}{100 \text{ mg}} = \frac{x \text{ tab}}{1 \text{ tab}}$$

Answer: 2 tabs. The dose ordered is greater than what is available. More than 1 tab will be needed to administer the dose.

13. a) 2 caps (1 g = 1000 mg)

500 mg × 2 = 1000 mg.

b) 1 caps (500 mg = 0.5 g)

1 caps of 500 mg

Initial dose: 500 mg : 1 caps = 1000 mg : x caps

Answer: 2 caps.

OR

$$\frac{1000 \text{ mg}}{500 \text{ mg}} \times 1 \text{ caps} = x \text{ caps};$$

$$\frac{1000 \text{ mg}}{500 \text{ mg}} = \frac{x \text{ caps}}{1 \text{ caps}}$$

Daily dose: 500 mg : 1 caps = 500 mg : x caps

OR

$$\frac{500 \text{ mg}}{500 \text{ mg}} \times 1 \text{ caps} = x \text{ caps};$$

$$\frac{500 \text{ mg}}{500 \text{ mg}} = \frac{x \text{ caps}}{1 \text{ caps}}$$

Answer: 1 caps

14. No conversion is necessary.

125 mg : 1 tab = 250 mg : x tab

OR

$$\frac{250 \text{ mg}}{125 \text{ mg}} \times 1 \text{ tab} = x \text{ tab}; \frac{250 \text{ mg}}{125 \text{ mg}} = \frac{x \text{ tab}}{1 \text{ tab}}$$

Answer: 2 tabs. The dose ordered is more than what is available. Therefore you will need more than 1 tab to administer the dose.

15. gr iss = 90 mg

a) 30-mg tablets

b) three 30-mg tablets. This strength will allow the client to take 3 tabs to achieve the desired dose, as opposed to six 15-mg tabs. This dose is logical since the maximum number of tablets administered is three.

30 mg : 1 tab = 90 mg : x tab

OR

$$\frac{90 \text{ mg}}{30 \text{ mg}} \times 1 \text{ tab} = x \text{ tab}; \frac{90 \text{ mg}}{30 \text{ mg}} = \frac{x \text{ tab}}{1 \text{ tab}}$$

Answer: 3 30 mg tabs

16. No conversion is needed.

The best strength to use is 1.5 mg. This would allow the client to swallow the least amount. 1.5 mg : 1 tab = 3 mg : x tab

OR

$$\frac{3 \text{ mg}}{1.5 \text{ mg}} \times 1 \text{ tab} = x \text{ tab}; \frac{3 \text{ mg}}{1.5 \text{ mg}} = \frac{x \text{ tab}}{1 \text{ tab}}$$

Answer: 2 1.5 mg tabs would be the least number of tablets; 0.75 mg would require the client to swallow 4 tabs to receive the dose ($0.75 \times 4 = 3$).

17. 50 mg : 1 tab = 100 mg : x tab

OR

$$\frac{100 \text{ mg}}{50 \text{ mg}} \times 1 \text{ tab} = x \text{ tab}; \frac{100 \text{ mg}}{50 \text{ mg}} = \frac{x \text{ tab}}{1 \text{ tab}}$$

Answer: You need 2 tabs to administer 100 mg.

2 tabs t.i.d. (3 times a day) = 6 tabs × 3 days = 18 tabs

18. It would be best to administer 1 of the 80-mg tablets and 1 of the 40-mg tablets (80 + 40 = 120 mg). This would be the least number of tablets.

19. The conversion to use here is 65 mg = gr 1.

gr x = 650 mg

325 mg : 1 tab = 650 mg : x tab

OR

$$\frac{650 \text{ mg}}{325 \text{ mg}} \times 1 \text{ tab} = x \text{ tab}; \frac{650 \text{ mg}}{325 \text{ mg}} = \frac{x \text{ tab}}{1 \text{ tab}}$$

Answer: 2 tabs. The dose ordered is larger than the required dose; therefore more than 1 tab will be required.

20. 0.5 mg : 1 tab = 1 mg : x tab

OR

$$\frac{1 \text{ mg}}{0.5 \text{ mg}} \times 1 \text{ tab} = x \text{ tab}; \frac{1 \text{ mg}}{0.5 \text{ mg}} = \frac{x \text{ tab}}{1 \text{ tab}}$$

$x = 2$ tabs $\qquad x = 2$ tabs

Answer: 2 tabs ($0.5 \times 2 = 1$)

21. 1 mg : 1 caps = 3 mg : x caps

OR

$$\frac{3 \text{ mg}}{1 \text{ mg}} \times 1 \text{ caps} = x \text{ caps}; \frac{3 \text{ mg}}{1 \text{ mg}} = \frac{x \text{ caps}}{1 \text{ caps}}$$

Answer: 3 caps. They are administered in whole numbers. The answer is logical. The maximum number of tablets or capsules administered is three.

22. Equivalent: 60 mg = gr 1. Therefore

$$\text{gr } \frac{1}{150} = 0.4 \text{ mg}$$

0.4 mg : 1 tab = 0.4 mg : x tab

OR

$$\frac{0.4 \text{ mg}}{0.4 \text{ mg}} \times 1 \text{ tab} = x \text{ tab}; \frac{0.4 \text{ mg}}{0.4 \text{ mg}} = \frac{x \text{ tab}}{1 \text{ tab}}$$

Answer: 1 tab. The label indicates gr $\frac{1}{150}$ = 0.4 mg. Therefore only 1 tab is needed to administer the dose.

23. Choose the 6-mg tab and give 1 tab, which allows the client to swallow the least number of tabs without scoring.

6 mg : 1 tab = 6 mg : x tab

OR

$$\frac{6 \text{ mg}}{6 \text{ mg}} \times 1 \text{ tab} = x \text{ tab}; \frac{6 \text{ mg}}{6 \text{ mg}} = \frac{x \text{ tab}}{1 \text{ tab}}$$

Answer: 1 6 mg tab

24. Conversion is required. Equivalent: 1000 mg = 1 g; therefore 0.2 g = 200 mg

100 mg : 1 tab = 200 mg : x tab

OR

$$\frac{200 \text{ mg}}{100 \text{ mg}} \times 1 \text{ tab} = x \text{ tab}; \frac{200 \text{ mg}}{100 \text{ mg}} = \frac{x \text{ tab}}{1 \text{ tab}}$$

Answer: 2 tabs: The dose ordered is larger than what is available, therefore more than 1 tab is needed.

25. 40 mg : 1 tab = 60 mg : x tab

OR

$$\frac{60 \text{ mg}}{40 \text{ mg}} \times 1 \text{ tab} = x \text{ tab}; \frac{60 \text{ mg}}{40 \text{ mg}} = \frac{x \text{ tab}}{1 \text{ tab}}$$

Answer: $1\frac{1}{2}$ tabs or 1.5 tabs. The tabs are scored, so 1 tab can be broken to administer the dose. (State as $1\frac{1}{2}$ tabs for administration purposes.)

26. No conversion is needed.

$$5 \text{ mg} : 1 \text{ tab} = 2.5 \text{ mg} : x \text{ tab}$$

OR

$$\frac{2.5 \text{ mg}}{5 \text{ mg}} \times 1 \text{ tab} = x \text{ tab}; \frac{2.5 \text{ mg}}{5 \text{ mg}} = \frac{x \text{ tab}}{1 \text{ tab}}$$

Answer: 0.5 tab or $\frac{1}{2}$ tab. This is an acceptable answer (0.5 tab or $\frac{1}{2}$ tab) since the tablets are scored. The dose ordered is less than what is available. You will need less than 1 tab to administer the required dose. (State as $\frac{1}{2}$ tab for administration purposes.)

27. No conversion is needed.

$$200 \text{ mg} : 1 \text{ tab} = 400 \text{ mg} : x \text{ tab}$$

OR

$$\frac{400 \text{ mg}}{200 \text{ mg}} \times 1 \text{ tab} = x \text{ tab}; \frac{400 \text{ mg}}{200 \text{ mg}} = \frac{x \text{ tab}}{1 \text{ tab}}$$

Answer: 2 tabs. The dose ordered is more than what is available. You will need more than 1 tab to administer the dose.

28. No conversion is needed.

$$75 \text{ mg} : 1 \text{ cap} = 150 \text{ mg} : x \text{ cap}$$

OR

$$\frac{150 \text{ mg}}{75 \text{ mg}} \times 1 \text{ cap} = x \text{ cap}; \frac{150 \text{ mg}}{75 \text{ mg}} = \frac{x \text{ cap}}{1 \text{ cap}}$$

Answer: 2 caps. The dose ordered is more than what is available. You will need more than 1 cap to administer the dose.

29. Change 1 g to 1000 mg (1000 mg = 1 g)

$$500 \text{ mg} : 1 \text{ tab} = 1000 \text{ mg} : x \text{ tab}$$

OR

$$\frac{1000 \text{ mg}}{500 \text{ mg}} \times 1 \text{ tab} = x \text{ tab}; \frac{1000 \text{ mg}}{500 \text{ mg}} = \frac{x \text{ tab}}{1 \text{ tab}}$$

Answer: 2 tabs. The dose ordered is greater than what is available. You will need more than 1 tab to administer the dose.

30. $25 \text{ mg} : 1 \text{ tab} = 12.5 \text{ mg} : x \text{ tab}$

OR

$$\frac{12.5 \text{ mg}}{25 \text{ mg}} \times 1 \text{ tab} = x \text{ tab}; \frac{12.5 \text{ mg}}{25 \text{ mg}} = \frac{x \text{ tab}}{1 \text{ tab}}$$

Answer: 0.5 tab or $\frac{1}{2}$ tab (2 quarters). The dose ordered is less than what is available. You will need less than 1 tab to administer the dose.

(State as $\frac{1}{2}$ tab for administration purposes.)

31. It would be best to administer one 75-mcg tablet and one 25-mcg tablet for a total of 100 mcg. This would be the least number of tablets (75 mcg + 25 mcg = 100 mcg).

32. $12.5 \text{ mg} : 1 \text{ tab} = 6.25 \text{ mg} : x \text{ tab}$

OR

$$\frac{6.25 \text{ mg}}{12.5 \text{ mg}} \times 1 \text{ tab} = x \text{ tab}; \frac{6.25 \text{ mg}}{12.5 \text{ mg}} = \frac{x \text{ tab}}{1 \text{ tab}}$$

Answer: 0.5 tab or $\frac{1}{2}$ (2 quarters). This is an acceptable answer since the tablet is scored in quarters. The better answer for administration purposes is $\frac{1}{2}$ tab.

33. $0.5 \text{ mg} : 1 \text{ tab} = 0.25 \text{ mg} : x \text{ tab}$

OR

$$\frac{0.25 \text{ mg}}{0.5 \text{ mg}} \times 1 \text{ tab} = x \text{ tab}; \frac{0.25 \text{ mg}}{0.5 \text{ mg}} = \frac{x \text{ tab}}{1 \text{ tab}}$$

Answer: 0.5 tab or $\frac{1}{2}$ tab. This is an acceptable answer since the tablet is scored. (State answer as $\frac{1}{2}$ tab for administration purposes.)

34. Conversion is necessary: 1000 mg = 1 g; therefore 0.25 g = 250 mg

$$250 \text{ mg} : 1 \text{ tab} = 250 \text{ mg} : x \text{ tab}$$

OR

$$\frac{250 \text{ mg}}{250 \text{ mg}} \times 1 \text{ tab} = x \text{ tab}; \frac{250 \text{ mg}}{250 \text{ mg}} = \frac{x \text{ tab}}{1 \text{ tab}}$$

Answer: 1 tab. 0.25 g = 250 mg, which is equal to 1 tab.

35. No conversion is necessary: Label indicates 0.025 mg = 25 mcg.

$$25 \text{ mcg} : 1 \text{ tab} = 25 \text{ mcg} : x \text{ tab}$$

OR

$$\frac{25 \text{ mcg}}{25 \text{ mcg}} \times 1 \text{ tab} = x \text{ tab}; \frac{25 \text{ mcg}}{25 \text{ mcg}} = \frac{x \text{ tab}}{1 \text{ tab}}$$

Answer: 1 tab. 0.025 mg is equal to 25 mcg. Therefore only 1 tab is needed to administer the dose.

36. 325 mg : 1 tab = 650 mg : x tab

OR

$$\frac{650 \text{ mg}}{325 \text{ mg}} \times 1 \text{ tab} = x \text{ tab}; \frac{650 \text{ mg}}{325 \text{ mg}} = \frac{x \text{ tab}}{1 \text{ tab}}$$

Answer: 2 tabs. The dose ordered is greater than what is available; you will need more than 1 tab to administer the dose.

37. Conversion is necessary. 1000 mg = 1 g; therefore 0.2 g = 200 mg

100 mg : 1 cap = 200 mg : x cap

OR

$$\frac{200 \text{ mg}}{100 \text{ mg}} \times 1 \text{ cap} = x \text{ cap}; \frac{200 \text{ mg}}{100 \text{ mg}} = \frac{x \text{ cap}}{1 \text{ cap}}$$

Answer: 2 caps. The dose ordered is greater than what is available. You will need more than 1 caps to administer the dose.

38. 400 mg : 1 tab = 800 mg : x tab

OR

$$\frac{800 \text{ mg}}{400 \text{ mg}} \times 1 \text{ tab} = x \text{ tab}; \frac{800 \text{ mg}}{400 \text{ mg}} = \frac{x \text{ tab}}{1 \text{ tab}}$$

Answer: 2 tabs. The dose ordered is greater than what is available. You will need more than 1 tab to administer the dose.

39. 30 mg : 1 tab = 60 mg : x tab

$$\frac{60 \text{ mg}}{30 \text{ mg}} \times 1 \text{ tab} = x \text{ tab}; \frac{60 \text{ mg}}{30 \text{ mg}} = \frac{x \text{ tab}}{1 \text{ tab}}$$

Answer: 2 tabs. The dose ordered is greater than what is available. You will need more than 1 tab to administer the dose.

40. Conversion: 1000 mg = 1 g. Therefore 0.3 g = 300 mg

100 mg : 1 tab = 300 mg : x tab

OR

$$\frac{300 \text{ mg}}{100 \text{ mg}} \times 1 \text{ tab} = x \text{ tab}; \frac{300 \text{ mg}}{100 \text{ mg}} = \frac{x \text{ tab}}{1 \text{ tab}}$$

Answer: 3 tabs. The dose ordered is greater than what is available. You will need more than 1 tab to administer the dose. Three tablets is the maximum number of tablets that should be given.

41. 80 mg : 1 cap = 160 mg : x cap

OR

$$\frac{160 \text{ mg}}{80 \text{ mg}} \times 1 \text{ cap} = x \text{ cap}; \frac{160 \text{ mg}}{80 \text{ mg}} = \frac{x \text{ cap}}{1 \text{ cap}}$$

Answer: 2 caps. The dose ordered is greater than what is available. You will need more than 1 cap to administer the dose.

Answers to Practice Problems on Oral Liquids

Note: The setup shown for problems that required conversions reflect converting of what the doctor ordered to what is available.

42. 20 mg : 5 mL = 100 mg : x mL

OR

$$\frac{100 \text{ mg}}{20 \text{ mg}} \times 5 \text{ mL} = x \text{ mL}; \frac{100 \text{ mg}}{20 \text{ mg}} = \frac{x \text{ mL}}{5 \text{ mL}}$$

Answer: 25 mL. In order to administer the dose required, more than 5 mL will be necessary. The dosage ordered is 5 times larger than what the available strength is.

43. Conversion is required. Equivalent: 1g = 1000 mg

500 mg : 10 mL = 1000 mg : x mL

OR

$$\frac{1000 \text{ mg}}{500 \text{ mg}} \times 10 \text{ mL} = x \text{ mL};$$

$$\frac{1000 \text{ mg}}{500 \text{ mg}} = \frac{x \text{ mL}}{10 \text{ mL}}$$

Answer: 20 mL. To administer the required dose, which is 2 times larger than the strength it is available in, more than 10 mL is required.

44. 40 mEq : 15 mL = 40 mEq : x mL

OR

$$\frac{40 \text{ mEq}}{40 \text{ mEq}} \times 15 \text{ mL} = x \text{ mL};$$

$$\frac{40 \text{ mEq}}{40 \text{ mEq}} = \frac{x \text{ mL}}{15 \text{ mL}}$$

Answer: 15 mL. The dose ordered is contained in 15 mL of the medication.

45. 80 mg : 15 mL = 120 mg : x mL

OR

$$\frac{120\text{ mg}}{80\text{ mg}} \times 15\text{ mL} = x\text{ mL};$$

$$\frac{120\text{ mg}}{80\text{ mg}} = \frac{x\text{ mL}}{15\text{ mL}}$$

Answer: 22.5 mL or 22½ mL. To administer the dose required, more than 15 mL will be necessary.

46. 200 mg : 5 mL = 250 mg : x mL

OR

$$\frac{250\text{ mg}}{200\text{ mg}} \times 5\text{ mL} = x\text{ mL}; \frac{250\text{ mg}}{200\text{ mg}} = \frac{x\text{ mL}}{5\text{ mL}}$$

Answer: 6.3 mL. The dose ordered is greater than what is available. The answer to the nearest tenth is 6.3 mL

47. 125 mg : 5 mL = 100 mg : x mL

OR

$$\frac{100\text{ mg}}{125\text{ mg}} \times 5\text{ mL} = x\text{ mL}; \frac{100\text{ mg}}{125\text{ mg}} = \frac{x\text{ mL}}{5\text{ mL}}$$

Answer: 4 mL. The amount ordered is less than what is available, so less than 5 mL will be needed to administer the required dose.

48. Use the mcg equivalent to calculate the dose.

50 mcg : 1 mL = 125 mcg : x mL

OR

$$\frac{125\text{ mcg}}{50\text{ mcg}} \times 1\text{ mL} = x\text{ mL};$$

$$\frac{125\text{ mcg}}{50\text{ mcg}} = \frac{x\text{ mL}}{1\text{ mL}}$$

Answer: 2.5 mL or $2\frac{1}{2}$ mL. ($2\frac{1}{2}$ mL is preferred for administration purposes.) The dose ordered is larger than what is available so you will need more than 1 mL to administer the dose.

49. 125 mg : 5 mL = 250 mg : x mL

OR

$$\frac{250\text{ mg}}{125\text{ mg}} \times 5\text{ mL} = x\text{ mL}; \frac{250\text{ mg}}{125\text{ mg}} = \frac{x\text{ mL}}{5\text{ mL}}$$

Answer: 10 mL. The dose ordered is more than what is available. You will need more than 5 mL to administer the dose.

50. Conversion is required. Equivalent: 1000 mg = 1 g.

Therefore 0.5 g = 500 mg

125 mg : 5 mL = 500 mg : x mL

OR

$$\frac{500\text{ mg}}{125\text{ mg}} \times 5\text{ mL} = x\text{ mL}; \frac{500\text{ mg}}{125\text{ mg}} = \frac{x\text{ mL}}{5\text{ mL}}$$

Answer: 20 mL. The dose ordered is 4 times larger than the available strength; therefore more than 5 mL will be needed to administer the dose.

51. 20 mg : 5 mL = 60 mg : x mL

$$\frac{20x}{20} = \frac{300}{20}$$

OR

$$\frac{60\text{ mg}}{20\text{ mg}} \times 5\text{ mL} = x\text{ mL}; \frac{60\text{ mg}}{20\text{ mg}} = \frac{x\text{ mL}}{5\text{ mL}}$$

Answer: 15 mL. The dose ordered is more than what is available. You will need more than 5 mL to administer the dose.

52. 30 mg : 1 mL = 150 mg : x mL

OR

$$\frac{150\text{ mg}}{30\text{ mg}} \times 1\text{ mL} = x\text{ mL}; \frac{150\text{ mg}}{30\text{ mg}} = \frac{x\text{ mL}}{1\text{ mL}}$$

Answer: 5 mL. The dose ordered is 5 times larger than the available strength. You will need more than 1 mL to administer the required dose.

53. 12.5 mg : 5 mL = 25 mg : x mL

OR

$$\frac{25\text{ mg}}{12.5\text{ mg}} \times 5\text{ mL} = x\text{ mL};$$

$$\frac{25\text{ mg}}{12.5\text{ mg}} = \frac{x\text{ mL}}{5\text{ mL}}$$

Answer: 10 mL. The dose needed is 2 times more than the available strength, so you will need more than 5 mL to administer the required dose.

54. The label indicates that 5 mL = 300 mg of the medication.

$$300 \text{ mg} : 5 \text{ mL} = 600 \text{ mg} : x \text{ mL}$$

OR

$$\frac{600 \text{ mg}}{300 \text{ mg}} \times 5 \text{ mL} = x \text{ mL}; \frac{600 \text{ mg}}{300 \text{ mg}} = \frac{x \text{ mL}}{5 \text{ mL}}$$

a) 10 mL. The dose ordered is 2 times more than the available strength. You will need more than 5 mL to administer the required dose.

b) Two containers are needed. One container delivers 300 mg.

55. $2 \text{ mg} : 1 \text{ mL} = 10 \text{ mg} : x \text{ mL}$

OR

$$\frac{10 \text{ mg}}{2 \text{ mg}} \times 1 \text{ mL} = x \text{ mL}; \frac{10 \text{ mg}}{2 \text{ mg}} = \frac{x \text{ mL}}{1 \text{ mL}}$$

Answer: 5 mL. The dose ordered is 5 times greater than the available strength. More than 1 mL will be needed to administer the required dose.

56. Conversion is required. Equivalent: 1000 mg = 1 g.

Therefore 0.5 g = 500 mg.

$$62.5 \text{ mg} : 5 \text{ mL} = 500 \text{ mg} : x \text{ mL}$$

OR

$$\frac{500 \text{ mg}}{62.5 \text{ mg}} \times 5 \text{ mL} = x \text{ mL};$$

$$\frac{500 \text{ mg}}{62.5 \text{ mg}} = \frac{x \text{ mL}}{5 \text{ mL}}$$

Answer: 40 mL. The dose ordered is larger than the available strength. You will need more than 5 mL to administer the required dose.

57. $200{,}000 \text{ U} : 5 \text{ mL} = 500{,}000 \text{ U} : x \text{ mL}$

OR

$$\frac{500{,}000 \text{ U}}{200{,}000 \text{ U}} \times 5 \text{ mL} = x \text{ mL};$$

$$\frac{500{,}000 \text{ U}}{200{,}000 \text{ U}} = \frac{x \text{ mL}}{5 \text{ mL}}$$

Answer: 12.5 mL or $12\frac{1}{2}$ mL. The amount ordered is greater than the strength available, you will need more than 5 mL to administer the required dose.

58. Conversion is required. Equivalent: 1g = 1000 mg.

$$125 \text{ mg} : 5 \text{ mL} = 1000 \text{ mg} : x \text{ mL}$$

OR

$$\frac{1000 \text{ mg}}{125 \text{ mg}} \times 5 \text{ mL} = x \text{ mL};$$

$$\frac{1000 \text{ mg}}{125 \text{ mg}} = \frac{x \text{ mL}}{5 \text{ mL}}$$

Answer: 40 mL. The dose ordered is more than the strength available. You will need more than 5 mL to administer the dose.

59. $16 \text{ mg} : 5 \text{ mL} = 24 \text{ mg} : x \text{ mL}$

OR

$$\frac{24 \text{ mg}}{16 \text{ mg}} \times 5 \text{ mL} = x \text{ mL}; \frac{24 \text{ mg}}{16 \text{ mg}} = \frac{x \text{ mL}}{5 \text{ mL}}$$

Answer: 7.5 mL or $7\frac{1}{2}$ mL. The dose ordered is greater than the available strength. You will need more than 5 mL to administer the required dose.

60. $325 \text{ mg} : 10.15 \text{ mL} = 650 \text{ mg} : x \text{ mL}$

OR

$$\frac{650 \text{ mg}}{325 \text{ mg}} \times 10.15 \text{ mL} = x \text{ mL};$$

$$\frac{650 \text{ mg}}{325 \text{ mg}} = \frac{x \text{ mL}}{10.15 \text{ mL}}$$

Answer: 20.3 mL. The dose ordered is 2 times greater than the available strength. You will need more than 10.15 mL to administer the dose.

61. $300 \text{ mg} : 5 \text{ mL} = 400 \text{ mg} : x \text{ mL}$

$$\frac{300\,x}{300} = \frac{2{,}000}{300}$$

OR

$$\frac{400 \text{ mg}}{300 \text{ mg}} \times 5 \text{ mL} = x \text{ mL}; \frac{400 \text{ mg}}{300 \text{ mg}} = \frac{x \text{ mL}}{5 \text{ mL}}$$

Answer: 6.66 = 6.7 mL to the nearest tenth. The dose ordered is more than what is available. You will need more than 5 cc to administer the dose.

62. $10 \text{ mg} : 1 \text{ mL} = 150 \text{ mg} : x \text{ mL}$

OR

$$\frac{150 \text{ mg}}{10 \text{ mg}} \times 1 \text{ mL} = x \text{ mL}; \frac{150 \text{ mg}}{10 \text{ mg}} = \frac{x \text{ mL}}{1 \text{ mL}}$$

Answer: 15 mL. The dose ordered is greater than the available strength, so you will need more than 1 mL to administer the required dose.

63. Conversion is necessary. 1000 mg = 1 g; therefore 0.3 g = 300 mg

$$50 \text{ mg} : 5 \text{ mL} = 300 \text{ mg} : x \text{ mL}$$

OR

$$\frac{300 \text{ mg}}{50 \text{ mg}} \times 5 \text{ mL} = x \text{ mL}; \frac{300 \text{ mg}}{50 \text{ mg}} = \frac{x \text{ mL}}{5 \text{ mL}}$$

Answer: 30 mL. The dosage ordered is greater than the available strength, so you will need more than 5 mL to administer the required dose.

64. 100,000 U : 1 mL = 200,000 U : x mL

OR

$$\frac{200{,}000 \text{ U}}{100{,}000 \text{ U}} \times 1 \text{ mL} = x \text{ mL};$$

$$\frac{200{,}000 \text{ U}}{100{,}000 \text{ U}} = \frac{x \text{ mL}}{1 \text{ mL}}$$

Answer: 2 mL. The dose ordered is greater than the available strength, so you will need more than 1 mL to administer the required dose.

65. 100 mg : 1 mL = 150 mg : x mL

OR

$$\frac{150 \text{ mg}}{100 \text{ mg}} \times 1 \text{ mL} = x \text{ mL}; \frac{150 \text{ mg}}{100 \text{ mg}} = \frac{x \text{ mL}}{1 \text{ mL}}$$

Answer: 1.5 mL or $1\frac{1}{2}$ mL. ($1\frac{1}{2}$ mL is the best answer for administration purposes.) The dosage ordered is greater than the available strength, so you will need more than 1 mL to administer the required dose.

66. Conversion is necessary. 1000 mg = 1 g; therefore 0.25 g = 250 mg

$$125 \text{ mg} : 5 \text{ mL} = 250 \text{ mg} : x \text{ mL}$$

OR

$$\frac{250 \text{ mg}}{125 \text{ mg}} \times 5 \text{ mL} = x \text{ mL}; \frac{250 \text{ mg}}{125 \text{ mg}} = \frac{x \text{ mL}}{5 \text{ mL}}$$

Answer: 10 mL. The dose ordered is greater than the available strength; therefore you will need more than 5 mL to administer the dose.

67. 200 mg : 5 mL = 200 mg : x mL

OR

$$\frac{200 \text{ mg}}{200 \text{ mg}} \times 5 \text{ mL} = x \text{ mL}; \frac{200 \text{ mg}}{200 \text{ mg}} = \frac{x \text{ mL}}{5 \text{ mL}}$$

Answer: 5 mL. The dose ordered is equivalent to what is available. Label indicates 200 mg = 5 mL.

68. 20 mg : 5 mL = 30 mg : x mL

OR

$$\frac{30 \text{ mg}}{20 \text{ mg}} \times 5 \text{ mL} = x \text{ mL}; \frac{30 \text{ mg}}{20 \text{ mg}} = \frac{x \text{ mL}}{5 \text{ mL}}$$

Answer: 7.5 mL. The dose ordered is greater than the available strength, so you will need more than 5 mL to administer the required dose.

69. 15 mg : 1 mL = 150 mg : x mL

OR

$$\frac{150 \text{ mg}}{15 \text{ mg}} \times 1 \text{ mL} = x \text{ mL}; \frac{150 \text{ mg}}{15 \text{ mg}} = \frac{x \text{ mL}}{1 \text{ mL}}$$

Answer: 10 mL. The dose ordered is 10 times more than the available strength, so you will need more than 1 mL to administer the required dose.

70. Conversion is necessary. 1 oz = 30 mL

$$1 \text{ oz} : 30 \text{ mL} = 1 \text{ oz} : x \text{ mL}$$

OR

$$\frac{1 \text{ oz}}{1 \text{ oz}} \times 30 \text{ mL} = x \text{ mL}; \frac{1 \text{ oz}}{1 \text{ oz}} = \frac{x \text{ mL}}{30 \text{ mL}}$$

Answer: 30 mL. The medication label indicates 30 mL; therefore you will need to administer 30 mL for the client to receive 1 oz.

71. 30 mg: 1 mL = 50 mg : x mL

OR

$$\frac{50 \text{ mg}}{30 \text{ mg}} \times 1 \text{ mL} = x \text{ mL}; \frac{50 \text{ mg}}{30 \text{ mg}} = \frac{x \text{ mL}}{1 \text{ mL}}$$

Answer: 1.7 mL (1.66 mL to the nearest tenth). The dose ordered is greater than the available strength, so you will need more than 1 mL to administer the required dose.

Chapter 16

Answers to Practice Problems

1.

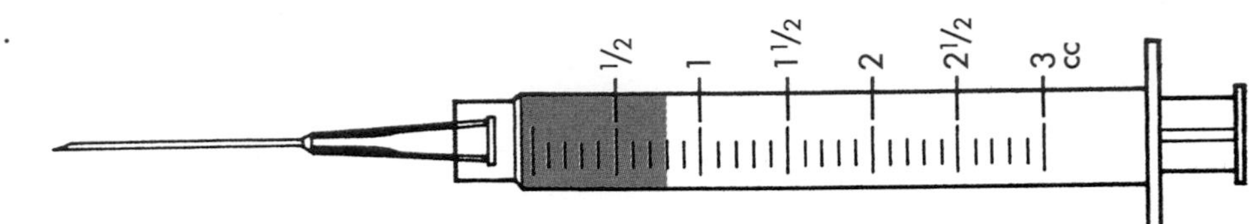

2.

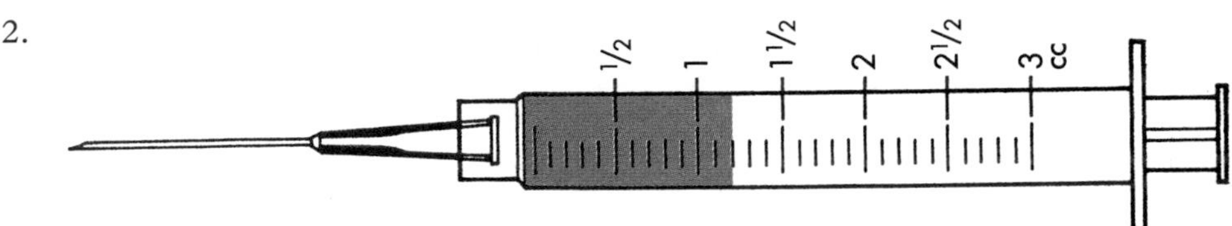

3.

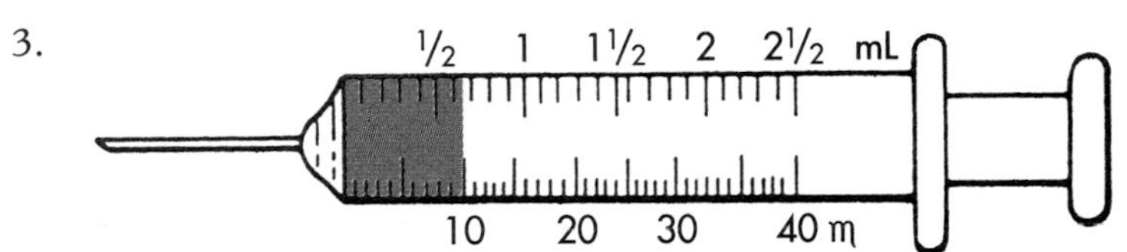

4.

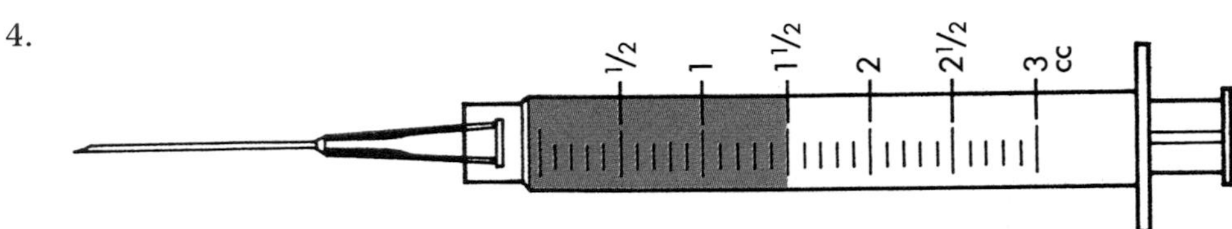

5.

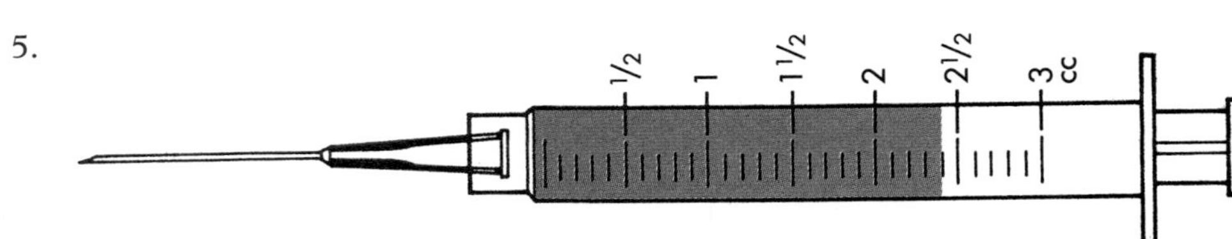

6. m 8
7. 1.4 cc
8. 1 cc
9. 0.9 cc
10. 0.4 cc
11. 4.4 cc
12. 7 cc
13. 3.2cc

Answers to Practice Problems: Reading Parenteral Labels

14. 20 mL
15. 25 mg/mL; 500 mg/20 mL is also correct.
16. 10 mL
17. 10 mL
18. 0.1 mg/mL
19. I.V. only
20. 10 mL
21. 25 mg/mL
22. 2 mL
23. 2 mL
24. 2 mg/2 mL
25. 1 mL
26. 20 mL
27. 2 mEq/mL
28. 50 mL
29. 84 mg/mL
30. 10 mL
31. 1000 U/mL
32. 10 mL
33. 100 U/mL
34. 100 mL
35. 200,000 U/5 mL

Answers to Chapter Review

Problems requiring conversion reflect converting of what the doctor ordered to what is available.

1. Conversion is required. Equivalent: 1000 mcg = 1 mg

   Therefore 0.05 mg = 50 mcg

$$100 \text{ mcg} : 1 \text{ mL} = 50 \text{ mcg} : x \text{ mL} \quad \text{OR} \quad \frac{50 \text{ mcg}}{100 \text{ mcg}} \times 1 \text{ mL} = x \text{ mL}; \frac{50 \text{ mcg}}{100 \text{ mcg}} = \frac{x \text{ mL}}{1 \text{ mL}}$$

   Answer: 0.5 mL or $\frac{1}{2}$ mL. The dose ordered is less than what is available. (Answer of $\frac{1}{2}$ mL is preferred for administration purposes.) Therefore you will need less than 1 mL to administer the dose.

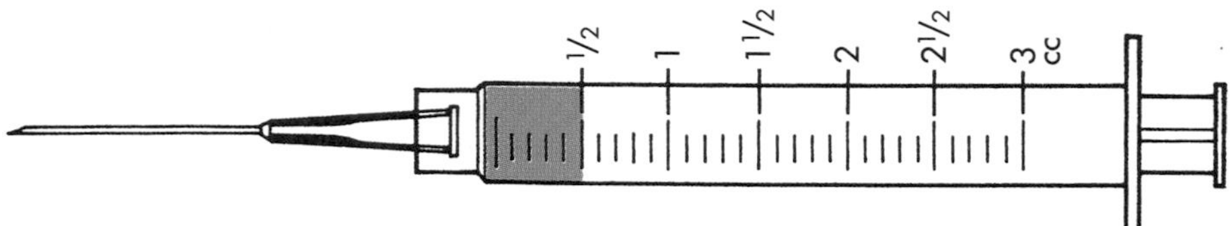

2. Demerol:

$$75 \text{ mg} : 1 \text{ mL} = 50 \text{ mg} : x \text{ mL} \quad \text{OR} \quad \frac{50 \text{ mg}}{75 \text{ mg}} \times 1 \text{ mL} = x \text{ mL}; \frac{50 \text{ mg}}{75 \text{ mg}} = \frac{x \text{ mL}}{1 \text{ mL}}$$

   Answer: 0.66 mL = 0.7 mL. The dose ordered is less than what is available. Therefore less than 1 mL would be required to administer the dose.

   Vistaril:

$$50 \text{ mg} : 1 \text{ mL} = 25 \text{ mg} : x \text{ mL} \quad \text{OR} \quad \frac{25 \text{ mg}}{50 \text{ mg}} \times 1 \text{ mL} = x \text{ mL}; \frac{25 \text{ mg}}{50 \text{ mg}} = \frac{x \text{ mL}}{1 \text{ mL}}$$

   Answer: 0.5 mL or $\frac{1}{2}$ mL. The dose ordered is less than what is available. Therefore you will need less than 1 mL to administer the dose. The total number of mL you will prepare to administer is 1.2 mL. This dose is measurable on the small hypodermics. These two medications are often administered in the same syringe. (0.7 mL + 0.5 mL = 1.2 mL)

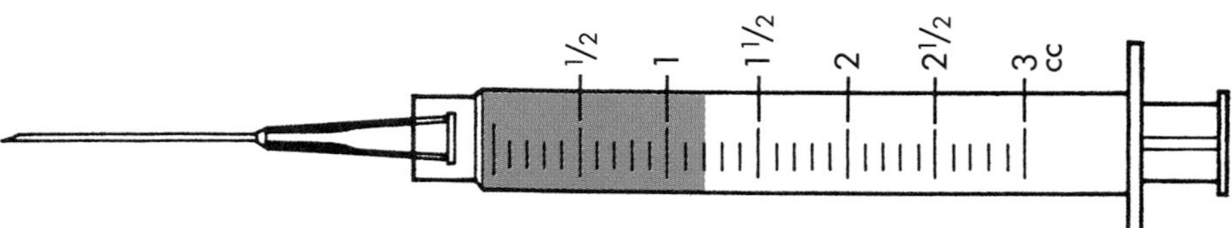

3. $10 \text{ mg} : 2 \text{ mL} = 5 \text{ mg} : x \text{ mL} \quad \text{OR} \quad \frac{5 \text{ mg}}{10 \text{ mg}} \times 2 \text{ mL} = x \text{ mL}; \frac{5 \text{ mg}}{10 \text{ mg}} = \frac{x \text{ mL}}{2 \text{ mL}}$

   x = 1 mL. The dose required is less than the dose available; therefore you will need less than 2 mL to administer the dose.

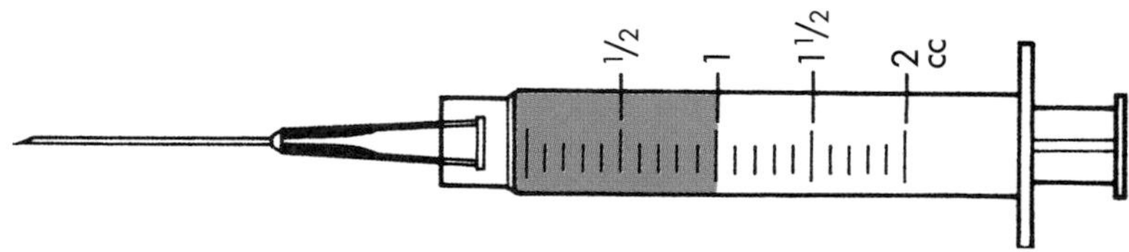

4. 20,000 U : 1 mL = 5,000 U : x mL OR $\frac{5{,}000 \text{ U}}{20{,}000 \text{ U}} \times 1 \text{ mL} = x \text{ mL}; \frac{5{,}000 \text{ U}}{20{,}000 \text{ U}} = \frac{x \text{ mL}}{1 \text{ mL}}$

Answer: 0.25 mL. The dose ordered is less than what is available; therefore you will need less than 1 mL to administer the dose. This dose can be measured accurately on the 1 cc (tuberculin) syringe, since it is measured in hundredths of a mL. The dose you are administering is $\frac{25}{100}$.

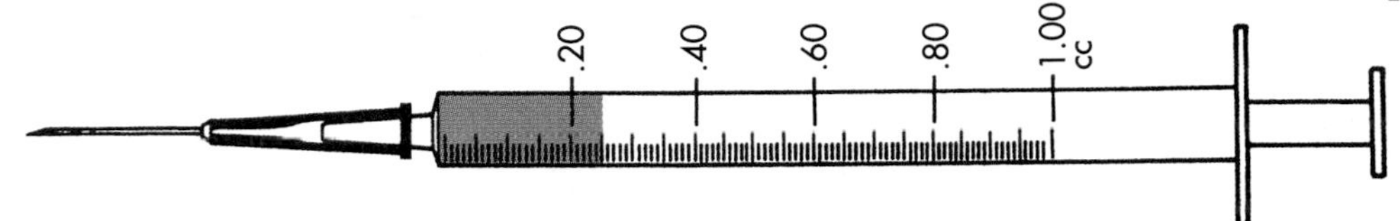

5. Conversion is required. Equivalent: 60 mg = gr 1

Therefore gr $\frac{1}{4}$ = 15 mg

10 mg : 1 mL = 15 mg : x mL OR $\frac{15 \text{ mg}}{10 \text{ mg}} \times 1 \text{ mL} = x \text{ mL}; \frac{15 \text{ mg}}{10 \text{ mg}} = \frac{x \text{ mL}}{1 \text{ mL}}$

Answer: 1.5 mL or $1\frac{1}{2}$ mL. The dose ordered is more than what is available; therefore you will need more than 1 mL to administer the dose. The preferred answer is $1\frac{1}{2}$ mL for administration purposes, and the syringe has fraction markings.

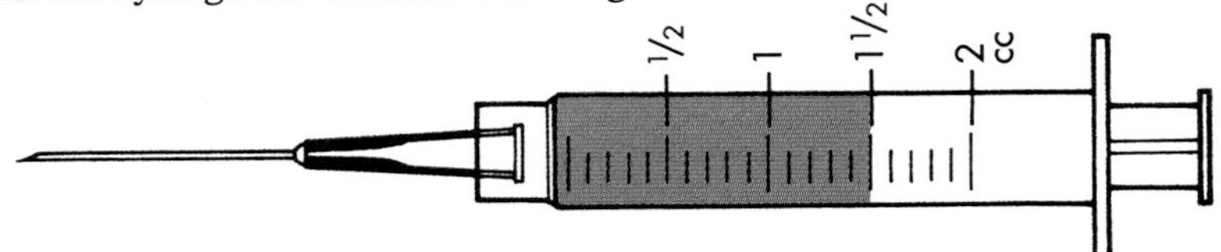

6. 10 mg : 1 mL = 20 mg : x mL OR $\frac{20 \text{ mg}}{10 \text{ mg}} \times 1 \text{ mL} = x \text{ mL}; \frac{20 \text{ mg}}{10 \text{ mg}} = \frac{x \text{ mL}}{1 \text{ mL}}$

Answer: 2 mL. The dose ordered is more than what is available; therefore you will need more than 1 mL to administer the required dose.

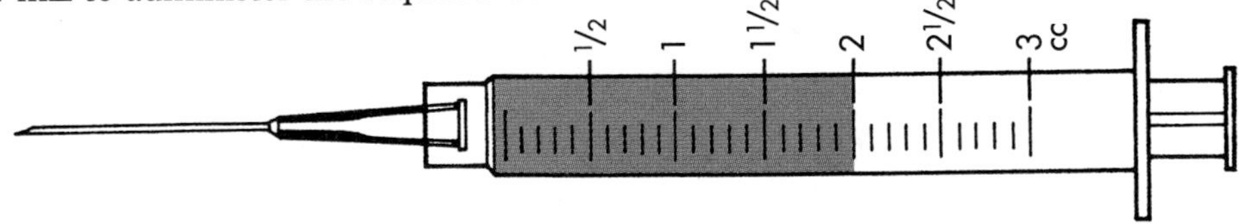

Alternate method for solving:

40 mg : 4 mL = 20 mg : x mL OR $\frac{20 \text{ mg}}{40 \text{ mg}} \times 4 \text{ mL} = x \text{ mL}; \frac{20 \text{ mg}}{40 \text{ mg}} = \frac{x \text{ mL}}{4 \text{ mL}}$

This setup still gives an answer of 2 mL.

7. Conversion is required. Equivalent: 1000 mg = 1 g

Therefore 0.3 g = 300 mg

150 mg : 1 mL = 300 mg : x mL OR $\frac{300 \text{ mg}}{150 \text{ mg}} \times 1 \text{ mL} = x \text{ mL}; \frac{300 \text{ mg}}{150 \text{ mg}} = \frac{x \text{ mL}}{1 \text{ mL}}$

Answer: 2 mL. The dose ordered is more than the dose available, therefore you will need more than 1 mL to administer the dose.

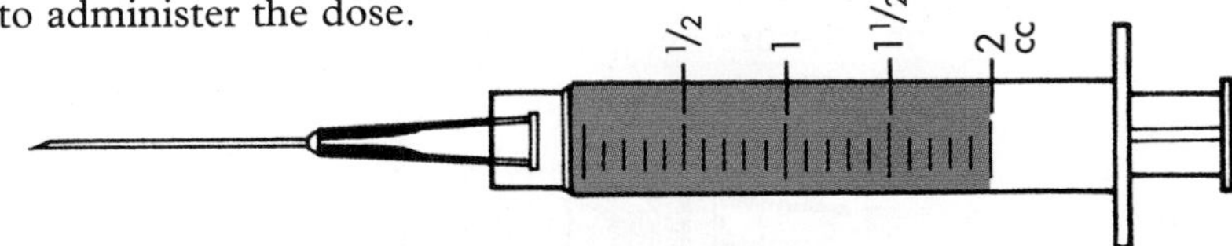

8. Conversion is required. Equivalent: 60 mg = gr 1.

Therefore gr $\frac{1}{150}$ = 0.4 mg

$$0.4\text{ mg} : 1\text{ mL} = 0.4\text{ mg} : x\text{ mL} \quad \text{OR} \quad \frac{0.4\text{ mg}}{0.4\text{ mg}} \times 1\text{ mL} = x\text{ mL}; \frac{0.4\text{ mg}}{0.4\text{ mg}} = \frac{x\text{ mL}}{1\text{ mL}}$$

Answer: 1 mL. After making the conversion, you can see that, although the dose ordered was in gr, it is equivalent to the same number of mL as what is available.

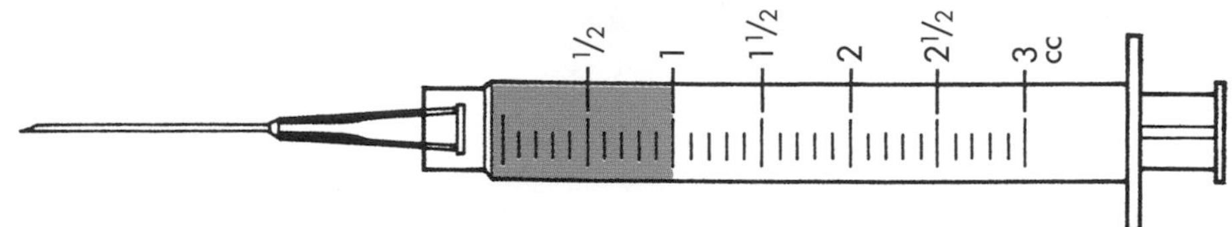

9. Conversion is required. Equivalent: 1000 mg = 1 g

Therefore 0.5 g = 500 mg

$$225\text{ mg} : 1\text{ mL} = 500\text{ mg} : x\text{ mL} \quad \text{OR} \quad \frac{500\text{ mg}}{225\text{ mg}} \times 1\text{ mL} = x\text{ mL}; \frac{500\text{ mg}}{225\text{ mg}} = \frac{x\text{ mL}}{1\text{ mL}}$$

Answer: 2.2 mL. The dose ordered is more than what is available; therefore you will need more than 1 mL. The dose here was rounded off to the nearest tenth of a mL. The small hypodermics are marked in tenths of a mL. To round to the nearest tenth, the math is carried to the hundredths place.

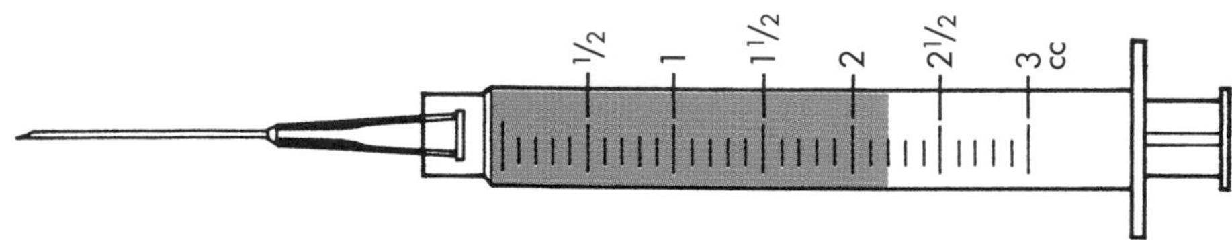

10. Conversion is required. Equivalent: 1000 mcg = 1 mg

Therefore 100 mcg = 0.1 mg

$$0.5\text{ mg} : 2\text{ mL} = 0.1\text{ mg} : x\text{ mL} \quad \text{OR} \quad \frac{0.1\text{ mg}}{0.5\text{ mg}} \times 2\text{ mL} = x\text{ mL}; \frac{0.1\text{ mg}}{0.5\text{ mg}} = \frac{x\text{ mL}}{2\text{ mL}}$$

Answer: 0.4 mL. The dose ordered is less than what is available. The dose required would be less than 2 mL.

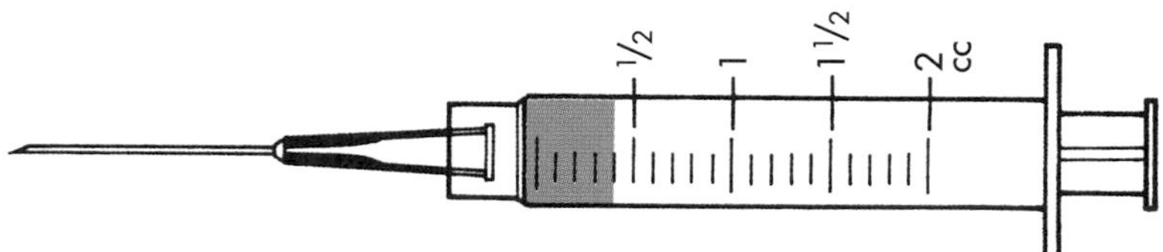

11. Conversion is required. Equivalent: 60 mg = gr 1

Therefore gr $\frac{1}{2}$ = 30 mg

$$120\text{ mg} : 1\text{ mL} = 30\text{ mg} : x\text{ mL} \quad \text{OR} \quad \frac{30\text{ mg}}{120\text{ mg}} \times 1\text{ mL} = x\text{ mL}; \frac{30\text{ mg}}{120\text{ mg}} = \frac{x\text{ mL}}{1\text{ mL}}$$

Answer: 0.3 mL. 0.25 mL is rounded off to the nearest tenth in order to administer the dose with the small hypodermic. The dose ordered is less than what is available.

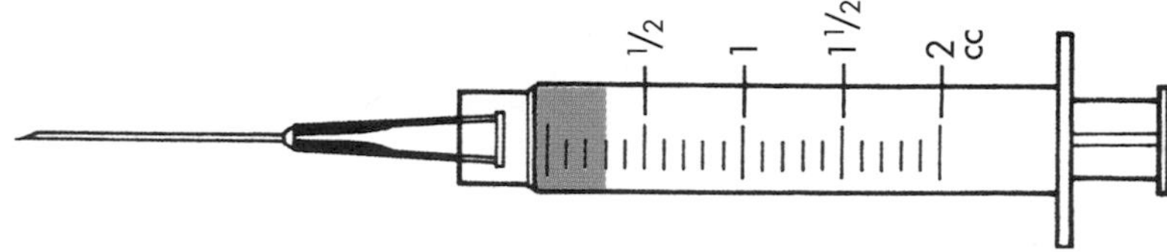

12. 4 mg : 1 mL = 2 mg : x mL OR $\frac{2 \text{ mg}}{4 \text{ mg}} \times 1 \text{ mL} = x \text{ mL}; \frac{2 \text{ mg}}{4 \text{ mg}} = \frac{x \text{ mL}}{1 \text{ mL}}$

Answer: 0.5 mL or $\frac{1}{2}$ mL. The dose ordered is less than what is available; therefore less than 1 mL is required to administer the dose. (The preferred answer for administration purposes is $\frac{1}{2}$ mL.)

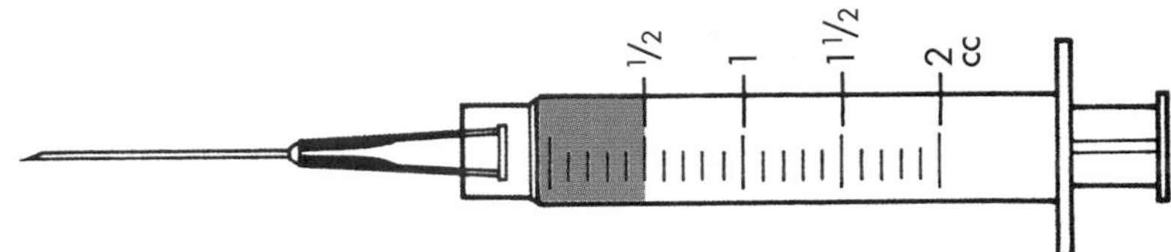

13. 300,000 U : 1 mL = 250,000 U : x mL OR $\frac{250{,}000 \text{ U}}{300{,}000 \text{ U}} \times 1 \text{ mL} = x \text{ mL}; \frac{250{,}000 \text{ U}}{300{,}000 \text{ U}} = \frac{x \text{ mL}}{1 \text{ mL}}$

Answer: 0.8 mL. 0.83 mL is rounded to the nearest tenth. The dose ordered is less than what is available; therefore you will need less than 1 mL to administer the dose.

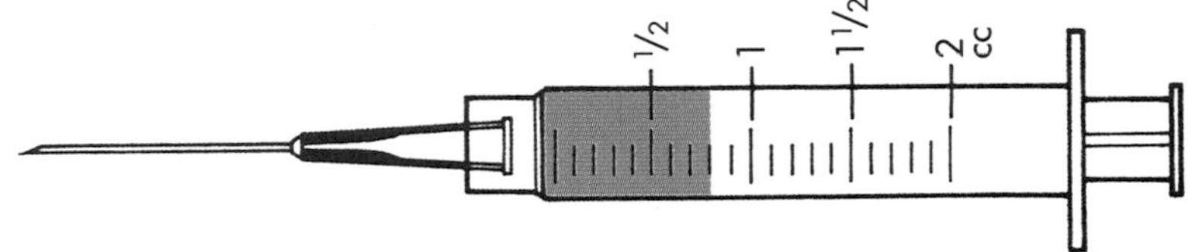

14. 125 mg : 2 mL = 100 mg : x mL OR $\frac{100 \text{ mg}}{125 \text{ mg}} \times 2 \text{ mL} = x \text{ mL}; \frac{100 \text{ mg}}{125 \text{ mg}} = \frac{x \text{ mL}}{2 \text{ mL}}$

Answer: 1.6 mL. The amount ordered is less than what is available; therefore you will need less than 2 mL to administer the required dose.

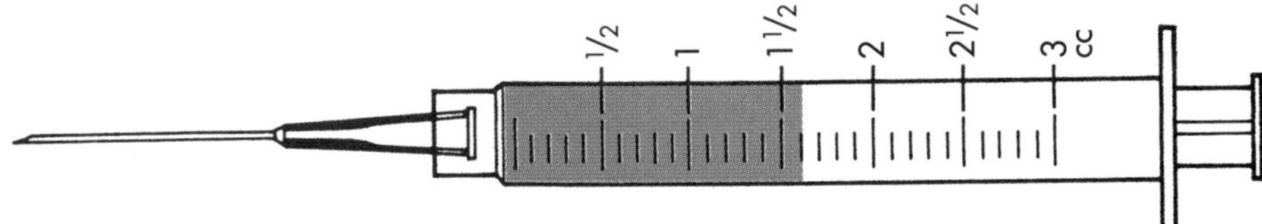

15. 0.2 mg : 1 mL = 0.4 mg : x mL OR $\frac{0.4 \text{ mg}}{0.2 \text{ mg}} \times 1 \text{ mL} = x \text{ mL}; \frac{0.4 \text{ mg}}{0.2 \text{ mg}} = \frac{x \text{ mL}}{1 \text{ mL}}$

Answer: 2 mL. The dose ordered is more than what is available; therefore you will need more than 1 mL to administer the required dose.

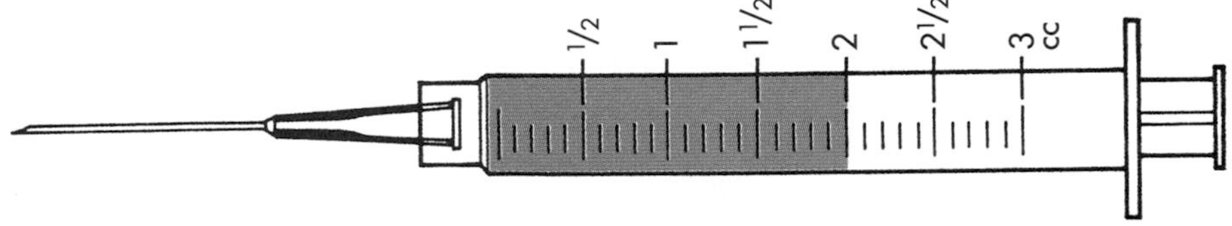

16. 10,000 U : 1 mL = 8,000 U : x mL OR $\frac{8{,}000 \text{ U}}{10{,}000 \text{ U}} \times 1 \text{ mL} = x \text{ mL}; \frac{8{,}000 \text{ U}}{10{,}000 \text{ U}} = \frac{x \text{ mL}}{1 \text{ mL}}$

Answer: 0.8 mL. The dose ordered is less than what is available. You will need less than 1 mL to administer the dose.

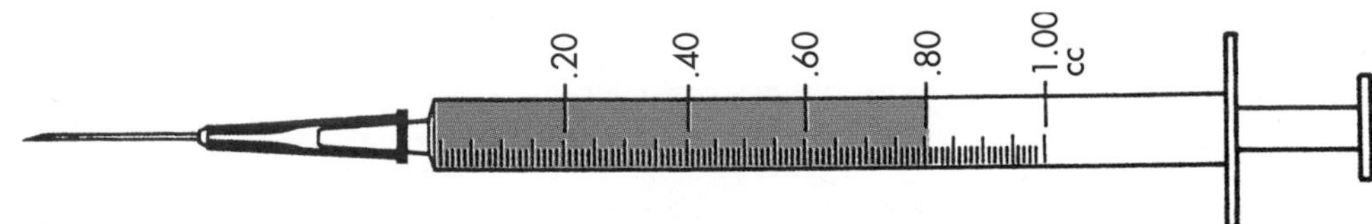

17. 10 mg : 1 mL = 4 mg : x mL OR $\frac{4 \text{ mg}}{10 \text{ mg}} \times 1 \text{ mL} = x \text{ mL}; \frac{4 \text{ mg}}{10 \text{ mg}} = \frac{x \text{ mL}}{1 \text{ mL}}$

Answer: 0.4 mL. The dose ordered is less than what is available; therefore you will need less than a mL to administer the dose.

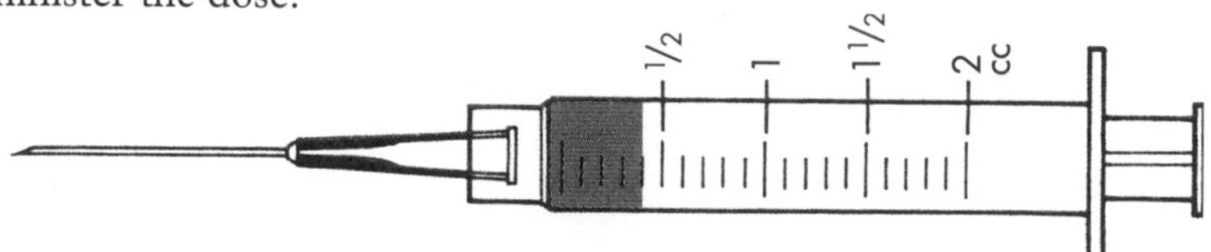

18. 5 mg : 1 mL = 10 mg : x mL OR $\frac{10 \text{ mg}}{5 \text{ mg}} \times 1 \text{ mL} = x \text{ mL}; \frac{10 \text{ mg}}{5 \text{ mg}} = \frac{x \text{ mL}}{1 \text{ mL}}$

Answer: 2 mL. The dose ordered is more than what is available; therefore you will need more than 1 mL to administer the dose.

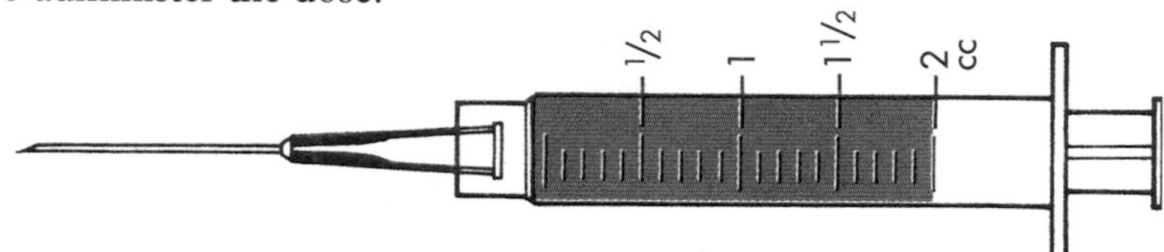

19. Conversion is required. Equivalent: 60 mg = gr 1

Therefore gr $\frac{1}{4}$ = 15 mg

30 mg : 1 mL = 15 mg : x mL OR $\frac{15 \text{ mg}}{30 \text{ mg}} \times 1 \text{ mL} = x \text{ mL}; \frac{15 \text{ mg}}{30 \text{ mg}} = \frac{x \text{ mL}}{1 \text{ mL}}$

gr $\frac{1}{2}$: 1 mL = gr $\frac{1}{4}$: x mL

If fractions are used:

$$\frac{\text{gr } \frac{1}{4}}{\text{gr } \frac{1}{2}} \times 1 \text{ mL} = x \text{ mL} \quad \text{OR} \quad \frac{\text{gr } \frac{1}{4}}{\text{gr } \frac{1}{2}} = \frac{x \text{ mL}}{1 \text{ mL}}$$

Answer: 0.5 mL or $\frac{1}{2}$ mL. The dose ordered is less than what is available; therefore you will need less than 1 mL to administer the dose. (The preferred answer is $\frac{1}{2}$ mL for administration purposes.)

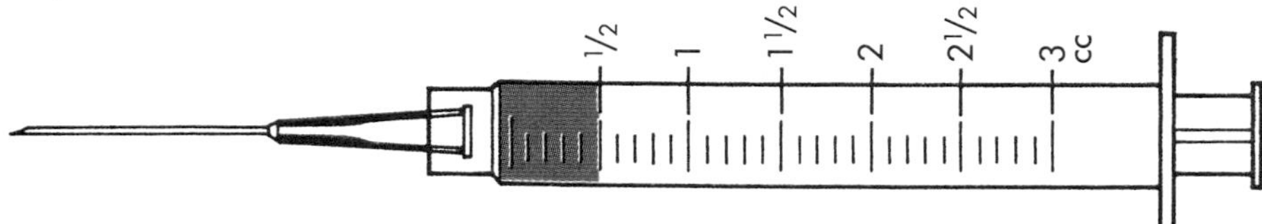

20. 50 mg : 1 mL = 25 mg : x mL OR $\frac{25 \text{ mg}}{50 \text{ mg}} \times 1 \text{ mL} = x \text{ mL}; \frac{25 \text{ mg}}{50 \text{ mg}} = \frac{x \text{ mL}}{1 \text{ mL}}$

Answer: 0.5 mL or $\frac{1}{2}$ mL. The dose ordered is less than what is available; therefore you will need less than 1 mL to administer the dose. (The preferred answer is $\frac{1}{2}$ mL for administration purposes.)

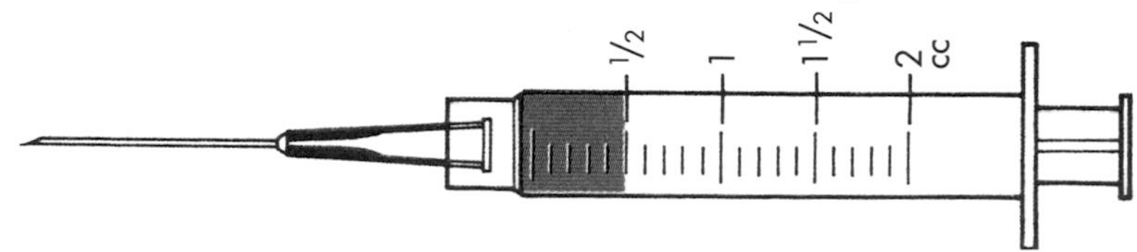

21. 2 mg : 1 mL = 1.5 mg : x mL OR $\frac{1.5 \text{ mg}}{2 \text{ mg}} \times 1 \text{ mL} = x \text{ mL}; \frac{1.5 \text{ mg}}{2 \text{ mg}} = \frac{x \text{ mL}}{1 \text{ mL}}$

Answer: 0.8 mL. 0.75 mL is rounded to nearest tenth. The dose ordered is less than what is available. You will need less than 1 mL to administer the dose.

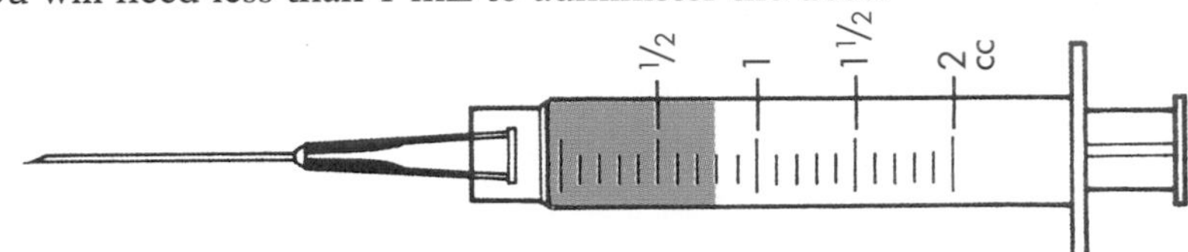

22. 4 mg : 1 mL = 3 mg : x mL OR $\frac{3 \text{ mg}}{4 \text{ mg}} \times 1 \text{ mL} = x \text{ mL}; \frac{3 \text{ mg}}{4 \text{ mg}} = \frac{x \text{ mL}}{1 \text{ mL}}$

Answer: 0.8 mL. 0.75 mL is rounded to nearest tenth. The dose ordered is less than what is available. You will need less than 1 mL to administer the dose.

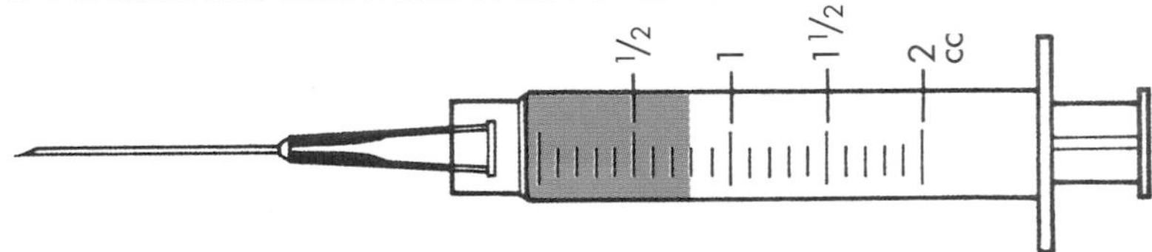

23. Conversion is required. Equivalent: gr 1 = 60 mg

Therefore gr $\frac{1}{300}$ = 0.2 mg

0.4 mg : 1 mL = 0.2 mg : x mL OR $\frac{0.2 \text{ mg}}{0.4 \text{ mg}} \times 1 \text{ mL} = x \text{ mL}; \frac{0.2 \text{ mg}}{0.4 \text{ mg}} = \frac{x \text{ mL}}{1 \text{ mL}}$

Answer: 0.5 mL or $\frac{1}{2}$ mL (The preferred answer is $\frac{1}{2}$ mL for administration purposes.)

The dose ordered is one half of what is available. You will need less than 1 mL to administer the dose.

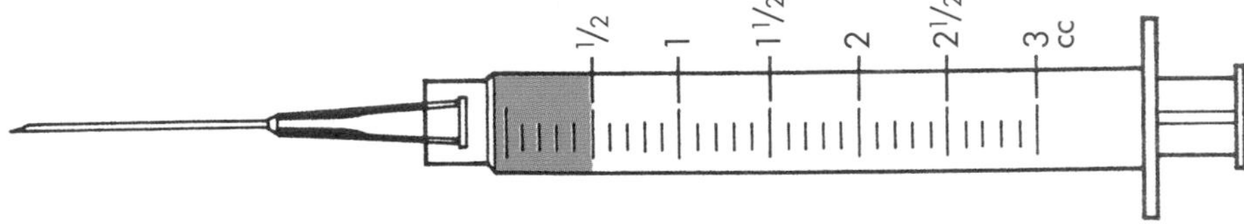

24. 5 mg : 1 mL = 3 mg : x mL OR $\frac{3 \text{ mg}}{5 \text{ mg}} \times 1 \text{ mL} = x \text{ mL}; \frac{3 \text{ mg}}{5 \text{ mg}} = \frac{x \text{ mL}}{1 \text{ mL}}$

Answer: 0.6 mL. The dose ordered is less than what is available. You will need less than 1 mL to administer the dose.

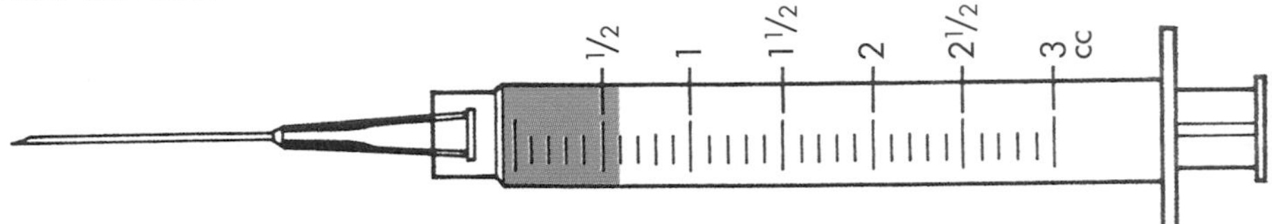

25. 50 mg : 1 mL = 90 mg : x mL OR $\frac{90 \text{ mg}}{50 \text{ mg}} \times 1 \text{ mL} = x \text{ mL}; \frac{90 \text{ mg}}{50 \text{ mg}} = \frac{x \text{ mL}}{1 \text{ mL}}$

Answer: 1.8 mL. The dose ordered is more than what is available. You will need more than 1 mL to administer the dose.

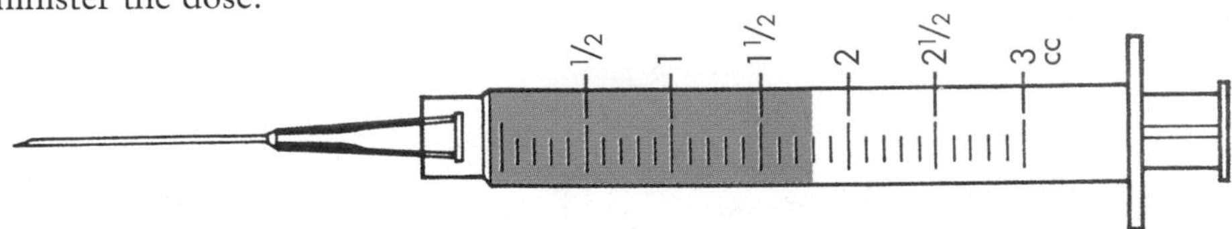

26. 250 mg : 2 mL = 400 mg : x mL OR $\frac{400 \text{ mg}}{250 \text{ mg}} \times 2 \text{ mL} = x \text{ mL}; \frac{400 \text{ mg}}{250 \text{ mg}} = \frac{x \text{ mL}}{2 \text{ mL}}$

Answer 3.2 mL. The dose ordered is more than what is available. You will need more than 2 mL to administer the dose.

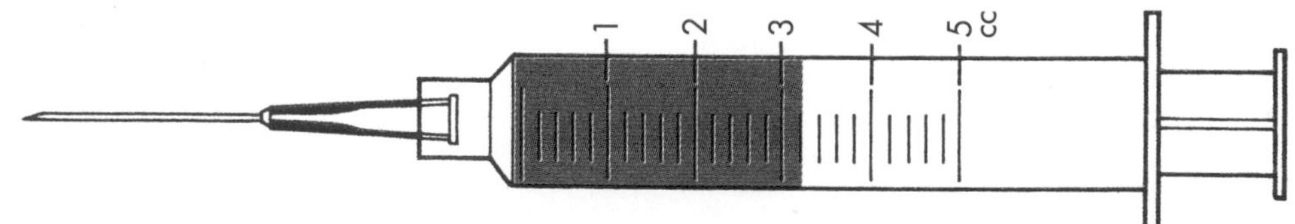

27. 125 mg : 2 mL = 40 mg : x mL OR $\frac{40 \text{ mg}}{125 \text{ mg}} \times 2 \text{ mL} = x \text{ mL}; \frac{40 \text{ mg}}{125 \text{ mg}} = \frac{x \text{ mL}}{2 \text{ mL}}$

Answer: 0.6 mL. 0.64 mL is rounded to nearest tenth. The dose ordered is less than what is available. You will need less than 1 mL to administer the dose.

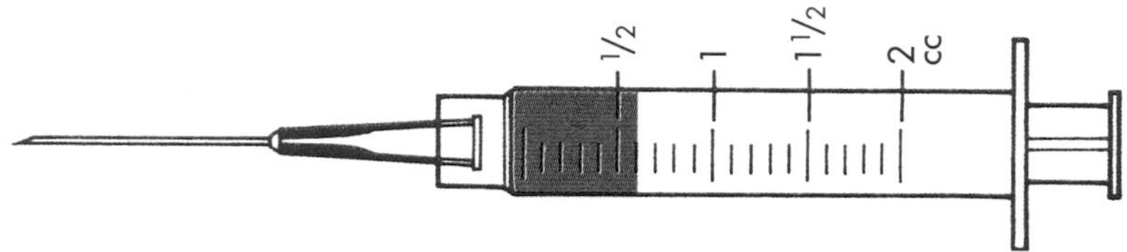

28. Conversion is needed. Equivalent: 1000 mcg = 1 mg

Therefore 200 mcg = 0.2 mg

0.2 mg : 1 mL = 0.2 mg : x mL OR $\frac{0.2 \text{ mg}}{0.2 \text{ mg}} \times 1 \text{ mL} = x \text{ mL}; \frac{0.2 \text{ mg}}{0.2 \text{ mg}} = \frac{x \text{ mL}}{1 \text{ mL}}$

Answer: 1 mL. Since 200 mcg = 0.2 mg, you will need 1 mL to administer the required dose.

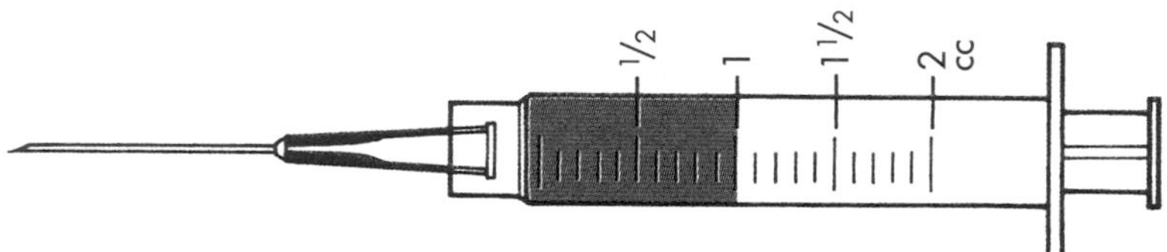

29. 5,000 U : 1 mL = 2,500 U : x mL OR $\frac{2{,}500 \text{ U}}{5{,}000 \text{ U}} \times 1 \text{ mL} = x \text{ mL}$ OR $\frac{2{,}500 \text{ U}}{5{,}000 \text{ U}} = \frac{x \text{mL}}{1 \text{mL}}$

Answer: 0.5 mL. The dose ordered is less than what is available. You will need less than 1 mL to administer the dose.

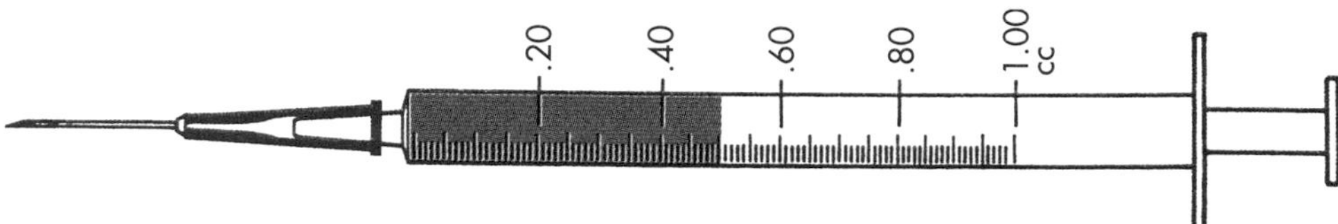

30. 50 mg : 1 mL = 35 mg : x mL OR $\frac{35 \text{ mg}}{50 \text{ mg}} \times 1 \text{ mL} = x \text{ mL}; \frac{35 \text{ mg}}{50 \text{ mg}} = \frac{x \text{ mL}}{1 \text{ mL}}$

Answer: 0.7 mL. The dose ordered is less than what is available. You will need less than 1 mL to administer the required dose.

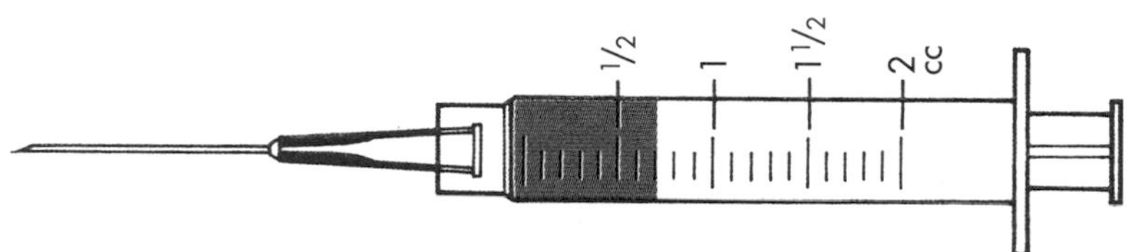

31. 75 mg : 1 mL = 60 mg : x mL OR $\frac{60\text{ mg}}{75\text{ mg}} \times 1\text{ mL} = x\text{ mL}; \frac{60\text{ mg}}{75\text{ mg}} = \frac{x\text{ mL}}{1\text{ mL}}$

Answer: 0.8 mL. The dose ordered is less than what is available. You will need less than 1 mL to administer the required dose.

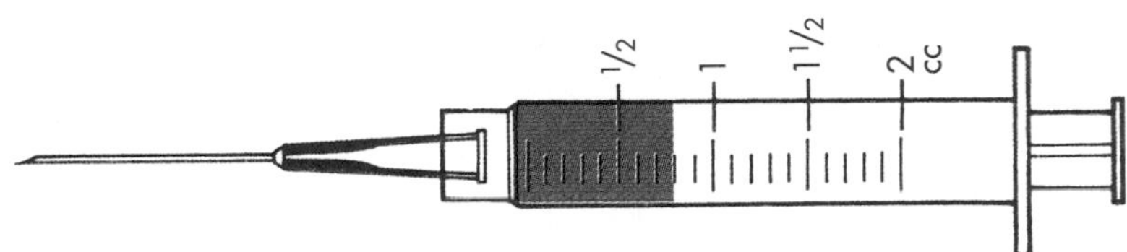

32. 300,000 U : 1 mL = 400,000 U : x mL OR $\frac{400{,}000\text{ U}}{300{,}000\text{ U}} \times 1\text{ mL} = x\text{ mL}; \frac{400{,}000\text{ U}}{300{,}000\text{ U}} = \frac{x\text{ mL}}{1\text{ mL}}$

Answer: 1.3 mL. 1.33 mL is rounded to the nearest tenth. The dose ordered is more than what is available. You will need more than 1 mL to administer the required dose.

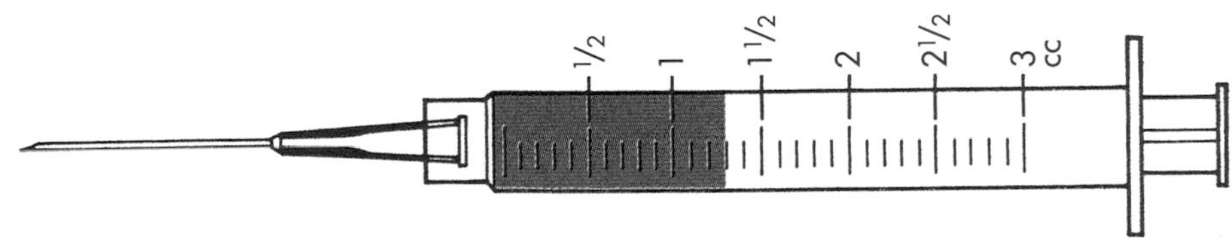

33. 0.5 mg : 2 mL = 0.4 mg : x mL OR $\frac{0.4\text{ mg}}{0.5\text{ mg}} \times 2\text{ mL} = x\text{ mL}; \frac{0.4\text{ mg}}{0.5\text{ mg}} = \frac{x\text{ mL}}{2\text{ mL}}$

Answer: 1.6 mL. The dose ordered is less than what is available. You will need less than 2 mL to administer the required dose.

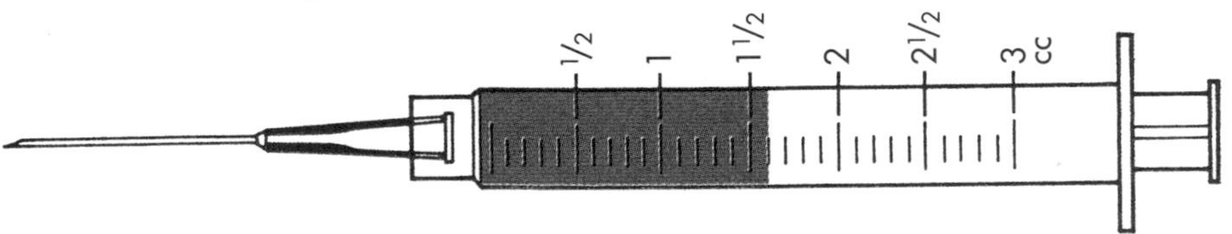

34. 500 mg : 2 mL = 100 mg : x mL OR $\frac{100\text{ mg}}{500\text{ mg}} \times 2\text{ mL} = x\text{ mL}; \frac{100\text{ mg}}{500\text{ mg}} = \frac{x\text{ mL}}{2\text{ mL}}$

Answer: 0.4 mL. The dose ordered is less than what is available. You will need less than 2 mL to administer the required dose.

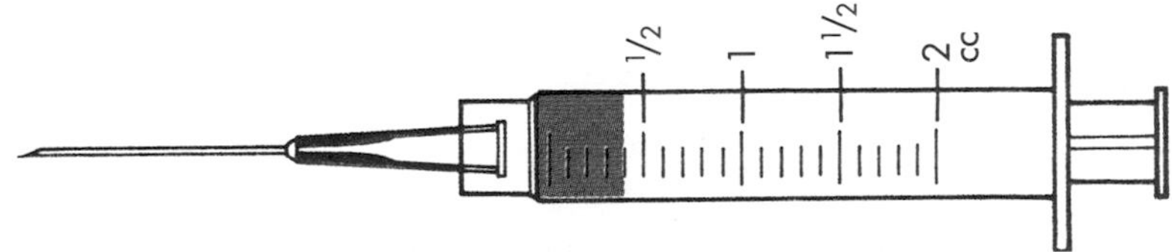

35. 80 mg : 1 mL = 60 mg : x mL OR $\frac{60\text{ mg}}{80\text{ mg}} \times 1\text{ mL} = x\text{ mL}; \frac{60\text{ mg}}{80\text{ mg}} = \frac{x\text{ mL}}{1\text{ mL}}$

Answer: 0.8 mL. 0.75 mL is rounded to the nearest tenth. The dose ordered is less than what is available. You will need less than 1 mL to administer the dose.

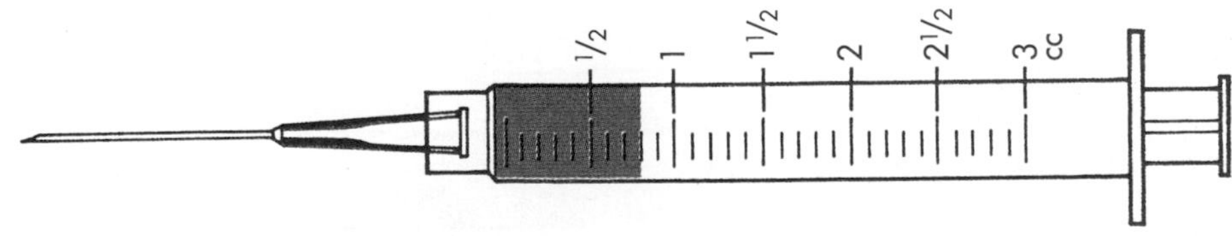

36. 4 mg : 1 mL = 2 mg : x mL OR $\frac{2 \text{ mg}}{4 \text{ mg}} \times 1 \text{ mL} = x \text{ mL}; \frac{2 \text{ mg}}{4 \text{ mg}} = \frac{x \text{ mL}}{1 \text{ mL}}$

Answer: 0.5 mL or $\frac{1}{2}$ mL. ($\frac{1}{2}$ mL is preferred for administration purposes.) The dose ordered is less than what is available. Therefore you will need less than 1 mL to administer the dose.

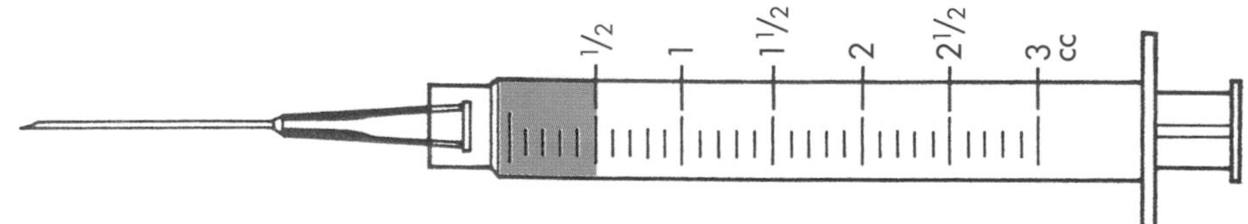

37. 25 mg : 1 mL = 75 mg : x mL OR $\frac{75 \text{ mg}}{25 \text{ mg}} \times 1 \text{ mL} = x \text{ mL}; \frac{75 \text{ mg}}{25 \text{ mg}} = \frac{x \text{ mL}}{1 \text{ mL}}$

Answer: 3 mL. The dose ordered is greater than what is available. Therefore you will need more than 1 mL to administer the dose.

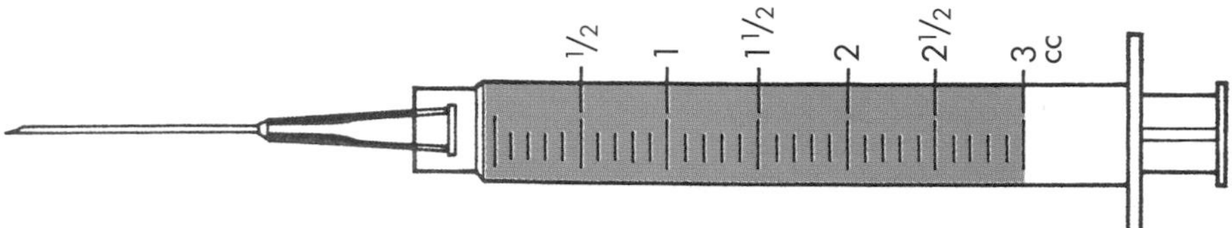

38. 50 mg : 1 mL = 120 mg : x mL OR $\frac{120 \text{ mg}}{50 \text{ mg}} \times 1 \text{ mL} = x \text{ mL}; \frac{120 \text{ mg}}{50 \text{ mg}} = \frac{x \text{ mL}}{1 \text{ mL}}$

Answer: 2.4 mL. The dose ordered is greater than what is available. Therefore you will need more than 1 mL to administer the dose.

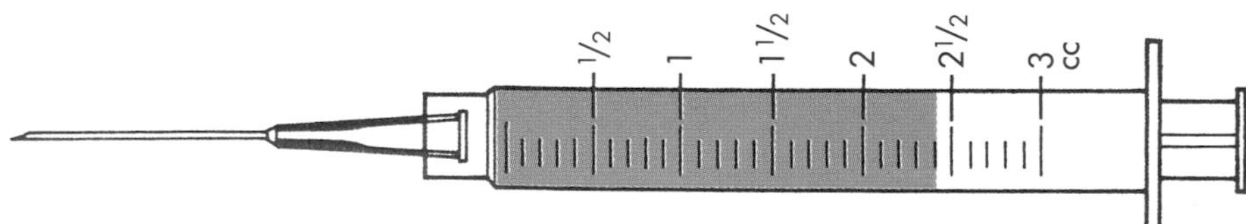

39. 2,000 U : 1 mL = 3,000 U : x mL OR $\frac{3{,}000 \text{ U}}{2{,}000 \text{ U}} \times 1 \text{ mL} = x \text{ mL}; \frac{3{,}000 \text{ U}}{2{,}000 \text{ U}} = \frac{x \text{ mL}}{1 \text{ mL}}$

Answer: 1.5 mL or $1\frac{1}{2}$ mL. The dose ordered is greater than what is available. Therefore you will need more than 1 mL to administer the dose. (The preferred answer is $1\frac{1}{2}$ mL for administration purposes.)

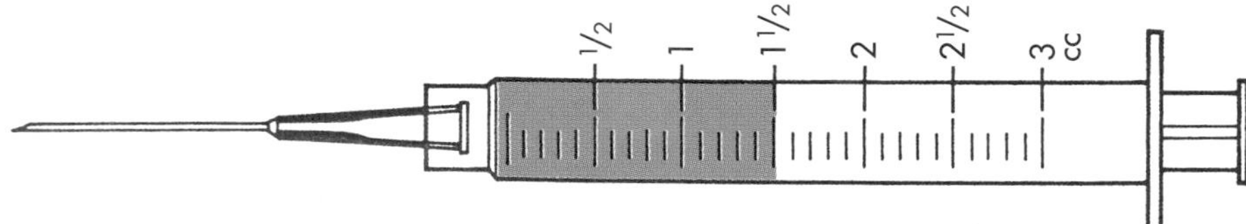

40. 25 mg : 1 mL = 50 mg : x mL OR $\frac{50 \text{ mg}}{25 \text{ mg}} \times 1 \text{ mL} = x \text{ mL}; \frac{50 \text{ mg}}{25 \text{ mg}} = \frac{x \text{ mL}}{1 \text{ mL}}$

Answer: 2 mL. The dose ordered is greater than what is available. Therefore you will need more than 1 mL to administer the dose.

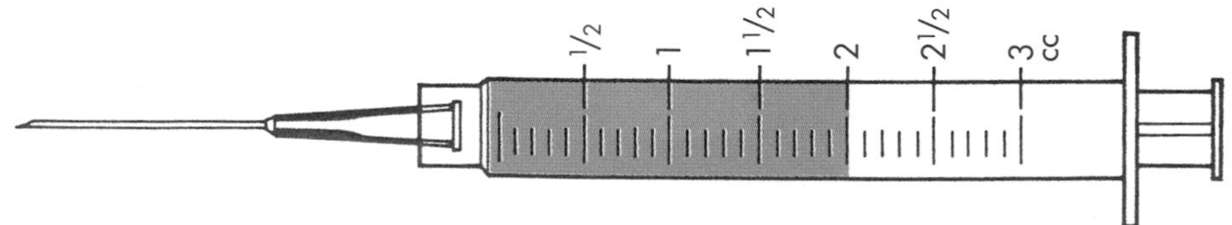

41. 30 mg : 0.3 mL = 30 mg : x mL OR $\frac{30 \text{ mg}}{30 \text{ mg}} \times 0.3 \text{ mL} = x \text{ mL}; \frac{30 \text{ mg}}{30 \text{ mg}} = \frac{x \text{ mL}}{0.3 \text{ mL}}$

Answer: 0.3 mL. The label indicates that the dose ordered, 30 mg, is contained in a volume of 0.3 mL.

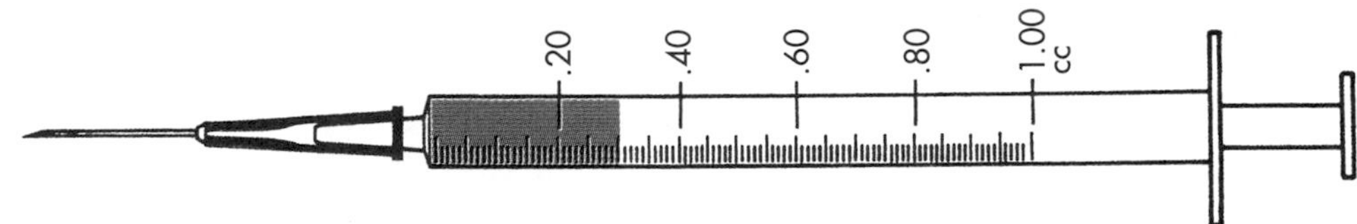

42. Conversion is required. Equivalent: 1000 mg = 1 g

Therefore 0.3 g = 300 mg

300 mg : 2 mL = 300 mg : x mL OR $\frac{300 \text{ mg}}{300 \text{ mg}} \times 2 \text{ mL} = x \text{ mL}; \frac{300 \text{ mg}}{300 \text{ mg}} = \frac{x \text{ mL}}{2 \text{ mL}}$

Answer: 2 mL. The label indicates that the dose ordered, 300 mg, is contained in a volume of 2 mL.

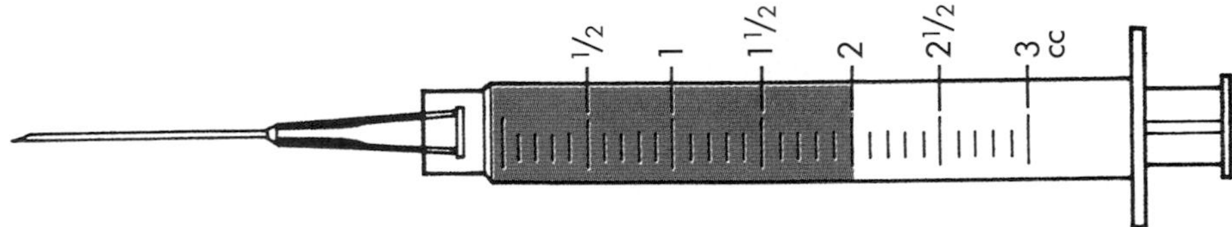

43. 5 mg : 1 mL = 7.5 mg : x mL OR $\frac{7.5 \text{ mg}}{5 \text{ mg}} \times 1 \text{ mL} = x \text{ mL}; \frac{7.5 \text{ mg}}{5 \text{ mg}} = \frac{x \text{ mL}}{1 \text{ mL}}$

Answer: 1.5 mL or $1\frac{1}{2}$ mL. ($1\frac{1}{2}$ mL is preferred for administration purposes.) The dose ordered is greater than what is available. Therefore you will need more than 1 mL to administer the dose.

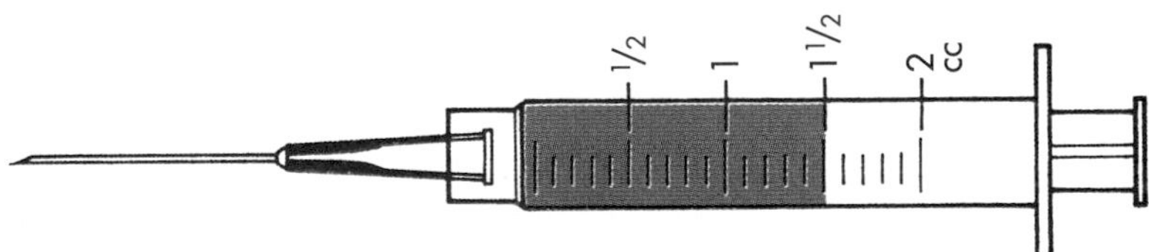

44. 1 mg : 1 mL = 1 mg : x mL OR $\frac{1 \text{ mg}}{1 \text{ mg}} \times 1 \text{ mL} = x \text{ mL}; \frac{1 \text{ mg}}{1 \text{ mg}} = \frac{x \text{ mL}}{1 \text{ mL}}$

Answer: 1 mL. The label indicates that the dose ordered, 1 mg, is contained in a volume of 1 mL.

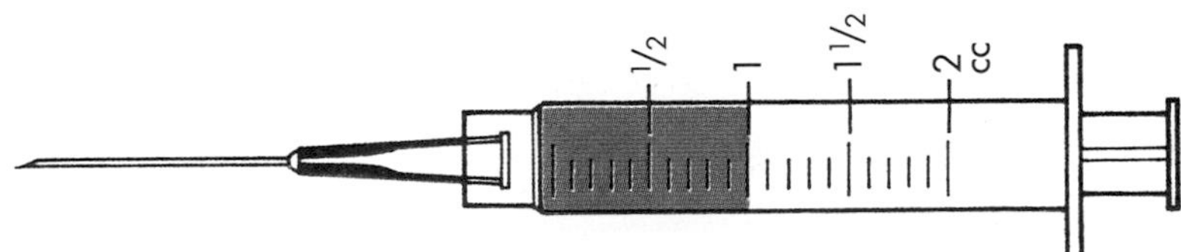

45. 20 mg : 2 mL = 30 mg : x mL OR $\frac{30 \text{ mg}}{20 \text{ mg}} \times 2 \text{ mL} = x \text{ mL}; \frac{30 \text{ mg}}{20 \text{ mg}} = \frac{x \text{ mL}}{2 \text{ mL}}$

Answer: 3 mL. The dose ordered is greater than what is available. Therefore you will need more than 2 mL to administer the dose.

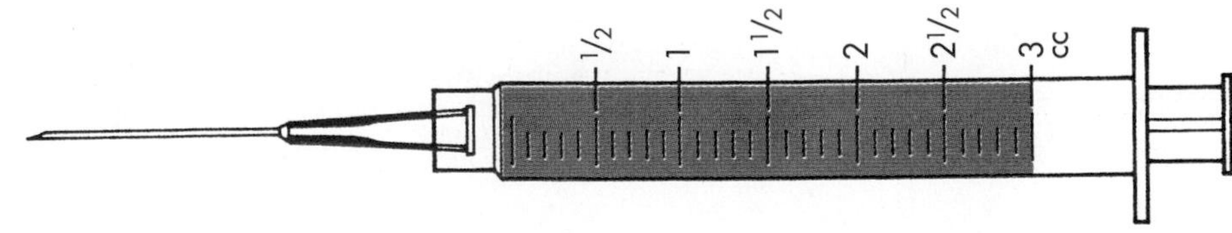

46. 4 mg : 1 mL = 12 mg : x mL OR $\frac{12 \text{ mg}}{4 \text{ mg}} \times 1 \text{ mL} = x \text{ mL}; \frac{12 \text{ mg}}{4 \text{ mg}} = \frac{x \text{ mL}}{1 \text{ mL}}$

Answer: 3 mL. The dose ordered is greater than what is available. Therefore you will need more than 1 mL to administer the dose.

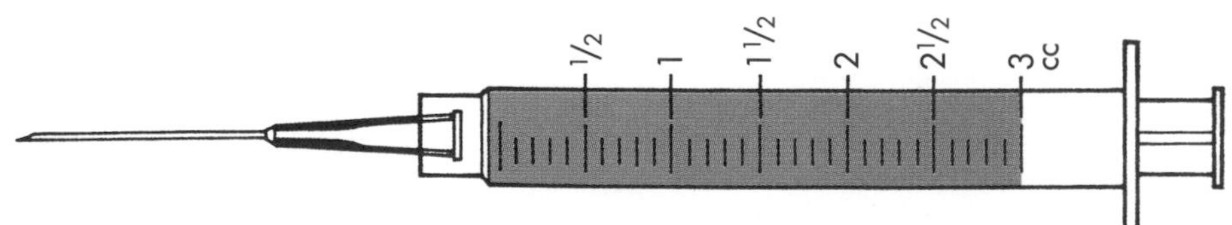

47. Conversion is required. Equivalent: 1000 mg = 1 g

Therefore 0.25 g = 250 mg

25 mg : 1 mL = 250 mg : x mL OR $\frac{250 \text{ mg}}{25 \text{ mg}} \times 1 \text{ mL} = x \text{ mL}; \frac{250 \text{ mg}}{25 \text{ mg}} = \frac{x \text{ mL}}{1 \text{ mL}}$

Answer: 10 mL. The dose ordered is greater than what is available. Therefore you will need more than 1 mL to administer the dose.

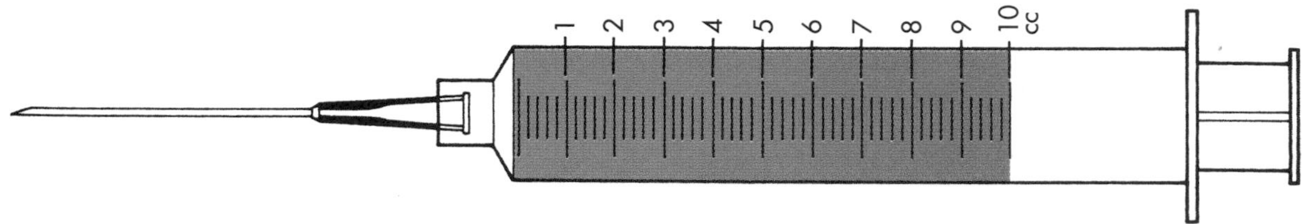

Alternate method for solving:

500 mg : 20 mL = 250 mg : x mL OR $\frac{250 \text{ mg}}{500 \text{ mg}} \times 20 \text{ mL} = x \text{ mL}; \frac{250 \text{ mg}}{500 \text{ mg}} = \frac{x \text{ mL}}{20 \text{ mL}}$

48. Conversion is required. Equivalent: 1000 mg = 1 g

Therefore 0.5 g = 500 mg

500 mg : 1 mL = 500 mg : x mL OR $\frac{500 \text{ mg}}{500 \text{ mg}} \times 1 \text{ mL} = x \text{ mL}; \frac{500 \text{ mg}}{500 \text{ mg}} = \frac{x \text{ mL}}{1 \text{ mL}}$

Answer: 1 mL. The dose ordered, 500 mg, is contained in a volume of 1 mL.

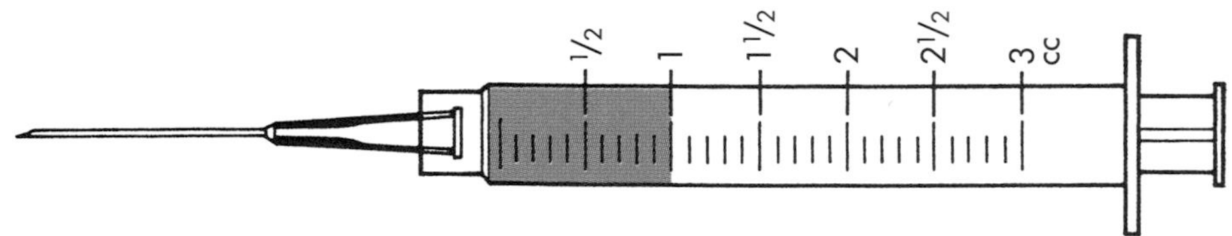

Chapter 17

Answers to Practice Problems

1. 3.5 mL
2. none stated
3. 250 mg/mL
4. 1 hr
5. 2 mL

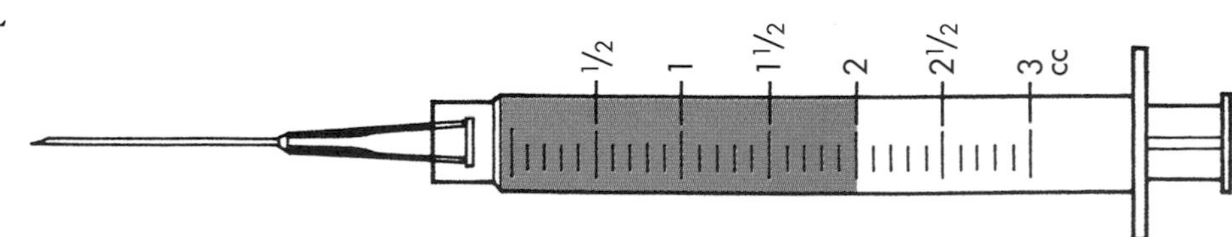

6. 2.7 mL
7. sterile water for injection
8. 250 mg per 1.5 mL
9. 3 days
10. 7 days
11. 2.4 mL

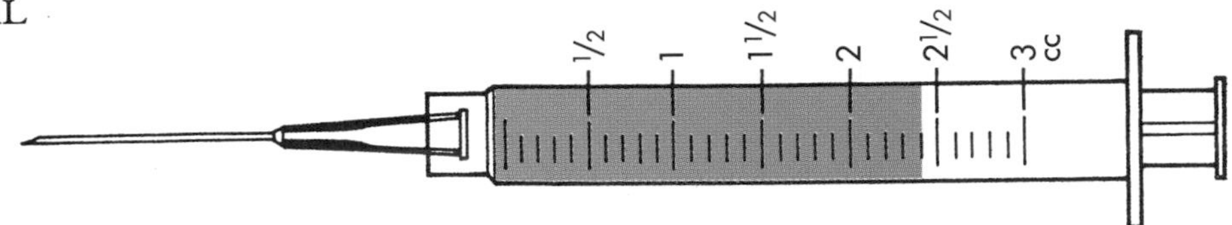

12. 2.5 mL
13. sterile water for injection
14. 330 mg/mL
15. 96 hours
16. 1.5 mL ($1\frac{1}{2}$ mL for administration purposes)

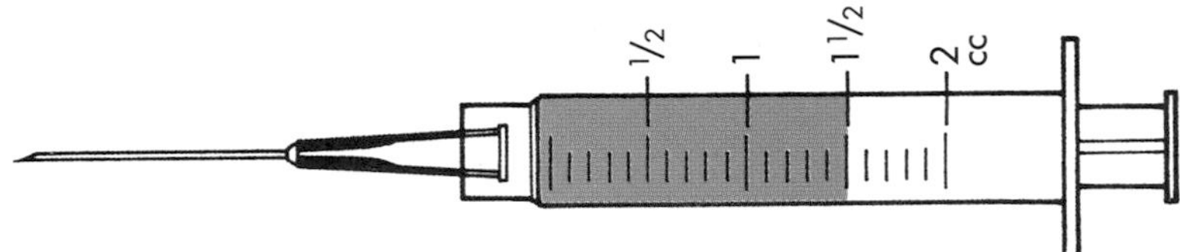

17. I.V.
18. 95 mL
19. sterile water for injection
20. 100 mg/mL
21. 24 hrs
22. 5 days
23. 10 mL

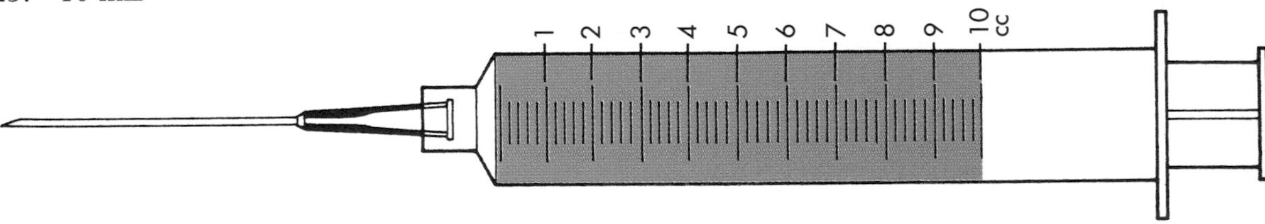

24. 5 mL; 1 tsp
25. water
26. 250 mg/5 mL
27. Refrigerate and keep tightly closed.
28. 20 mL
29. sterile water
30. 50 mg/mL
31. I.V.

32. 140 mL
33. 200 mL
34. 200 mg/5 mL
35. 10 days
36. 20,000,000 U
37. 500,000 U/mL
38. 1,000,000 U/mL—This strength is closest to what is ordered.
39. a week (7 days)
40. 1,000,000 U
41. 500,000 U/mL
42. refrigerator
43. 7 days
44. 500,000 U/mL
45. 7 days

Answers to Chapter Review

1. 250 mg : 1 mL = 400 mg : x mL

OR

$$\frac{400 \text{ mg}}{250 \text{ mg}} \times 1 \text{ mL} = x \text{ mL}; \frac{400 \text{ mg}}{250 \text{ mg}} = \frac{x \text{ mL}}{1 \text{ mL}}$$

$$\frac{250x}{250} = \frac{400}{250}$$

$$x = 1.6 \text{ mL}$$

$$\frac{400}{250} = x \qquad \frac{400}{250} = x$$

Answer: 1.6 mL. The dose ordered is more than what is available. You will need more than 1 mL to administer the dose.

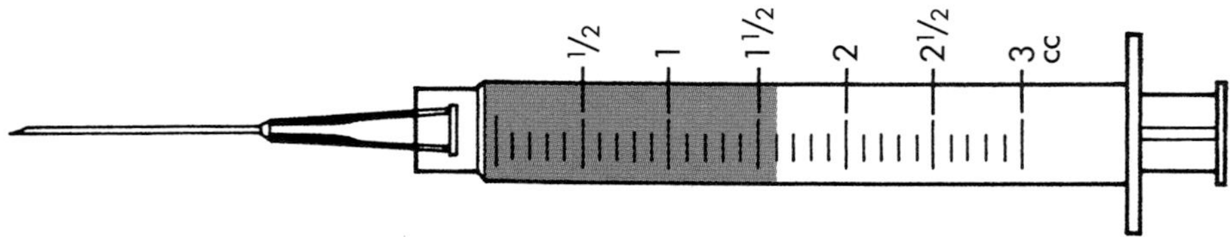

2. 1 g : 10 mL = 1 g : x mL OR $\frac{1 \text{ g}}{1 \text{ g}} \times 10 \text{ mL} = x \text{ mL}; \frac{1 \text{ g}}{1 \text{ g}} = \frac{x \text{ mL}}{10 \text{ mL}}$

$\frac{10}{1} = x \qquad x = 10 \text{ mL} \qquad \frac{10}{1} = x$

Answer: 10 mL. The dose ordered is equal to the volume of the reconstituted solution. Large volumes of I.V. solution may be administered; thus 10 mL I.V. is acceptable.

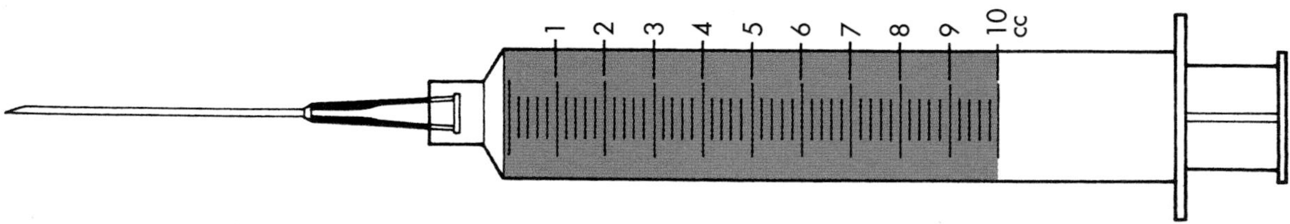

3. 250 mg : 1.5 mL = 300 mg : x mL OR $\frac{300 \text{ mg}}{250 \text{ mg}} \times 1.5 \text{ mL} = x \text{ mL}$; $\frac{300 \text{ mg}}{250 \text{ mg}} = \frac{x \text{ mL}}{1.5 \text{ mL}}$

$$\frac{250x}{250} = \frac{450}{250} \qquad \frac{300 \times 1.5}{250} = x \qquad \frac{450}{250} = x$$

$$x = 1.8 \text{ mL} \qquad \frac{450}{250} = x$$

Answer: 1.8 mL. The dose ordered is greater than what is available; you will need more than 1.5 mL to administer the dose.

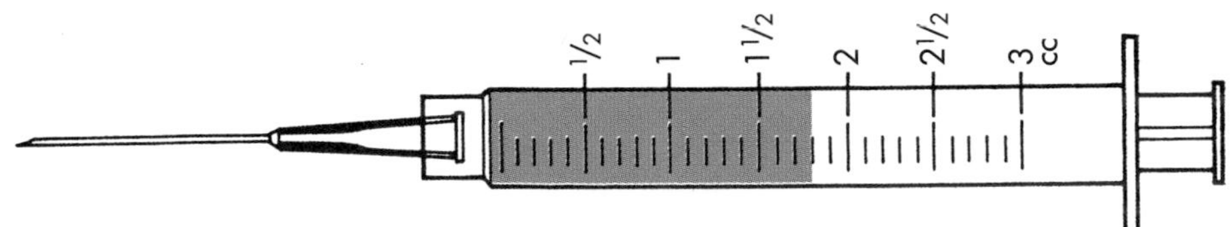

4. 3 g : 30 mL = 1.5 g : x mL OR $\frac{1.5 \text{ g}}{3.0 \text{ g}} \times 30 \text{ mL} = x \text{ mL}$; $\frac{1.5 \text{ g}}{3 \text{ g}} = \frac{x \text{ mL}}{30 \text{ mL}}$

$$\frac{3x}{3} = \frac{45}{3} \qquad \frac{1.5 \times 30}{3.0} = x \qquad \frac{45}{3} = x$$

$$x = 15 \text{ mL} \qquad \frac{45}{3.0} = x$$

Answer: 15 mL. The dose ordered is less than the available dose. You will need less than 30 mL to administer the dose; 15 mL I.V. can be administered.

5. a) 2 mL

   b) sterile water or lidocaine 1% HCl

   c) 1 g = 2.6 mL; 1g/ 2.6 mL

1 g : 2.6 mL = 1 g : x mL OR $\frac{1 \text{ g}}{1 \text{ g}} \times 2.6 \text{ mL} = x \text{ mL}$; $\frac{1 \text{ g}}{1 \text{ g}} = \frac{x \text{ mL}}{2.6 \text{ mL}}$

$$x = 2.6 \text{ mL} \qquad \frac{1 \times 2.6}{1} = x \qquad \frac{2.6}{1} = x$$

Answer: 2.6 mL. When mixed according to directions, the solution gives 1 g in 2.6 mL. Therefore you will need to administer 2.6 mL to give 1 g.

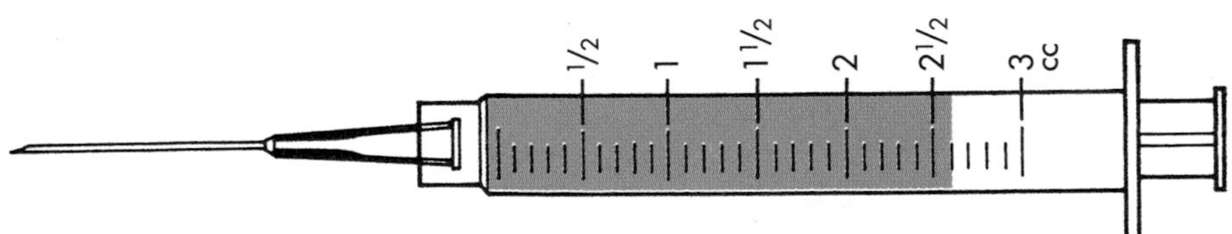

6. a) 500,000 U/mL

   b) 1.6 mL

500,000 U : 1 mL = 600,000 U : x mL OR $\frac{600{,}000 \text{ U}}{500{,}000 \text{ U}} \times 1 \text{ mL} = x \text{ mL}$; $\frac{600{,}000 \text{ U}}{500{,}000 \text{ U}} = \frac{x \text{ mL}}{1 \text{ mL}}$

$$\frac{500{,}000x}{500{,}000} = \frac{600{,}000}{500{,}000} \qquad \frac{600{,}000 \times 1}{500{,}000} = x \qquad \frac{600{,}000}{500{,}000} = x$$

$$\frac{600{,}000}{500{,}000} \qquad \frac{600{,}000}{500{,}000} = x$$

$$x = 1.2 \text{ mL} \qquad x = 1.2 \text{ mL}$$

Answer: 1.2 mL.

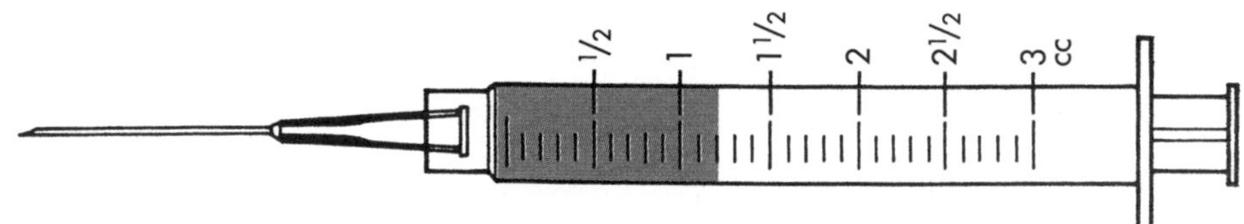

7. a) 250 mg/2 mL

$250 \text{ mg} : 2 \text{ mL} = 200 \text{ mg} : x \text{ mL}$ OR $\frac{200 \text{ mg}}{250 \text{ mg}} \times 2 \text{ mL} = x \text{ mL}; \frac{200 \text{ mg}}{250 \text{ mg}} = \frac{x \text{ mL}}{2 \text{ mL}}$

$\frac{250x}{250} = \frac{400}{250}$ $\quad \frac{200 \times 2}{250} = x \quad \frac{400}{250} = x$

$x = 1.6 \text{ mL}$ $\quad \frac{400}{250} = x$

Answer: 1.6 mL. The dose ordered is less than what is available. You will need less than 2 mL to administer the dose.

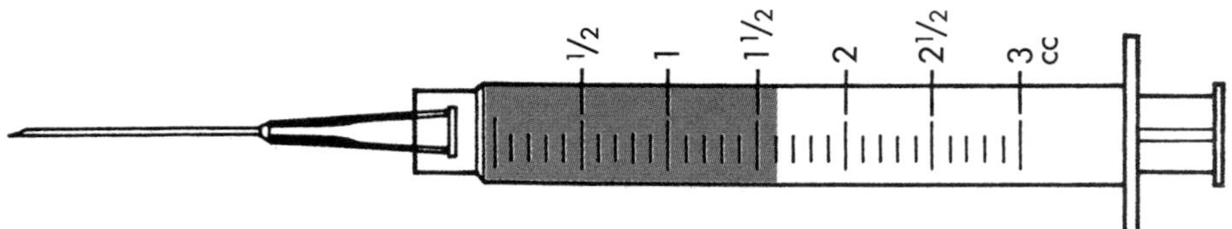

8. a) sterile water for injection

b) $1 \text{ g} : 2.5 \text{ mL} = 1 \text{ g} : x \text{ mL}$ OR $\frac{1 \text{ g}}{1 \text{ g}} \times 2.5 \text{ mL} = x \text{ mL}; \frac{1 \text{ g}}{1 \text{ g}} = \frac{x \text{ mL}}{2.5 \text{ mL}}$

$x = 2.5 \text{ mL} \left(2\frac{1}{2} \text{ mL}\right)$ $\quad \frac{1 \times 2.5}{1} = x \quad \frac{2.5}{1} = x$

$\frac{2.5}{1} = x$

Answer: 2 1/2 mL (for administration purposes). When mixed according to directions, 1 g will be contained in 2.5 mL. Administer 2 1/2 mL.

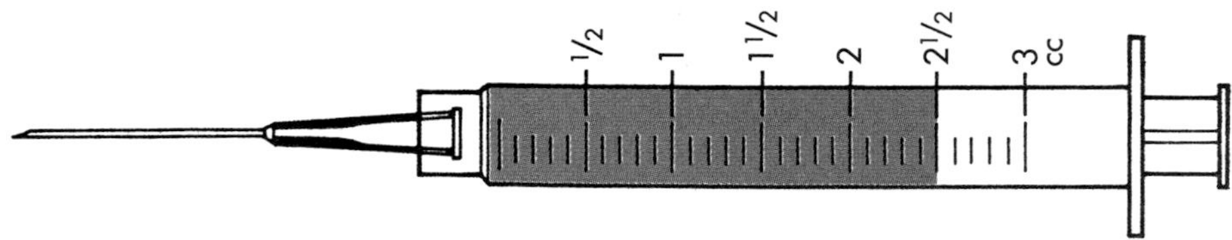

9. a) 78 mL

b) 125 mg per 5 mL

c) 20 mL

$125 \text{ mg} : 5 \text{ mL} = 500 \text{ mg} : x \text{ mL}$ OR $\frac{500 \text{ mg}}{125 \text{ mg}} \times 5 \text{ mL} = x \text{ mL}; \frac{500 \text{ mg}}{125 \text{ mg}} = \frac{x \text{ mL}}{5 \text{ mL}}$

$\frac{125x}{125} = \frac{2{,}500}{125}$ $\quad \frac{500 \times 5}{125} = x \quad \frac{2{,}500}{125} = x$

$x = 20 \text{ mL}$ $\quad \frac{2{,}500}{125} = x$

Answer: 20 mL. The dose ordered is more than what is available. You will need more than 5 mL to give the dose. Since it's a p.o. liquid and sometimes large volumes are administered, 20 mL p.o. can be administered.

10. a) 5.7 mL of sterile water or sodium chloride for injection

$1 \text{ g} : 2 \text{ mL} = 1 \text{ g} : x \text{ mL}$ OR $\frac{1 \text{ g}}{1 \text{ g}} \times 2 \text{ mL} = x \text{ mL}; \frac{1 \text{ g}}{1 \text{ g}} = \frac{x \text{ mL}}{2 \text{ mL}}$

$x = 2 \text{ mL}$ $\quad \frac{1 \times 2}{1} = x \quad \frac{2}{1} = x$

$\frac{2}{1} = x$

Answer: 2 mL. If mixed according to directions, 2 mL would contain 1 g of the medication.

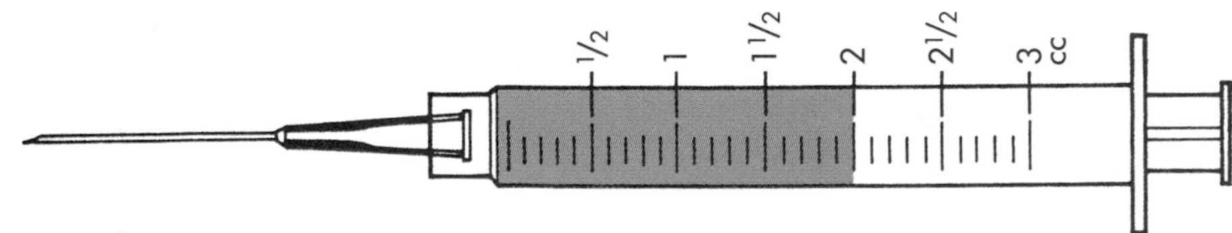

11. a) 2.5 mL of sterile water
    b) 330 mg/mL

$330 \text{ mg} : 1 \text{ mL} = 500 \text{ mg} : x \text{ mL}$ OR $\frac{500 \text{ mg}}{330 \text{ mg}} \times 1 \text{ mL} = x \text{ mL}; \frac{500 \text{ mg}}{330 \text{ mg}} = \frac{x \text{ mL}}{1 \text{ mL}}$

Answer: 1.5 mL. ($1\frac{1}{2}$ mL for administration purposes). The dose ordered is more than what is available. You will need more than 1 mL to administer the dose.

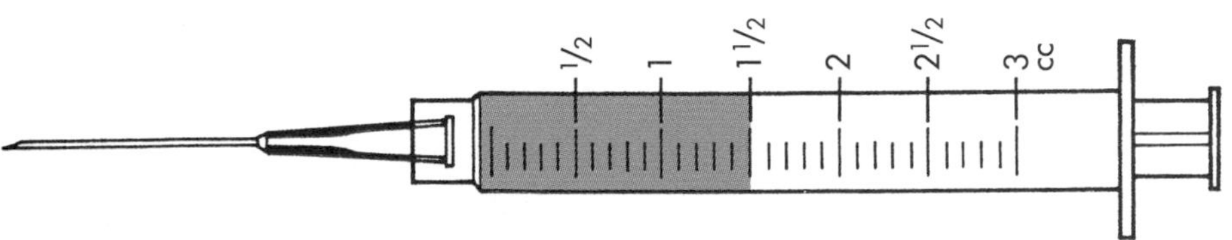

12. a) 250 mg/mL

A conversion is necessary.

$1000 \text{ mg} = 1\text{g}$

$250 \text{ mg} : 1 \text{ mL} = 1000 \text{ mg} : x \text{ mL}$ OR $\frac{1000 \text{ mg}}{250 \text{ mg}} \times 1 \text{ mL} = x \text{ mL}; \frac{1000 \text{ mg}}{250 \text{ mg}} = \frac{x \text{ mL}}{1 \text{ mL}}$

Answer: 4 mL. The dose ordered is more than what is available. You will need more than 1 mL to administer the dose.

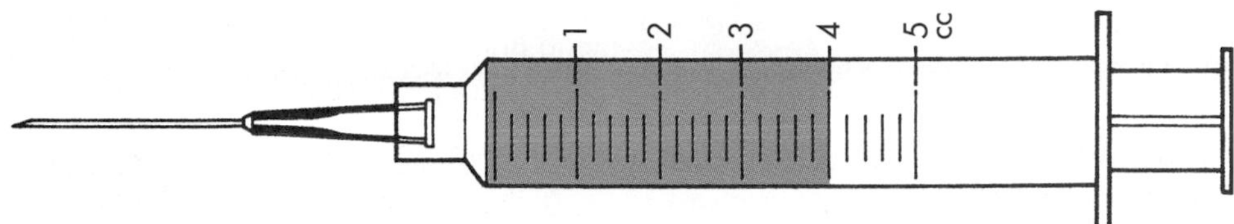

13. a) 1 g
    b) 3 mL
    c) 300 mg/mL

$300 \text{ mg} : 1 \text{ mL} = 750 \text{ mg} : x \text{ mL}$ OR $\frac{750 \text{ mg}}{300 \text{ mg}} \times 1 \text{ mL} = x \text{ mL}; \frac{750 \text{ mg}}{300 \text{ mg}} = \frac{x \text{ mL}}{1 \text{ mL}}$

Answer: 2.5 mL. ($2\frac{1}{2}$ mL for administration purposes). The dose ordered is more than what is available; therefore you will need more than 1 mL to administer the dose.

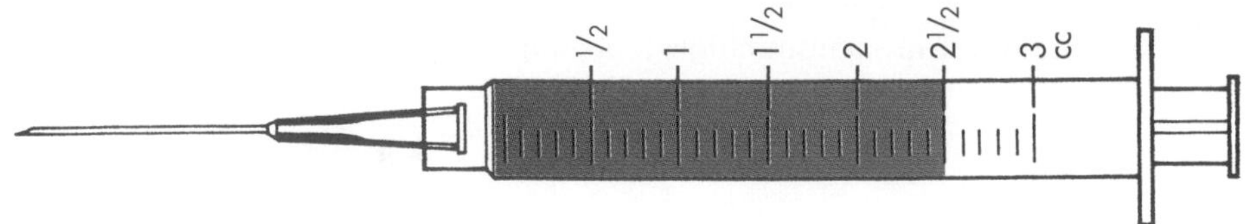

14. a) 5 g

    b) 9 mL

    c) 400 mg/mL

    Conversion: 1000 mg = 1 g; therefore 0.5 g = 500 mg

    $$400 \text{ mg} : 1 \text{ mL} = 500 \text{ mg} : x \text{ mL} \quad \text{OR} \quad \frac{500 \text{ mg}}{400 \text{ mg}} \times 1 \text{ mL} = x \text{ mL}; \frac{500 \text{ mg}}{400 \text{ mg}} = \frac{x \text{ mL}}{1 \text{ mL}}$$

    Answer: 1.3 mL. 1.25 mL is rounded to the nearest tenth. The dose ordered is more than what is available per mL; therefore more than 1 mL is required. The small hypodermics are marked in tenths of a mL. To round to the nearest tenth, the math is carried to the hundredths' place.

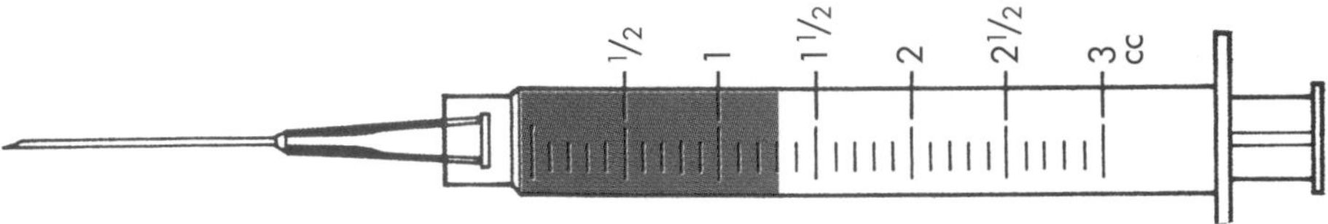

15. a) 10 mL

    b) 100 mg/mL

    Conversion: 1000 mg = 1 g; therefore 0.5 g = 500 mg

    $$100 \text{ mg} : 1 \text{ mL} = 500 \text{ mg} : x \text{ mL} \quad \text{OR} \quad \frac{500 \text{ mg}}{100 \text{ mg}} \times 1 \text{ mL} = x \text{ mL}; \frac{500 \text{ mg}}{100 \text{ mg}} = \frac{x \text{ mL}}{1 \text{ mL}}$$

    Answer: 5 mL. The dose ordered is more than what is available, therefore you will need more than 1 mL to administer the dose.

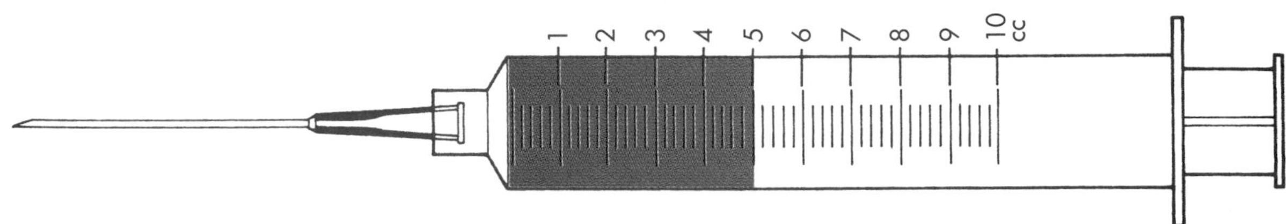

16. $$500{,}000 \text{ U} : 1 \text{ mL} = 400{,}000 \text{ U} : x \text{ mL} \quad \text{OR} \quad \frac{400{,}000 \text{ U}}{500{,}000 \text{ U}} \times 1 \text{ mL} = x \text{ mL}; \frac{400{,}000 \text{ U}}{500{,}000 \text{ U}} = \frac{x \text{ mL}}{1 \text{ mL}}$$

    Answer: 0.8 mL. The dose ordered is less than what is available. You will need less than 1 mL to administer the dose.

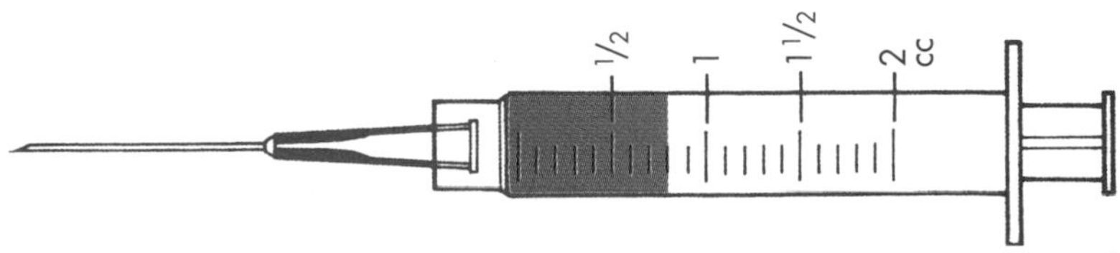

17. a) 500,000 U/mL. It is closer to the doctor's order; client will receive less volume.

    b) 1.6 mL

$$500{,}000\text{ U} : 1\text{ mL} = 600{,}000\text{ U} : x\text{ mL} \quad \text{OR} \quad \frac{600{,}000\text{ U}}{500{,}000\text{ U}} \times 1\text{ mL} = x\text{ mL}; \frac{600{,}000\text{ U}}{500{,}000\text{ U}} = \frac{x\text{ mL}}{1\text{ mL}}$$

Answer: 1.2 mL. The dose ordered is greater than what is available. You will need more than 1 mL to administer the dose.

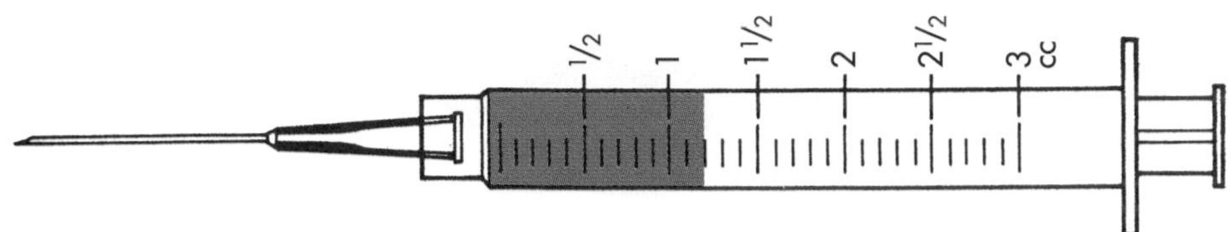

18. $$300\text{ mg} : 1\text{ mL} = 250\text{ mg} : x\text{ mL} \quad \text{OR} \quad \frac{250\text{ mg}}{300\text{ mg}} \times 1\text{ mL} = x\text{ mL}; \frac{250\text{ mg}}{300\text{ mg}} = \frac{x\text{ mL}}{1\text{ mL}}$$

Answer: 0.8 mL. 0.83 is rounded to the nearest tenth. The dose ordered is less than what is available; therefore you will need less than 1 mL to administer the dose.

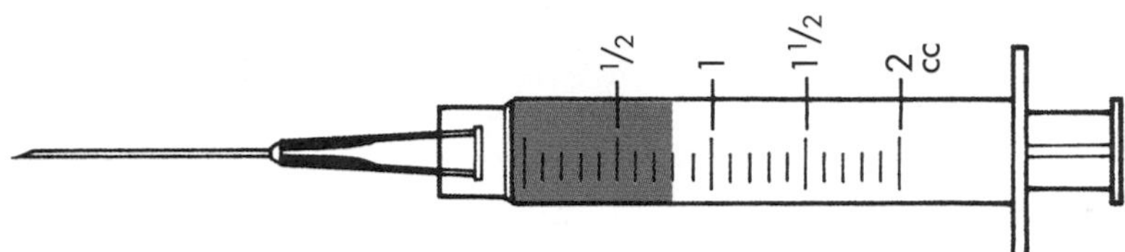

19. a) 2 mL

    b) 1 g = 2.6 mL; 1g/2.6 mL

$$1\text{ g} : 2.6\text{ mL} = 0.5\text{ g} : x\text{ mL} \quad \text{OR} \quad \frac{0.5\text{ g}}{1\text{ g}} \times 2.6\text{ mL} = x\text{ mL}; \frac{0.5\text{ g}}{1\text{ g}} = \frac{x\text{ mL}}{2.6\text{ mL}}$$

Answer: 1.3 mL. The dose ordered is one half of the dose available. You will need less than 2.6 mL to administer the dose.

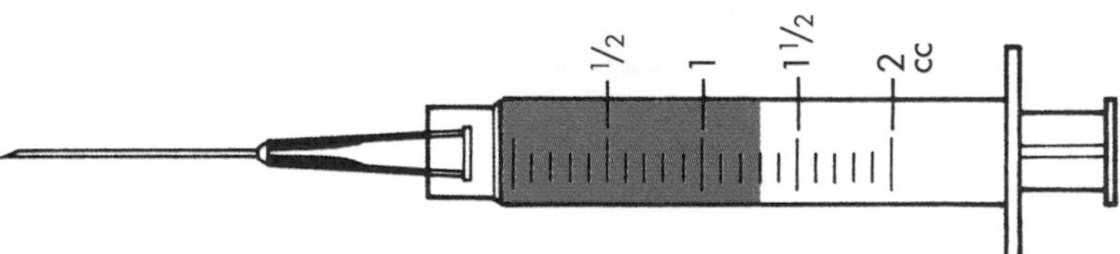

20. a) 5.7 mL

    b) 1 g = 2 mL; 1 g/2 mL

$$1\text{ g} : 2\text{ mL} = 1\text{ g} : x\text{ mL} \quad \text{OR} \quad \frac{1\text{ g}}{1\text{ g}} \times 2\text{ mL} = x\text{ mL}; \frac{1\text{ g}}{1\text{ g}} = \frac{x\text{ mL}}{2\text{ mL}}$$

Answer: 2 mL. The dose ordered is equivalent to 2 mL; therefore you will need 2 mL to administer the dose.

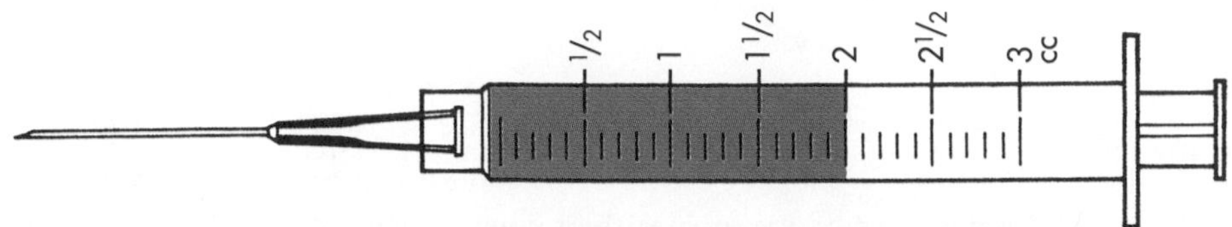

21. Conversion is required. Equivalent: 1000 mg = 1 g; therefore 0.4 g = 400 mg

$$95 \text{ mg} : 1 \text{ mL} = 400 \text{ mg} : x \text{ mL} \quad \text{OR} \quad \frac{400 \text{ mg}}{95 \text{ mg}} \times 1 \text{ mL} = x \text{ mL}; \frac{400 \text{ mg}}{95 \text{ mg}} = \frac{x \text{ mL}}{1 \text{ mL}}$$

Answer: 4.2 mL. 4.21 mL is rounded to the nearest tenth. The dose ordered is greater than what is available. Therefore you will need more than 1 mL to administer the dose. (Syringe is calibrated in 0.2 increments.)

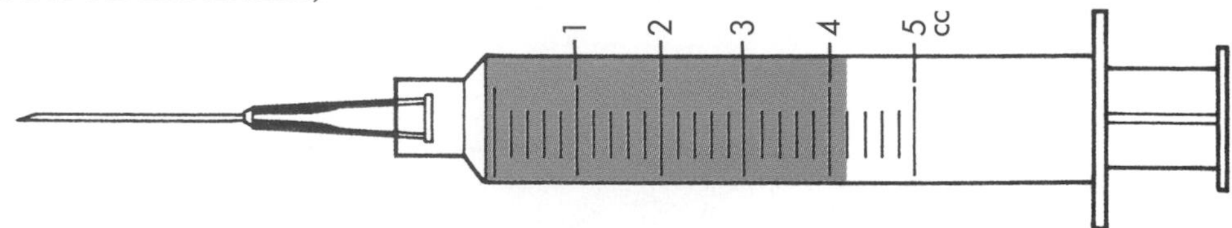

22. Conversion is required. Equivalent: 1000 mg = 1 g

Therefore 0.5 g = 500 mg

$$50 \text{ mg} : 1 \text{ mL} = 500 \text{ mg} : x \text{ mL} \quad \text{OR} \quad \frac{500 \text{ mg}}{50 \text{ mg}} \times 1 \text{ mL} = x \text{ mL}; \frac{500 \text{ mg}}{50 \text{ mg}} = \frac{x \text{ mL}}{1 \text{ mL}}$$

Answer: 10 mL. The dose ordered is greater than what is available. Therefore you will need more than 1 mL to administer the dose.

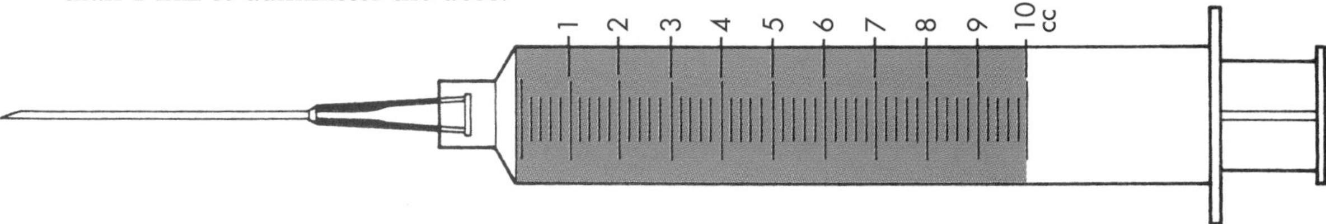

23. Conversion is required. Equivalent: 1000 mcg = 1 mg; therefore 0.05 mg = 50 mcg

$$200 \text{ mcg} : 5 \text{ mL} = 50 \text{ mcg} : x \text{ mL} \quad \text{OR} \quad \frac{50 \text{ mcg}}{200 \text{ mcg}} \times 5 \text{ mL} = x \text{ mL}; \frac{50 \text{ mcg}}{200 \text{ mcg}} = \frac{x \text{ mL}}{5 \text{ mL}}$$

Answer: 1.3 mL. 1.25 mL is rounded to the nearest tenth. The dose ordered is less than what is available. Therefore you will need less than 5 mL to administer the dose.

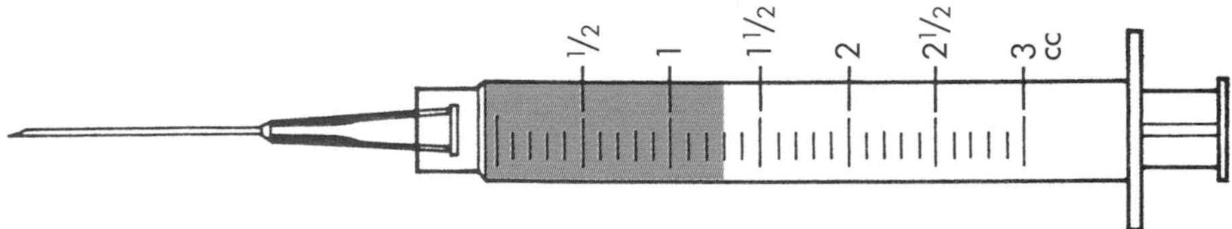

24. Conversion is required. Equivalent: 1000 mg = 1 g; therefore 0.25 g = 250 mg

$$50 \text{ mg} : 1 \text{ mL} = 250 \text{ mg} : x \text{ mL} \quad \text{OR} \quad \frac{250 \text{ mg}}{50 \text{ mg}} \times 1 \text{ mL} = x \text{ mL}; \frac{250 \text{ mg}}{50 \text{ mg}} = \frac{x \text{ mL}}{1 \text{ mL}}$$

Answer: 5 mL. The dose ordered is more than what is available. Therefore you will need more than 1 mL to administer the dose.

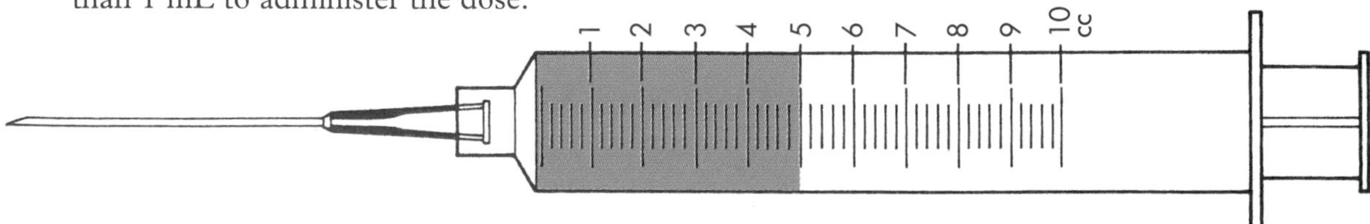

25. a) 80 mL
    b) 20 mL

$$100 \text{ mg} : 5 \text{ mL} = 400 \text{ mg} : x \text{ mL} \quad \text{OR} \quad \frac{400 \text{ mg}}{100 \text{ mg}} \times 5 \text{ mL} = x \text{ mL}; \frac{400 \text{ mg}}{100 \text{ mg}} = \frac{x \text{ mL}}{5 \text{ mL}}$$

Answer: 20 mL. The dose ordered is greater than what is available. Therefore you will need more than 5 mL to administer the dose.

Chapter 18

Answers to Practice Problems

1. Lente; human
2. protamine zinc; beef and pork
3. NPH; beef and pork
4. Ultralente; human
5. 22 U
6. 41 U
7.

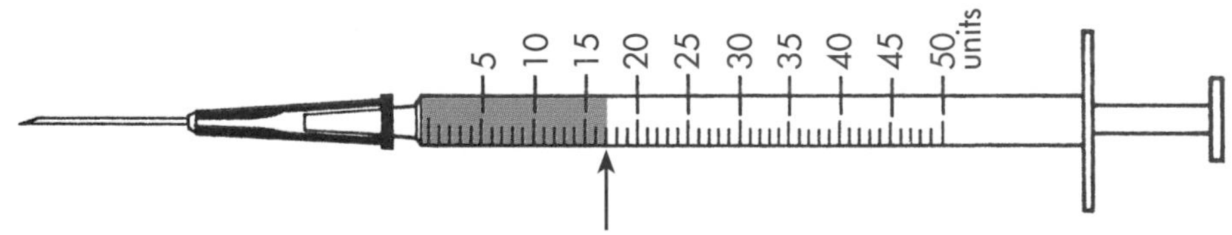

8.

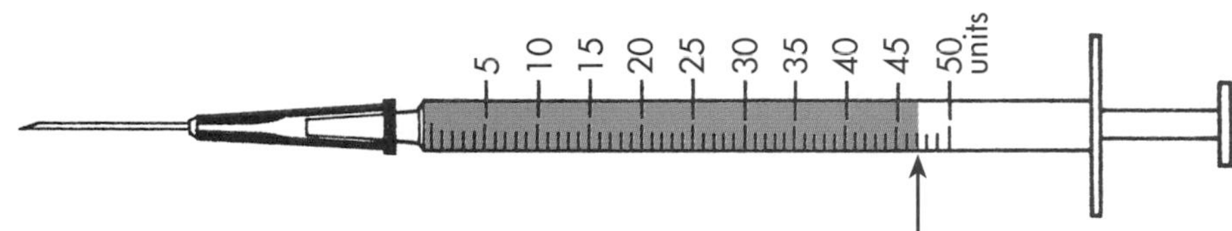

9. 40 U
10. 27 U
11. 53 U
12. 14 U
13.

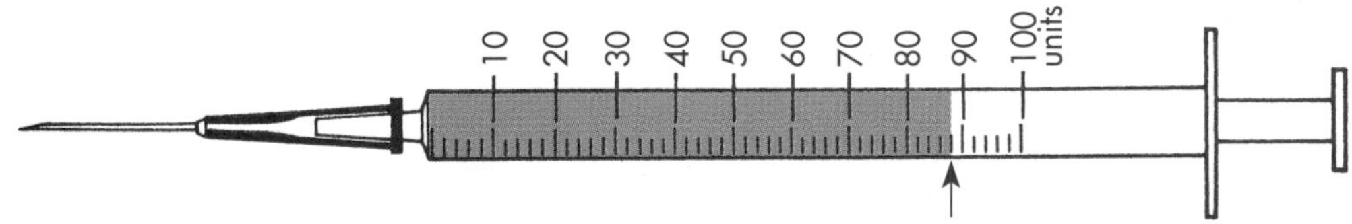

14.

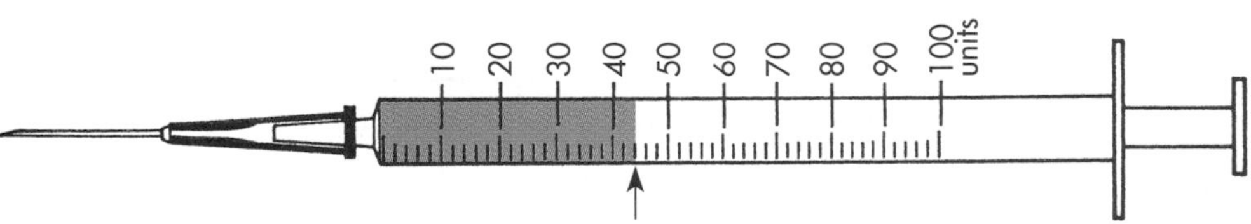

15.

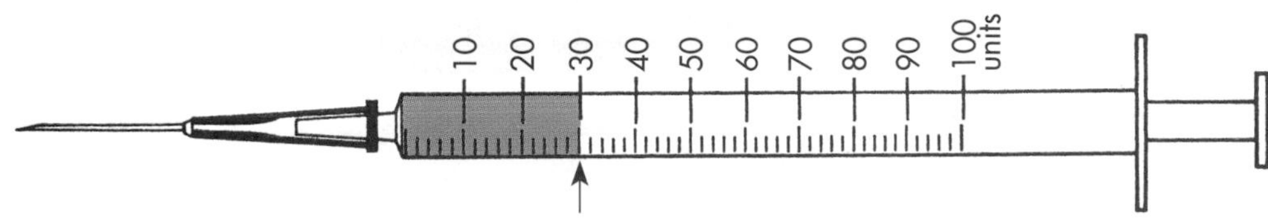

Answers to Chapter Review

1.

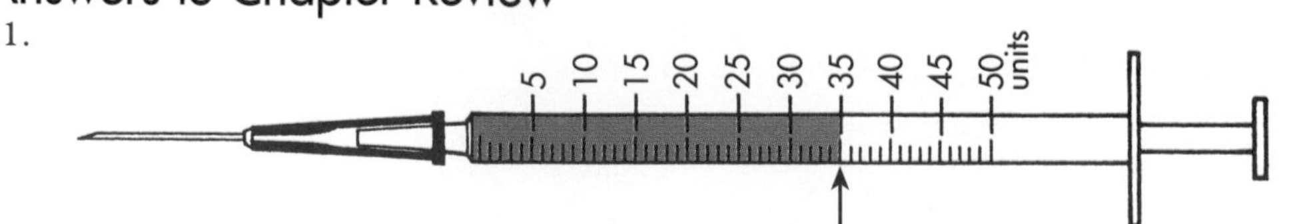

2.

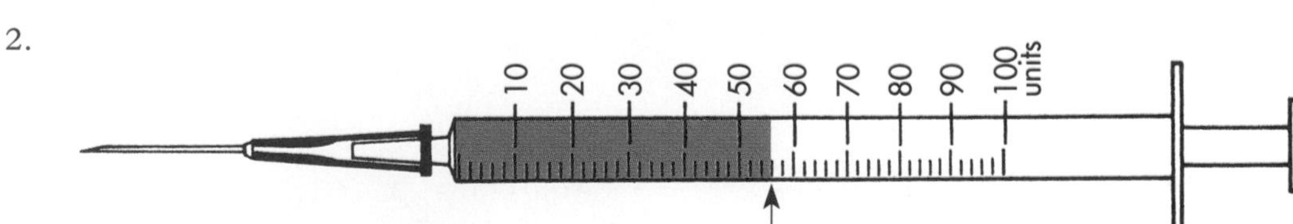

3.

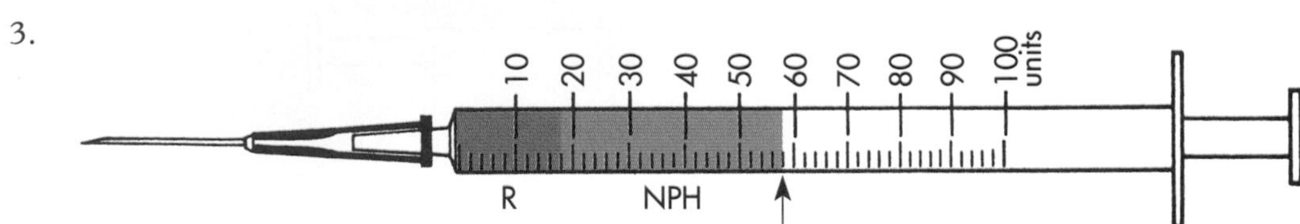

4.

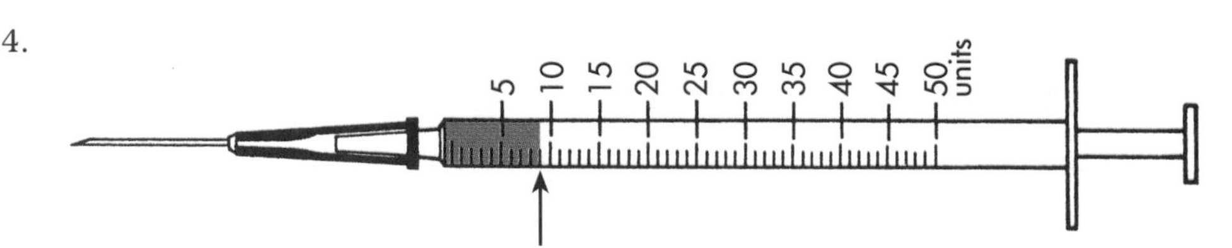

5. 15 U
6. 26 U
7. 16 U
8. 52 U
9. 38 U
10. 65 U
11. 15 U
12.

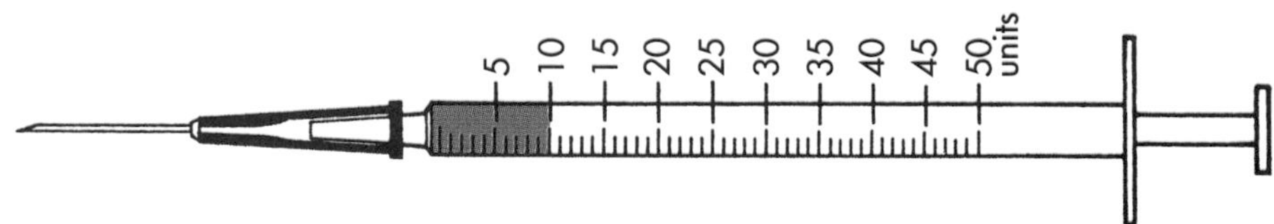

13.

14.

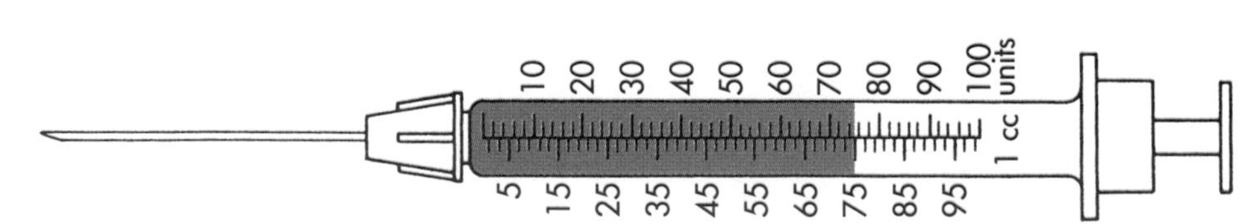

15.

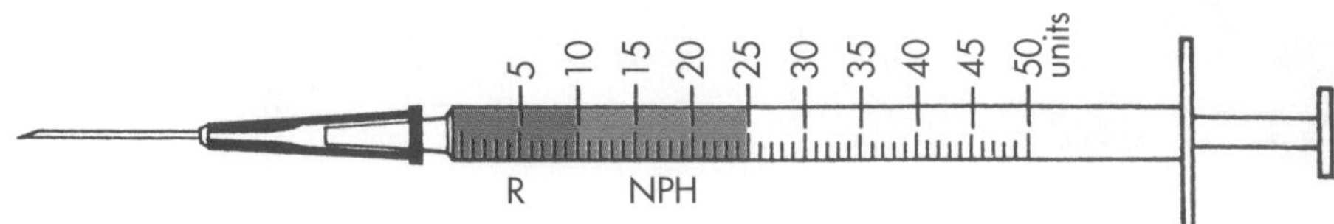

16.

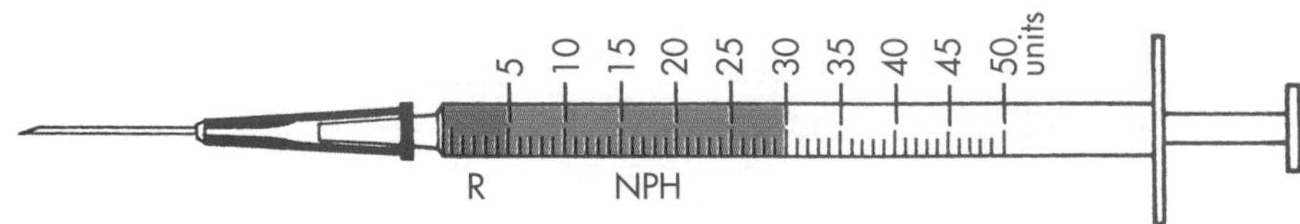

17.

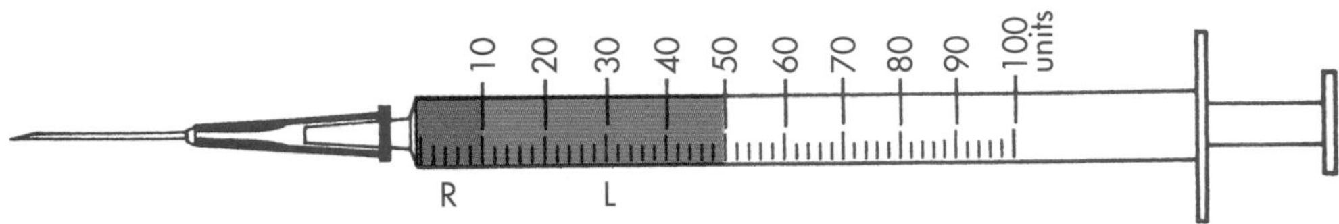

18.

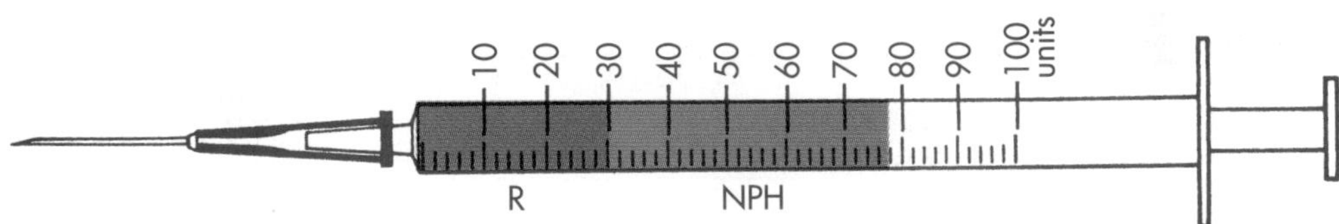

19.

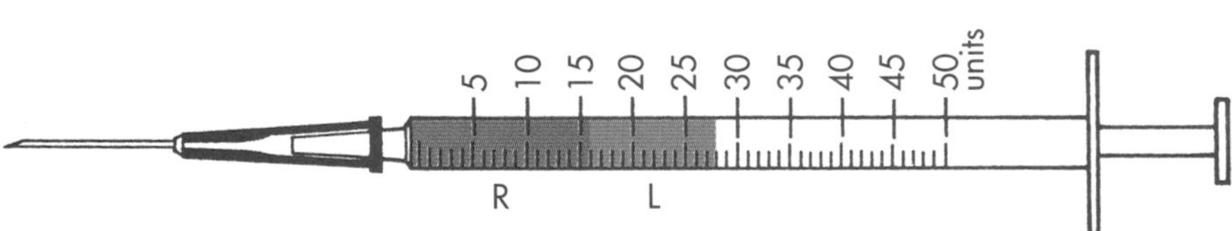

20.

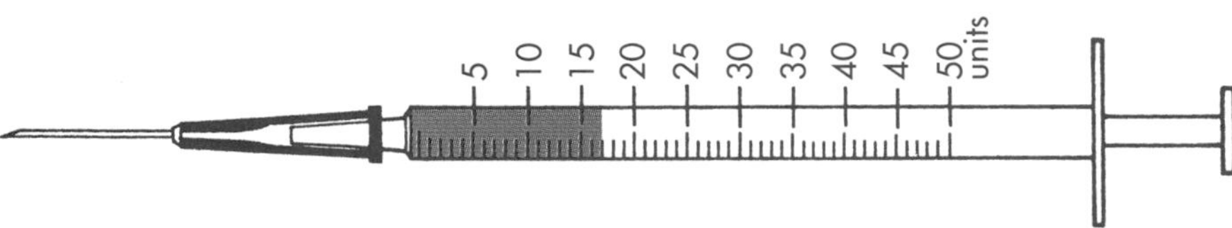

21.

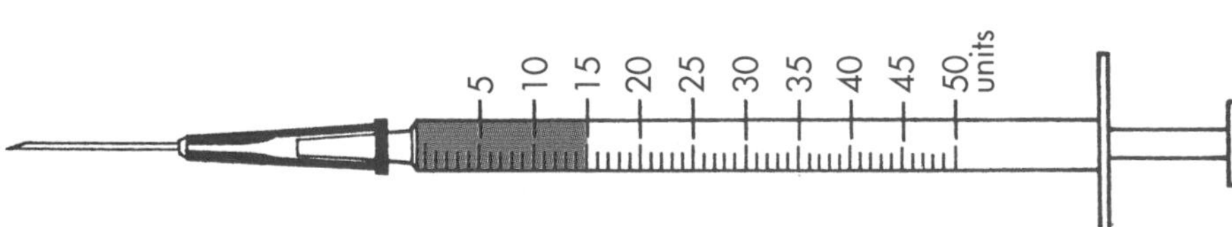

22.

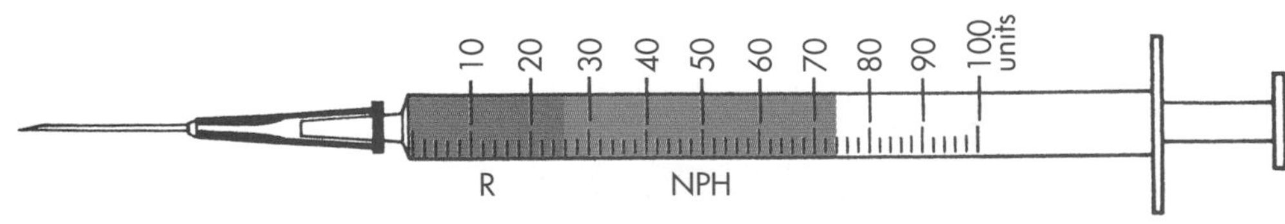

23.

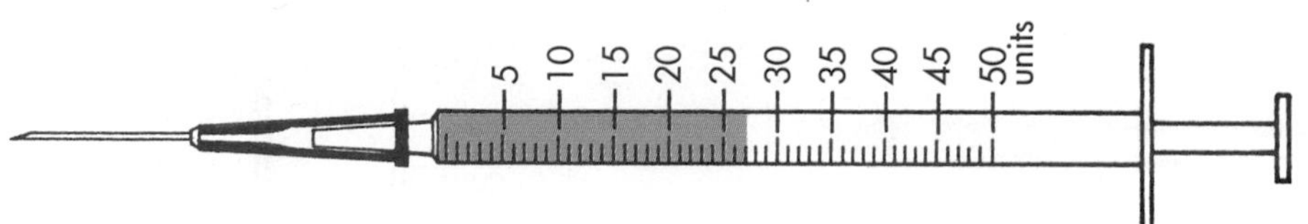

24.

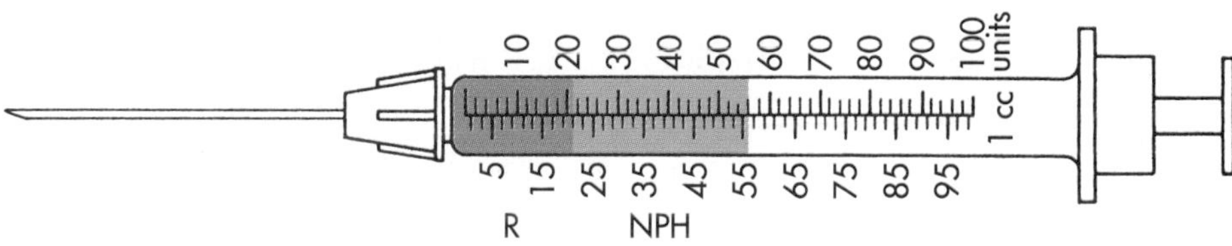

25.

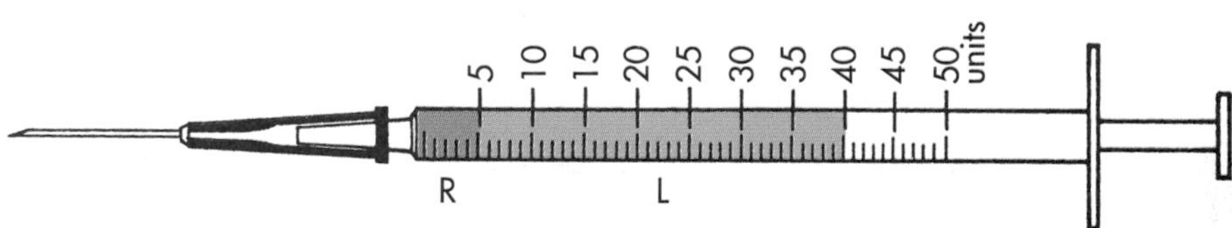

26.

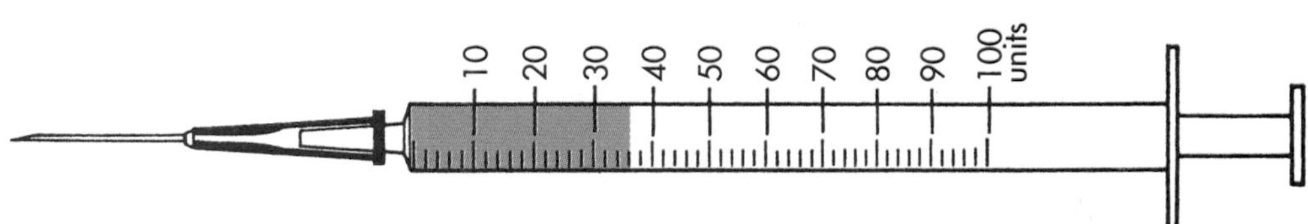

27.

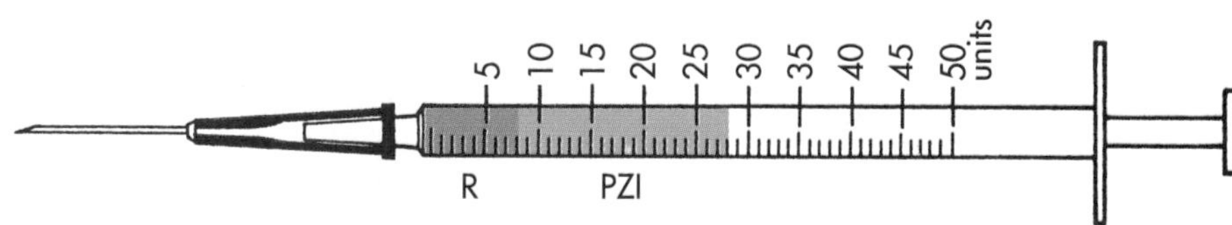

28. 6 U for blood sugar level of 364

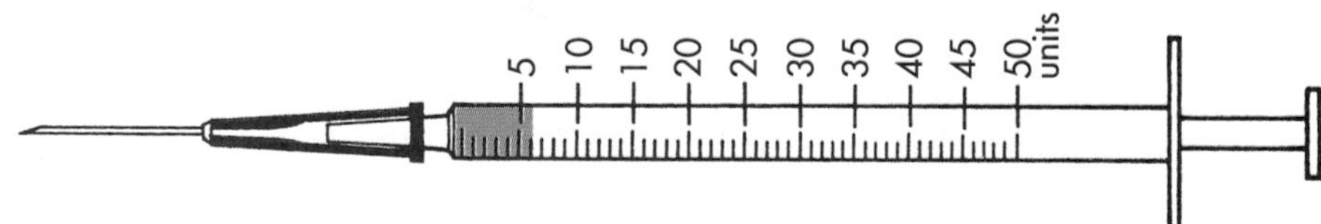

29.

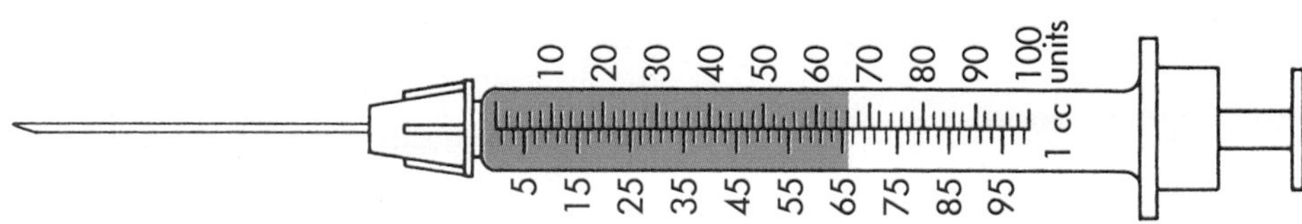

30.

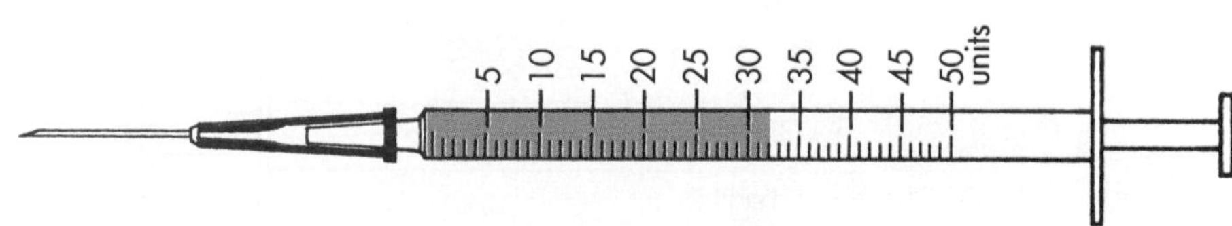

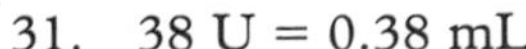

31. 38 U = 0.38 mL

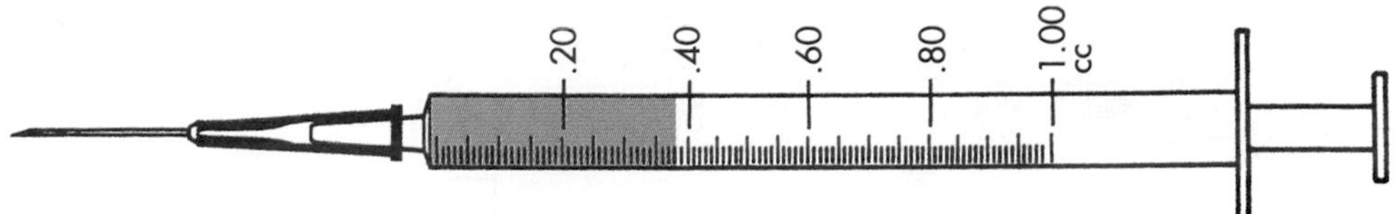

32. 12 U = 0.12 mL

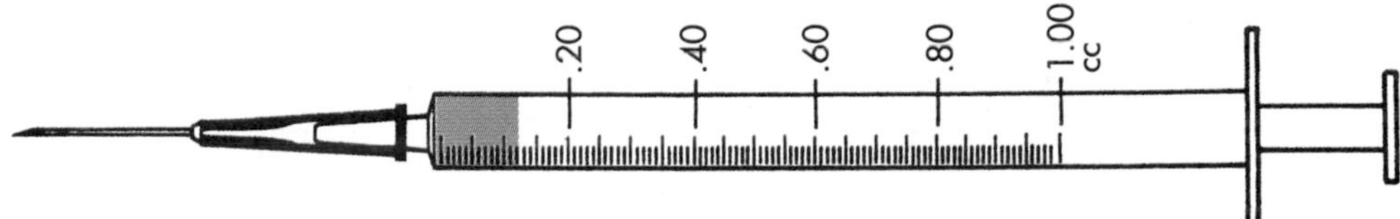

33. 60 U = 0.60 mL

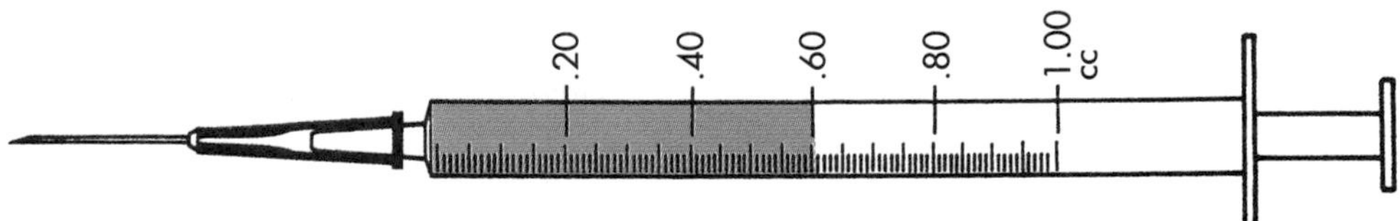

34. 64 U = 0.64 mL

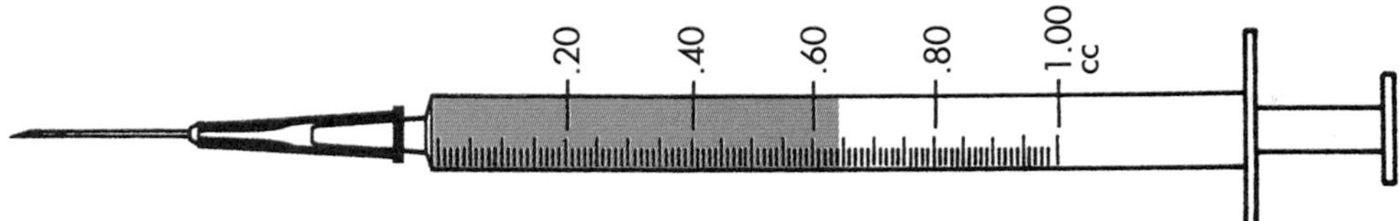

35. 35 U

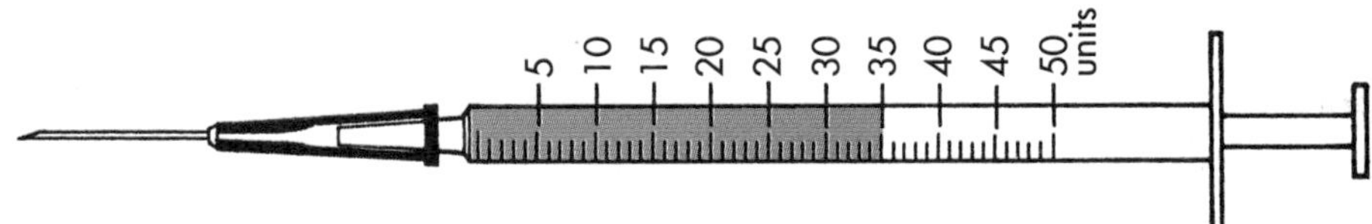

36. 9 U

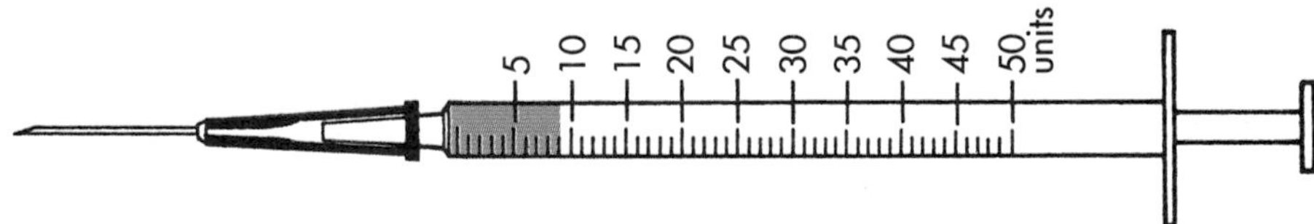

37. 24 U

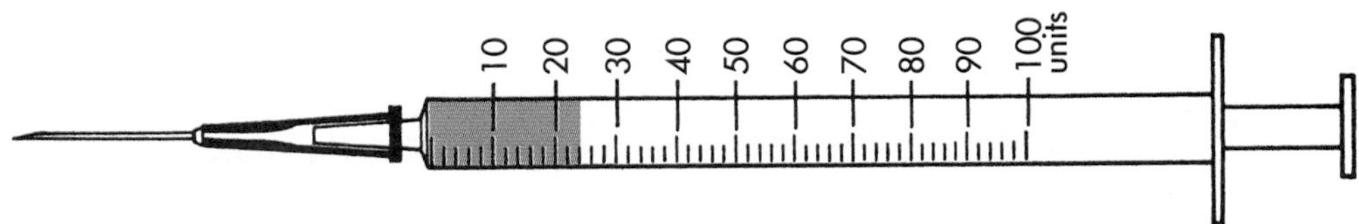

38. 26 U total

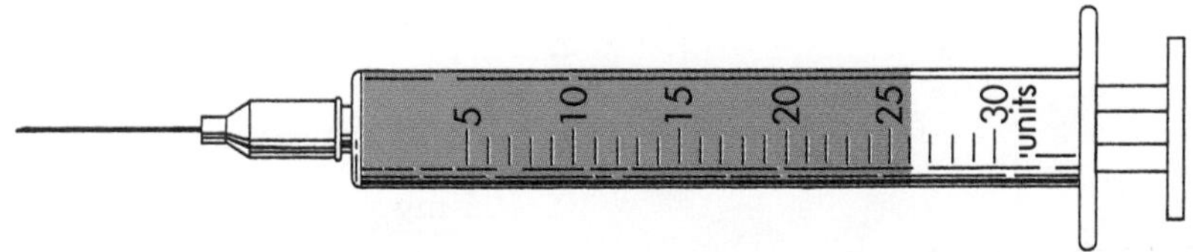

39. 11 U total

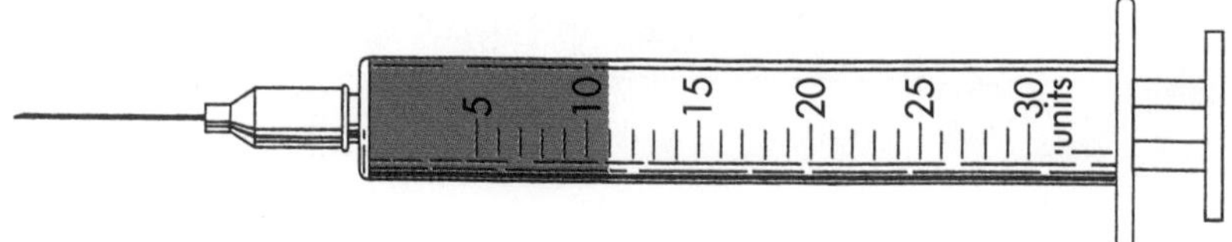

40. 20 U total

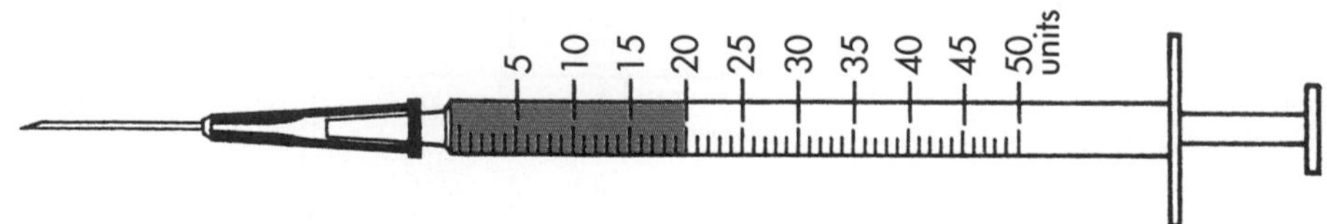

Chapter 19

Answers to Practice Problems

1. 9.1 kg
2. 29.1 kg
3. 10 kg
4. 23.6 kg
5. 32.3 kg
6. 5.5 kg
7. 3.8 kg
8. 2.5 kg
9. 44 lb
10. 101.2 lb
11. 48.4 lb
12. 33 lb
13. 74.8 lb
14. 50.6 lb
15. 160.6 lb
16. 215.6 lb

Answers to Practice Problems: Calculating According to mg/kg

17. a) 25–50 mg/kg/day

b) Convert weight first (2.2 lb = 1 kg).
$35 \div 2.2 = 15.9$ kg

$$\frac{25 \text{ mg}}{x \text{ mg}} = \frac{1 \text{ kg}}{15.9 \text{ kg}} \; x = 25 \times 15.9$$

or

$$25 \text{ mg} \times 15.9 = 397.5 \text{ mg}$$

$$\frac{50 \text{ mg}}{x \text{ mg}} = \frac{1 \text{ kg}}{15.9 \text{ kg}} \; x = 50 \times 15.9$$

OR

$$50 \text{ mg} \times 15.9 \text{ kg} = 795 \text{ mg}$$

Dose range is 397.5–795 mg.

c) The dose ordered falls within the range that is safe.

$$(150 \text{ mg} \times 4 = 600 \text{ mg})$$

d) $125 \text{ mg} : 5 \text{ mL} = 150 \text{ mg} : x \text{ mL}$

OR

$$\frac{150 \text{ mg}}{125 \text{ mg}} \times 5 \text{ mL} = x \text{ mL}; \frac{150 \text{ mg}}{125 \text{ mg}} = \frac{x \text{ mL}}{5 \text{ mL}}$$

$$x = 6 \text{ mL}$$

18. a) $\frac{15 \text{ mg}}{x \text{ mg}} = \frac{1 \text{ kg}}{35 \text{ kg}}$

$x = 35 \times 15$

$x = 525$ mg—maximum dose for 24 hr

OR

$$35 \text{ kg} \times 15 \text{ mg} = 525 \text{ mg}$$

b) $\frac{525 \text{ mg}}{3} = 175 \text{ mg}$

c) No, not safe. $200 \text{ mg} \times 3 = 600$ mg. This is greater than the maximum dose. Check order with doctor.

19. a) $\frac{8 \text{ mg}}{x \text{ mg}} = \frac{1 \text{ kg}}{40 \text{ kg}} = 320 \text{ mg}$

OR

$$8 \text{ mg} \times 40 \text{ kg} = 320 \text{ mg}$$

$$\frac{25 \text{ mg}}{x \text{ mg}} = \frac{1 \text{ kg}}{40 \text{ kg}} = 1000 \text{ mg}$$

OR

$$25 \text{ mg} \times 40 \text{ kg} = 1000 \text{ mg}$$

Answer: 1000 mg is maximum dose.

b) four divided doses

$$320 \text{ mg} \div 4 = 80 \text{ mg}$$

$$1000 \text{ mg} \div 4 = 250 \text{ mg}$$

Answer: 80–250 mg (250 mg is maximum divided dose)

20. a) Weight conversion (2.2 lb = 1 kg)
$9 \div 2.2 = 4.1$ kg

b) $$\frac{3 \text{ mg}}{x \text{ mg}} = \frac{1 \text{ kg}}{4.1 \text{ kg}} = 12.3 \text{ mg}$$

OR

$$3 \text{ mg} \times 4.1 \text{ kg} = 12.3 \text{ mg}$$

$$\frac{5 \text{ mg}}{x \text{ mg}} = \frac{1 \text{ kg}}{4.1 \text{ kg}} = 20.5 \text{ mg}$$

OR

$$5 \text{ mg} \times 4.1 \text{ kg} = 20.5 \text{ mg}$$

Safety range for the child for a day is 12.3 mg–20.5 mg. The divided dose is 6.2 mg–10.3 mg

c) The dose ordered is safe.

$10 \text{ mg} \times 2 = 20$ mg. The maximum dose per day is 20.5 mg.

d) $20 \text{ mg} : 5 \text{ mL} = 10 \text{ mg} : x \text{ mL}$

OR

$$\frac{10 \text{ mg}}{20 \text{ mg}} \times 5 \text{ mL} = x \text{ mL}; \frac{10 \text{ mg}}{20 \text{ mg}} = \frac{x \text{ mL}}{5 \text{ mL}}$$

$$x = 2.5 \text{ mL}$$

You need to give 2.5 mL to administer the ordered dose of 10 mg. (State as 2 1/2 mL for administration purposes.)

21. a) Convert weight to kg (2.2 lb = 1 kg).
$84 \text{ lb} \div 2.2 = 38.2$ kg

$$\frac{0.1 \text{ mg}}{x \text{ mg}} = \frac{1 \text{ kg}}{38.2 \text{ kg}} = 3.8 \text{ mg}$$

OR

$$38.2 \text{ kg} \times 0.1 \text{ mg} = 3.82 \text{ mg} = 3.8 \text{ mg}$$

OR

$$\frac{0.2 \text{ mg}}{x \text{ mg}} = \frac{1 \text{ kg}}{38.2 \text{ kg}} = 7.6 \text{ mg}$$

$$0.2 \text{ mg} \times 38.2 \text{ kg} = 7.64 \text{ mg} = 7.6 \text{ mg}$$

The dose ordered is safe.

b) You would administer 0.5 mL.

$15 \text{ mg} : 1 \text{ mL} = 7.5 \text{ mg} : x \text{ mL}$

OR

$$\frac{7.5 \text{ mg}}{15 \text{ mg}} \times 1 \text{ mL} = x \text{ mL}; \frac{7.5 \text{ mg}}{15 \text{ mg}} = \frac{x \text{ mL}}{1 \text{ mL}}$$

$x = 0.5$ mL (State as 1/2 mL for administration purposes.)

22. a) Convert weight to kg (2.2 lb = 1 kg).

$$11 \text{ lb} \div 2.2 = 5 \text{ kg}$$

$$\frac{4 \text{ mg}}{x \text{ mg}} = \frac{1 \text{ kg}}{5 \text{ kg}} = 20 \text{ mg}$$

OR

$$4 \text{ mg} \times 5 \text{ kg} = 20 \text{ mg}$$

$$\frac{8 \text{ mg}}{x \text{ mg}} = \frac{1 \text{ kg}}{5 \text{ kg}} = 40 \text{ mg}$$

OR

$$8 \text{ mg} \times 5 \text{ kg} = 40 \text{ mg}$$

The dose that is ordered is safe. It falls within the safe range. $15 \text{ mg} \times 2 = 30$ mg.

b) $30 \text{ mg} : 5 \text{ mL} = 15\text{mg} : x \text{ ml}$

OR

$$\frac{15 \text{ mg}}{30 \text{ mg}} \times 5 \text{ mL}; \frac{15 \text{ mg}}{30 \text{ mg}} = \frac{x \text{ mL}}{5 \text{ mL}}$$

You would give 2.5 mL (2 1/2 mL for administration purposes).

23. Convert the child's weight to kg (2.2 lb = 1 kg).

$44 \text{ lbs} \div 2.2 = 20$ kg

$$\frac{2.5 \text{ mg}}{x \text{ mg}} = \frac{1 \text{ kg}}{20 \text{ kg}}$$

OR

$$20 \text{ kg} \times 2.5 \text{ mg}$$

$$x = 50 \text{ mg/day}$$

24. a) Convert weight (2.2 lb = 1 kg).

$$38 \text{ lb} \div 2.2 = 17.3 \text{ kg}$$

b) $$\frac{40 \text{ mg}}{x \text{ mg}} = \frac{1 \text{ kg}}{17.3 \text{ kg}}$$

OR

$40 \text{ mg} \times 17.3 \text{ kg}$

$x = 692 \text{ mg/day}$

c) $\frac{692 \text{ mg}}{4} = 173 \text{ mg}$

d) The dose ordered is not safe.
$200 \text{ mg} \times 4 = 800 \text{ mg}$

25. a) 20–40 mg/kg/day

b) Convert weight (2.2 lb = 1 kg).

$16 \text{ lb} \div 2.2 = 7.27 \text{ kg}$; round to 7.3 kg

$$\frac{20 \text{ mg}}{x \text{ mg}} = \frac{1 \text{ kg}}{7.3 \text{ kg}} = 146 \text{ mg}$$

OR

$$20 \text{ mg} \times 7.3 \text{ kg} = 146 \text{ mg}$$

$$\frac{40 \text{ mg}}{x \text{ mg}} = \frac{1 \text{ kg}}{7.3 \text{ kg}} = 292 \text{ mg}$$

OR

$$40 \text{ mg} \times 7.3 \text{ kg} = 292 \text{ mg}$$

Safe dose range for the child is 146–292 mg

c) The dose ordered is not safe.
$125 \text{ mg} \times 3 = 375 \text{ mg}$.

26. Convert weight (2.2 lb = 1 kg).

$44 \text{ lb} \div 2.2 = 20 \text{ kg}$

$$\frac{30 \text{ mg}}{x \text{ mg}} = \frac{1 \text{ kg}}{20 \text{ kg}} = 600 \text{ mg}$$

OR

$$30 \text{ mg} \times 20 \text{ kg} = 600 \text{ mg}$$

$$\frac{50 \text{ mg}}{x \text{ mg}} = \frac{1 \text{ kg}}{20 \text{ kg}} = 1000 \text{ mg}$$

OR

$$50 \text{ mg} \times 20 \text{ kg} = 1000 \text{ mg}$$

The dose ordered is safe.
$250 \text{ mg} \times 4 = 1000 \text{ mg}$

27. No weight conversion is required.

$$\frac{0.25 \text{ mg}}{x \text{ mg}} = \frac{1 \text{ kg}}{66.3 \text{ kg}}$$

OR

$$0.25 \text{ mg} \times 66.3 \text{ kg} = 16.6 \text{ mg}$$

$$x = 16.6 \text{ mg}$$

28. Weight conversion is required (2.2 lb = 1 kg).

$200 \text{ lb} \div 2.2 = 90.9 \text{ kg}$

$$\frac{150 \text{ mg}}{x \text{ mg}} = \frac{1 \text{ kg}}{90.9 \text{ kg}}$$

OR

$$150 \text{ mg} \times 90.9 \text{ kg} = 13{,}635 \text{ mg}$$

$$x = 13{,}635 \text{ mg}$$

$$\frac{200 \text{ mg}}{x \text{ mg}} = \frac{1 \text{ kg}}{90.9 \text{ kg}}$$

OR

$$200 \text{ mg} \times 90.9 \text{ kg}$$

$$x = 18{,}180 \text{ mg}$$

To determine the number of g, convert the mg obtained to g (1000 mg = 1 g).

$13{,}635 \text{ mg} \div 1000 = 13.63 \text{ g}$
(13.6 g to nearest tenth)

$18{,}180 \text{ mg} \div 1000 = 18.18 \text{ g}$
(18.2 g to nearest tenth)

The daily dose range in g is 13.6–18.2 g.

29. Convert weight (2.2 lb = 1 kg, 16 oz = 1 lb).

$6 \text{ oz} \div 16 = 0.37 \text{ lb} = 0.4 \text{ lb}$ (to nearest tenth)

Total weight in lb = 12.4 lb

$12.4 \text{ lb} \div 2.2 = 5.63 \text{ kg}$ (5.6 to nearest tenth)

$$\frac{15 \text{ mg}}{x \text{ mg}} = \frac{1 \text{ kg}}{5.6 \text{ kg}}$$

OR

$$15 \text{ mg} \times 5.6 \text{ kg} = 84 \text{ mg}$$

$$x = 84 \text{ mg}$$

$$\frac{50 \text{ mg}}{x \text{ mg}} = \frac{1 \text{ kg}}{5.6 \text{ kg}}$$

OR

$$50 \text{ mg} \times 5.6 \text{ kg} = 280 \text{ mg}$$

$$x = 280 \text{ mg}$$

The safe dose range is 84–280 mg/day.

30. 0.60 m^2

31. 0.27 m^2

32. $0.90\ m^2$

33. $0.8\ m^2$

34. $0.28\ m^2$

35. $0.52\ m^2$

36. $0.45\ m^2$

37. $0.9\ m^2$

38. $0.3\ m^2$

39. $0.60\ m^2$

40. $0.51\ m^2$

Answers to Practice Problems: Determining the Dose Using the Formula

41. a) $0.52\ m^2$

b) $\frac{0.52}{1.7} \times 25 = \frac{0.52 \times 25}{1.7} = \frac{13}{1.7} = 7.64$

Answer: 7.6 mg

42. a) $0.52\ m^2$

b) $\frac{0.52}{1.7} \times 200 = \frac{0.52 \times 200}{1.7} = \frac{104}{1.7}$

$\frac{104}{1.7} = 61.17 = 61.2$ mg

$\frac{0.52}{1.7} \times 400 = \frac{208}{1.7} = 122.35$

122.35 mg = 122.4 mg

Answer: 61.2–122.4 mg

43. $\frac{1.5}{1.7} \times 5\ \text{mg} = \frac{1.5 \times 5}{1.7} = \frac{7.5}{1.7}$

$\frac{7.5}{1.7} = 4.41\ \text{mg} = 4.4\ \text{mg}$

$\frac{1.5}{1.7} \times 15\ \text{mg} = \frac{22.5}{1.7} = 13.23$

13.23 mg = 13.2 mg

Answer: 4.4–13.2 mg

44. $\frac{0.8}{1.7} \times 20\ \text{mg} = \frac{0.8 \times 20}{1.7} = \frac{16}{1.7}$

$\frac{16}{1.7} = 9.41\ \text{mg} = 9.4\ \text{mg}$

Answer: No; the correct dose is 9.4 mg.

45. $\frac{0.92}{1.7} \times 25\ \text{mg} = \frac{0.92 \times 25}{1.7} = \frac{23}{1.7}$

$\frac{23}{1.7} = 13.52\ \text{mg} = 13.5\ \text{mg}$

Answer: The dose is incorrect. The correct dose is 13.5 mg.

46. $\frac{1.5}{1.7} \times 250\ \text{mg} = \frac{1.5 \times 250}{1.7} = \frac{375}{1.7}$

$\frac{375}{1.7} = 220.58\ \text{mg}$

Answer: 220.6 mg

47. $0.74 \times 20 = 14.8$ mg

$0.74 \times 30 = 22.2$ mg

Answer: 14.8–22.2 mg

48. $\frac{0.67}{1.7} \times 20\ \text{mg} = \frac{13.4}{1.7} = 7.88\ \text{mg} = 7.9\ \text{mg}.$

The dose is correct.

49. $\frac{0.94}{1.7} \times 10 = 5.5$ mg

$\frac{0.94}{1.7} \times 20 = 11.1$ mg

Range: 5.5–11.1 mg

50. a) $0.45\ m^2$

b) $\frac{0.45}{1.7} \times 500\ \text{mg} = \frac{225}{1.7} = 132.35$

Answer: 132.4 mg

51. $\frac{1.3}{1.7} \times 500 = \frac{1.3 \times 500}{1.7} = \frac{650}{1.7} = 382.35$

Answer: 382.4 mg

52. a) $0.55\ m^2$

b) $\frac{0.55}{1.7} \times 25 = \frac{0.55 \times 25}{1.7} = \frac{13.75}{1.7}$

$\frac{13.75}{1.7} = 8.08$

Answer: 8.1 mg

53. $\frac{0.52}{1.7} \times 15 = \frac{0.52 \times 15}{1.7} = \frac{7.8}{1.7} = 4.58$

Answer: 4.6 mg

54. $\frac{1.10}{1.7} \times 150 = \frac{1.10 \times 150}{1.7} = \frac{165}{1.7} = 97.05$

Answer: 97.1 mg

55. $\sqrt{\frac{95.5 \text{ (kg)} \times 180 \text{ (cm)}}{3600}}$

$\sqrt{4.775} = 2.185 = 2.19 \text{ m}^2$

Answer: 2.19 m²

56. $\sqrt{\frac{10 \text{ (kg)} \times 70 \text{ (cm)}}{3600}}$

$\sqrt{0.194} = 0.44 \text{ m}^2$

Answer: 0.44 m²

57. $\sqrt{\frac{4.8 \text{ (lb)} \times 21 \text{ (in)}}{3131}}$

$\sqrt{0.032} = 0.178 = 0.18 \text{ m}^2$

Answer: 0.18 m²

58. $\sqrt{\frac{170 \text{ (lb)} \times 67 \text{ (in)}}{3131}}$

$\sqrt{3.637} = 1.907 = 1.91 \text{ m}^2$

Answer: 1.91 m²

Answers to Chapter Review

1. Convert weight (2.2 lb = 1 kg).

   22 lb = 2.2 ÷ 2.2 = 10 kg

   1 mg × 10 kg = 10 mg

   The dose ordered for this child is safe.

2. Convert weight (2.2 lb = 1 kg).

   a) 23 lb = 23 ÷ 22 = 10.5 kg

   b) 20 mg × 10.5 kg = 210 mg/day

   40 mg × 10.5 kg = 420 mg/day

   The safety range for this 10.5 kg child is 210–420 mg/day.

   c) The drug is given in divided doses q8h.

   q8h = 24 ÷ 8 = 3 doses per day

   210 mg ÷ 3 = 70 mg per dose

   420 mg ÷ 3 = 140 mg per dose

   The dose range is 70–140 mg per dose q8h.

   d) The dose ordered is not safe since 150 mg × 3 = 450 mg.

   Notify the doctor and question the order.

3. a) Convert child's weight in kg to lb. The recommended dose is stated in lb.

   2.2 lb = 1 kg

   17 kg = 17 × 2.2 = 37.4 lb.

   The dose range is stated as

   2.2–3.2 mg/lb/day.

   2.2 mg × 37.4 lb = 82.28 mg = 82.3 mg

   3.2 mg × 37.4 lb = 119.68 mg = 119.7 mg

   The dose range is 82.3–119.7 mg.

   q6h = 4 doses

   82.3 mg ÷ 4 = 20.57 mg = 20.6 mg

   119.7 mg ÷ 4 = 29.92 mg = 29.9 mg

   The dose range is 20.6–29.9 mg per dose.

   The dose ordered: 25 mg q6h.

   This dose is safe because 25 mg × 4 = 100 mg.

   b) 5 mg : 1 mL = 25 mg : x mL

   OR

   $\frac{25 \text{ mg}}{5 \text{ mg}} \times 1 \text{ mL} = x \text{ mL}$

   $x = 5$ mL

   $\frac{25 \text{ mg}}{5 \text{ mg}} = \frac{x \text{ mL}}{5 \text{ mL}}$

   $x = 5$ mL

   Give 5 mL per dose.

4. No conversion of weight is required. The child's weight is in kg, and the recommended dose is expressed in kg (12.5 mg/kg).

   12.5 mg × 35 kg = 437.5 mg/day

   q6h = 4 doses

   437.5 mg ÷ 4 =

   109.37 = 109.4 mg per dose

   Dose ordered is safe because 100 mg × 4 = 400 mg.

Alternate ways of doing problems 1-10 in the Chapter Review are possible.

5. No conversion of weight is required. The child's weight is in lb, and the recommended dose is expressed in lb (2 mg/lb).

$$2 \text{ mg} \times 30 \text{ lb} = 60 \text{ mg/day}$$

$$q12 = 2 \text{ doses}$$

$$60 \text{ mg} \div 2 = 30 \text{ mg per dose}$$

75 mg × 2 = 150 mg. This dose is too high; notify the doctor.

6. Convert the child's weight in lb to kg. The recommended dose is expressed in kg (60 mg/kg).

$$2.2 \text{ lb} = 1 \text{ kg}$$

$$42 \text{ lb} = 42 \div 2.2 = 19.1 \text{ kg}$$

$$60 \text{ mg} \times 19.1 \text{ kg} = 1{,}146 \text{ mg/day}$$

$$q6h = 4 \text{ doses}$$

$$1{,}146 \text{ mg} \div 4 = 286.5 \text{ mg per dose}$$

The dose ordered is safe because 250 mg × 4 = 1000 mg

7. Convert the child's weight in lbs to kg. The recommended dose is stated in kg (10 to 25 mg/kg).

$$36 \text{ lb} = 36 \div 2.2 = 16.4 \text{ kg}$$

$$10 \text{ mg} \times 16.4 \text{ kg} = 164 \text{ mg/day}$$

$$25 \text{ mg} \times 16.4 \text{ kg} = 410 \text{ mg/day}$$

The safety range is 164–410 mg/day.

The drug is given q6-8h. The dose in this problem is ordered q8h.

$$24 \div 8 = 3 \text{ doses}$$

$$164 \text{ mg} \div 3 = 54.7 \text{ mg/dose}$$

$$410\text{mg} \div 3 = 136.7 \text{ mg/dose}$$

The dose ordered is 150 mg q8h.

$$150 \text{ mg} \times 3 = 450 \text{ mg}$$

Notify the doctor; the dose is high.

8. a) Convert the child's weight in lb to kg. The recommended dose is expressed in kg (25–50 mg/kg).

$$66 \text{ lbs} = 66 \div 2.2 = 30 \text{ kg}$$

$$25 \text{ mg} \times 30 \text{ kg} = 750 \text{ mg/day}$$

$$50 \text{ mg} \times 30 \text{ kg} = 1{,}500 \text{ mg/day}$$

The safety range is 750–1,500 mg/day.

The drug is given in divided doses (4).

The dosage ordered is q6h.

$$24 \div 6 = 4 \text{ doses}$$

$$750 \text{ mg} \div 4 = 187.5 \text{ mg/per dose}$$

$$1{,}500 \text{ mg} \div 4 = 375 \text{ mg/per dose}$$

The dose range is 187.5–375 mg per dose q6h. 250 mg × 4 = 1000 mg. This is a safe dose since the total dose falls within the safety range for 24 hr, and the divided dose also falls within the safe range.

b) You would give 10 mL for one dose.

$$125 \text{ mg} : 5 \text{ mL} = 250 \text{ mg} : x \text{ mL}$$

OR

$$\frac{250 \text{ mg}}{125 \text{ mg}} \times 5 \text{ mL} = x \text{ mL};$$

$$\frac{250 \text{ mg}}{125 \text{ mg}} = \frac{x \text{ mL}}{5 \text{ mL}}$$

$$x = 10 \text{ mL}$$

9. a) No conversion of weight is required. The child's weight is stated in kg, and the recommended dose is (20–40 mg/kg).

$$20 \text{ mg} \times 35 = 700 \text{ mg}$$

$$40 \text{ mg} \times 35 = 1{,}400 \text{ mg}$$

The safety range is 700–1,400 mg/day.

The drug is given in divided doses q12h.

$$24 \div 12 = 2 \text{ doses}$$

$$700 \text{ mg} \div 2 = 350 \text{ mg}$$

$$1{,}400 \text{ mg} \div 2 = 700 \text{ mg}$$

350–700 mg per dose is safe.

The doctor ordered 400 mg I.M. q12h.

This dose is safe.

$$400 \text{ mg} \times 2 = 800 \text{ mg}$$

b) Administer 1 mL.

$$400 \text{ mg} : 1 \text{ mL} = 400 \text{ mg} : x \text{ mL}$$

OR

$$\frac{400 \text{ mg}}{400 \text{ mg}} \times 1 \text{ mL} = x \text{ mL};$$

$$\frac{400 \text{ mg}}{400 \text{ mg}} = \frac{x \text{ mL}}{1 \text{ mL}}$$

$$x = 1 \text{ mL}$$

10. Convert the child's weight in lb to kg. The recommended dose is expressed in kg (120 mg/kg).

$$46 \text{ lb} = 46 \div 2.2 = 20.9 \text{ kg}$$

$$120 \text{ mg} \times 20.9 \text{ kg} = 2{,}508 \text{ mg/day}$$

The drug is given in four equally divided doses.

The dose for this child is ordered q6h.

$$24 \div 6 = 4 \text{ doses.}$$

$$2{,}508 \text{ mg} \div 4 = 627 \text{ mg per dose}$$

$$250 \text{ mg} \times 4 = 1000 \text{ mg}$$

The dose ordered is low. Notify the doctor. 250 mg each dose is less than 627 mg.

11. a) 0.45 m^2

b) $\frac{0.45}{1.7} \times 500 \text{ mg} = 132.4 \text{ mg}$

12. a) 0.54 m^2

b) $\frac{0.54}{1.7} \times 25 \text{ mg} = 7.9 \text{ mg}$

13. a) 1.2 m^2

b) $\frac{1.2}{1.7} \times 250 \text{ mg} = 176.5 \text{ mg}$

14. a) 1.1 m^2

b) $\frac{1.1}{1.7} \times 30 \text{ mg} = 19.4 \text{ mg}$

15. a) 1.05 m^2

b) $\frac{1.05}{1.7} \times 150 \text{ mg} = 92.6 \text{ mg}$

16. $\frac{0.70}{1.7} \times 50 \text{ mg} = 20.6 \text{ mg}$

17. $\frac{0.66}{1.7} \times 10 \text{ mg} = 3.9 \text{ mg}$

$$\frac{0.66}{1.7} \times 20 \text{ mg} = 7.8 \text{ mg}$$

The dose range is 3.9–7.8 mg.

18. $\frac{0.55}{1.7} \times 2{,}000 \text{ U} = 647.1 \text{ U}$

19. $\frac{0.55}{1.7} \times 200 \text{ mg} = 64.7 \text{ mg}$

$$\frac{0.55}{1.7} \times 250 \text{ mg} = 80.9 \text{ mg}$$

The dose range is 64.7–80.9 mg.

20. $\frac{0.22}{1.7} \times 150 \text{ mg} = 19.4 \text{ mg}$

21. Dose is incorrect; the child's dose is 17.3 mg.

$$\frac{0.49}{1.7} \times 60 \text{ mg} = 17.3 \text{ mg}$$

The dose of 25 mg is too high.

22. $\frac{0.32}{1.7} \times 10 \text{ mg} = 1.9 \text{ mg}$

The dose of 4 mg is too high.

23. Dose is correct.

$$\frac{0.68}{1.7} \times 125 \text{ mg} = 50 \text{ mg}$$

$$\frac{0.68}{1.7} \times 150 \text{ mg} = 60 \text{ mg}$$

The dose of 50 mg falls within the range of 50–60 mg.

24. Dose is incorrect.

$$\frac{0.55}{1.7} \times 25 \text{ mg} = 8.1 \text{ mg}$$

The dose of 5 mg is too low.

25. The dose is correct.

$$\frac{1.2}{1.7} \times 75 \text{ mg} = 52.9 \text{ mg}$$

$$\frac{1.2}{1.7} \times 100 \text{ mg} = 70.6 \text{ mg}$$

The dose ordered is 60 mg and falls within the dose range of 52.9–70.6 mg.

26. $\sqrt{\frac{100 \text{ (lb)} \times 55 \text{ (in)}}{3131}} = \frac{5500}{3131} = 1.756$

$$\sqrt{1.756} = 1.325$$

Answer: 1.33 m^2

27. $\sqrt{\frac{60.9 \text{ (kg)} \times 130 \text{ (cm)}}{3600}} = \frac{7{,}917}{3{,}600} = 2.199$

$$\sqrt{2.199} = 1.482$$

Answer: 1.48 m^2

28. $\sqrt{\frac{55 \text{ (lb)} \times 45 \text{ (in)}}{3131}} = \frac{2{,}475}{3{,}131} = 0.790$

$$\sqrt{0.790} = 0.888$$

Answer: 0.89 m^2

29. $\sqrt{\frac{60 \text{ (lb)} \times 35 \text{ (in)}}{3131}} = \frac{2{,}100}{3{,}131} = 0.670$

$$\sqrt{0.670} = 0.818$$

Answer: 0.82 m^2

30. $$\sqrt{\frac{65\ (\text{kg}) \times 132\ (\text{cm})}{3600}} = \frac{8{,}580}{3{,}600} = 2.383$$

$$\sqrt{2.383} = 1.543$$

Answer: 1.54 m^2

31. $$\sqrt{\frac{24\ (\text{lb}) \times 28\ (\text{in})}{3131}} = \frac{672}{3{,}131} = 0.214$$

$$\sqrt{0.214} = 0.462$$

Answer: 0.46 m^2

32. $$\sqrt{\frac{6\ (\text{kg}) \times 55\ (\text{cm})}{3600}} = \frac{330}{3{,}600} = 0.091$$

$$\sqrt{0.091} = 0.301$$

Answer: 0.30 m^2

33. $$\sqrt{\frac{42\ (\text{lb}) \times 45\ (\text{in})}{3131}} = \frac{1{,}890}{3{,}131} = 0.603$$

$$\sqrt{0.603} = 0.776$$

Answer: 0.78 m^2

34. $$\sqrt{\frac{8\ (\text{kg}) \times 70\ (\text{cm})}{3600}} = \frac{560}{3{,}600} = 0.155$$

$$\sqrt{0.155} = 0.393$$

Answer: 0.39 m^2

35. $$\sqrt{\frac{74\ (\text{kg}) \times 160\ (\text{cm})}{3600}} = \frac{11{,}840}{3{,}600} = 3.288$$

$$\sqrt{3.288} = 1.813$$

Answer: 1.81 m^2

36. 10 mg : 1 mL = 7 mg : x mL

OR

$$\frac{7\text{ mg}}{10\text{ mg}} \times 1\text{ mL} = x\text{ mL}$$

OR

$$\frac{7\text{ mg}}{10\text{ mg}} = \frac{x\text{ mL}}{1\text{ mL}}$$

Answer: 0.7 mL. The dose ordered is less than what is available. Therefore you will need less than 1 mL to administer the dose.

37. 10 mg : 1 mL = 150 mg : x mL

OR

$$\frac{150\text{ mg}}{10\text{ mg}} \times 1\text{ mL} = x\text{ mL};\ \frac{150\text{ mg}}{10\text{ mg}} = \frac{x\text{ mL}}{1\text{ mL}}$$

Answer: 15 mL. The dose ordered is more than what is available. Therefore you will need more than 1 mL to administer the dose.

38. 0.05 mg : 1 mL = 0.1 mg : x mL

OR

$$\frac{0.1\text{ mg}}{0.05\text{ mg}} \times 1\text{ mL} = x\text{ mL};\ \frac{0.1\text{ mg}}{0.05\text{ mg}} = \frac{x\text{ mL}}{1\text{ mL}}$$

Answer: 2 mL. The dose ordered is more than what is available. Therefore you will need more than 1 mL to administer the dose.

39. 50 mg : 5 mL = 80 mg : x mL

OR

$$\frac{80\text{ mg}}{50\text{ mg}} \times 5\text{ mL} = x\text{ mL};\ \frac{80\text{ mg}}{50\text{ mg}} = \frac{x\text{ mL}}{5\text{ mL}}$$

Answer: 8 mL. The dose ordered is greater than what is available. Therefore you will need more than 5 mL to administer the dose.

40. 125 mg : 5 mL = 250 mg : x mL

OR

$$\frac{250\text{ mg}}{125\text{ mg}} \times 5\text{ mL} = x\text{ mL};\ \frac{250\text{ mg}}{125\text{ mg}} = \frac{x\text{ mL}}{5\text{ mL}}$$

Answer: 10 mL. The dose ordered is greater than what is available. Therefore you will need more than 5 mL to administer the dose.

41. Conversion is required:
Equivalent: 1000 mg = 1 g

Therefore 0.25 g = 250 mg

100 mg : 5 mL = 250 mg : x mL

OR

$$\frac{250\text{ mg}}{100\text{ mg}} \times 5\text{ mL} = x\text{ mL};\ \frac{250\text{ mg}}{100\text{ mg}} = \frac{x\text{ mL}}{5\text{ mL}}$$

Answer: 12.5 mL. The dose ordered is greater than what is available. Therefore, you would need more than 5 mL to administer the dose.

42. 250 mg : 5 mL = 100 mg : x mL

OR

$$\frac{100\text{ mg}}{250\text{ mg}} \times 5\text{ mL} = x\text{ mL};\ \frac{100\text{ mg}}{250\text{ mg}} = \frac{x\text{ mL}}{5\text{ mL}}$$

Answer: 2 mL. The dose ordered is less than what is available. Therefore you will need less than 5 mL to administer the dose.

43. 20 mg : 2 mL = 7.3 mg : x mL

OR

$$\frac{7.3\text{mg}}{20\text{ mg}} \times 2\text{ mL} = x\text{ mL}; \frac{7.3\text{ mg}}{20\text{ mg}} = \frac{x\text{ mL}}{2\text{ mL}}$$

Answer: 0.73 mL. The dose ordered is less than what is available. Therefore you will need less than 2 mL to administer the dose.

44. 0.4 mg : 1 mL = 0.1 mg : x mL

OR

$$\frac{0.1\text{ mg}}{0.4\text{ mg}} \times 1\text{ mL} = x\text{ mL}; \frac{0.1\text{ mg}}{0.4\text{ mg}} = \frac{x\text{ mL}}{1\text{ mL}}$$

Answer: 0.25 mL. The dose ordered is less than what is available. Therefore you would need less than 1 mL to administer the dose.

45. 250 mg : 1 mL = 160 mg : x mL

OR

$$\frac{160\text{ mg}}{250\text{ mg}} \times 1\text{ mL} = x\text{ mL}; \frac{160\text{ mg}}{250\text{ mg}} = \frac{x\text{ mL}}{1\text{ mL}}$$

Answer: 0.64 mL. The dose ordered is less than what is available. Therefore you will need less than 1 mL to administer the dose.

46. 15 mg : 1 mL = 3.5 mg : x mL

OR

$$\frac{3.5\text{ mg}}{15\text{ mg}} \times 1\text{ mL} = x\text{ mL}; \frac{3.5\text{ mg}}{15\text{ mg}} = \frac{x\text{ mL}}{1\text{ mL}}$$

Answer: 0.23 mL. The dose ordered is less than what is available. Therefore you will need less than 1 mL to administer the dose.

Chapter 20

Answers to Practice Problems

1. $75\text{ mL} \times \frac{10\text{ gtt/mL}}{60\text{ min}} = 75 \times \frac{1}{6} =$

$\frac{75}{6} = 12.5 = 13$ gtt/min; 13 macrogtt/min

2. $\frac{30\text{ mL}}{1\text{ hr}} \times \frac{60\text{ gtt/mL}}{60\text{ min}} = \frac{30}{1} =$

$\frac{30}{1} = 30$ gtt/min; 30 microgtt/min

3. $\frac{125\text{ mL}}{1\text{ hr}} \times \frac{15\text{ gtt/mL}}{60\text{ min}} = \frac{125}{1} \times \frac{1}{4} =$

$\frac{125}{4} = 31.2$

Answer: 31 gtt/min; 31 macrogtt/min

4. $\frac{1000\text{ mL}}{6\text{ hr}} \times \frac{15\text{ gtt/mL}}{60\text{ min}} = \frac{1000}{6} \times \frac{1}{4} =$

$\frac{1000}{24} = 41.6$

Answer: 42 gtt/min; 42 macrogtt/min

5. $60\text{ mL} \times \frac{60\text{ gtt/mL}}{45\text{ min}} = 60 \times \frac{4}{3} =$

$\frac{240}{3} = 80$ gtt/min; 80 microgtt/min

6. $\frac{1000\text{ mL}}{16\text{ hr}} \times \frac{15\text{ gtt/mL}}{60\text{ min}} = \frac{1000}{16} \times \frac{1}{4} =$

$\frac{1000}{64} = 15.6$

Answer: 16 gtt/min; 16 macrogtt/min

7. $\frac{150\text{ mL}}{2\text{ hr}} \times \frac{20\text{ gtt/mL}}{60\text{ min}} = \frac{150}{2} \times \frac{1}{3} =$

$\frac{150}{6} = 25$ gtt/min; 25 macrogtt/min

8. $\frac{3{,}000\text{ mL}}{24\text{ hr}} \times \frac{10\text{ gtt/mL}}{60\text{ min}} = \frac{3{,}000}{24} \times \frac{1}{6} =$

$\frac{3{,}000}{144} = 20.8$

Answer: 21 gtt/minute; 21 macrogtt/min

9. $\frac{2{,}000\text{ mL}}{12\text{ hr}} \times \frac{15\text{ gtt/mL}}{60\text{ min}} = \frac{2{,}000}{12} \times \frac{1}{4} =$

$\frac{2{,}000}{48} = 41.6$

Answer: 42 gtt/min; 42 macrogtt/min

10. $60\text{ mL} \times \frac{60\text{ gtt/mL}}{30\text{ min}} = 60 \times 2 =$

120 gtt/min; 120 microgtt/min

11. $\frac{125\text{ mL}}{1\text{ hr}} \times \frac{15\text{ gtt/mL}}{60\text{ min}} = \frac{125}{1} \times \frac{1}{4} =$

$\frac{125}{4} = 31.2$

Answer: 31 gtt/min; 31 macrogtt/min

12. $\frac{2{,}500 \text{ mL}}{16 \text{ hrs}} \times \frac{10 \text{ gtt/mL}}{60 \text{ min}} = \frac{2{,}500}{16} \times \frac{1}{6} =$

$\frac{2{,}500}{96} = 26.0$

Answer: 26 gtt/min; 26 macrogtt/min

13. $\frac{100 \text{ mL}}{1 \text{ hr}} \times \frac{60 \text{ gtt/mL}}{60 \text{ min}} = \frac{100}{1} \times \frac{1}{1} =$

$\frac{100}{1} = 100$ gtt/min

Answer: 100 gtt/min; 100 microgtt/min

14. 1 L = 1000 mL

2 L = 2,000 mL

$\frac{2{,}000 \text{ mL}}{10 \text{ hr}} \times \frac{15 \text{ gtt/mL}}{60 \text{ min}} = \frac{2{,}000}{10} \times \frac{1}{4} =$

$\frac{2{,}000}{40} = 50$ gtt/min

Answer: 50 gtt/min; 50 macrogtt/min

15. $\frac{130 \text{ mL}}{1 \text{ hr}} \times \frac{15 \text{ gtt/mL}}{60 \text{ min}} = \frac{130}{1} \times \frac{1}{4} =$

$\frac{130}{4} = 32.5$

Answer: 33 gtt/min; 33 macrogtt/min

16. $\frac{250 \text{ mL}}{1 \text{ hr}} \times \frac{10 \text{ gtt/mL}}{60 \text{ min}} = \frac{250}{1} \times \frac{1}{6} =$

$\frac{250}{6} = 41.6$

Answer: 42 gtt/min; 42 macrogtt/min

17. $50 \text{ mL} \times \frac{10 \text{ gtt/mL}}{45 \text{ min}} = 50 \times \frac{10}{45} =$

$\frac{500}{45} = 11.1$

Answer: 11 gtt/min; 11 macrogtt/min

18. $75 \text{ mL} \times \frac{10 \text{ gtt/mL}}{30 \text{ min}} = 75 \times \frac{1}{3} =$

$\frac{75}{3} = 25$ gtt/min; 25 macrogtt/min

19. $50 \text{ mL} \times \frac{10 \text{ gtt/mL}}{30 \text{ min}} = 50 \times \frac{1}{3} =$

$\frac{50}{3} = 16.6$

Answer: 17 macrogtt/min, or 17 gtt/min

20. a) 50 mg : 1 mL = 500 mg : x mL

OR

$\frac{500 \text{ mg}}{50 \text{ mg}} \times 1 \text{ mL} = x \text{ mL};$

$\frac{500 \text{ mg}}{50 \text{ mg}} = \frac{x \text{ mL}}{1 \text{ mL}}$

Answer: 10 mL

b) $\frac{100 \text{ mL}}{1 \text{ hr}} \times \frac{15 \text{ gtt/mL}}{60 \text{ min}} = 100 \times \frac{1}{4} =$

$\frac{100}{4} = 25$

Answer: 25 macrogtt/min; 25 gtt/min

21. a) 50 mg : 10 mL = 20 mg : x mL

OR

$\frac{20 \text{ mg}}{50 \text{ mg}} \times 10 \text{ mL} = x \text{ mL};$

$\frac{20 \text{ mg}}{50 \text{ mg}} = \frac{x \text{ mL}}{10 \text{ mL}}$

Answer: 4 mL

b) $\frac{300 \text{ mL}}{6 \text{ hr}} \times \frac{60 \text{ gtt/mL}}{60 \text{ min}} = \frac{300}{6} = 50$

Answer: 50 microgtt/min; 50 gtt/min

22. a) 16 mg : 1 mL = 300 mg : x mL

OR

$\frac{300 \text{ mg}}{16 \text{ mg}} \times 1 \text{ mL} = x \text{ mL};$

$\frac{300 \text{ mg}}{16 \text{ mg}} = \frac{x \text{ mL}}{1 \text{ mL}}$

Answer: 18.75 mL, rounded to 18.8 mL to nearest tenth

Alternate method for calculating dose:

320 mg : 20 mL = 300 mg : x mL

OR

$\frac{300 \text{ mg}}{320 \text{ mg}} \times 20 \text{ mL} = x \text{ mL};$

$\frac{300 \text{ mg}}{320 \text{ mg}} = \frac{x \text{ mL}}{20 \text{ mL}}$

Answer: 18.75 mL, rounded to 18.8 mL to nearest tenth

b) $\frac{300 \text{ mL}}{1 \text{ hr}} \times \frac{10 \text{ gtt/mL}}{60 \text{ min}} = 300 \times \frac{1}{6} =$

$\frac{300}{6} = 50$

Answer: 50 macrogtt/min; 50 gtt/min

23. $\frac{100 \text{ mL}}{1 \text{ hr}} \times \frac{10 \text{ gtt/mL}}{60 \text{ min}} = 100 \times \frac{1}{6} =$

$\frac{100}{6} = 16.6$

Answer: 17 macrogtt/min; 17 gtt/min

24. a) 15 mEq : 1000 mL = 4 mEq : x mL

$$\frac{15x}{15} = \frac{4{,}000}{15} = 266.6$$

x = 267 mL/hr to deliver 4 mEq of potassium chloride

b) $\frac{267 \text{ mL}}{1 \text{ hr}} \times \frac{10 \text{ gtt/mL}}{60 \text{ min}} = 44.5 \text{ gtt/min}$

Answer: 45 gtt/min; 45 macrogtt/min

45 gtt/min or 45 macrogtt/min would deliver 4 mEq of potassium chloride each hour.

25. a) 50 U : 250 mL = 10 U : x mL

$$\frac{50x}{50} = \frac{2{,}500}{50} = 50 \text{ mL/hr}$$

50 mL/hr must be administered for client to receive 10 U/hr.

b) $\frac{50 \text{ mL}}{1 \text{ hr}} \times \frac{15 \text{ gtt/mL}}{60 \text{ min}} = 12.5 \text{ gtt/min}$

Answer: 13 gtt/min; 13 macrogtt/min

13 gtt/min (13 macrogtt/min) of this solution would deliver 10 U/hr.

26. a) 40 U : 250 mL = 15 U : x mL

$$\frac{40x}{40} = \frac{3750}{40} = 93.7 = 94 \text{ mL/hr}$$

b) $\frac{94 \text{ mL}}{1 \text{ hr}} \times \frac{60}{60} = 94$ gtt/min; 94 microgtt/min

Answer: 94 gtt/min; 94 gtt/microgtt/min
94 gtt/min of this solution would deliver 15 U/hr.

27. $\frac{150 \text{ mL}}{x \text{ hr}} \times \frac{60 \text{ gtt/mL}}{60 \text{ min}} = 60$

$$\frac{150}{x} \times \frac{1}{1} = 60$$

$$\frac{150}{x} = \frac{60}{1}$$

$$\frac{60x}{60} = \frac{150}{60} = 2.5 \text{ hr } \left(2\frac{1}{2} \text{ hr}\right)$$

28. $\frac{x \text{ mL}}{5 \text{ hr}} \times \frac{15 \text{ gtt/mL}}{60 \text{ min}} = 35$ gtt/min; 35 macrogtt/min

$$\frac{x}{5} \times \frac{1}{4} = 35$$

$$\frac{x}{20} = \frac{35}{1}$$

$$x = 35 \times 20$$

$$x = 700 \text{ mL}$$

29. $\frac{180 \text{ mL}}{x \text{ hr}} \times \frac{15 \text{ gtt/mL}}{60 \text{ min}} = 45$ gtt/min; 45 macrogtt/min

$$\frac{180}{x} \times \frac{1}{4} = 45$$

$$\frac{180}{4x} = \frac{45}{1}$$

$$\frac{180x}{180} = \frac{180}{180}$$

Answer: 1 hr

30. $\frac{x \text{ mL}}{8 \text{ hr}} \times \frac{15 \text{ gtt/mL}}{60} = 45$ gtt/min; 45 macrogtt/min

$$\frac{x}{8} \times \frac{1}{4} = 45$$

$$\frac{x}{32} = \frac{45}{1}$$

$$x = 45 \times 32$$

Answer: 1,440 mL

31. $\frac{90 \text{ cc}}{x \text{ hr}} \times \frac{60 \text{ gtt/mL}}{60 \text{ min}} = 60 \text{ gtt/min}$

$$\frac{90}{x} \times \frac{60}{60} = 60$$

$$\frac{90}{x} = \frac{60}{1}$$

$$\frac{60x}{60} = \frac{90}{60}$$

Answer: 1.5 hr $\left(1\frac{1}{2} \text{ hr}\right)$

32. $\frac{250 \text{ mL}}{3 \text{ hr}} \times \frac{15 \text{ gtt/mL}}{60 \text{ min}} = \frac{83}{1} \times \frac{1}{4} =$

$\frac{83}{4} = 20.7$

Answer: 21 gtt/min; 21 macrogtt/min

33. $\frac{200 \text{ mL}}{1.5 \text{ hr}} \times \frac{15 \text{ gtt/mL}}{60 \text{ min}} = \frac{133}{1} \times \frac{1}{4} =$

$\frac{133}{4} = 33.2$

Answer: 33 gtt/min; 33 macrogtt/min

34. $\frac{500 \text{ mL}}{60 \text{ mL/hr}} = 8.33 \text{ hr}$

$0.33 \times 60 = 19.8 = 20$ minutes

a) Answer: 8 hr + 20 minutes = infusion time

b) Answer: 6:20 AM (10:00 PM + 8 hr + 20 minutes)

35. $\frac{250 \text{ mL}}{80 \text{ mL/hr}} = 3.12$

$0.12 \times 60 = 7.2 = 7$ minutes

a) Answer: 3 hr + 7 minutes = infusion time

b) Answer: 5:07 AM (2 AM + 3 hr + 7 minutes)

36. $\frac{1000 \text{ mL}}{40 \text{ mL/hr}} = 25$ hours

a) Answer: 25 hr = infusion time

b) Answer: 3:10 PM August 27 (2:10 PM on August 26 + 25 hr)

37. Step 1: 60 gtt : 1 mL = 25 gtt : x mL

$60x = 25$

$x = 25 \div 60 = 0.41$ mL/min

Step 2: 0.41 mL/min × 60 (min) = 24.6 = 25 mL/hr

Step 3: $\frac{1000 \text{ mL}}{25 \text{ mL/hr}} = 40 \text{ hr}$

Answer: 40 hr = infusion time

38. Step 1: 15 gtt : 1 mL = 17 gtt : x mL

$15x = 17$

$x = 17 \div 15 = 1.13 = 1.1$ mL/min

Step 2: 1.1 mL/min × 60 (min) = 66 mL/hr

Step 3: $\frac{250 \text{ mL}}{66 \text{ mL/hr}} = 3.78$

$60 \times 0.78 = 46.8 = 47$ minutes

Answer: 3 hr and 47 minutes = infusion time

39. Step 1: 20 gtt : 1 mL = 30 gtt : x mL

$20x = 30$

$x = 30 \div 20 = 1.5$ mL/min

Step 2: 1.5 mL/min × 60 (min) = 90 mL/hr

Step 3: $\frac{1000 \text{ mL}}{90 \text{ mL/hr}} = 11.11$

$60 \times 0.11 = 6.6 = 7$ minutes

Answer: 11 hr and 7 minutes = infusion time

40. a) Dilution volume: 27 mL

b) $\frac{30 \text{ mL (diluted drug)} + 15 \text{ mL flush}}{1} \times \frac{60 \text{ gtt/mL}}{50 \text{ min}} = \frac{45}{1} \times \frac{60}{50} = \frac{2{,}700}{50} =$
54 gtt/min

Answer: 54 microgtt/min; 54 gtt/min

c) 54 mL/hr

41. a) Dilution volume: 13 mL

b) $\frac{15 \text{ mL (diluted drug)} + 15 \text{ mL flush}}{1} \times \frac{60 \text{ gtt/mL}}{45 \text{ min}} = \frac{30}{1} \times \frac{60}{45} = \frac{1{,}800}{45} =$
40 microgtt/min

Answer: 40 microgtt/min; 40gtt/min

c) 40 mL/hr

Answers to Chapter Review

1. $\frac{1000 \text{ mL}}{8 \text{ hr}} \times \frac{20 \text{ gtt/mL}}{60 \text{ min}} =$
42 gtt/min; 42 macrogtt/min

2. $\frac{2{,}500 \text{ mL}}{24 \text{ hr}} \times \frac{10 \text{ gtt/mL}}{60 \text{ min}} =$
17 gtt/min; 17 macrogtt/min

3. $\frac{500 \text{ mL}}{4 \text{ hr}} \times \frac{15 \text{ gtt/mL}}{60 \text{ min}} = 31$ gtt/min;
31 macrogtt/min

Some answers in the Chapter Review reflect the number of gtt rounded to the nearest whole number.

4. $\frac{300 \text{ mL}}{6 \text{ hr}} \times \frac{60 \text{ gtt/mL}}{60 \text{ min}} = 50 \text{ gtt/min;}$
50 microgtt/min

5. $\frac{1000 \text{ mL}}{24 \text{ hr}} \times \frac{60 \text{ gtt/mL}}{60 \text{ min}} = 42 \text{ gtt/min;}$
42 microgtt/min

6. $\frac{1000 \text{ mL}}{12 \text{ hr}} \times \frac{10 \text{ gtt/mL}}{60 \text{ min}} = 14 \text{ gtt/min;}$
14 macrogtt/min

7. $\frac{1000 \text{ mL}}{10 \text{ hr}} \times \frac{20 \text{ gtt/mL}}{60 \text{ min}} = 33 \text{ gtt/min;}$
33 macrogtt/min

8. $\frac{1{,}500 \text{ mL}}{12 \text{ hr}} \times \frac{10 \text{ gtt/mL}}{60 \text{ min}} = 21 \text{ gtt/min;}$
21 macrogtt/min

9. $\frac{500 \text{ mL}}{4 \text{ hr}} \times \frac{10 \text{ gtt/mL}}{60 \text{ min}} = 21 \text{ gtt/min;}$
21 macrogtt/min

10. $\frac{250 \text{ mL}}{3 \text{ hr}} \times \frac{10 \text{ gtt/mL}}{60 \text{ min}} = 14 \text{ gtt/min;}$
14 macrogtt/min

11. $\frac{1{,}500 \text{ mL}}{8 \text{ hr}} \times \frac{20 \text{ gtt/mL}}{60 \text{ min}} = 63 \text{ gtt/min;}$
63 macrogtt/min

12. $\frac{3{,}000 \text{ mL}}{24 \text{ hr}} \times \frac{15 \text{ gtt/mL}}{60 \text{ min}} = 31 \text{ gtt/min;}$
31 macrogtt/min

13. Note: 1 L = 1000 mL; therefore
2 L = 2,000 mL

$\frac{2{,}000 \text{ mL}}{24 \text{ hr}} \times \frac{15 \text{ gtt/mL}}{60 \text{ min}} = 21 \text{ gtt/min;}$
21 macrogtt/min

14. $\frac{1000 \text{ mL}}{7 \text{ hr}} \times \frac{10 \text{ gtt/mL}}{60 \text{ min}} = 24 \text{ gtt/min;}$
24 macrogtt/min

15. $\frac{500 \text{ mL}}{4 \text{ hr}} \times \frac{60 \text{ gtt/mL}}{60 \text{ min}} = 125 \text{ gtt/min;}$
125 microgtt/min

16. $\frac{1000 \text{ mL}}{6 \text{ hr}} \times \frac{20 \text{ gtt/mL}}{60 \text{ min}} = 56 \text{ gtt/min;}$
56 macrogtt/min

17. $\frac{250 \text{ mL}}{8 \text{ hr}} \times \frac{60 \text{ gtt/mL}}{60 \text{ min}} = 31 \text{ gtt/min;}$
31 microgtt/min

18. $\frac{50 \text{ mL}}{1 \text{ hr}} \times \frac{60 \text{ gtt/mL}}{60 \text{ min}} = 50 \text{ gtt/min;}$
50 microgtt/min

19. $\frac{150 \text{ mL}}{1 \text{ hr}} \times \frac{15 \text{ gtt/mL}}{60 \text{ min}} = 38 \text{ gtt/min;}$
38 macrogtt/min

20. $\frac{500 \text{ mL}}{6 \text{ hr}} \times \frac{12 \text{ gtt/mL}}{60 \text{ min}} = 17 \text{ gtt/min;}$
17 macrogtt/min

21. $\frac{1{,}500 \text{ mL}}{12 \text{ hr}} \times \frac{10 \text{ gtt/mL}}{60 \text{ min}} = 21 \text{ gtt/min;}$
21 macrogtt/min

22. $\frac{1{,}500 \text{ mL}}{24 \text{ hr}} \times \frac{12 \text{ gtt/mL}}{60 \text{ min}} = 13 \text{ gtt/min;}$
13 macrogtt/min

23. $\frac{2{,}000 \text{ mL}}{16 \text{ hr}} \times \frac{20 \text{ gtt/mL}}{60 \text{ min}} = 42 \text{ gtt/min;}$
42 macrogtt/min

24. $\frac{500 \text{ mL}}{8 \text{ hr}} \times \frac{15 \text{ gtt/mL}}{60 \text{ min}} = 16 \text{ gtt/min;}$
16 macrogtt/min

25. $\frac{250 \text{ mL}}{10 \text{ hr}} \times \frac{60 \text{ gtt/mL}}{60 \text{ min}} = 25 \text{ gtt/min;}$
25 microgtt/min

26. $\frac{75 \text{ mL}}{1 \text{ hr}} \times \frac{60 \text{ gtt/mL}}{60 \text{ min}} = 75 \text{ gtt/min;}$
75 microgtt/min

27. $\frac{125 \text{ mL}}{1 \text{ hr}} \times \frac{20 \text{ gtt/mL}}{60 \text{ min}} = 42 \text{ gtt/min;}$
42 macrogtt/min

28. $\frac{40 \text{ mL}}{1 \text{ hr}} \times \frac{60 \text{ gtt/mL}}{60 \text{ min}} = 40 \text{ gtt/min;}$
40 microgtt/min

29. $50 \text{ mL} \times \frac{60 \text{ gtt/mL}}{45 \text{ min}} = 67 \text{ gtt/min;}$
67 microgtt/min

30. $\frac{90 \text{ mL}}{1 \text{ hr}} \times \frac{15 \text{ gtt/mL}}{60 \text{ min}} = 23 \text{ gtt/min;}$
23 macrogtt/min

31. $\frac{150 \text{ mL}}{1 \text{ hr}} \times \frac{10 \text{ gtt/mL}}{60 \text{ min}} = 25 \text{ gtt/min;}$
25 macrogtt/min

32. $\frac{3{,}000 \text{ mL}}{24 \text{ hr}} \times \frac{15 \text{ gtt/mL}}{60 \text{ min}} = 31 \text{ gtt/min;}$
31 macrogtt/min

33. $50 \text{ mL} \times \frac{10 \text{ gtt/mL}}{40 \text{ min}} = 13 \text{ gtt/min;}$
13 macrogtt/min

34. $100 \text{ mL} \times \dfrac{20 \text{ gtt/mL}}{30 \text{ min}} = 67 \text{ gtt/min};$
67 macrogtt/min

35. $\dfrac{250 \text{ mL}}{5 \text{ hr}} \times \dfrac{20 \text{ gtt/mL}}{60 \text{ min}} = 17 \text{ gtt/min};$
17 macrogtt/min

36. $\dfrac{80 \text{ mL}}{1 \text{ hr}} \times \dfrac{20 \text{ gtt/mL}}{60 \text{ min}} = 27 \text{ gtt/min};$
27 macrogtt/min

37. $150 \text{ mL} \times \dfrac{12 \text{ gtt/mL}}{30 \text{ min}} = 60 \text{ gtt/min};$
60 macrogtt/min

38. $50 \text{ mL} \times \dfrac{60 \text{ gtt/mL}}{30 \text{ min}} = 100 \text{ gtt/min};$
100 microgtt/min

39. $\dfrac{500 \text{ mL}}{3 \text{ hr}} \times \dfrac{10 \text{ gtt/mL}}{60 \text{ min}} = 28 \text{ gtt/min};$
28 macrogtt/min

40. $\dfrac{250 \text{ mL}}{2 \text{ hr}} \times \dfrac{15 \text{ gtt/mL}}{60 \text{ min}} = 31 \text{ gtt/min};$
31 macrogtt/min

41. $\dfrac{1{,}750 \text{ mL}}{24 \text{ hr}} \times \dfrac{10 \text{ gtt/mL}}{60 \text{ min}} = 12 \text{ gtt/min};$
12 macrogtt/min

42. $\dfrac{150 \text{ mL}}{1.5 \text{ hr}} \times \dfrac{60 \text{ gtt/mL}}{60 \text{ min}} = 100 \text{ gtt/min};$
100 microgtt/min

43. Note: 1 L = 1000 mL; therefore,
2 L = 2,000 mL

$\dfrac{2{,}000 \text{ mL}}{16 \text{ hr}} = 125 \text{ mL/hr}$

44. $\dfrac{500 \text{ mL}}{4 \text{ hr}} = 125 \text{ mL/hr}$

45. $\dfrac{200 \text{ mL}}{2 \text{ hr}} = 100 \text{ mL/hr}$

46. $\dfrac{500 \text{ mL}}{8 \text{ hr}} = 63 \text{ mL/hr}$

47. $\dfrac{500 \text{ mL}}{6 \text{ hr}} \times \dfrac{10 \text{ gtt/mL}}{60 \text{ min}} = 14 \text{ gtt/min};$
14 macrogtt/min

48. $\dfrac{1{,}100 \text{ mL}}{12 \text{ hr}} \times \dfrac{20 \text{ gtt/mL}}{60 \text{ min}} = 31 \text{ gtt/min};$
31 macrogtt/min

49. $\dfrac{3{,}000 \text{ mL}}{20 \text{ hr}} \times \dfrac{20 \text{ gtt/mL}}{60 \text{ min}} = 50 \text{ gtt/min};$
50 macrogtt/min

50. $\dfrac{500 \text{ mL}}{6 \text{ hr}} \times \dfrac{10 \text{ gtt/mL}}{60 \text{ min}} = 14 \text{ gtt/min};$
14 macrogtt/min

51. Time remaining = 7 hr

Volume remaining = 300 mL

$\dfrac{300 \text{ mL}}{7 \text{ hr}} \times \dfrac{15 \text{ gtt/mL}}{60 \text{ min}} = 11 \text{ gtt/min};$
11 macrogtt/min

Slow the IV rate from 13 gtt/min (13 macrogtt/min) to 11 gtt/min (11 macrogtt/min).

52. Time remaining = 4 hr

Volume remaining = 600 mL

$\dfrac{600 \text{ mL}}{4 \text{ hr}} \times \dfrac{20 \text{ gtt/mL}}{60 \text{ min}} = 50 \text{ gtt/min};$
50 macrogtt/min

Increase IV rate from 42 gtt/min (42 macrogtt/min) to 50 gtt/min (50 macrogtt/min).

53. Time remaining = 4 hr

Volume remaining = 400 mL

$\dfrac{400 \text{ mL}}{4 \text{ hr}} = 100 \text{ mL/hr}$

The hourly rate must be adjusted first; then gtt/min recalculated:

$\dfrac{100 \text{ mL}}{1 \text{ hr}} \times \dfrac{15 \text{ gtt/mL}}{60 \text{ min}} = 25 \text{ gtt/min};$
25 macrogtt/min

The I.V. was ahead. Slow the I.V. from 31 gtt/min (31 macrogtt/min) to 25 gtt/min (25 macrogtt/min). The original I.V. order of 125 mL/hr = 31 gtt/min (31 macrogtt/min).

54. Time remaining = 5 hr

Volume remaining = 250 mL

$\dfrac{250 \text{ mL}}{5 \text{ hr}} \times \dfrac{10 \text{ gtt/mL}}{60 \text{ min}} = 8 \text{ gtt/min};$
8 macrogtt/min

The I.V. is ahead of time. The rate must be slowed to 8 gtt/min (8 macrogtt/min).

55. Time remaining = 4 hr

Volume remaining = 600 mL

The I.V. is behind time.

$\dfrac{1000 \text{ mL}}{10 \text{ hr}} \times \dfrac{15 \text{ gtt/mL}}{60 \text{ min}} = 25 \text{ gtt/min};$
25 macrogtt/min

Recalculating the I.V.

$$\frac{600\text{ mL}}{4\text{ hr}} \times \frac{15\text{ gtt/mL}}{60\text{ min}} = 37.5\text{ gtt/min} =$$

38 macrogtt/min; 38 gtt/min

The I.V. will have to be increased from 25 gtt/min (25 macrogtt/min) to 38 gtt/min (38 macrogtt/min).

56. $\frac{900\text{ mL}}{x\text{ hr}} \times \frac{15\text{ gtt/mL}}{60\text{ min}} = 80\text{ gtt/min;}$
80 macrogtt/min

Time: 2.81 hr. Since .81 represents a fraction of an additional hour, convert it to minutes—multiply by 60 minutes.

Answer: 2 hr and 49 minutes

57. $\frac{1000\text{ mL}}{100\text{ cc/hr}} = 10\text{ hr}$

58. $\frac{1000\text{ mL}}{x\text{ hr}} \times \frac{10\text{ gtt/mL}}{60\text{ min}} = 20\text{ gtt/min;}$
20 macrogtt/min

Time: 8.33 hr

$0.33 \times 60 = 19.8 = 20$ minutes

Answer: 8 hr and 20 minutes

59. $\frac{450\text{ mL}}{x\text{ hr}} \times \frac{20\text{ gtt/mL}}{60\text{ min}} = 25\text{ gtt/min;}$
25 macrogtt/min

Answer: 6 hr

60. $\frac{100\text{ mL}}{x\text{ hr}} \times \frac{15\text{ gtt/mL}}{60\text{ min}} = 10\text{ gtt/min;}$
10 macrogtt/min

Answer: 2.5 hr = $2\frac{1}{2}$ hr

61. $\frac{x\text{ mL}}{8\text{ hr}} \times \frac{15\text{ gtt/mL}}{60\text{ min}} = 25\text{ gtt/min;}$
25 macrogtt/min

800 mL

62. $\frac{x\text{ mL}}{10\text{ hr}} \times \frac{60\text{ gtt/mL}}{60\text{ min}} = 40\text{ gtt/min;}$
40 microgtt/min

400 mL

63. $\frac{x\text{ mL}}{5\text{ hr}} \times \frac{15\text{ gtt/mL}}{60\text{ min}} = 30\text{ gtt/min;}$
30 macrogtt/min

600 mL

64. a) $10\text{ mEq} : 500\text{ mL} = 2\text{ mEq} : x\text{ mL}$

$$10x = 500 \times 2$$

$$\frac{10x}{10} = \frac{1000}{10}$$

$$x = 100\text{ mL}$$

Therefore 100 mL of fluid would be needed to administer 2 mEq of potassium chloride.

b) $\frac{100\text{ mL}}{1\text{ hr}} \times \frac{20\text{ gtt/mL}}{60\text{ min}} = 33\text{ gtt/min}$
33 macrogtt/min

33 gtt/min (33 macrogtt/min) would deliver 2 mEq of potassium chloride each hour.

65. a) $30\text{ mEq} : 1000\text{ mL} = 4\text{ mEq} : x\text{ mL}$

$$\frac{30x}{30} = \frac{4000}{30} = 133.3$$

133 mL would deliver 4 mEq of potassium chloride.

b) $\frac{133\text{ mL}}{1\text{ hr}} \times \frac{15\text{ gtt/mL}}{60\text{ min}} = 33\text{ gtt/min}$
33 macrogtt/min

33 gtt/min (33 macrogtt/min) would deliver 4 mEq of potassium chloride each hour.

66. $50\text{ U} : 250\text{ mL} = 7\text{ U} : x\text{ mL}$

$$\frac{50x}{50} = \frac{1750}{50} = 35\text{ mL/hr}$$

Answer: 35 mL/hr

67. $100\text{ U} : 250\text{ mL} = 18\text{ U} : x\text{ mL}$

$$\frac{100x}{100} = \frac{4{,}500}{100} = 45\text{ mL/hr}$$

Answer: 45 mL/hr

68. $100\text{ U} : 100\text{ mL} = 11\text{ U} : x\text{ mL}$

$$\frac{100x}{100} = \frac{1{,}100}{100} = 11\text{ mL/hr}$$

Answer: 11 mL/hr

69. $\frac{150\text{ mL}}{1\text{ hr}} \times \frac{10\text{ gtt/mL}}{60\text{ min}} = 25\text{ gtt/min;}$
25 macrogtt/min

70. $40\text{ mL} \times \frac{60\text{ gtt/mL}}{40\text{ min}} = 60\text{ gtt/min;}$
60 microgtt/min

71. $35 \text{ mL} \times \frac{60 \text{ gtt/mL}}{30 \text{ min}} = 70 \text{ gtt/min}$;
70 microgtt/min

72. $80 \text{ mL} \times \frac{15 \text{ gtt/mL}}{40 \text{ min}} = 30 \text{ gtt/min}$;
30 macrogtt/min

73. $50 \text{ mL} \times \frac{10 \text{ gtt/mL}}{25 \text{ min}} = 20 \text{ gtt/min}$;
20 macrogtt/min

74. $\frac{65 \text{ mL}}{1 \text{ hr}} \times \frac{15 \text{ gtt/mL}}{60 \text{ min}} = 16 \text{ gtt/min}$;
16 macrogtt/min

75. Step 1: 60 gtt : 1 mL = 50 gtt : x mL

$60x = 50$

$x = 50 \div 60$; $x = 0.83$ mL/min

Step 2: 0.83 mL × 60 (min) = 49.8 = 50 mL/hr

Step 3: $\frac{50 \text{ mL}}{50 \text{ mL/hr}} = 1 \text{ hr}$

Answer: Infusion time = 1 hr

76. Step 1: $\frac{500 \text{ mL}}{80 \text{ mL/hr}} = 6.25$

Step 2: 60 × 0.25 = 15 minutes

Infusion time is 6 hrs and 15 minutes.

Step 3: (7 PM + 6 hrs + 15 minutes)

Answer: 1:15 AM

77. $\frac{150 \text{ mL}}{25 \text{ mL/hr}} = 6 \text{ hr}$

a) Infusion time = 6 hr

b) (3:10 AM + 6 hrs = 9:10 AM) I.V. will be completed at 9:10 AM

78. Conversion is required. Equivalent: 1 L = 1000 mL

Therefore 2.5 L = 2,500 mL

Step 1: $\frac{2{,}500 \text{ mL}}{150 \text{ mL/hr}} = 16.66$

Step 2: 60 × 0.66 = 39.6 = 40 minutes

Infusion time is 16 hr and 40 minutes.

*79. $\frac{30 \text{ mL (dd)} + 20 \text{ mL (F)}}{1} \times \frac{60 \text{ gtt/mL}}{20 \text{ min}}$

$= \frac{50 \text{ mL}}{1} \times \frac{60 \text{ gtt/mL}}{20 \text{ min}}$

$= \frac{3{,}000}{20} = 150 \text{ gtt/min}$

a) 150 gtt/min; 150 microgtt/min

b) 150 mL/hr

*80. $\frac{80 \text{ mL (dd)} + 15 \text{ mL (F)}}{1} \times \frac{60 \text{ gtt/mL}}{60 \text{ min}}$

$= \frac{95 \text{ mL}}{1} \times \frac{60 \text{ gtt/mL}}{60 \text{ min}}$

$= \frac{5{,}700}{60} = 95 \text{ gtt/min}$

a) 95 gtt/min; 95 microgtt/min

b) 95 mL/hr

*81. $\frac{40 \text{ mL (dd)} + 15 \text{ mL (F)}}{1} \times \frac{60 \text{ gtt/mL}}{45 \text{ min}}$

$= \frac{55 \text{ mL}}{1} \times \frac{60 \text{ gtt/mL}}{45 \text{ min}}$

$= \frac{3{,}300}{45} = 73 \text{ gtt/min}$

a) 73 gtt/min; 73 microgtt/min

b) 73 mL/hr

**dd* stands for diluted drug; *F* stands for flush.

Chapter 21

Answers to Chapter Review

1. 10,000 U : 1 mL = 3,500 U : x mL OR $\frac{3{,}500 \text{ U}}{10{,}000 \text{ U}} \times 1 \text{ mL} = x \text{ mL}$; $\frac{3{,}500 \text{ U}}{10{,}000 \text{ U}} = \frac{x \text{ mL}}{1 \text{ mL}}$

$x = 0.35$ mL. The dose ordered is less than what is available. Therefore you will need less than 1 mL to administer the dose.

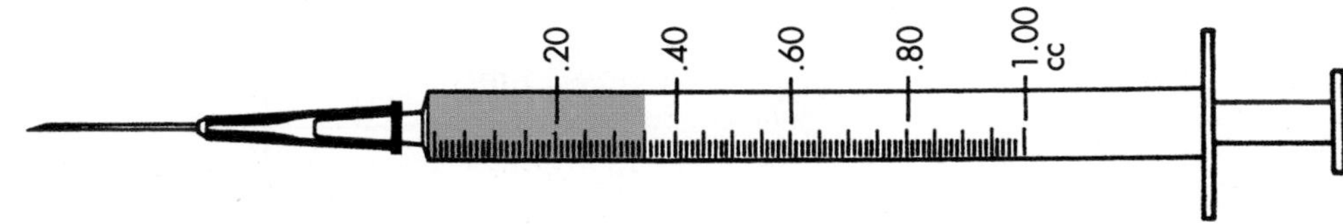

2. $20{,}000\text{ U} : 1\text{ mL} = 16{,}000\text{ U} : x\text{ mL}$ OR $\frac{16{,}000\text{ U}}{20{,}000\text{ U}} \times 1\text{ mL} = x\text{ mL}; \frac{16{,}000\text{ U}}{20{,}000\text{ U}} = \frac{x\text{ mL}}{1\text{ mL}}$

   Answer: 0.8 mL. The dose ordered is less than what is available. Therefore you will need less than 1 mL to administer the dose.

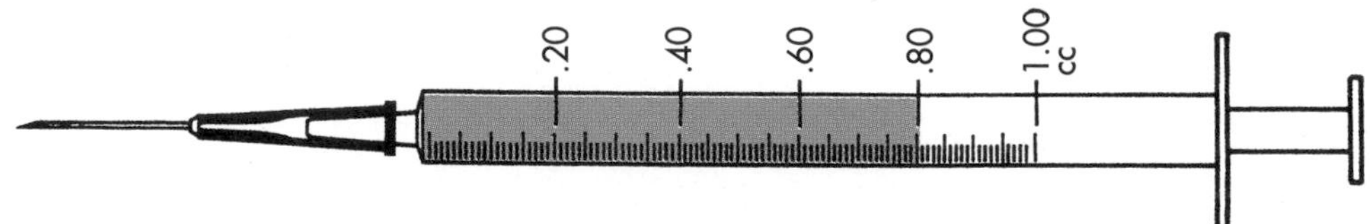

3. $2{,}500\text{ U} : 1\text{ mL} = 2{,}000\text{ U} : x\text{ mL}$ OR $\frac{2{,}000\text{ U}}{2{,}500\text{ U}} \times 1\text{ mL} = x\text{ mL}; \frac{2{,}000\text{ U}}{2{,}500\text{ U}} = \frac{x\text{ mL}}{1\text{ mL}}$

   Answer: 0.8 mL. The dose ordered is less than what is available. Therefore you will need less than 1 mL to administer the dose.

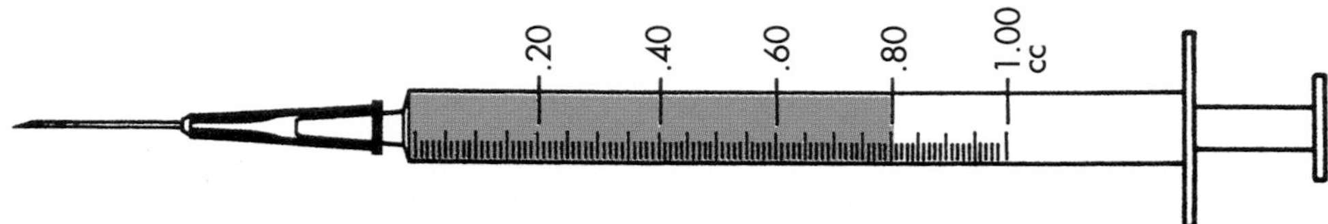

4. $5{,}000\text{ U} : 1\text{ mL} = 2{,}000\text{ U} : x\text{ mL}$ OR $\frac{2{,}000\text{ U}}{5{,}000\text{ U}} \times 1\text{ mL} = x\text{ mL}; \frac{2{,}000\text{ U}}{5{,}000\text{ U}} = \frac{x\text{ mL}}{1\text{ mL}}$

   Answer: 0.4 mL. The dose ordered is less than what is available. Therefore you will need less than 1 mL to administer the dose.

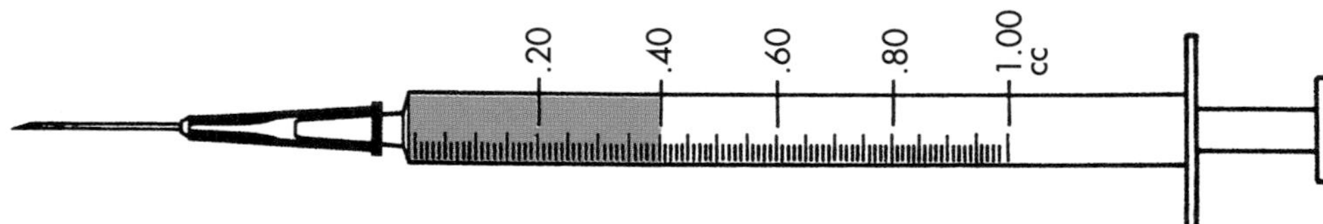

5. $1000\text{ U} : 1\text{ mL} = 500\text{ U} : x\text{ mL}$ OR $\frac{500\text{ U}}{1000\text{ U}} \times 1\text{ mL} = x\text{ mL}; \frac{500\text{ U}}{1000\text{ U}} = \frac{x\text{ mL}}{1\text{ mL}}$

   Answer: 0.5 mL. The dose ordered is less than what is available. Therefore you will need less than a mL to administer the dose.

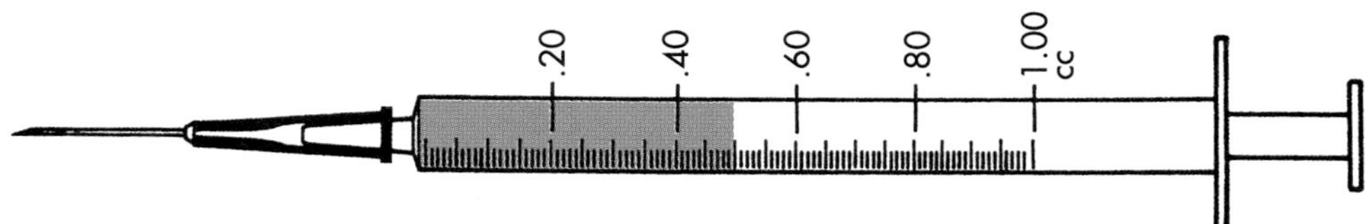

6. $10\text{ U} : 1\text{ mL} = 10\text{ U} : x\text{ mL}$ OR $\frac{10\text{ U}}{10\text{ U}} \times 1\text{ mL} = x\text{ mL}; \frac{10\text{ U}}{10\text{ U}} = \frac{x\text{ mL}}{1\text{ mL}}$

   1 mL contains 10 U, so you will need 1 mL to administer the dose.

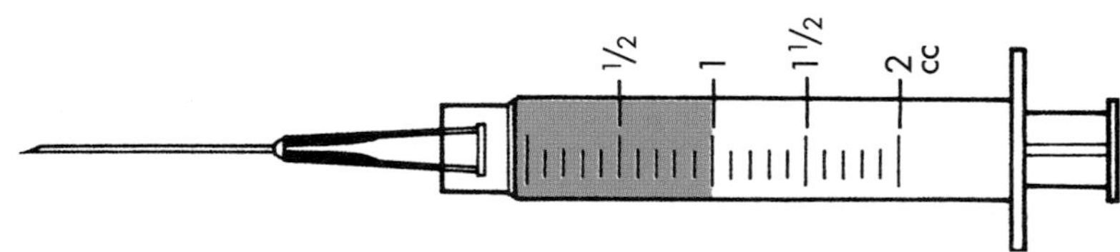

7. 10,000 U : 1 mL = 50,000 U : x mL $\quad \dfrac{50{,}000\ \text{U}}{10{,}000\ \text{U}} \times 1\ \text{mL} = x\ \text{mL}; \dfrac{50{,}000\ \text{U}}{10{,}000\ \text{U}} = \dfrac{x\ \text{mL}}{1\ \text{mL}}$

Answer: 5 mL would be needed to administer the dose. The dose ordered is greater than what is available. Therefore you will need more than a mL to administer the dose.

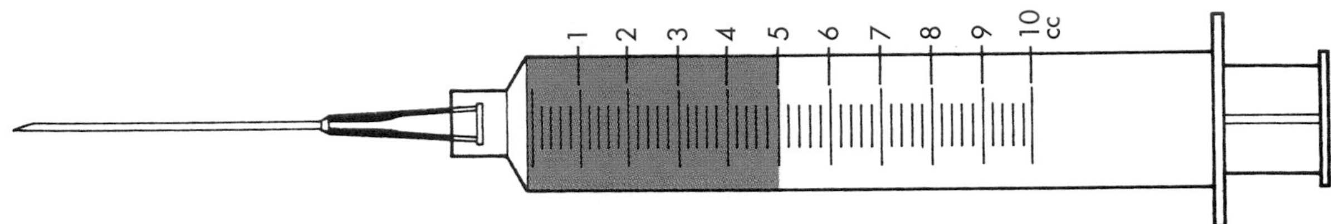

8. 20,000 U : 1 mL = 15,000 U : x mL OR $\dfrac{15{,}000\ \text{U}}{20{,}000\ \text{U}} \times 1\ \text{mL} = x\ \text{mL}; \dfrac{15{,}000\ \text{U}}{20{,}000\ \text{U}} = \dfrac{x\ \text{mL}}{1\ \text{mL}}$

Answer: 0.75 mL. The dose ordered is less than what is available. Therefore you will need less than 1 mL to administer the dose.

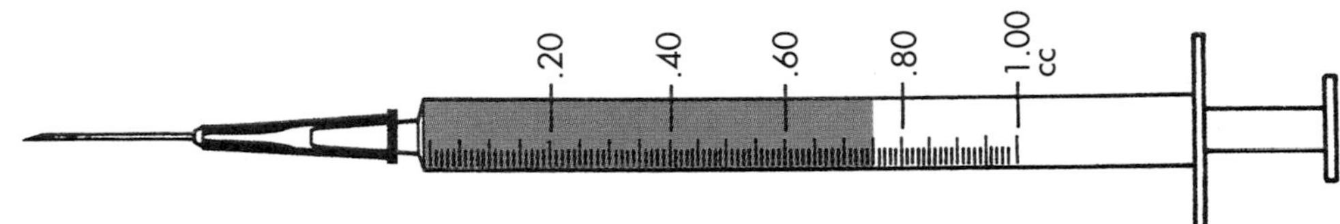

9. 2,500 U : 1 mL = 3,000 U : x mL OR $\dfrac{3{,}000\ \text{U}}{2{,}500\ \text{U}} \times 1\ \text{mL} = x\ \text{mL}; \dfrac{3{,}000\ \text{U}}{2{,}500\ \text{U}} = \dfrac{x\ \text{mL}}{1\ \text{mL}}$

Answer: 1.2 mL. The dose ordered is more than what is available. Therefore you will need more than 1 mL to administer the dose.

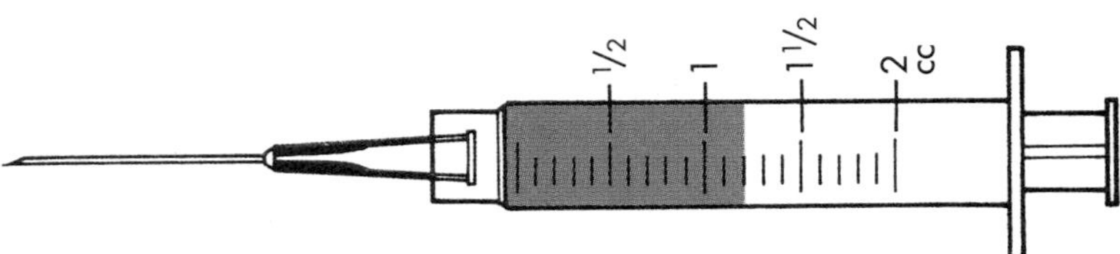

10. 20,000 U : 1 mL = 17,000 U : x mL OR $\dfrac{17{,}000\ \text{U}}{20{,}000\ \text{U}} \times 1\ \text{mL} = x\ \text{mL}; \dfrac{17{,}000\ \text{U}}{20{,}000\ \text{U}} = \dfrac{x\ \text{mL}}{1\ \text{mL}}$

Answer: 0.85 mL. The dose ordered is less than what is available. You will need less than 1 mL to administer the dose.

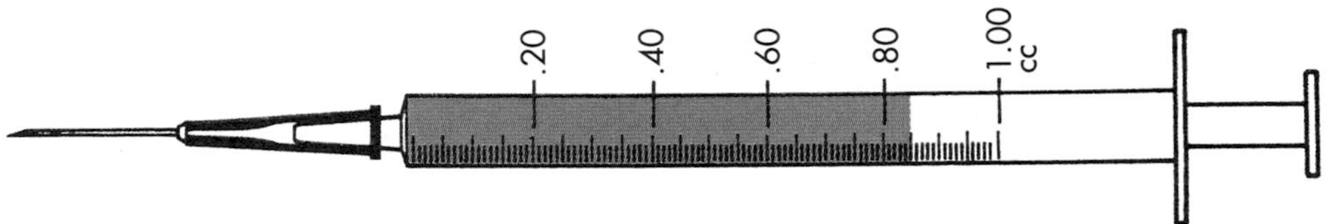

11. 10,000 U : 1 mL = 8,500 U : x mL OR $\dfrac{8{,}500\ \text{U}}{10{,}000\ \text{U}} \times 1\ \text{mL} = x\ \text{mL}; \dfrac{8{,}500\ \text{U}}{10{,}000\ \text{U}} = \dfrac{x\ \text{mL}}{1\ \text{mL}}$

Answer: 0.85 mL. The dose ordered is less than what is available. Therefore you will need less than 1 mL to administer the dose.

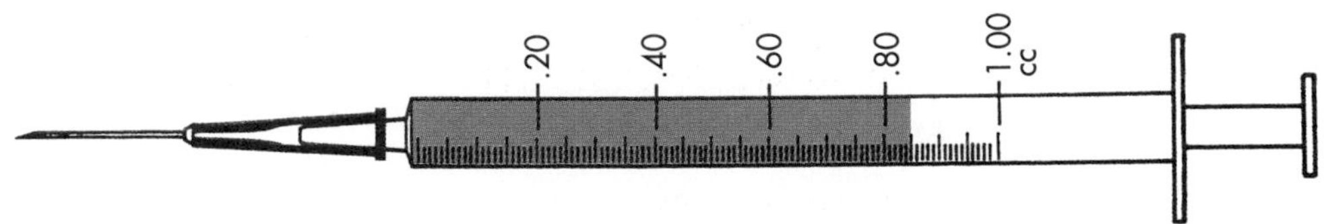

12. 10,000 U:1 mL = 2,500 U : x mL OR $\frac{2{,}500 \text{ U}}{10{,}000 \text{ U}} \times 1 \text{ mL} = x \text{ mL}; \frac{2{,}500 \text{ U}}{10{,}000} \text{U} = \frac{x \text{ mL}}{1 \text{ mL}}$

Answer: 0.25 mL. The dose ordered is less than what is available. Therefore you will need less than 1 mL to administer the dose.

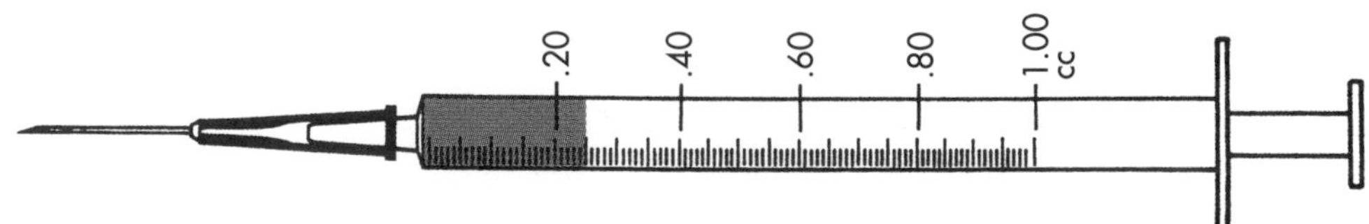

13. 25,000 U : 1000 mL = 2,000 U : x mL

$$\frac{25{,}000x}{25{,}000} = \frac{2{,}000{,}000}{25{,}000}$$

$$x = \frac{2{,}000{,}000}{25{,}000}$$

x = 80 mL/hr. To administer 2,000 U of heparin per hour, 80 mL/hr must be given.

14. 25,000 U : 500 mL = 1,500 U : x mL

$$\frac{25{,}000x}{25{,}000} = \frac{750{,}000}{25{,}000}$$

$$x = \frac{750{,}000}{25{,}000}$$

x = 30 mL/hr. To administer 1,500 U of heparin per hour 30 mL/hr must be given.

15. 25,000 U : 250 mL = 1,800 U : x mL

$$\frac{25{,}000x}{25{,}000} = \frac{450{,}000}{25{,}000}$$

x = 18 mL/hr. To administer 1,800 U of heparin per hour, 18 mL/hr must be given.

16. 40,000 U : 1000 mL = x U : 25 mL

$$\frac{1000x}{1000} = \frac{1{,}000{,}000}{1000}$$

$$x = \frac{1{,}000{,}000}{1000}$$

x = 1000 U/hr

17. 25,000 U : 250 mL = x U : 11 mL

$$\frac{250x}{250} = \frac{275{,}000}{250}$$

x = 1,100 U/hr

18. 40,000 U : 500 mL = x U : 30 mL

$$\frac{500x}{500} = \frac{1{,}200{,}000}{500}$$

Answer: 2,400 U/hr

19. 20,000 U : 500 mL = x U : 12 mL

$$\frac{500x}{500} = \frac{240{,}000}{500}$$

Answer: 480 U/hr

20. 25,000 U : 500 mL = x U : 15 mL

$$\frac{500x}{500} = \frac{375{,}000}{500}$$

Answer: 750 U/hr

21. 1 L = 1000 mL

a) $\frac{1000 \text{ mL}}{24 \text{ hr}} = 41.6 = 42 \text{ mL/hr}$

40,000 U : 1000 mL = x U : 42 mL

$$\frac{1000x}{1000} = \frac{1{,}680{,}000}{1000}$$

$$x = \frac{1{,}680{,}000}{1000}$$

x = 1,680 U/hr

b) $\frac{42 \text{ mL}}{1 \text{ hr}} \times \frac{15 \text{ gtt/mL}}{60 \text{ min}} = 10.5 =$ 11 gtt/min

22. 1 L = 1000 mL

a) Calculate mL/hr.

$$\frac{1000 \text{ mL}}{10 \text{ hr}} = 100 \text{ mL/hr}$$

b) Calculate U/hr.

15,000 U : 1000 mL = x U : 100 mL

$$\frac{1000x}{1000} = \frac{1{,}500{,}000}{1000}$$

$$x = \frac{1{,}500{,}000}{1000}$$

x = 1,500 U/hr

23. a) 35,000 U : 1000 mL = x U : 20 mL

$$\frac{1000x}{1000} = \frac{700{,}000}{1000}$$

$$x = \frac{700{,}000}{1000}$$

$$x = 700 \text{ U/hr}$$

b) $\frac{20 \text{ mL}}{1 \text{ hr}} \times \frac{60 \text{ gtt/mL}}{60 \text{ min}} = 20 \text{ gtt/min}$

24. a) Convert gtt/min to mL/min.

10 gtt : 1 mL = 20 gtt : x mL

$$\frac{10x}{10} = \frac{20}{10}$$

$$x = 2 \text{ mL/min}$$

Convert mL/min to mL/hr.

2 mL × 60 min = 120 mL/hr

b) 10,000 U : 500 mL = x U : 120 mL

$$\frac{500x}{500} = \frac{1{,}200{,}000}{500}$$

$$x = \frac{1{,}200{,}000}{500}$$

$$x = 2{,}400 \text{ U/hr}$$

25. 25,000 U : 500 mL = x U : 25 mL

$$\frac{500x}{500} = \frac{625{,}000}{500}$$

Answer: 1,250 U/hr

26. 20,000 U : 500 mL = x U : 40 mL

$$\frac{500x}{500} = \frac{800{,}000}{500}$$

Answer: 1,600 U/hr

27. a) Calculate mL/hr to be administered.

40,000 U : 1000 mL = 1,400 U : x mL

$$\frac{40{,}000x}{40{,}000} = \frac{1{,}400{,}000}{40{,}000}$$

$$x = 35 \text{ mL/hr}$$

b) Calculate gtt/min.

$$\frac{35 \text{ mL}}{1 \text{ hr}} \times \frac{15 \text{ gtt/mL}}{60 \text{ min}} = 8.7 = 9 \text{ gtt/min}$$

28. a) 40,000 U : 1000 mL = 1000 U : x mL

$$\frac{40{,}000x}{40{,}000} = \frac{1{,}000{,}000}{40{,}000}$$

$$x = \frac{1{,}000{,}000}{40{,}000}$$

$$x = 25 \text{ mL/hr}$$

b) $\frac{25 \text{ mL}}{1 \text{ hr}} \times \frac{15 \text{ gtt/mL}}{60 \text{ min}} = 6.2 = 6 \text{ gtt/min}$

29. 25,000 U : 500 mL = 1000 U : x mL

$$\frac{25{,}000x}{25{,}000} = \frac{500{,}000}{25{,}000}$$

$$x = \frac{500{,}000}{25{,}000}$$

$$x = 20 \text{ mL/hr}$$

$$\frac{20 \text{ mL}}{1 \text{ hr}} \times \frac{60 \text{ gtt/mL}}{60 \text{ min}} = 20 \text{ gtt/min}$$

30. 25,000 U : 1000 mL = 2,000 U : x mL

$$\frac{25{,}000x}{25{,}000} = \frac{2{,}000{,}000}{25{,}000}$$

$$x = \frac{2{,}000{,}000}{25{,}000}$$

$$x = 80 \text{ mL/hr}$$

$$\frac{80 \text{ mL}}{1 \text{ hr}} \times \frac{15 \text{ gtt/mL}}{60 \text{ min}} = 20 \text{ gtt/min}$$

31. Step 1: Convert gtt/min to mL/min.

15 gtt : 1 mL = 15 gtt : x mL

$$\frac{15x}{15} = \frac{15}{15}$$

$$x = 1 \text{ mL/min}$$

Step 2: Convert mL/min to mL/hr.

1 mL/min × 60 min = 60 mL/hr

Step 3: Calculate units per hour.

50,000 U : 1000 mL = x U : 60 mL

$$\frac{1000x}{1000} = \frac{3{,}000{,}000}{1000}$$

$$x = \frac{3{,}000{,}000}{1000}$$

$$x = 3{,}000 \text{ U/hr}$$

32. Step 1: Convert gtt/min to mL/min.

10 gtt : 1 mL = 20 gtt : x mL

$$\frac{10x}{10} = \frac{20}{10}$$

$$x = 2 \text{ mL/min}$$

Step 2: Convert mL/min to mL/hr.

$$2 \text{ mL/min} \times 60 \text{ min} = 120 \text{ mL/hr}$$

Step 3: Calculate units per hour.

$$25{,}000 \text{ U} : 250 \text{ mL} = x \text{ U} : 120 \text{ mL}$$
$$\frac{250x}{250} = \frac{3{,}000{,}000}{250}$$
$$x = \frac{3{,}000{,}000}{250}$$
$$x = 12{,}000 \text{ U/hr}$$

33. Step 1: Convert gtt/min to mL/min.

$$60 \text{ gtt} : 1 \text{ mL} = 20 \text{ gtt} : x \text{ mL}$$
$$\frac{60x}{60} = \frac{20}{60}$$
$$x = 0.33 \text{ mL/min}$$

Step 2: Convert mL/min to mL/hr.

$$0.33 \text{ mL/min} \times 60 \text{ min} = 19.8 \text{ mL/hr} = 20 \text{ mL/hr}$$

Step 3: Calculate units per hour.

$$20{,}000 \text{ U} : 500 \text{ mL} = x \text{ U} : 20 \text{ mL}$$
$$\frac{500x}{500} = \frac{400{,}000}{500}$$
$$x = \frac{400{,}000}{500}$$
$$x = 800 \text{ U/hr}$$

34. Step 1: Convert gtt/min to mL/min.

$$15 \text{ gtt} : 1 \text{ mL} = 14 \text{ gtt} : x \text{ mL}$$
$$\frac{15x}{15} = \frac{14}{15}$$
$$x = 0.93 \text{ mL/min}$$

Step 2: Convert mL/min to mL/hr.

$$0.93 \text{ mL/min} \times 60 \text{ min} = 55.8 = 56 \text{ mL/hr}$$

Step 3: Calculate units per hour.

$$25{,}000 \text{ U} : 1000 \text{ mL} = x \text{ U} : 56 \text{ mL}$$
$$\frac{1000x}{1000} = \frac{1{,}400{,}000}{1000}$$
$$x = \frac{1{,}400{,}000}{1000}$$
$$x = 1{,}400 \text{ U/hr}$$

35. Step 1: Convert gtt/min to mL/min:

$$10 \text{ gtt} : 1 \text{ mL} = 24 \text{ gtt} : x \text{ mL}$$
$$\frac{10x}{10} = \frac{24}{10}$$
$$x = 2.4 \text{ mL/min}$$

Step 2: Convert mL/min to mL/hr.

$$2.4 \text{ mL/min} \times 60 \text{ min} = 144 \text{ mL/hr}$$

Step 3: Calculate units per hour:

$$20{,}000 \text{ U} : 1000 \text{ mL} = x \text{ U} : 144 \text{ mL}$$
$$\frac{1000x}{1000} = \frac{2{,}880{,}000}{1000}$$
$$x = \frac{2{,}880{,}000}{1000}$$
$$x = 2{,}880 \text{ U/hr}$$

36. $30{,}000 \text{ U} : 500 \text{ mL} = x \text{ U} : 25 \text{ mL}$

$$\frac{500x}{500} = \frac{750{,}000}{500}$$
$$x = \frac{750{,}000}{500}$$
$$x = 1{,}500 \text{ U/hr}$$

37. $20{,}000 \text{ U} : 1000 \text{ mL} = x \text{ U} : 40 \text{ mL}$

$$\frac{1000x}{1000} = \frac{800{,}000}{1000}$$
$$x = \frac{800{,}000}{1000}$$
$$x = 800 \text{ U/hr}$$

38. $40{,}000 \text{ U} : 500 \text{ mL} = x \text{ U} : 25 \text{ mL}$

$$\frac{500x}{500} = \frac{1{,}000{,}000}{500}$$
$$x = \frac{1{,}000{,}000}{500}$$
$$x = 2{,}000 \text{ U/hr}$$

39. $35{,}000 \text{ U} : 1000 \text{ mL} = x \text{ U} : 20 \text{ mL}$

$$\frac{1000x}{1000} = \frac{700{,}000}{1000}$$
$$x = \frac{700{,}000}{1000}$$
$$x = 700 \text{ U/hr}$$

40. $25{,}000 \text{ U} : 1000 \text{ mL} = x \text{ U} : 30 \text{ mL}$

$$\frac{1000x}{1000} = \frac{750{,}000}{1000}$$
$$x = \frac{750{,}000}{1000}$$
$$x = 750 \text{ U/hr}$$

41. $40{,}000 \text{ U} : 1000 \text{ mL} = x \text{ U} : 30 \text{ mL}$

$$\frac{1000x}{1000} = \frac{1{,}200{,}000}{1000}$$
$$x = 1{,}200 \text{ U/hr}$$

42. 20,000 U : 1000 mL = x U : 80 mL

$$\frac{1000x}{1000} = \frac{1,600,000}{1000}$$

x = 1,600 U/hr

43. 50,000 U : 1000 mL = x U : 70 mL

$$\frac{1000x}{1000} = \frac{3,500,000}{1000}$$

x = 3,500 U/hr

44. 20,000 U : 500 mL = x U : 30 mL

$$\frac{500x}{500} = \frac{600,000}{500}$$

x = 1,200 U/hr

45. 30,000 U : 1000 mL = x U : 25 mL

$$\frac{1000x}{1000} = \frac{750,000}{1000}$$

x = 750 U/hr

Chapter 22

Answers to Practice Problems

1. a) Step 1: Conversion: Equivalent: 1000 mcg = 1 mg

Therefore 250 mg = 250,000 mcg

Step 2: 250,000 mcg : 500 mL = x mcg : 1 mL

$$\frac{500x}{500} = \frac{250,000}{500} = 500 \text{ mcg/mL}$$

Concentration of solution is 500 mcg/mL.

Step 3: Calculate dose range.

Lower dose:
2.5 mcg × 50 kg = 125 mcg/min

Upper dose:
5 mcg × 50 kg = 250 mcg/min

Step 4: Convert dosage range to mL/min.

Lower dose:
500 mcg : 1 mL = 125 mcg : x mL

$$\frac{500x}{500} = \frac{125}{500}$$

x = 0.25 mL/min

Upper dose:
500 mcg : 1 mL = 250 mcg : x mL

$$\frac{500x}{500} = \frac{250}{500}$$

x = 0.5 mL/min

Step 5: Convert mL/min to mL/hr.

Lower dose: 0.25 mL × 60 min = 15 mL/hr (gtt/min)

Upper dose: 0.5 mL × 60 min = 30 mL/hr (gtt/min)

a) A dose range of 2.5–5 mcg/kg/min is equal to a flow rate of 15–30 mL/hr (gtt/min).

b) Determine dose infusing per minute at 25 mL/hr:

500 mcg : 1 mL = x mcg : 25 mL
x = 12,500 mcg/hr

12,500 mcg ÷ 60 min = 208.3 mcg/min

2. a) 2 mg : 250 mL = x mg : 30 mL

$$\frac{250x}{250} = \frac{60}{250}$$

x = 0.24 mg/hr

b) Convert mg to mcg (1000 mcg = 1 mg).

0.24 mg = 240 mcg/hr

c) Convert mcg/hr to mcg/min.

240 mcg/hr ÷ 60 min = 4 mcg/min

3. a) Change g to mg. (Note you were asked mg/min and mg/hr.)

0.25 g = 250 mg

Calculate mg/hr.

250 mg : 8 hr = x mg : 1 hr

$$\frac{8x}{8} = \frac{250}{8}$$

x = 31.25 = 31.3 mg/hr

Answer: 31.3 mg/hr

b) Convert mg/hr to mg/min:

31.3 mg/hr ÷ 60 = 0.52 mg/min

4. Note: Calculate units per hour only.

Step 1: 60 gtt : 1 mL : 15 gtt : x mL

$$\frac{60x}{60} = \frac{15}{60}$$

x = 0.25 mL/min

Step 2: 0.25 mL/min × 60 = 15 mL/hr

Step 3: 10 U : 1000 cc = x U : 15 mL

$$\frac{1000x}{1000} = \frac{150}{1000}$$

$$x = 0.15 \text{ U/hr}$$

5. Step 1: Determine the dose per minute.

60 kg × 3 mcg/kg = 180 mcg/min

Step 2: Convert to dose per hour.

180 mcg/min × 60 = 10,800 mcg/hr

Step 3: Convert to like units.

10,800 mcg = 10.8 mg

Calculate flow rate (mL/hr).

50 mg : 250 mL = 10.8 mg : x mL

$$50x = 250 \times 10.8$$

$$\frac{50x}{50} = \frac{2{,}700}{50}$$

$$x = 54 \text{ mL/hr}$$

6. a) 50 mg : 250 mL = x mg : 3 mL

$$\frac{250x}{250} = \frac{150}{250}$$

$$x = 0.6 \text{ mg/hr}$$

Convert to mcg (1000 mcg = 1 mg).

0.6 mg = 600 mcg/hr

b) Convert mcg/hr to mcg/min.

600 mcg/hr ÷ 60 min = 10 mcg/min

Answers to Chapter Review

1. a) Calculate the dose per hr.

2 mg : 250 mL = x mg : 30 mL

$$\frac{250x}{250} = \frac{60}{250}$$

$$x = \frac{60}{250}$$

$$x = 0.24 \text{ mg/hr}$$

b) Convert mg to mcg (1000 mcg = 1 mg).

1000 × 0.24 mg/hr = 240 mcg/hr

c) Convert mcg/hr to mcg/min.

240 mcg/hr ÷ 60 min = 4 mcg/min.

2. a) Calculate dose per hr.

4 mg : 500 mL = x mg : 40 mL

$$\frac{500x}{500} = \frac{160}{500}$$

$$x = \frac{160}{500}$$

$$x = 0.32 \text{ mg/hr}$$

b) Convert to mcg (1000 mcg = 1 mg).

1000 × 0.32 mg/hr = 320 mcg/hr

c) Convert mcg/hr to mcg/min.

320 mcg/hr ÷ 60 min = 5.33 = 5.3 mcg/min

3. Step 1: Determine dose per hour.

800 mg : 500 mL = x mg : 30 mL

$$\frac{24{,}000}{500} = \frac{500x}{500}$$

$$x = \frac{24{,}000}{500} = 48 \text{ mg/hr}$$

Step 2: Convert mg to mcg (1000 mcg = 1 mg).

48 mg/hr × 1000 = 48,000 mcg/hr

Step 3: Convert mcg/hr to mcg/min.

48,000 mcg/hr ÷ 60 min = 800 mcg/min

200 mg : 5 mL = 800 mg : x mL

OR

$$\frac{800 \text{ mg}}{200 \text{ mg}} \times 5 \text{ mL} = x \text{ mL};$$

$$\frac{800 \text{ mg}}{200 \text{ mg}} = \frac{x \text{ mL}}{5 \text{ mL}}$$

Answer: 20 mL. The dose ordered is greater than what is available.

4. a) Determine dose per hour.

50 mg : 250 mL = x mg : 30 mL

$$\frac{1{,}500}{250} = \frac{250x}{250}$$

$$x = \frac{1{,}500}{250}$$

$$x = 6 \text{ mg/hr}$$

Convert mg to mcg (1000 mcg = 1 mg).

6 mg/hr × 1000 = 6,000 mcg/hr

b) Convert mcg/hr to mcg/min.

6,000 mcg/hr ÷ 60 min = 100 mcg/min

5. a) Calculate mg/hr.

$$100 \text{ mg} : 250 \text{ mL} = x \text{ mg} : 25 \text{ mL}$$
$$\frac{250x}{250} = \frac{2{,}500}{250}$$
$$x = \frac{2{,}500}{250}$$
$$x = 10 \text{ mg/hr}$$

Convert mg to mcg.
(1000 mcg = 1 mg)

10 mg = 10,000 mcg/hr

b) Convert mcg/hr to mcg/min.

10,000 mcg/hr ÷ 60 min = 166.66 = 166.7 mcg/min

6. a) Convert metric weight to the same as answer request.

$$1 \text{ g} = 1000 \text{ mg}$$
$$2{,}000 \text{ mg} : 250 \text{ mL} = x \text{ mg} : 60 \text{ mL}$$
$$\frac{250x}{250} = \frac{120{,}000\ x}{250}$$
$$x = \frac{120{,}000}{250}$$
$$x = 480 \text{ mg/hr}$$

b) Convert mg/hr to mg/min

480 mg/hr ÷ 60 min = 8 mg/min

7. Step 1: Convert g to mg (1000 mg = 1 g).

0.25 g = 250 mg

Step 2: Calculate mg/hr.

$$250 \text{ mg} : 6 \text{ hr} = x \text{ mg} : 1 \text{ hr}$$
$$\frac{250}{6} = \frac{6x}{6}$$
$$x = \frac{250}{6}$$
$$x = 41.66 = 41.7 \text{ mg/hr.}$$

8. a) Convert g to mg (1000 mg = 1 g).

2 g = 2,000 mg

b) Calculate mg/hr.

$$2{,}000 \text{ mg} : 250 \text{ mL} = x \text{ mg} : 30 \text{ mL}$$
$$\frac{250x}{250} = \frac{60{,}000}{250}$$
$$x = \frac{60{,}000}{250}$$
$$x = 240 \text{ mg/hr}$$

c) Convert mg/hr to mg/min.

240 mg ÷ 60 min = 4 mg/min

9. a) Step 1: Calculate gtt/min to mL/min.

$$60 \text{ gtt} : 1 \text{ mL} = 45 \text{ gtt} : x \text{ mL}$$
$$\frac{60x}{60} = \frac{45}{60}$$
$$x = \frac{45}{60}$$
$$x = 0.75 \text{ mL/min}$$

Step 2: Calculate U/min.

$$20 \text{ U} : 1000 \text{ mL} = x \text{ units} : 0.75 \text{ mL}$$
$$\frac{15}{1000} = \frac{1000x}{1000}$$
$$x = \frac{15}{1000}$$
$$x = 0.015 \text{ U/min}$$

b) Calculate U/hr.

0.015 U/min × 60 min = 0.9 U/hr

10. 30 U : 1000 mL = x U : 40 mL

$$\frac{1{,}200}{1000} = \frac{1000x}{1000}$$
$$x = \frac{1{,}200}{1000}$$
$$x = 1.2 \text{ U/hr}$$

11. 30 U : 500 mL = x U : 45 mL

$$\frac{1{,}350}{500} = \frac{500x}{500}$$
$$x = \frac{1{,}350}{500}$$
$$x = 2.7 \text{ U/hr}$$

12. a) Change metric measures to same as question. 1 g = 1000 mg; therefore 2 g = 2,000 mg

Calculate mg/hr.

$$2{,}000 \text{ mg} : 500 \text{ mL} : x \text{ mg} : 30 \text{ mL}$$
$$\frac{60{,}000}{500} = \frac{500x}{500}$$
$$x = \frac{60{,}000}{500}$$
$$x = 120 \text{ mg/hr}$$

b) Change mg/hr to mg/min.

120 mg/hr ÷ 60 min = 2 mg/min

13. a) Change metric measures to same as question.

$$2 \text{ g} = 2{,}000 \text{ mg}$$

Calculate mg/hr:

$$2{,}000 \text{ mg} : 500 \text{ mL} = x \text{ mg} : 45 \text{ mL}$$

$$\frac{90{,}000}{500} = \frac{500x}{500}$$

$$x = \frac{90{,}000}{500}$$

$$x = 180 \text{ mg/hr}$$

b) Change mg/hr to mg/min

$$180 \text{ mg/hr} \div 60 \text{ min} = 3 \text{ mg/min}$$

14. Determine dose per hour:

$$500 \text{ mcg/min} \times 60 \text{ min} = 30{,}000 \text{ mcg/hr}$$

Convert mcg to mg.

$$1000 \text{ mcg} = 1 \text{ mg}$$

$$30{,}000 \text{ mcg/hr} = 30 \text{ mg/hr}$$

Calculate flow rate in mL/hr.

$$50 \text{ mg} : 250 \text{ mL} = 30 \text{ mg} : x \text{ mL}$$

$$\frac{50x}{50} = \frac{7{,}500}{50}$$

$$x = 150 \text{ mL/hr}$$

Set at 150 mL/hr to deliver 30 mg/hr.

15. 400 mg : 500 mL = x mg : 35 mL

$$\frac{500x}{500} = \frac{14{,}000}{500}$$

$$x = 28 \text{ mg/hr}$$

16. a) Calculate mg/hr.

$$2 \text{ mg} : 250 \text{ mL} = x \text{ mg} : 30 \text{ mL}$$

$$\frac{60}{250} = \frac{250x}{250}$$

$$x = \frac{60}{250}$$

$$x = 0.24 \text{ mg/hr}$$

b) Convert mg to mcg. (1000 mcg = 1 mg)

$$0.24 \text{ mg} \times 1000 = 240 \text{ mcg/hr}$$

c) Convert mcg/hr to mcg/min.

$$240 \text{ mcg} \div 60 \text{ min} = 4 \text{ mcg/min}$$

17. Convert metric weight to same as question.

$$1000 \text{ mg} = 1 \text{ g}$$

Calculate mg/hr.

$$1000 \text{ mg} : 10 \text{ hr} = x \text{ mg} : 1 \text{ hr}$$

$$\frac{10x}{10} = \frac{1000}{10}$$

$$x = 100 \text{ mg/hr}$$

18. 150 mg : 500 mL = x mg : 30 mL

$$\frac{500x}{500} = \frac{4{,}500}{500}$$

$$x = \frac{4{,}500}{500}$$

$$x = 9 \text{ mg/hr}$$

19. a) Convert metric weights g to mg.

$$2 \text{ g} = 2{,}000 \text{ mg } (1000 \text{ mg} = 1 \text{ g})$$

$$2{,}000 \text{ mg} : 250 \text{ mL} = x \text{ mg} : 22\text{mL}$$

$$\frac{250x}{250} = \frac{44{,}000\,x}{250}$$

$$x = \frac{44{,}000}{250}$$

$$x = 176 \text{ mg/hr}$$

b) Change mg/hr to mg/min.

176 mg/hr ÷ 60 min = 2.93 = 2.9 mg/min

20. a) Calculate dose per hour

$$4 \text{ mg} : 250 \text{ mL} = x \text{ mg} : 8 \text{ mL}$$

$$\frac{250x}{250} = \frac{32}{250}$$

$$x = \frac{32}{250}$$

$$x = 0.128 \text{ mg/hr}$$

Convert mg to mcg.

$$0.128 \text{ mg} \times 1000 = 128 \text{ mcg/hr}$$

b) Convert mcg/hr to mcg/min.

128 mcg/hr ÷ 60 min = 2.13 mcg/min = 2.1 mcg/min

21. a) 500 mg : 250 mL = x mg : 30 mL

$$\frac{250x}{250} = \frac{15{,}000}{250}$$

$$x = \frac{15{,}000}{250}$$

$$x = 60 \text{ mg/hr}$$

b) Convert mg/hr to mg/min.

60 mg/hr ÷ 60 min = 1 mg/min

22. a) Calculate mg/hr.

500 mg : 500 mL = x mg : 30 mL

$$\frac{500x}{500} = \frac{15{,}000}{500}$$

$$x = \frac{15{,}000}{500}$$

x = 30 mg/hr

Convert mg to mcg. (1000 mcg = 1 mg)

30 mg = 30,000 mcg/hr

b) Convert mcg/hr to mcg/min.

30,000 mcg/hr ÷ 60 min = 500 mcg/min

23. 25 g : 300 mL = 2 g : x mL

$$\frac{25x}{25} = \frac{600}{25}$$

$$x = \frac{600}{25}$$

x = 24 mL/hr to administer 2 g

24. Determine dose per hour.

200 mcg/min × 60 min = 12,000 mcg/hr

Convert mcg to mg.

(1000 mcg = 1 mg)

12,000 mcg ÷ 1000 = 12 mg/hr

Calculate the mL/hr.

400 mg : 500 mL = 12 mg : x mL

$$\frac{400x}{400} = \frac{6{,}000}{400}$$

x = 15 mL/hr

25. 25 g : 300 mL = 3 g : x mL

$$\frac{25x}{25} = \frac{900}{25}$$

$$x = \frac{900}{25}$$

x = 36 mL/hr to administer 3 g

26. Convert dose per min to dose per hour.

10 mcg/min × 60 = 600 mcg/hr

Convert measures to like units (mcg to mg). 1000 mcg = 1 mg

600 mcg = 600 ÷ 1000 = 0.6 mg

c) Calculate mL/hr.

50 mg : 250 mL = 0.6 mg : x mL

$$\frac{50x}{50} = \frac{150}{50}$$

x = 3 mL/hr

Calculate the flow rate in gtt/min.

To deliver 10 mcg/min, the I.V. is to infuse at 3 gtt/min (3 microgtt/min).

27. Convert weight in lb to kg.

120 lb = 54.54 = 54.5 kg

Calculate dose per minute.

54.5 kg × 2 mcg = 109 mcg/min

28. No conversion of weight is required.

80 kg × 3 mcg = 240 mcg/minute

29. No conversion of weight is required.

73.5 kg × 0.7 mg = 51.45 mg/hr

30. a) Convert weight in lb to kg.

110 lb ÷ 2.2 = 50 kg

Calculate the dose per hour.

50 kg × 0.7 mg = 35 mg/hr

b) Calculate the dose per minute.

35 mg/hr ÷ 60 min = 0.58 mg/min = 0.6 mg/min

c) The dose is safe; it falls within the safe range.

31. Step 1: Convert to like units.

Equivalent: 1000 mcg = 1 mg

Therefore 2 mg = 2,000 mcg

Step 2: Calculate the concentration of solution in mcg/mL.

2,000 mcg : 500 mL = x mcg : 1 mL

$$\frac{500x}{500} = \frac{2{,}000}{500}$$

x = 4 mcg/mL

Lower dose: 4 mcg : 1 mL = 2 mcg : x mL

$$\frac{4x}{4} = \frac{2}{4}$$

x = 0.5 mL/min

Upper dose: 4 mcg : 1 mL = 6 mcg : x mL

$$\frac{4x}{4} = \frac{6}{4}$$

$$x = 1.5 \text{ mL/min}$$

Step 3: Convert mL/min to mL/hr.

Lower dose: 0.5 mL × 60 min = 30 mL/hr (gtt/min)

Upper dose: 1.5 mL × 60 min = 90 mL/hr (gtt/min)

A dose range of 2–6 mcg/min is equal to a flow rate of 30–90 mL/hr (gtt/min).

32. Determine the dose per hour:

$$0.15 \text{ mg/min} \times 60 \text{ min} = 9 \text{ mg/hr}$$

Calculate the flow rate (mL/hr, gtt/min).

$$150 \text{ mg} : 500 \text{ mL} = 9 \text{ mg} : x \text{ mL}$$

$$\frac{150x}{150} = \frac{4{,}500}{150} = 30 \text{ mL/hr}$$

To infuse 0.15 mg/min set the flow rate at 30 mL/hr (gtt/min).

33. Step 1: Convert to like units.

Equivalent: 1000 mcg = 1 mg

Therefore 5,000 mg = 5,000,000 mcg

Step 2: Calculate the concentration of solution in mcg/mL.

5,000,000 mcg : 500 mL = x mcg : 1 mL

$$\frac{500x}{500} = \frac{5{,}000{,}000}{500}$$

$$x = 10{,}000 \text{ mcg/mL}$$

The concentration of solution is 10,000 mcg/mL.

Step 3: Calculate the dose range.

Lower dose: 50 mcg × 60 kg = 3,000 mcg/min

Upper dose: 75 mcg × 60 kg = 4,500 mcg/min

Step 4: Convert the dose range to mL/min.

Lower dose: 10,000 mcg : 1 mL = 3,000 mcg : x mL

$$\frac{10{,}000x}{10{,}000} = \frac{3{,}000}{10{,}000}$$

$$x = 0.3 \text{ mL/min}$$

Upper dose: 10,000 mcg : 1 mL = 4,500 mcg : x mL

$$\frac{10{,}000x}{10{,}000} = \frac{4{,}500}{10{,}000}$$

$$x = 0.45 \text{ mL/min}$$

Step 5: Convert mL/min to mL/hr.

Lower dose: 0.3 mL × 60 min = 18 mL/hr (gtt/min)

Upper dose: 0.45 mL × 60 min = 27 mL/hr (gtt/min)

a) A dose range of 50–75 mcg is equal to a flow rate of 18–27 mL/hr (gtt/min).

b) Determine the dose per minute infusing at 30 mL/hr.

$$10{,}000 \text{ mcg} : 1 \text{ mL} = x \text{ mcg} : 30 \text{ mL}$$

$$x = 10{,}000 \times 30 = 300{,}000 \text{ mcg/hr}$$

300,000 mcg/hr ÷ 60 min = 5,000 mcg/min

34. Calculate the dose per minute for client.

$$65 \text{ kg} \times 10 \text{ mcg} = 650 \text{ mcg/min}$$

Determine the dose per hour.

$$650 \text{ mcg/min} \times 60 \text{ min} = 39{,}000 \text{ mcg/hr}$$

Convert to like units.

$$1000 \text{ mcg} = 1 \text{ mg}$$

$$39{,}000 \text{ mcg} = 39 \text{ mg/hr}$$

Calculate mL/hr flow rate:

$$500 \text{ mg} : 250 \text{ mL} = 39 \text{ mg} : x \text{ mL}$$

$$x = 19.5 = 20 \text{ mL/hr}$$

Answer: To deliver a dose of 10 mcg/kg set the flow rate at 20 mL/hr (gtt/min).

35. Convert g to mg.

$$1000 \text{ mg} = 1 \text{ g}$$

$$0.25 \text{ g} = 250 \text{ mg}$$

Calculate mg/hr.

$$250 \text{ mg} \div 6 = 41.6 = 42 \text{ mg/hr}$$

Answer: The client is receiving 42 mg/hr of aminophylline.

36. a) Convert g to mg.

$$1 \text{ g} = 1000 \text{ mg}$$

Calculate mg/hr.

$$1000 \text{ mg} : 500 \text{ mL} = x \text{ mg} : 20 \text{ mL}$$

$$x = 40 \text{ mg/hr}$$

b) Convert mg/hr to mg/min.

40 mg/hr ÷ 60 min = 0.66 mg/min = 0.7 mg

Answer: At the rate of 20 mL/hr the client is receiving a dose of 40 mg/hr or 0.7 mg/min.

37. a) Convert gtt/min to mL/min.

$$60 \text{ gtt} : 1 \text{ mL} = 15 \text{ gtt} : x \text{ mL}$$
$$x = 0.25 = 0.3 \text{ mL/min}$$

Determine mg/min.

$$300 \text{ mg} : 500 \text{ mL} = x \text{ mg} : 0.3 \text{ mL}$$
$$x = 0.18 = 0.2 \text{ mg/min}$$

b) Calculate mg/hr.

$$0.2 \text{ mg/min} \times 60 \text{ min} = 12 \text{ mg/hr}$$

Answer: At 15 gtt/min the client is receiving a dose of 0.2 mg/min and 12 mg/hr.

Answers to Comprehensive Posttest

1. 200 mg : 5 mL = 300 mg : x mL

OR

$$\frac{300 \text{ mg}}{200 \text{ mg}} \times 5 \text{ mL} = x \text{ mL}; \frac{300 \text{ mg}}{200 \text{ mg}} = \frac{x \text{ mL}}{5 \text{ mL}}$$

Answer: 7.5 mL or $7\frac{1}{2}$ mL

2. Conversion is required.

Equivalent: 1000 mg = 1 g

500 mg : 1 tab = 1000 mg : x tab

OR

$$\frac{1000 \text{ mg}}{500 \text{ mg}} \times 1 \text{ tab} = x \text{ tab}; \frac{1000 \text{ mg}}{500 \text{ mg}} = \frac{x \text{ tab}}{1 \text{ tab}}$$

Answer: 2 tabs

3. 0.1 mg : 1 cap = 0.2 mg : x cap

OR

$$\frac{0.2 \text{ mg}}{0.1 \text{ mg}} \times 1 \text{ caps} = x \text{ caps}; \frac{0.2 \text{ mg}}{0.1 \text{ mg}} = \frac{x \text{ caps}}{1 \text{ caps}}$$

Answer: 2 caps

4. Tablets B Septra DS. The doctor's order indicates DS, which means double strength; therefore the client should be given the tabs that are labeled DS.

5. 0.1 mg : 1 mL = 1 mg : x mL

OR

$$\frac{1 \text{ mg}}{0.1 \text{ mg}} \times 1 \text{ mL} = x \text{ mL}; \frac{1 \text{ mg}}{0.1 \text{ mg}} = \frac{x \text{ mL}}{1 \text{ mL}}$$

Answer: 10 mL

6. 10,000 U : 1 mL = 6,500 U : x mL

OR

$$\frac{6{,}500\text{ U}}{10{,}000\text{ U}} \times 1\text{ mL} = x\text{ mL}; \quad \frac{6{,}500\text{ U}}{10{,}000\text{ U}} = \frac{x\text{ mL}}{1\text{ mL}}$$

Answer: 0.65 mL

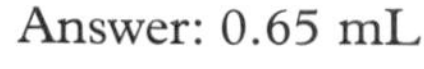

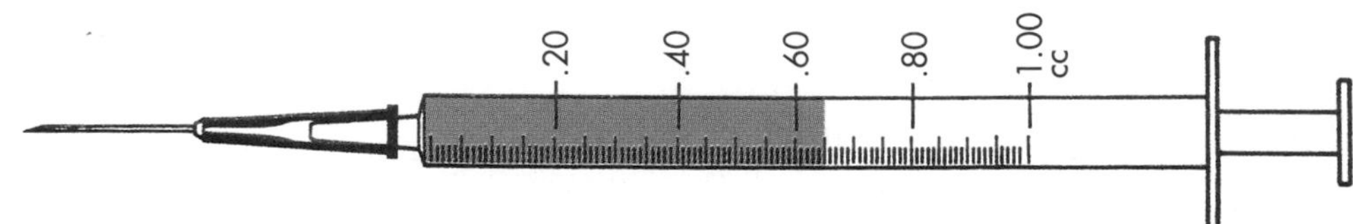

7. Conversion is required.

Equivalent: 1000 mg = 1g

Therefore 0.75 g = 750 mg

1,200 mg : 120 mL = 750 mg : x mL

OR

$$\frac{750\text{ mg}}{1{,}200\text{ mg}} \times 120\text{ mL} = x\text{ mL}; \quad \frac{750\text{ mg}}{1{,}200\text{ mg}} = \frac{x\text{ mL}}{120\text{ mL}}$$

Answer: 75 mL

8. a) 50 mg : 10 mL = 75 mg : x mL

OR

$$\frac{75\text{ mg}}{50\text{ mg}} \times 10\text{ mL} = x\text{ mL}; \quad \frac{75\text{ mg}}{50\text{ mg}} = \frac{x\text{ mL}}{10\text{ mL}}$$

Answer: 15 mL

b) $$\frac{1000\text{ mL}}{6\text{ hr}} \times \frac{10\text{ gtt/min}}{60\text{ min}} = \frac{1000}{6} \times \frac{1}{6} = \frac{1000}{36} = 27.7$$

Answer: 28 macrogtt/min; 28 gtt/min

9. Convert weight (lb) to kg.

Equivalent: 2.2 lb = 1 kg

Therefore 110 ÷ 2.2 = 50 kg

50 kg × 1 mg = 50 mg

Answer: 50 mg

10. Conversion is required.

Equivalent: 1000 mg = 1g

Therefore 0.3 g = 300 mg

150 mg : 1 tab = 300 mg : x tab

OR

$$\frac{300\text{ mg}}{150\text{ mg}} \times 1\text{ tab} = x\text{ tab}; \quad \frac{300\text{ mg}}{150\text{ mg}} = \frac{x\text{ tab}}{1\text{ tab}}$$

Answer: 2 tabs

11. a) 95 mg/mL (Vial is 1 g.)

b) Conversion is required. 1000 mg = 1 g

Therefore 0.25 g = 250 mg

95 mg : 1 mL = 250 mg : x mL

OR

$$\frac{250 \text{ mg}}{95 \text{ mg}} \times 1 \text{ mL} = x \text{ mL}; \frac{250 \text{ mg}}{95 \text{ mg}} = \frac{x \text{ mL}}{1 \text{ mL}}$$

Answer: 2.63 mL = 2.6 mL to nearest tenth

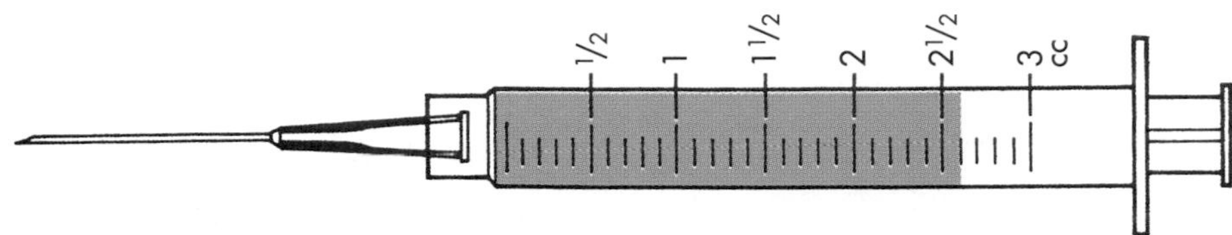

12. Answer: 2 tabs (one 50-mg tab and one 25-mg tab)

    Total = 75 mg

    Administer the least number of tablets to client.

13. $\frac{250 \text{ mL}}{3 \text{ hr}} \times \frac{20 \text{ gtt/mL}}{60 \text{ min}} = \frac{250}{3} \times \frac{1}{3} = \frac{250}{9} = 27.7$

    Answer: 28 macrogtt/min; 28 gtts/min

14. $\frac{80 \text{ mL}}{1 \text{ hr}} \times \frac{15 \text{ gtt/mL}}{60 \text{ min}} = \frac{80}{1} \times \frac{1}{4} = \frac{80}{4} = 20$

    Answer: 20 macrogtt/min; 20 gtt/min

15. $100 \text{ mL} \times \frac{10 \text{ gtt/mL}}{45 \text{ min}} = 100 \times \frac{2}{9} = \frac{200}{9} = 22.2$

    Answer: 22 macrogtt/min; 22 gtt/min

16. $\frac{1000 \text{ mL}}{60 \text{ mL/hr}} = 16.66$

    $60 \times 0.66 = 39.6 = 40$ min

    Answer: 16 hr + 40 min

17. 6 mg TMP × 12 kg = 72 mg/day

    12 mg TMP × 12 kg = 144 mg/day

    Divided dose: 72 mg/day ÷ 2 = 36 mg q12h

    144 mg/day ÷ 2 = 72 mg q12h

    The safe dose range is 72–144 mg/day

    The divided dose is 36–72 mg q12h

    Answer: The doctor ordered 60 mg q12h. The dose is safe (60 mg × 2 = 120 mg).

18. $\frac{100 \text{ mL}}{50 \text{ mL/hr}} = 2 \text{ hr}$

    a) 2 hr

    b) 12 noon or 12 PM (10:00 AM and 2 hours)

19. Determine the dose per hour:

    10 mcg/min × 60 min = 600 mcg/hr

    Convert to like units:

    1000 mcg = 1 mg, therefore

600 mcg = 0.6 mg

Calculate mL/hr:

50 mg : 250 mL = 0.6 mg : x mL

x = 3 mL/hr

Answer: To deliver 10 mcg/min set the flow rate at 3 mL/hr (gtt/min).

20. a) 22 units

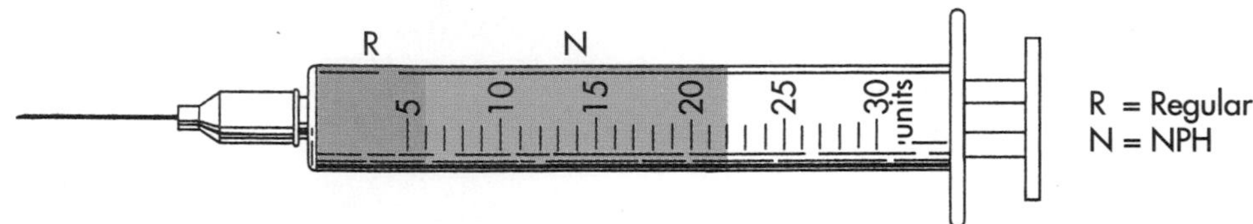

21. a) 52 mL

b) $$\frac{55 \text{ mL (diluted drug)} + 20 \text{ mL (flush)}}{1} \times \frac{60 \text{ gtt/mL}}{50 \text{ min}} = \frac{75}{1} \times \frac{60}{50} = 75 \times \frac{6}{5} = \frac{450}{5} =$$

90 gtt/min; 90 microgtt/min

c) 90 mL/hr (gtt/min with a microdrip = mL/hr)

22. 250 mg : 5 mL = 125 mg : x mL

OR

$$\frac{125 \text{ mg}}{250 \text{ mg}} \times 5 \text{ mL} = x \text{ mL}; \frac{125 \text{ mg}}{250 \text{ mg}} = \frac{x \text{ mL}}{5 \text{ mL}}$$

Answer: $2\frac{1}{2}$ mL or 2.5 mL. (The better answer for administration purposes is $2\frac{1}{2}$ mL.)

23. $$\sqrt{\frac{102 \text{ (lb)} \times 51 \text{ (in)}}{3131}} = \sqrt{1.66} = 1.288 = 1.29 \text{ m}^2$$

Answer: 1.29 m^2

24. a) $$\sqrt{\frac{13.6 \text{ (kg)} \times 60 \text{ cm}}{3600}} = \sqrt{0.226} = 0.475 = 0.48 \text{ m}^2$$

Answer: 0.48 m^2

b) 0.48 m^2 × 500 mg/m^2 = 240

Answer: 240 mg

c) 50 mg : 1 mL = 240 mg : x mL

OR

$$\frac{240 \text{ mg}}{50 \text{ mg}} \times 1 \text{ mL} = x \text{ mL}; \frac{240 \text{ mg}}{50 \text{ mg}} = \frac{x \text{ mL}}{1 \text{ mL}}$$

Answer: 4.8 mL

25. a) 25 mg : 1 tab = 50 mg : x tab

OR

$$\frac{50 \text{ mg}}{25 \text{ mg}} \times 1 \text{ tab} = x \text{ tab}; \frac{50 \text{ mg}}{25 \text{ mg}} = \frac{x \text{ tab}}{1 \text{ tab}}$$

Answer: 2 tabs

b) Hold the medication since the systolic b/p (top number) is less than 100 and notify the doctor.

Index

G

H

I

Medication Administration Abbreviations

Abbreviation	Meaning	Abbreviation	Meaning
$\overline{a}$	before	OU	both eyes
aa, $\overline{aa}$	of each	p	after
a.c.	before meals	p.c.	after meals
A.D., AD	right ear	per	through or by
ad.lib.	as desired, freely	per os, p.o.	by or through mouth
A.S., AS	left ear	p.r.	by rectum
A.U., AU	both ears	p.r.n.	when necessary/required
b.i.d., bid	twice a day	q.	every, each
b.i.w.	twice a week	q.a.m.	every morning
c	with	q.d.	every day
cap, caps	capsule	q.h.	every hour
d.c., D/C	discontinue	q2h, q4h	every two hours, every four hours
dil.	dilute		
DS	double strength	qhs, q.h.s.	every night at bedtime
EC	enteric coated	q.i.d.	four times a day
elix.	elixir	q.n.	every night
fl, fld.	fluid	q.o.d.	every other day
gtt	drop	q.s.	a sufficient amount/as much as needed
h, hr	hour		
h.s.	hour of sleep, at bedtime	$\overline{s}$	without
ID	intradermal	$\overline{ss}$, ss	one half
I.M.	intramuscular	s.c., S.C., s.q.	subcutaneous
I.V.	intravenous	sl, SL	sublingual
IVPB	intravenous piggyback	sol, soln	solution
IVSS	intravenous soluset	s.o.s.	once if necessary
LA	long-acting	SR	slow-release
LOS	length of stay	stat, STAT	immediately, at once
NGT, ng	nasogastric tube	supp	suppository
n.p.o., NPO	nothing by mouth	susp	suspension
NS, N/S	normal saline	syp, syr	syrup
o.d.	once a day	tab	tablet
OD	right eye	t.i.d.	three times a day
o.n.	every night	t.i.w.	three times a week
os	mouth	tr., tinct	tincture
OS	left eye	ung., oint	ointment